AF781500

Animal Health and Veterinary Medicine

Animal Health and Veterinary Medicine

Edited by Andrea Santoro

SYRAWOOD
PUBLISHING HOUSE
New York

Published by Syrawood Publishing House,
750 Third Avenue, 9th Floor,
New York, NY 10017, USA
www.syrawoodpublishinghouse.com

Animal Health and Veterinary Medicine
Edited by Andrea Santoro

© 2018 Syrawood Publishing House

International Standard Book Number: 978-1-68286-625-2 (Hardback)

This book contains information obtained from authentic and highly regarded sources. Copyright for all individual chapters remain with the respective authors as indicated. All chapters are published with permission under the Creative Commons Attribution License or equivalent. A wide variety of references are listed. Permission and sources are indicated; for detailed attributions, please refer to the permissions page and list of contributors. Reasonable efforts have been made to publish reliable data and information, but the authors, editors and publisher cannot assume any responsibility for the validity of all materials or the consequences of their use.

The publisher's policy is to use permanent paper from mills that operate a sustainable forestry policy. Furthermore, the publisher ensures that the text paper and cover boards used have met acceptable environmental accreditation standards.

Trademark Notice: Registered trademark of products or corporate names are used only for explanation and identification without intent to infringe.

Cataloging-in-Publication Data

Animal health and veterinary medicine / edited by Andrea Santoro.
p. cm.
Includes bibliographical references and index.
ISBN 978-1-68286-625-2
1. Animal health. 2. Veterinary medicine. 3. Animals--Diseases. I. Santoro, Andrea.
SF745 .A55 2018
636.089--dc23

Printed in China.

TABLE OF CONTENTS

PREFACE

Veterinary medicine studies methods that seek to diagnose, treat and prevent diseases and disorders in animals. This branch of medicine has various sub-specialties like veterinary physicians, paraveterinary workers and specializations such as osteopaths, physiotherapists and chiropractors. Veterinary medicine also extends to the prevention and regulation of zoonotic diseases, which are harmful to animals and human beings. This book strives to provide a fair idea about this discipline and to help develop a better understanding of the latest advances within this field. It is appropriate for students seeking detailed information in this area as well as for experts.

Significant researches are present in this book. Intensive efforts have been employed by authors to make this book an outstanding discourse. This book contains the enlightening chapters which have been written on the basis of significant researches done by the experts.

Finally, I would also like to thank all the members involved in this book for being a team and meeting all the deadlines for the submission of their respective works. I would also like to thank my friends and family for being supportive in my efforts.

Editor

1

Mapping the Global Distribution of Livestock

Timothy P. Robinson[1,2]*, G. R. William Wint[3], Giulia Conchedda[2], Thomas P. Van Boeckel[4,5,6,7], Valentina Ercoli[2], Elisa Palamara[2], Giuseppina Cinardi[2], Laura D'Aietti[2], Simon I. Hay[8,9], Marius Gilbert[4,5]

1 Livestock Systems and Environment Research Theme (LSE), International Livestock Research Institute (ILRI), Nairobi, Kenya, **2** Animal Production and Health Division (AGA), Food and Agriculture Organization of the United Nations (FAO), Rome, Italy, **3** Environmental Research Group Oxford (ERGO) - Department of Zoology, University of Oxford, Oxford, United Kingdom, **4** Biological Control and Spatial Ecology, Université Libre de Bruxelles, Brussels, Belgium, **5** Fonds National de la Recherche Scientifique, Brussels, Belgium, **6** Department of Ecology and Evolutionary - Biology Department, Princeton University, Princeton, New Jersey, United States of America, **7** Princeton Environmental Institute, Princeton, New Jersey, United States of America, **8** Spatial Ecology and Epidemiology Group - Department of Zoology, University of Oxford, Oxford, United Kingdom, **9** Fogarty International Center, National Institutes of Health, Bethesda, Maryland, United States of America

Abstract

Livestock contributes directly to the livelihoods and food security of almost a billion people and affects the diet and health of many more. With estimated standing populations of 1.43 billion cattle, 1.87 billion sheep and goats, 0.98 billion pigs, and 19.60 billion chickens, reliable and accessible information on the distribution and abundance of livestock is needed for a many reasons. These include analyses of the social and economic aspects of the livestock sector; the environmental impacts of livestock such as the production and management of waste, greenhouse gas emissions and livestock-related land-use change; and large-scale public health and epidemiological investigations. The Gridded Livestock of the World (GLW) database, produced in 2007, provided modelled livestock densities of the world, adjusted to match official (FAOSTAT) national estimates for the reference year 2005, at a spatial resolution of 3 minutes of arc (about 5×5 km at the equator). Recent methodological improvements have significantly enhanced these distributions: more up-to date and detailed sub-national livestock statistics have been collected; a new, higher resolution set of predictor variables is used; and the analytical procedure has been revised and extended to include a more systematic assessment of model accuracy and the representation of uncertainties associated with the predictions. This paper describes the current approach in detail and presents new global distribution maps at 1 km resolution for cattle, pigs and chickens, and a partial distribution map for ducks. These digital layers are made publically available via the Livestock Geo-Wiki (http://www.livestock.geo-wiki.org), as will be the maps of other livestock types as they are produced.

Editor: Matthew Baylis, University of Liverpool, United Kingdom

Funding: TPR is funded by the following Consultative Group on International Agricultural Research (CGIAR) Research Programmes: Humidtropics; Climate Change, Agriculture and Food Security (CCAFS); and Agriculture for Nutrition and Health (A4NH). MG & TPVB are funded by the 'Fonds National de la Recherche Scientifique' (FNRS). SIH is funded by a Senior Research Fellowship from the Wellcome Trust (#095066) and receives support from the Li Ka Shing Foundation. SIH also acknowledges funding support from the Research and Policy for Infectious Disease Dynamics (RAPIDD) program of the Science & Technology Directorate, Department of Homeland Security, and the Fogarty International Center (FIC), National Institutes of Health (NIH). The bulk of this work was funded through various programmes and projects within the Animal Production and Health Division (AGA) of the Food and Agriculture Organization (FAO) of the United Nations: in particular the UK Department for International Development (DFID)-funded Pro-Poor Livestock Policy Initiative and the USAID-funded Emerging Pandemic Threats Plus (EPT+) programme. Other contributors include the United States NIH FIC grants: 3R01TW007869-03 and 1R56TW009502-01 and the FNRS Projet de Recherche (PDR) T.0073.13. The funders had no role in study design, data collection and analysis, decision to publish, or preparation of the manuscript.

Competing Interests: The authors have declared that no competing interests exist.

* E-mail: t.robinson@cgiar.org

Introduction

Livestock contributes directly to the livelihoods and food security of almost a billion people [1–2]. In recent decades, the world food economy has seen a shift towards increased consumption of animal-source foods. In developing countries, the meat and dairy sectors have grown at average yearly rates of 5.1 percent and 3.6 percent respectively since 1970 [3]. Most of this increase has been to supply expanding urban areas and has been primarily driven by population growth and increasing incomes, closely linked to urbanisation, making livestock one of the fastest-growing sectors in agriculture [1]. Globally, as human population growth slows and relatively high consumption levels of animal-source foods are reached in some of the countries that have seen the more rapid increases, Brazil and China in particular, growth in demand for meat, milk and eggs is also expected to slow down [4]. Notwithstanding regional reductions in growth, in many developing countries *per capita* consumption of animal-source foods is projected to continue rising and even to accelerate [3]. As well as the economic benefits that a growing livestock sector confers on the economies of these countries, and the potential improvements in food security and nutrition among the world's poor, some 766 million poor (<US$ 2 per day) livestock keepers could benefit directly [5]. This is particularly the case in mixed farming systems where livestock serve many socio-economic functions and promote arable agriculture through manure and draft power [6].

Much of this demand-led growth, and particularly that stemming from the burgeoning urban centres, is likely to be supplied by intensification of production and will generally not be met by small-holders except in particular circumstances where small-holders are well-connected to markets and do not suffer from poor economies of scale, such as the small-holder dairy sector in

India [7]. Whilst livestock sector growth presents economic opportunities, in cases where competition from integrated, industrial producers and increasingly tight sanitary standards marginalise the livestock-dependent poor and other small-scale farmers by forcing them out of markets [4,8–9], its main social effects on low-income populations may be negative if not carefully managed.

The growing livestock sector also places increased pressure on natural resources and the environment; making a significant contribution to global environmental change [10–11]. Also of concern are the public health implications of livestock production and intensification. As pressure on our global resources increases, people and their livestock are pushed into ever-closer proximity with natural areas and the habitats of wild fauna [12]. This increases the chances of emergence and spread, in livestock and people, of infectious zoonotic pathogens originating in wild animals [13–15].

To address these and other such issues requires accurate and accessible and information on the distribution and abundance of livestock. Analyses based on reliable livestock sector data can then be used for targeting and impact assessment, epidemiological evaluation, and to inform planning and policy formulation to promote safe, sustainable and equitable livestock sector development.

Until now, the only global estimates mapped at sub-national resolution have been the 2007 Gridded Livestock of the World (GLW) [16], though the distributions of some species have been modelled over more restricted areas. Neumann and colleagues, for example, modelled and validated the distribution of livestock in Europe by downscaling harmonised livestock statistics through a series of explanatory factors [17]. Other studies have modelled the distribution of poultry species in China and of ducks in Monsoon Asia [18–19].

The GLW provided modelled livestock densities of the world at a spatial resolution of 3 minutes of arc (about 5×5 km at the equator). The estimated densities were based on statistical relationships between observed densities within administrative units ('training data') derived from survey and census data, and several explanatory variables, including a time-series of remotely-sensed satellite data relating to climate and the environment, and other spatial data relating to demography, land cover and terrain. Reported sub-national statistics were thus spatially disaggregated and gaps where none were available filled with predictions to provide a complete global distribution map for each species.

The GLW maps have been put to a wide variety of uses. They were the fundamental inputs for mapping current and projected estimates of consumption and production of animal-source foods [7]. They have been applied to the analysis of land use dynamics [20] and of global ecosystem services [21] and have contributed to the estimates of the environmental impacts of livestock [22–24] and to the characterization of livestock production systems in Eastern Africa [25]. The GLW data have been used in several epidemiological and ecological studies of livestock disease distributions, including trypanosomosis [26–27], highly pathogenic avian influenza [28–29] and foot-and-mouth disease [30]. The livestock densities have been combined with information on livestock production systems and on production parameters, to estimate the impacts livestock disease and the economic benefits of removing these constraints to production. Examples from cattle in Africa include brucellosis [31] and trypanosomosis [32–33].

Since the GLW datasets were first published, considerable advances have been made to improve a) the sub-national statistics on which livestock distributions are based, b) the predictor variables, masks and stratification layers used in the modelling process, c) the modelling methodology itself, and d) the statistical evaluation of modelled results. Some of initial improvements were described in relation to poultry distributions in Asia [18,19] and methods have since been further developed. Here, we describe the current revised approach in detail and present new global distribution maps, at 1 km spatial resolution, for cattle, pigs and chickens and a partial duck distribution map.

Materials and Methods

Producing the global livestock distributions for the GLW was a labour-intensive and time-consuming process. Whilst the majority of time is taken in the laborious and painstaking work of acquiring, cleaning and standardising sub-national statistics and registering these to geospatial files of often-changing sub-national boundaries and international borders, it was clear that to become sustainable the data management and livestock mapping processes had to be automated as far as possible. Improvement in data management has been achieved by the development of GLIMS: the Global Livestock Impact Mapping System [34]. Significant advances in livestock distribution modelling have been made possible through the development of a suite of sequentially-implemented R-scripts that produce GLW version 2. The overall workflow from the collection of input data to post-processing and dissemination of outputs is illustrated in Fig. 1.

GLIMS and sub-national livestock data

Wint and Robinson [16] listed and described the variety of sources for sub-national livestock statistics. These data are collected and cross-referenced against other sources (such as earlier statistics and FAOSTAT national totals). They are then linked to Geographical Information System (GIS) files of the administrative areas at the level to which the livestock statistics are reported. The hierarchical structure and nomenclature of these administrative units varies from country to country but typically includes units such as regions, provinces or districts. This involves a careful process of matching place names, often in different languages, and editing the digital boundaries to account for the merging and splitting of administrative areas, as well as the assignation of livestock numbers to newly defined administrative units. Where possible the FAO Global Administrative Unit Layers (GAUL) files are used as source of national boundary files (http://www.fao.org/geonetwork/srv/en/main.home).

The resulting GIS files of administrative areas and attributed sub-national livestock statistics are then entered into GLIMS. The GLIMS data warehouse, hosted at FAO headquarters in Rome, provides a repository and the tools to edit, explore, search and retrieve the collated data. GLIMS is used to manage a variety of data pertaining to the livestock sector, which are then processed and distributed through various channels and in numerous formats [36]. A module has been specifically developed in GLIMS to extract data for a specified livestock species and aggregation of countries, which are then offered as training data, in the form of a geospatial polygon vector file containing livestock numbers, to the modelling procedures.

GLW 2: a revised livestock distribution modelling system

The procedure builds on the method developed by Wint and Robinson [16] for disaggregating livestock statistics, based on environmental and other spatial data. Spatially stratified, statistical regression models are developed using data from a series of sample points within each training data polygon and these models are then applied to the entire one-kilometre resolution set of predictor variables in order to estimate livestock densities, disaggregated

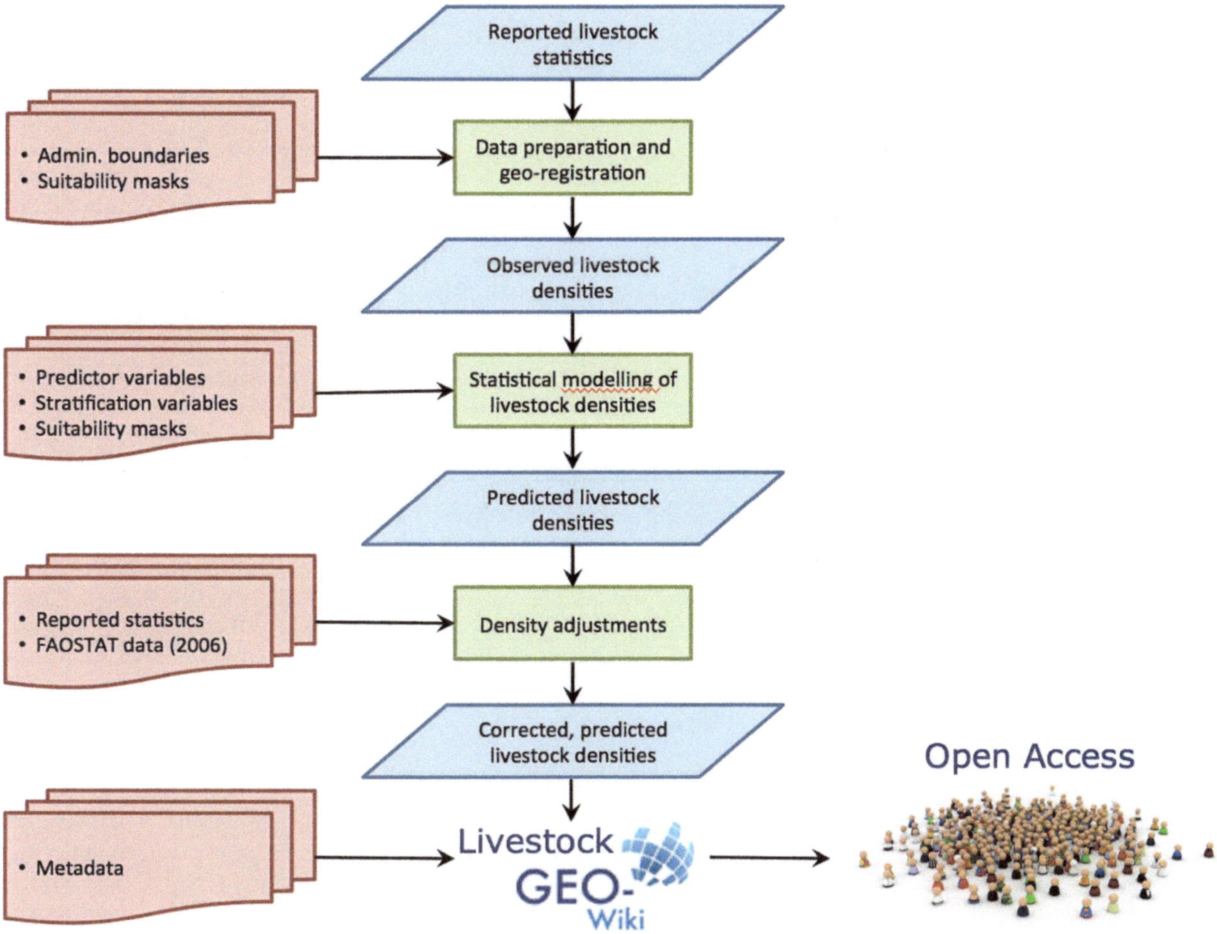

Figure 1. Overall workflow of GLW modelling.

over a defined study area. For GLW 2, this basic methodology has been revised and improved in a number of ways and was first assessed by Van Boeckel et al. [19] and Prosser et al. [18] in a detailed analysis of its performances for modelling domestic ducks in Asia and poultry in China respectively. Van Boeckel et al. (2011) looked at how downscaling performance was influenced by the aggregation level of input domestic duck data in Thailand (no data for the country, only one value for the country, administrative level 1 data, and administrative level 2 data) and comparing the predictions to actual admin level 3 data. The result was that downscaling based on the method outlined below was giving relatively good results provided that the training data were available at administrative level 1, and were degraded with coarser (national-level data) input data. In a separate study, Prosser et al. (2011) compared land-use based downscaling with the GLW 2 methodology to predict chicken ducks and geese in China, and found land-use based methods to give lower performances. In another previous study, though based on a non-stratified implementation of regression methods, Newmann et al. (2009) found comparable results between land-use and regression based downscaling [17]. In human population mapping, the AfriPop and AsiaPop databases are still largely based on land-use weighting of human population density per land use class [35–36], whereas new developments of the WorldPop consortium (www.worldpop.org.uk) are moving toward the use of machine learning methods such as random forest or boosted regression trees (Andy Tatem, comm. pers).

The stratified regressions are repeated a specified number of times using random selections of pixels from which to extract dependent and independent variables (bootstraps). This produces multiple models from which the variability as well as the mean values of the model predictions can be calculated for each pixel.

- The procedures for the statistical transformation of variables and their subsequent selection in the regression models has been revised, better to account for non-linearity and to provide a more flexible process of predictor variable selection.
- A method has been developed to combine the results from a number of stratification schemes; choosing for each location the predictions from the best models for that location. This results in an aggregate, mosaic prediction.
- The entire modelling procedure has been streamlined as a suite of scripts that allow new gridded livestock distributions to be produced relatively quickly using the programming language R [37] when updated input data become available. Automation also facilitates the evaluation of the effects of adjusting model parameters.

Because of the sheer volume of input and covariate data, the modelling must be broken down into continental tiles. Whilst bespoke geographic tiles can be created for specific tasks or projects, there are six continental tiles that are processed independently, and the global dataset is updated every time a new continental tile is processed (see file S1).

Data layers

The GIS data layers used in the modelling process fall into 3 categories: 1) masks and pixel area files; 2) the predictor covariates; and 3) the stratification layers. All variables are un-projected, using latitude and longitude coordinates and the WGS84 datum. The images have a pixel resolution of 30 minutes of arc (0.00833 degrees) – a nominal pixel resolution of approximately 1 km×1 km at the equator. All imagery is maintained and used as scaled integer data in Idrisi format [38].

Suitability masking is an important step of the modelling process; firstly for adjusting the reported livestock numbers into the densities used as dependent variables in the regression models, and secondly for masking out unsuitable areas with densities of zero in the modelled results. If, for example, an administrative area of 100 km^2 is reported to contain 100 cattle, but half of its area is deemed unsuitable for raising cattle, the effective density of cattle on 'usable' land is not 1 but 2 head km^{-2}. Suitability masking in this version is more conservative that it was in the original GLW [16]; areas of forest and desert are no longer explicitly excluded – it is left for the model to determine the suitability of these – so a single mask is used for both ruminant and monogastric species. Land pixels with elevations higher than 4,750 m above sea level or at a slope of gradient higher than 40 percent are deemed unsuitable as well as urban areas and pixels permanently covered with snow or ice. The digital elevation model (DEM) GTOPO30 of the US Geological Survey (USGS) is the source for elevation data and for derived slope information (https://lta.cr.usgs.gov/GTOPO30). The GLC2000 land cover classification developed by the Joint Research Centre (JRC) of the European Commission (EC) is the source for the land cover categories of urban areas and snow and ice [39].

Areas unsuitable for reasons that are not biological or environmental, for example protected areas, are treated differently in the modelling procedure, and are therefore masked separately. A global mask of protected areas is derived from the 2010 version of the World Database on Protected Areas (WDPA)(www.wdpa.org). The International Union for the Conservation of Nature (IUCN) categories Ia and Ib, II, and III were masked as unsuitable as these are characterised by stringent conservation measures and tight regulation of human activity – the encroachment of roaming cattle and other grazing activities is therefore less likely in these than in other areas [40]. Any sample point falling in an area masked for environmental or biological reasons is maintained as a sample point in the model, with a livestock density of zero. If, however a sample point falls in an area deemed unsuitable for legislative reasons, it is dropped from the analysis. The area may, in fact, be quite suitable for livestock, and a zero value for livestock density would mislead the statistical model. A simple land mask is also employed in the modelling process and a file containing the area of each pixel is required for converting livestock numbers into densities, and vice versa. The independent predictor variables offered to the regression analyses are drawn from a spatial data set that allows the modelling process to take advantage of any relationship between livestock densities and climatic, environmental, demographic or topographic factors. The mainstay of these is a Fourier-processed, decadal time series of geo-physical variables derived from Moderate Resolution Imaging Spectroradiometer (MODIS) satellite data (http://modis.gsfc.nasa.gov) from 2001 to 2008. The variables include two vegetation indices, the land surface temperature and the band 3 middle-infra-red, which is particularly suitable for vegetation mapping. Rogers and associates have described the Fourier processing of satellite data in several studies [41–44], while a description specific to the MODIS data series is provided by Scharlemann and colleagues [45]. The use of Fourier-processed time-series data is central to the modelling process since the Fourier variables reveal the seasonal characteristics of the environment. Each multi-temporal series is reduced to seven separate, and quite independent, data layers: the mean, and the phases and amplitudes of the annual, biannual and tri-annual cycles of change. Three additional variables combine the amplitude and phase of the three cycles of change and report the contribution of this combination to the total variance in the seasonal phenology. These are further supplemented by the maximum, the minimum and the variance of the satellite-derived geo-physical variables. Two other MODIS-derived products are included as predictor variables: 'green-up' and 'senescence', derived by Boston University from the NASA MOD12Q2 MODIS tiled phenology layers (http://www.bu.edu/lcsc/research/land-cover-dynamics) [46]. These represent the dates when new green vegetation is first detected at the beginning of a growth cycle, and the onset of senescence at the end of that cycle. Detailed information on the MODIS-derived predictor variables is available on file S2. Two climate-related variables are also used: the length of growing period (LGP), which has been modelled to 1 km spatial resolution [47–48] and the annual precipitation data (synoptic period 1950 to 2000) from the WorldClim climate dataset [49]. Since human activities are associated with livestock distributions, two demographic variables are also included. The first is the human population density in 2006, for which the source is the Global Rural-Urban Mapping Project (GRUMP) [50] (http://sedac.ciesin.columbia.edu/data/collection/grump-v1), with country totals adjusted to match the United Nations population values in 2006. The second is the travel time to areas populated by 50,000 people or more [51]. Finally, the GTOPO30 dataset is the source for elevation and slope information [52]. Table 1 provides a list of primary variables used in the analysis.

A given predictor variable may be associated quite differently with livestock densities in different ecological zones. For instance, daytime temperature may have a negative association with livestock densities in an ecological zone describing arid environments, whilst it may have a positive association in temperate regions. In GLW 2 the analyses are therefore spatially stratified using three stratification layers selected to represent different types of spatial zonation. The first of these comprises 25 discrete ecological zones (EZ25) and is the result of an unsupervised classification of some of the Fourier-processed MODIS data, achieved by first reducing the data using a principal component analysis (PCA), followed by clustering using the ADDAPIX programme [53]. The zonation is based on the mean values of the temperature and vegetation variables, as well as elevation and a vegetation seasonality index derived from the Fourier processed time-series of the satellite imagery to distinguish zones in each hemisphere. This is very similar to the stratification scheme that was used to produce the 2007 livestock densities. A second stratification scheme, that has proved very useful, is the map of global livestock production systems (GLPS version 5) [5]. This distinguishes livestock-only, mixed irrigated and mixed rain-fed farming areas, based on land cover, human population densities and data on irrigation. Each of the three categories is then subdivided, using data on temperature, elevation and LGP, into four sub-categories: hyper-arid; arid and semi-arid; humid and subhumid; and temperate and tropical highland. A third stratification scheme is provided by a published dataset on the biomes of the world [54]. Olson and associates subdivided the terrestrial world

Table 1. Summary of the predictor variables.

Type of variable	Predictor variables	Source
Vegetation and climate	14 Fourier-derived variables from MIR*	Scharlemann et al. (2008) [45]
	14 Fourier-derived variables from LSTday and 14 from LSTnight**	
	14 Fourier-derived variables from NDVI*** and 14 from EVI****	
	Green-up (annual cycle 1 and 2)	Zhang et al. (2003) [46]
	Senescence (annual cycle 1 and 2)	
	Length of Growing Period (LGP)	Jones & Thornton (2009) [48]
	Precipitation	Hijmans et al. (2005) [49]
Topography	GTOPO30 Elevation	USGS-EROS (1996) [52]
	GTOPO30 Slope	
Demography	Human population in 2006	CIESIN et al. (2004)**** [50]
	Travel time to places with >50,000 inhabitants	Nelson (2008) [51]

*Middle Infra-Red;
**Land Surface Temperature;
***Normalized Difference Vegetation Index;
****Enhanced Vegetation Index;
****Country totals adjusted to UN values in 2006 (http://www.un.org/esa/population/).

into 867 ecoregions, nested within 14 biomes. The ecoregions were evaluated as a stratification layer but proved too detailed, resulting in many strata failing to contain sufficient sample points to produce models. The biomes, however, have proved to be a useful means of stratification.

Modelling procedure

The polygon vector data containing the reported livestock numbers derived from GLIMS is combined with the masks and pixel area image and converted to pixel values of animal densities in areas defined as suitable. These observed densities are then converted to $\log_{10}$ (n+1) values in order to normalise the distribution of the dependent variable [55]. A set of sample points is randomly selected at a density of 30 per 10,000 km^2 (though this sometimes needs to be reduced for very large regions), with the constraint that at least one sample point must be selected per input polygon (i.e. if a polygon is smaller than 333 square kilometres). 75% of these points are used to train models and the remaining 25% are used to test their goodness of fit. The number of bootstraps to be used is specified in terms of the number of sample files and the number of point selections within each. Normally, 25 bootstraps are prepared by creating five different files of sample points and, within each, five different selections of the 75% to be used to train the models. Values for the suitability adjusted livestock densities, predictor variables, and stratification layers are extracted for each sample point in each of the five files.

Regressions are then run for each bootstrap, grouping data points according to each stratification scheme and using data points from each stratum of each stratification scheme. A constraint is imposed that a model can only be developed for a stratum if there are at least 30 unique observations for it. Unique, in this context, means from different polygons, each of which represents a single value for the dependent variable (suitability-corrected livestock density). For large polygons, many points may be included in the sample file but all will share the same livestock suitability-corrected density value and are therefore considered a single observation. An un-stratified model is also produced for each continental tile and this is used in areas where there are insufficient data points in any stratum to create a model for it.

Within each stratum a forward stepwise regression is applied. In contrast to standard stepwise regressions though, variables are entered in pairs; each variable being entered simultaneously with its quadratic term. This is intended to account for non-linearity in the relationship between dependent and independent variables. At each step, the pair of variables that best reduces the model Akaike information criterion (AIC) is maintained. In order to avoid over-fitting by including an excessive number of predictor variables, the procedure is halted when the difference in AIC drops below 1 percent in relative terms or when 2 * loglikelihood is below 6 in absolute terms (which corresponds to a p-value of 0.05 of the loglikelihood ratio test for the inclusion of a pair of variables). For the same reason, the maximum number of variables to be entered in a model is estimated by dividing the number of observations by 15. Then, for each bootstrap, the regression models for each stratum (given sufficient points) in each stratification scheme are applied to the predictor variables selected for inclusion in each model. This results in an image of predicted log10 densities for each stratification scheme plus an additional image of predicted log10 densities with no stratification employed.

The next step is to produce a composite of predicted values for each bootstrap by selecting, for each pixel, the prediction resulting from the best performing stratification scheme. Two options are available for choosing the best performing model: the one with the best (highest) R^2 value or the one with the best (lowest) residual standard error (RSE). The RSE provides information on the accuracy of predictions regardless of the slope of the regression line. In a single model, a poor R^2 value may be found concomitantly with a very low (good) RSE around a nearly horizontal line, which would in fact correspond to good prediction. An additional image is produced for each bootstrap, which shows, for each pixel, which of the stratification schemes (if any) contributed the predicted livestock density value used in the composite prediction. The correspondence between the observed and predicted livestock densities for the 25% of sample points reserved for testing is then compared for: a) the un-stratified model; b) the composite models based on best R^2; c) the composite model based on best RSE; and d) the models based on each of the single stratification schemes included. The statistics used for comparison are the simple Pearson correlation coefficient and the root mean square error (RMSE) between the predicted and observed densities. It is normally the case that the best R^2 or best RSE composite models out-perform all other models (and of these the best RSE model is preferred for the reasons given above). Sometimes, however, a single stratification scheme consistently performs comparably. In such cases, where there is no significant improvement to be had by using a composite model, the predictions from the single stratification are taken; following the principles of parsimony.

Based on either an individual stratification or an aggregate prediction for each bootstrap the predicted (log10) densities are then averaged across the 25 bootstraps to give the mean and standard deviation of modelled predictions. It is this mean value on which the final predicted densities are based, and the standard deviation of this mean shows the consistency in predictions of the bootstraps.

The first step in post-processing is to adjust the predicted densities within polygons for which observations were available such that the predicted totals (of livestock numbers) match those of the reported statistics in the input polygon data (where no observed data are indicated for a polygon by a value of −9,999 the predicted density is retained). In a second post-processing stage the polygon-corrected density maps are further adjusted to match FAO's official national statistics (from FAOSTAT, accessed in 2013), providing a time-standardised datasets for the year 2006. The year 2006 was selected for these livestock distribution maps since it is the base year from which FAO's revised agricultural projections to 2030 and 2050 have been made [3].

Further corrections are made to the predicted densities for pigs, for which a value of zero is applied to all pixels in countries where Islam is the majority religion. Masking only occurs in countries where all of the following conditions are met: 1) more than 50 percent of the population is Muslim; 2) sub-national GLIMS data indicate zero or no data; and 3) FAOSTAT indicates zero or no data for pigs but does report data for other livestock species (see file S3).

Accuracy of predictions

Beyond the intrinsic ability of the available variables to explain the variance in livestock densities, the goodness of fit of the regression models depends on the level of detail in the input data. Better model performances are expected with more observed data obtained at a lower administrative level [19]. To illustrate this, two tests were undertaken. The first example analysed the predictive accuracy of separate models for cattle in South America by degrading the input data from Brazil to increasingly coarse levels. Recent statistics (2009) are available for Brazil at municipality level (administrative level 2). Brazil accounts for 5,510 out of 7,217 total input polygons in South America so it is expected strongly to influence the continental model for cattle. A similar approach was used in the second test by evaluating the impact of using increasingly coarse training data from Thailand to predict chicken distributions in the country. Sub-district level (locally called *tambon*, corresponding to administrative level 3) statistics on chicken distributions are available for Thailand and, at this level, the country accounts for nearly one third of all the input polygons of the Asia tile. In both examples, the goodness of fit of predicted models was calculated against the input data at the highest administrative level.

Results

Figure 2 shows the global distributions of cattle, pigs and chickens and the partial distribution of ducks respectively; created by merging the results from the continental tiles for each species. These global maps represent the predicted data, first corrected to match the polygon values of the observed data and then to match the FAOSTAT country values in 2006. The highest cattle densities (Figure 2a) are found in India, in the East African highlands (particularly in Ethiopia), in Northern Europe and in South America. Desert areas and the tropical rain forests of Amazonia and of the Congo Basin have practically no cattle. The highest concentrations of pigs are found in China and in other Eastern Pacific countries (Figure 2b). Pigs are also densely distributed in European countries while only a few countries in Africa (e.g. Uganda, Burkina Faso, Ghana, Nigeria and Togo) have significant densities. Relatively high concentrations are also found in Central America and in Brazil. The distribution of chickens (Figure 2c) closely follows that of the human population. The highest concentrations are found in eastern China, in Pakistan and India, and in western Europe. In Africa, the countries facing the Gulf of Guinea and Madagascar also have high chicken densities. The densely populated east coast of the United States also shows high numbers whilst chickens are only sparsely distributed in the central and western states. The heavily populated areas of southern Brazil also show high concentrations of chickens. The distribution of ducks (Figure 2d), for those regions for which sub-national statistics were available, adds information to previous national and regional duck mapping efforts [18,19]. Ducks are far less common than chickens worldwide although high densities are to be found in South-East Asia and China where duck production is often integrated with rice cropping and fish farming [56–57]. Though to a lesser extent, duck densities are also quite high in a few European countries (e.g. France). file S4 provides a summary of the sub-national statistics used for the modelling and file S5 provides detailed metadata for the sub-national statistics used to develop the livestock distribution models. file S6 provides two graphic summaries of data availability for the modelled species (a) the average spatial resolution of the training data and (b) administrative level of the training data.

The thematic detail in GLW 2 has been significantly improved compared to the previous version; GLW 2007. Figure 3 zooms in on Thailand and its neighbouring countries and compares the original 2005-corrected distribution of poultry (a) with the new 2006-corrected maps of chickens (b) and ducks (c). Such thematic disaggregation is particularly important in this region because of the abundance of ducks and their important role in farming systems in this part of the world. The figure also illustrates that whilst GLW 2007 explicitly excluded the unsuitable areas based on expert opinion, GLW 2 applies a more conservative approach and leaves to the model to predict the livestock distribution. The two approaches however agree substantially in their mapping of areas with low or zero densities.

The finer spatial resolution of the GLW 2 maps (approximate cell size of 1 km^2 at the equator) also significantly increases the detail of predictions compared to the original version (approximate cell size of 5 km^2 at the equator). Figure 4 helps to illustrate this with an example from central Uganda. In this case, the finer pixel size combines with a higher disaggregation of the training data; input data were at administrative levels 1 and 4 respectively in the GLW 2007 and GLW 2.

As so very often the case, it is the gathering and processing of primary data – the sub-national statistics on livestock numbers – that is the most arduous and time-consuming part of the process. This operation is necessarily very labour-intensive and usually requires cases-by-case judgements to be made, in particular regarding the linking of reported statistics to geographical units. Few advances could be made, therefore, with respect to earlier

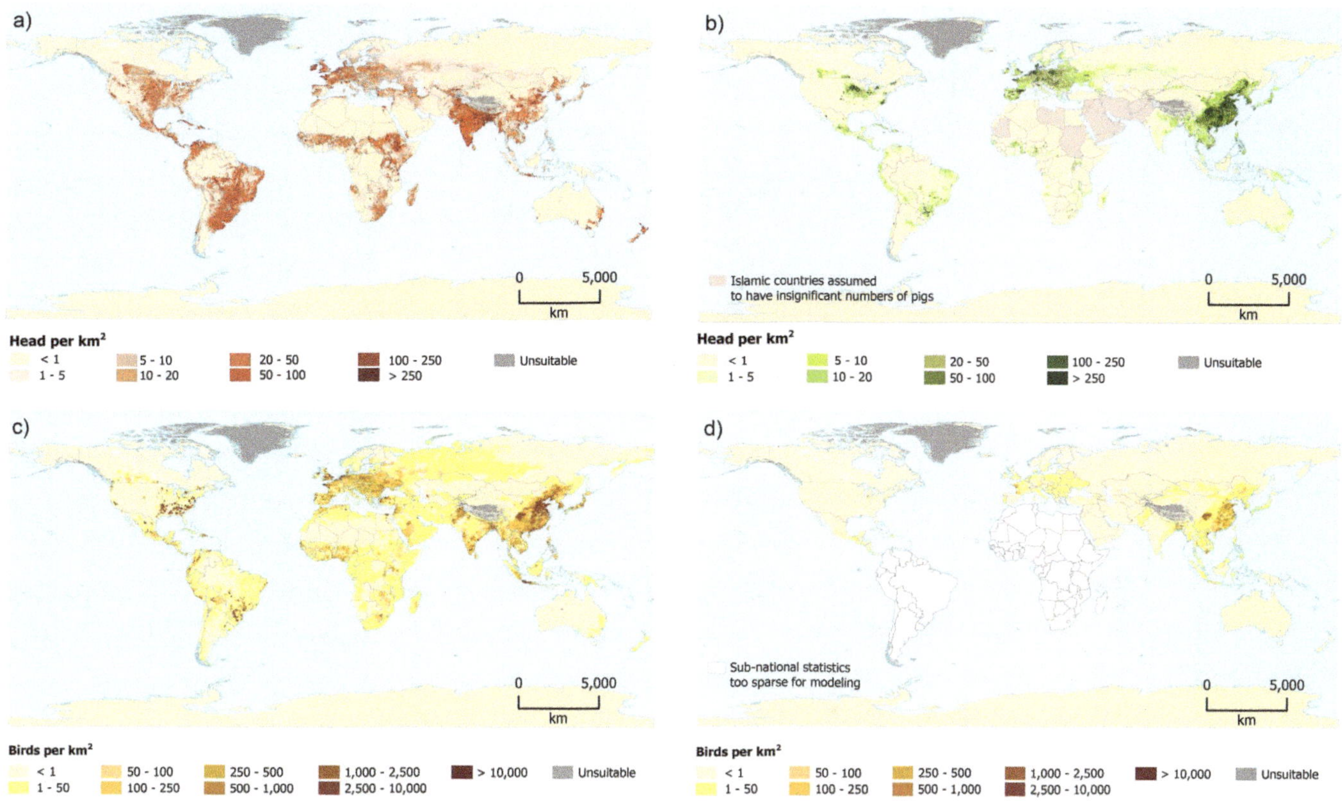

Figure 2. GLW 2 global distributions of a) cattle; b) pigs; c) chickens; and d) distribution of ducks, excluding South America and Africa.

approaches. The development of GLIMS, however, has greatly reduced the time and effort needed to store, query and prepare the livestock statistics for modelling. More importantly, the modelling procedure is easily repeated; the suite of R scripts is readily adapted to modelling recurrent updates, different species, different geographical tiles and different technical specifications for statistical modelling and aggregation of results. Automated post-processing activities further allow the rapid production of country-corrected maps for any specified year, global merging of continental tiles, and aggregation to coarser spatial resolutions, as needed.

Computer processing time was primarily a function of the extent of the continental window (i.e. the number of pixels), of the number of polygons contained in the input shape file and of the technical characteristics of the machines used for modelling. Processing time varied from a minimum of 17 hours for the duck model in Europe to a maximum of 210 hours (or 8.7 days) for the cattle model in Asia. file S7 reports the running times for each species and tile, the number of polygons processed in the input training data and the technical specifications of the computers that were used.

Table 2 summarises the fitting metrics for each tile, species and stratification scheme. It reports both the correlation coefficients and the RMSE between observed and predicted values in the validation data sets. The correlation coefficient is an indication of the precision of the predictions, i.e. the extent to which the observed and predicted values are proportional to each other. However, even with a nearly perfect correlation, the predicted values can be wrong in absolute terms if, for example, they systematically overestimate the population. The RMSE, in contrast, is an indicator of the accuracy of the predictions, i.e. how far they are, on average, from the observed values. The highest correlation coefficients between observed and predicted values are typically found for the species and tiles for which observed data are at a higher spatial resolution and are evenly distributed within the modelling window. The models for the Asian tile had the best correlation coefficients compared to models for other continents: pigs and ducks (0.81), chickens (0.74), and cattle (0.63). Better accuracy of predictions was generally found for cattle compared to other species with RMSE values as low as 0.33 and 0.35 in South and North America respectively. RMSE values for cattle and pigs were consistently lower than they were for chickens. Results in Table 2 also indicated, for a given species, that the best stratification differed across the six continental tiles. For the duck models, the biomes stratification scheme gave the lowest RMSE values in the European and North American tiles and performed similarly to the GLPS stratification in Oceania. Composite stratifications had the lowest RMSE values for all species in Asia, but this was the only tile for which the composite prediction performed consistently better than one of the individual stratification schemes. The biomes stratification performed the best in the North American tile, regardless of the species being modelled, and the EZ25 stratification consistently best in South America.

The results of the tests carried out to evaluate the influence of the administrative level of input data on the accuracy of the predictions are presented in Figure 5. In both countries and species tested, the accuracy of the predictions decreased (increasing RMSE values) as the administrative level of the input data became coarser. It is notable also that the RMSE values for the

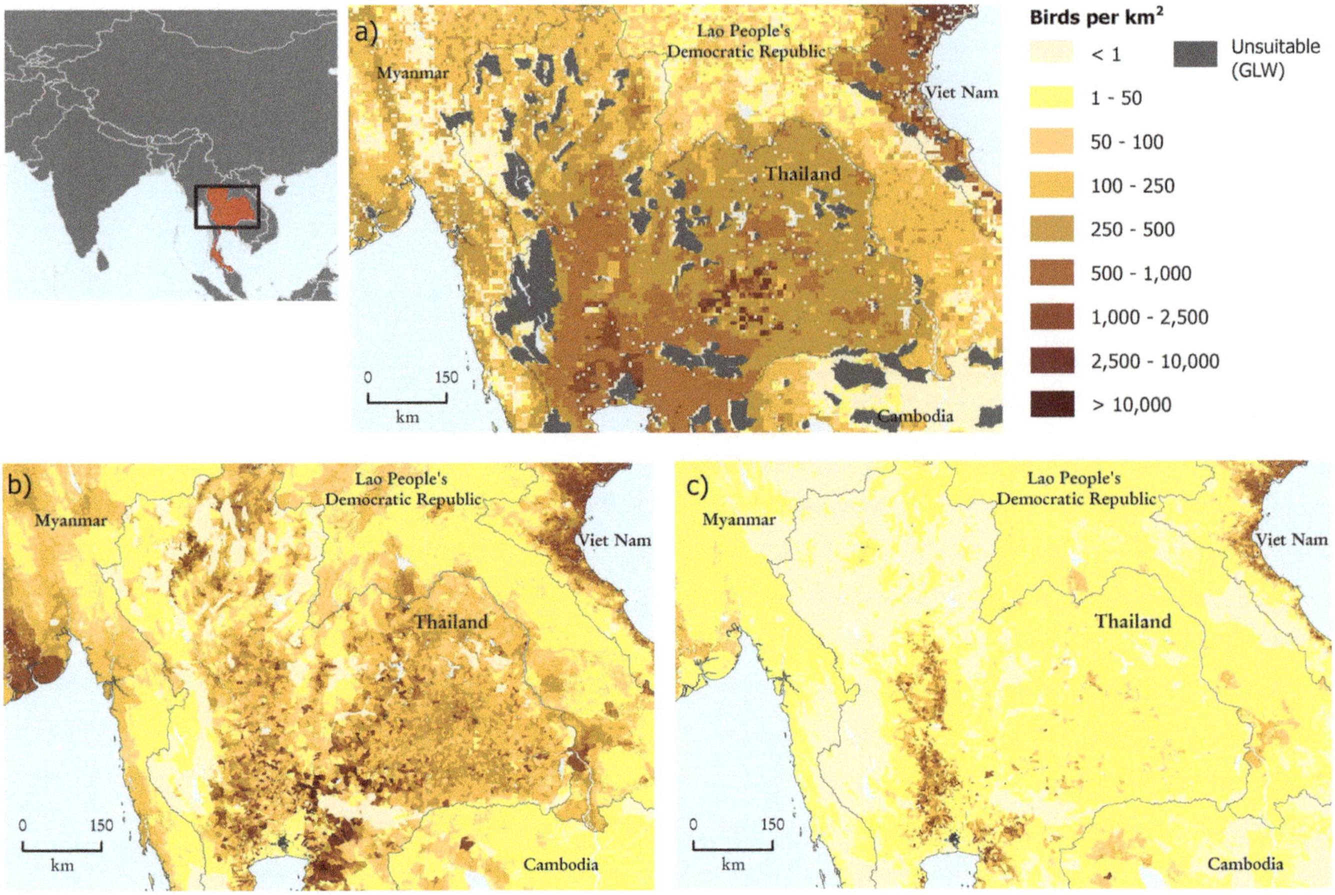

Figure 3. Thailand, visual comparison of a) poultry distribution as mapped in GLW at 5 km; against b) chicken and c) duck distributions mapped separately in GLW 2 at 1 km spatial resolution.

cattle predictions in Brazil were lower at all administrative levels than those for the chicken predictions in Thailand.

Discussion

The new GLW 2 livestock density maps described above provide a timely update of the GLW 2007 livestock distributions [16] and the enhnaced methods and automated procedures mean that updates will, in future, be more frequent than they have been to date. The differences in the modelling procedures, the type and resolution of predictor variables and the different unsuitability masks prevent an explicit, quantitative assessment of change between the livestock densities as mapped by the old and new GLW version. However, we can discuss the improvements that have been made over the original GLW, the accuracy of the predictions and areas where further advances could be made.

Improvements

The first and most obvious improvement is that GLW 2 provides more contemporary data on the distribution of livestock. The original GLW was published in 2007, but many of the reported statistics on which the predictions were based dated back to the 1990's. Whilst some data in the current set of reported statistics remain relatively old, especially in poor countries where censuses have not been carried out for many years, the median year for which livestock statistics have been obtained is much more recent, with most input data dating being more recent than 2000 (see file S4).

The second important improvement is in the spatial resolution of the training data, allowing the full potential of the higher spatial resolution (1 km) in the predictor variables to be availed. This is clearly shown in Figures 5, which illustrates how the use of higher resolution training data and predictor variables have allowed the spatial disaggregation of livestock census data at an unprecedented spatial resolution. Whilst the 1 km resolution may not be required for many applications, such as for example risk or impact assessments at global or continental scales, the higher resolution provides more opportunities for analysis and modelling to be carried out at the scale of individual countries; greatly extending the use of GLW 2. In some countries, the level of detail in the input data is so fine as to bring into question the usefulness of further disaggregating livestock densities to pixel-level. The reasons for continuing with the modelling, even for small polygons, are four in number. Firstly, even small administrative units are rarely homogeneous in terms of land use and farming so, provided that the covariates are accurate at the finer resolution, the data can still be spatially disaggregated in a meaningful way. Secondly, the training data come in heterogeneous administrative units, which would be otherwise difficult to compare between countries. Spatial disaggregation to pixel level harmonises the spatial scale of the estimates and thus facilitates comparison. Thirdly, even fine-scale input data often have gaps, caused for example by administrative units where no census data are available or are of restricted access.

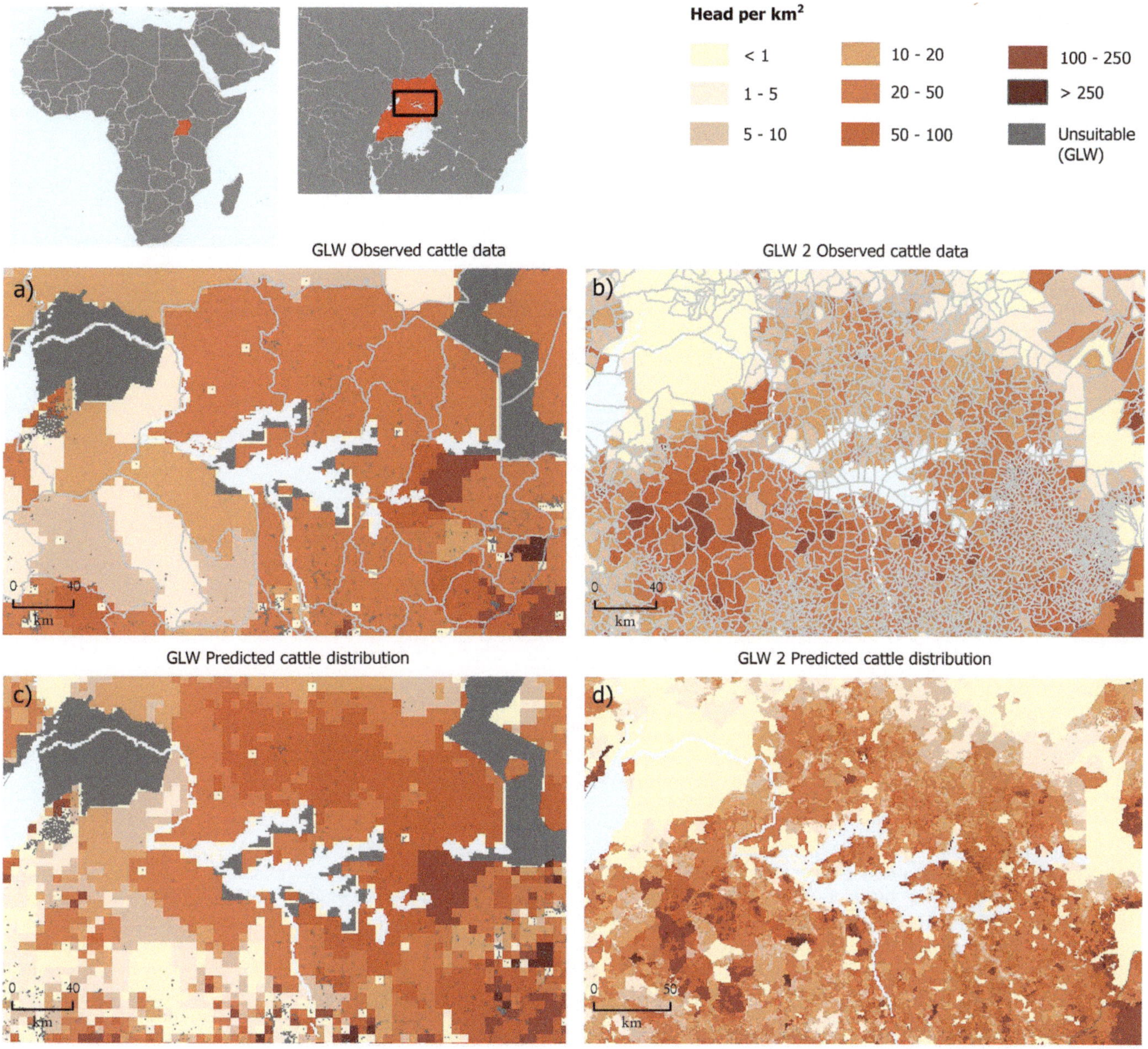

Figure 4. Uganda, visual comparison of observed cattle data a) in GLW 2007 (level 1) and b) in GLW 2 (level 4), and the resulting predicted distribution c) for GLW 2007 and d) for GLW 2.

The modelled distributions allow prediction of livestock densities to be made in those areas. The fourth reason is possibly the most important. Statistical models based on smaller administrative units will capture more of the underlying environmental variability, and are statistically more robust.

A third important improvement in GLW 2 is the estimation of uncertainty around the predicted livestock densities. Whilst the modelling procedure does not provide a full and explicit integration of uncertainty based on a Bayesian framework, the bootstrapping procedure allows coefficients of variation to be calculated around the mean estimates; provides an indicative estimate of the degree of consensus among the different models around the mean estimate.

Finally, the breakdown of species and species groups has also been changed. For example, the previous estimates of poultry densities have been replaced by separate estimates for chickens and ducks. Whilst only cattle, pigs, chicken and ducks have been presented here, GLW 2 is currently being applied to produce distribution maps for other species including goats, sheep and buffaloes, as well as regional maps of camels and equines. This level of species detail is essential for some epidemiological investigations, for example in understanding the geographical distribution of highly pathogenic avian influenza (HPAI) H5N1, where treating chickens and ducks separately has greatly enhanced our ability to predict risk [29].

These new GLW 2 outputs are already finding applications in diverse fields. The new pig distribution maps are currently being applied to a global analysis of current and future pig production, in which the pig distributions are further disaggregated by production system. The latest version (5) of the GLPS [5], which is based

Table 2. Summary of the fitting metrics for each continental tile and species modelled.

Tile	Species	Coefficient of correlation	Stratification	RMSE
Africa	Cattle	0.63	GLPS	0.42
	Chickens	0.66	GLPS	0.45
	Pigs	0.60	EZ25	0.40
	Ducks	n.a.	n.a.	n.a.
Asia	Cattle	0.63	Best RSE	0.46
	Chickens	0.74	Best RSE	0.51
	Pigs	0.81	Best RSE	0.45
	Ducks	0.81	Best RSE	0.57
Europe	Cattle	0.77	EZ25	0.42
	Chickens	0.42	EZ25	1.00
	Pigs	0.57	GLPS	0.67
	Ducks	0.55	Biomes	0.54
North America	Cattle	0.63	Biomes	0.35
	Chickens	0.59	Biomes	0.88
	Pigs	0.66	Biomes	0.45
	Ducks	0.57	Biomes	0.22
Oceania	Cattle	0.50	Biomes	0.48
	Chickens	0.63	Best RSE	0.59
	Pigs	0.72	Biomes	0.54
	Ducks	0.54	GLPS	0.59
South America	Cattle	0.73	EZ25	0.33
	Chickens	0.56	EZ25	0.77
	Pigs	0.64	EZ25	0.41
	Ducks	n.a.	n.a.	n.a.

on land cover data and agro-ecological conditions, maps potential systems rather than actual livestock systems. Integrating these livestock distribution maps with the GLPS will help bring these estimates closer to reality by showing where livestock actually are,

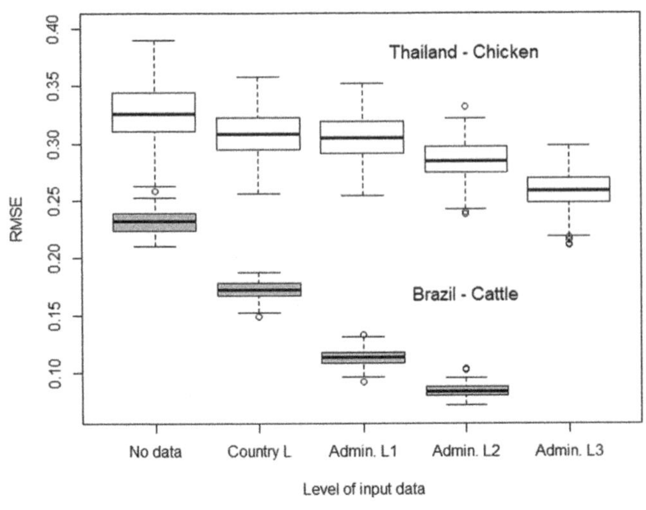

Figure 5. Residual Mean Square Error (RMSE) for predicted versus observed cattle distributions in Brazil, and chicken distributions in Thailand, by administrative level of training data.

rather than where we think conditions are suitable for them to occur. In combination with the revised agricultural projections to 2030 and 2050, recently released by the Agricultural Development and Economic Division (ESA) of FAO [3], these new maps are proving important inputs for further efforts to map the demand and supply of animal-source foods [7]. Likewise, updated global maps of livestock distributions will continue to support analyses that quantify greenhouse gas (GHG) emissions from both the ruminant and monogastric livestock sectors [58]. Finally, the revised maps will find many important epidemiological applications to study disease risk and estimate the impacts of diseases not only in livestock but also for those zoonotic diseases that spill over into the human population. The poultry distributions have already been incorporated into a number of HPAI H5N1 risk assessments [35,59], and their importance has been highlighted in assessing the risk of spread of the recently emerged H7N9 virus in China and beyond [60–61].

Future updates of GLW 2 to include new data as they become available will be greatly facilitated by the integration of the modelling procedure into a fully scripted workflow. The post-processing is part of this automated workflow and allows a variety of outputs to be derived with relative ease and speed. The reference output presented here is a global map of animal densities at 1 km resolution adjusted at the country level to match FAOSTAT 2006 totals. However, outputs expressed in absolute numbers (rather than densities), aggregated to different spatial resolutions (5 km, 10 km or 20 km), or matching different FAOSTAT country totals can also be derived.

Prediction accuracy

The accuracy of the predictions varied significantly according to species and the level of detail in the input training data, and were comparable to those found by Van Boeckel et al. (2011) in Asia, Van Boeckel et al. (2012) in Thailand, and Prosser et al. (2011) in Asia. The administrative level of the training data had a strong influence on model accuracy; with greater accuracy observed with higher administrative levels of training data for both cattle in Brazil and chickens in Thailand (Figure 5). The modifiable areal unit problem (MAUP), well known to quantitative geographers [62], has been demonstrated to have varying effects with different levels of aggregation of input data. Even though the absolute levels of accuracy in prediction for chickens in Thailand and cattle in Brazil were quite different, the fact that we found a positive association between model accuracy and the administrative level at which the training data were used suggests that, wherever possible, data should be sought and collected at the highest possible resolution to train models, even if this results in heterogeneity in administrative levels used to train models, a result comparable to the one found by Van Boeckel et al. (2011) for domestic ducks in Thailand.

Another observation is that the predictions in Europe and North America for cattle and ducks, whose distributions are conditional on presence of suitable pasture and access to water, were consistently better (i.e. had lower RMSE values) than those for chickens and pigs, whose production is highly intensive in these parts of the world (Table 2). In contrast, in a continent like Africa, where the majority of chicken and pig production is extensive, the accuracies of the models for cattle, pigs and chicken were comparable. These observations relate to the influence of the intensity of livestock production on the accuracy of the predictions. As production intensifies it becomes increasingly detached from the land resource base (for example as feeds are brought in that are grown in completely different places) and thus more difficult to predict based on spatial, agro-ecological variables. This effect is particularly marked for chickens and pigs, where the locations of intensive farming units often have more to do with accessibility to markets or to inputs of one sort or another, than to the agro-ecological characteristics of the land that can be quantified through remotely sensed variables. In support of this, Van Boeckel and colleagues [63] found significantly lower predictability for models of intensive chicken production than for models of extensive chicken production in Thailand. As chicken production becomes intensified in many countries, chicken distributions will become increasingly difficult to predict geographically using largely agro-environmental predictors. This inverse relationship between predictability and the level of intensification is well illustrated by the case of chickens in Europe (the model which performed least well, with an RMSE value of 1.0). The regression statistics suggest that the environmental predictors can only partially explain the distribution of chickens and that other factors that are not currently included in the regression models, relating to policy and economics, for example, are likely to be relatively more important in determining the distributions of chickens in such settings. With general trends toward intensified production, the modelling could be improved in the future by incorporating a wider set of anthropogenic, socio-economic and perhaps demand- or trade-related predictor variables. For intensive production systems, the intrinsic variability is also expected to be higher. A chicken production unit, falling into a single 1 km^2 pixel, may contain up to a million birds. The characteristics of that pixel, in all covariates, may be identical to those of a neighbouring pixel where an equivalent production plant was not installed. However, the difference in numbers will be so high that the stochastic decision to place the plant in one pixel rather than the other equivalent one will increase the variability that the model cannot capture, even with the most pertinent covariates.

Validation

A true validation of the predictive accuracy of these models would involve field observation of livestock densities in different pixels and testing those observations against predicted values. However, livestock census data are generally collected and distributed by area (administrative units) and so validation would have to be done on re-aggregated model predictions. Moreover, such validation would be extremely costly and time-consuming. Aside from artificially degrading the training data contributing to models, as we have done here (Figure 5), to make an internal validation of the disaggregation efficiency, there are few options for validation. One possibility which is being explored is the Livestock Geo-Wiki, currently under development along similar lines to the Geo-Wiki produced by the International Institute for Applied Systems Analysis (IIASA) [64–65]. Geo-Wiki uses Internet crowd-sourcing to validate and modify land cover information. It is a web-based application with Google Earth as a backdrop, over which various global land cover datasets are draped. Discrepancies in land cover assignation among the datasets can be highlighted and values may be either corroborated or changed by users logged onto the wiki. The development of the Livestock Geo-Wiki was proposed by Robinson and colleagues [5] as a way to validate livestock production systems information and it is hoped that some form of validation will also be possible for livestock distributions. The roles of the Livestock Geo-Wiki for the livestock distribution data described here are, however, in viewing and providing open access to the data.

Dissemination and future developments

An important objective of the Livestock Geo-Wiki is to disseminate the data. Currently, data on livestock production systems and livestock densities are disseminated via the Gridded Livestock of the World (GLW) website, hosted by FAO (http://www.fao.org/ag/againfo/resources/en/glw/home.html). Whilst this has provided a valuable information resource it is not interactive so the opportunities for users to provide feedback are limited. The Livestock Geo-Wiki has several advantages over more static ways of disseminating data, including, for example: (a) providing a central repository where many different aspects of livestock information may be explored in a highly interactive way; (b) publicising and disseminating open-access livestock sector data at a range of spatial scales; (c) using crowd-sourcing approaches to validate and improve livestock data; and (d) providing innovative data visualisation and analysis tools that will facilitate the investigation of dependencies among the data sets and address specific requirements of diverse groups of users. Instructions on the procedure to download the livestock data from the Livestock Geo-Wiki (http://www.livestock.geo-wiki.org) are provided in file S8.

The improvements to global livestock distribution data, presented here, have been motivated by the pressing need for higher resolution and more contemporary outputs than provided by the original GLW 2007 livestock distributions. Although the methodology has been considerably revised in many aspects, it remains similar to that developed by Wint and Robinson for GLW 2007 [16], involving the use of several stratified multiple regressions linking observed livestock densities to environmental data. New machine-learning methods such as Boosted Regression Trees, or Random Forests have recently demonstrated their increased predictive capacities over more standard statistical methods for species distribution modelling [66]. These methods can better account for non-monotonic relationships between dependent and predictor variables, and can better incorporate the effects of interactions among predictors. Currently, the comparative strength of the stratified regressions lies in the relatively fast fitting of models, and their rapid application to large data sets. However, with the advent of parallelised computing, the use of such machine-learning techniques for modelling livestock distributions is becoming a realistic prospect. These approaches should be investigated in relation to their potential superiority in terms of predictive capacity. In addition, alongside the current set of predictor variables, which are principally environmental in nature, incorporating more socio-economic and anthropogenic predictor variables may confer considerable improvements to models for which the livestock distributions are dominated by more intensified modes of production.

Considerable progress has been made in advancing the spatial modelling of livestock distributions, and there are clearly areas where further improvements can be made. No matter how good the predictive model though, it will always be limited by the quality of the training data on which is based. With this in mind, efforts must be made to identify areas where reported statistics on livestock distributions are out-dated, of low spatial resolution or of doubtful quality, and steps must be taken to address these shortfalls.

Supporting Information

Information S1 Specifications for the continental tiles.

Information S2 Detailed information on MODIS-derived predictor variables (source, derived Fourier variables, image values and rescaling if applicable).

Information S3 Islamic countries in relation to modelling the distributions of pigs. Countries emboldened in red are those flagged with zero values in modelling the distribution of pigs. (Source: Adapted from Wikipedia http://en.wikipedia.org/wiki/List_of_Muslim-majority_countries).

Information S4 Aggregate information on sub-national statistics (year and level of observation) by continental tile and species.

Information S5 5a. Country details on sub-national statistics for cattle (year and level of observation) by continental tile. (file SI5.pdf) Supplementary information 5b. Country details on sub-national statistics for pigs (year and level of observation) by continental tile. (file SI5.pdf) Supplementary information 5c. Country details on sub-national statistics for chickens (year and level of observation) by continental tile. (file SI5.pdf) Supplementary information 5d. Country details on sub-national statistics for ducks (year and level of observation) by continental tile.

Information S6 6a. Average Spatial Resolution (ASR) of the training data used to model a) cattle; b) pigs; c) chickens and d) ducks distributions. The ASR measures the effective resolution of input administrative units in kilometers. It is calculated as the square root of the land area divided by the number of administrative units [1,2]. (file SI6.pdf) Supplementary information 6b. Country level of detail for the training data of a) cattle; b) pigs; c) chickens and d) ducks.

Information S7 Polygon details and processing time for each continental tile and species.

Information S8 Procedure to download the output raster data.

Acknowledgments

The work presented here is the culmination of many years of collaboration between FAO, ILRI, the University of Oxford and the Université Libre de Bruxelles. The work has been facilitated in different ways by numerous colleagues and we would like in particular to acknowledge contributions from Samuel Jutzi, Joachim Otte, Henning Steinfeld, Jan Slingenbergh, Pierre Gerber, Jeroen Dijkman, Giuliano Cecchi, Russ Kruska, Philip Thornton, David Bourne, David Rogers, Steffen Fritz, Martina Duerauer and Christoph Perger.

Author Contributions

Conceived and designed the experiments: TR MG WW TPVB. Performed the experiments: TPR MG GRWW VE EP G. Conchedda G. Cinardi SIH. Analyzed the data: TPR MG GRWW TPVB VE EP G. Conchedda LDA G. Cinardi SIH. Contributed reagents/materials/analysis tools: TPR MG GRWW SIH. Wrote the paper: TPR MG GRWW TPVB G. Conchedda.

References

1. FAO (2009) The State of Food and Agriculture. Livestock in the Balance. Rome, Italy: Food and Agriculture Organization of the United Nations (FAO).
2. FAO (2011) World Livestock 2011 - Livestock in food security. Rome, Italy: Food and Agriculture Organization of the United Nations (FAO).
3. Alexandratos N, Bruinsma J (2012) World Agriculture Towards 2030/2050. The 2012 Revision. Global Perspective Studies Team. ESA Working Paper No. 12-03. Rome, Italy FAO, Food and Agriculture Organization of the United Nations.
4. de Haan C, Gerber P, Opio C (2010) Structural Change in the Livestock Sector. In: Steinfeld H, Mooney HA, Schneider F and Neville LE, editors. Livestock in a Changing Landscape. Drivers, Consequences, and Responses. Volume 1. Washington D.C., USA: Island Press. pp. 35–51.
5. Robinson TP, Thornton PK, Franceschini G, Kruska RL, Chiozza F, et al. (2011) Global livestock production systems. Rome: Food and Agriculture Organization of the United Nations (FAO) and International Livestock Research Institute (ILRI). pp. 152.
6. Otte J, Costales A, Dijkman J, Pica-Ciamarra U, Robinson T, et al. (2012) Livestock sector development for poverty reduction: an economic and policy perspective. Livestock's many virtues. Rome: Food and Agriculture Organization of the United Nations (FAO). 161 p.
7. Robinson TP, Pozzi F (2011) Mapping supply and demand for animal-source foods to 2030. Animal Production and Health Working Paper No. 2. Rome: Food and Agriculture Organisation (FAO) of the United Nations. pp. 164.
8. Narrod C, Tiongco M, Delgado C (2010) Socioeconomic Implications of the Livestock Industrialization Process. In: Steinfeld H, Mooney HA, Schneider F and Neville LE, editors. Livestock in a Changing Landscape. Drivers, Consequences, and Responses. Volume 1. Washington D.C., USA: Island Press. pp. 269–285.
9. World Bank (2005) Managing the livestock revolution. Report no. 32725-GLB. Washington D.C. USA: World Bank. pp. 63.
10. Solomon S, Qin D, Manning M, Chen Z, Marquis M, et al. (2007) Climate Change 2007: The physical science basis: Contribution of Working Group I to the Fourth Assessment Report of the Intergovernmental Panel on Climate Change. In: Solomon S, Qin D, Manning M, Chen Z, Marquis M, Averyt KB, Tignor M and Miller HL, editors. Cambridge, United Kingdom and New York, NY, USA: Cambridge University Press pp. 996.
11. Steinfeld H, Mooney HA, Schneider F, Neville LE (2010) Livestock in a Changing Landscape. Drivers, Consequences, and Responses. Volume 1. Washington D.C., USA: Island Press. pp. 396.
12. Bonfoh B, Schwabenbauer K, Wallinga D, Hartung J, Schelling E, et al. (2010) Human Health Hazards Associated with Livestock Production. In: Steinfeld H, Mooney HA, Schneider F and Neville LE, editors. Livestock in a Changing Landscape. Drivers, Consequences, and Responses. Volume 1. Washington D.C., USA: Island Press. pp. 197–221.

13. Herrero M, Thornton PK, Notenbaert AM, Wood S, Msangi S, et al. (2010) Smart Investments in Sustainable Food Production: Revisiting Mixed Crop-Livestock Systems. Science 327: 822–825.
14. Ito T, Couceiro JN, Kelm S, Baum LG, Krauss S, et al. (1998) Molecular basis for the generation in pigs of influenza A viruses with pandemic potential. J Virol: 7367–7373.
15. Ma W, Kahn RE, Richt JA (2009) The pig as a mixing vessel for influenza viruses: Human and veterinary implications. J Mol Genet Med: 158–166.
16. FAO (2007) Gridded Livestock of the World, 2007, by G.R.W. Wint and T.P. Robinson. Food and Agriculture Organization of the United Nations, Rome. 131 p.
17. Neumann K, Elbersen BS, Verburg PH, Staritsky I, Pérez-Soba M, et al. (2009) Modelling the spatial distribution of livestock in Europe. Landsc Ecol 24: 1207–1222.
18. Prosser DJ, Wu J, Ellis EC, Gale F, Van Boeckel TP, et al. (2011) Modelling the distribution of chickens, ducks, and geese in China. Agric Ecosyst Environ 141: 381–389.
19. Van Boeckel TP, Prosser D, Franceschini G, Biradar C, Wint W, et al. (2011) Modelling the distribution of domestic ducks in Monsoon Asia. Agric Ecosyst Environ 141: 373–380.
20. Letourneau A, Verburg PH, Stehfest E (2012) A land-use systems approach to represent land-use dynamics at continental and global scales. Environ Model Softw 33: 61–79.
21. Naidoo R, Balmford A, Costanza R, Fisher B, Green RE, et al. (2008) Global mapping of ecosystem services and conservation priorities. Proc Natl Acad Sci U S A 105: 9495–9500.
22. Herrero M, Thornton PK, Kruska R, Reid RS (2008) Systems dynamics and the spatial distribution of methane emissions from African domestic ruminants to 2030. Agric Ecosyst Environ 126: 122–137.
23. Steinfeld H, Gerber P, Wassenar T, Castel V, Rosales M, et al. (2006) Livestock's long shadow: Environmental issues and options. Rome, Italy: Food and Agriculture Organization (FAO).
24. Thornton PK, van de Steeg J, Notenbaert A, Herrero M (2009) The impacts of climate change on livestock and livestock systems in developing countries: A review of what we know and what we need to know. Agric Syst 101: 113–127.
25. Cecchi G, Wint W, Shaw A, Marletta A, Mattioli R, et al. (2010) Geographic distribution and environmental characterization of livestock production systems in Eastern Africa. Agric Ecosyst Environ 135: 98–110.
26. Cecchi G, Mattioli R (2009) Geospatial datasets and analyses for an environmental approach to African trypanosomiasis. PAAT (Programme Against African Trypanosomiasis). Technical and Scientific Series. No. 9. Rome: Food and Agriculture Organization of the United Nations. pp. 80.
27. Cecchi G, Mattioli RC, Slingenbergh J, de la Rocque S (2008) Land cover and tsetse fly distributions in sub-Saharan Africa. Med Vet Entomol 22: 364–373.
28. Gilbert M, Xiao X, Pfeiffer DU, Epprecht M, Boles S, et al. (2008) Mapping H5N1 highly pathogenic avian influenza risk in Southeast Asia. Proc Natl Acad Sci U S A 105: 4769–4774.
29. Muzaffar SB, Takekawa JY, Prosser DJ, Newman SH, Xiao X (2010) Rice Production Systems and Avian Influenza: Interactions between Mixed-Farming Systems, Poultry and Wild Birds. Waterbirds 33: 219–230.
30. Sumption K, Rweyemamu M, Wint W (2008) Incidence and Distribution of Foot-and-Mouth Disease in Asia, Africa and South America; Combining Expert Opinion, Official Disease Information and Livestock Populations to Assist Risk Assessment. Transbound Emerg Dis 55: 5–13.
31. Mangen MJ, Otte J, Pfeiffer D, Chilonda P (2002) Bovine brucellosis in sub-Saharan Africa: estimation of sero-prevalence and impact on meat and milk offtake potential. Livestock Policy Discussion Paper No. 8 Rome: Food and Agriculture of the United Nations - Livestock Information and Policy Branch, AGAL. pp. 58.
32. Hendrickx G, de La Rocque S, Reid R, Wint W (2001) Spatial trypanosomosis management: from data-layers to decision making. Trends Parasitol 17: 35–41.
33. Shaw A, Cecchi G, Wint G, Mattioli R, Robinson T (2014) Mapping the economic benefits to livestock keepers from intervening against bovine trypanosomosis in Eastern Africa. Prev Vet Med 113: 197–210.
34. Franceschini G, Robinson TP, Morteo K, Dentale D, Wint GRW, et al. (2009) The Global Livestock Impact Mapping System (GLIMS) as a tool for animal health applications. Vet Ital: 491–499.
35. Gaughan AE, Stevens FR, Linard C, Jia P, Tatem AJ (2013) High Resolution Population Distribution Maps for Southeast Asia in 2010 and 2015. PLoS ONE 8: e55882.
36. Linard C, Gilbert M, Snow RW, Noor AM, Tatem AJ (2012) Population Distribution, Settlement Patterns and Accessibility across Africa in 2010. PLoS ONE 7: e31743.
37. R Core Team (2012) R: A language and environment for statistical computing. R Foundation for Statistical Computing, Vienna, Austria. ISBN 3-900051-07-0, URL http://www.R-project.org/.
38. Eastman JR (2009) IDRISI Taiga (Worcester, MA: Clark University).
39. European Commission Joint Research Centre (2003) Global Land Cover 2000 database. Available: http://bioval.jrc.ec.europa.eu/products/glc2000/glc2000.php. Accessed 2014 April 16.
40. Dudley N (2008) Guidelines for Applying Protected Area Management Categories. International Union for the Conservation of Nature (IUCN). Gland, Switzerland. pp. 106.
41. Rogers DJ (1997) Satellite Imagery and the Prediction of Tsetse Distributions in East Africa. In Diagnosis and Control of Livestock Diseases using Nuclear and related techniques Vienna, Austria: International Atomic Energy Agency. pp. 397–420.
42. Rogers DJ (2000) Satellites, space, time and the African trypanosomiases. Adv Parasitol 47: 129–171.
43. Rogers DJ, Hay SI, Packer MJ (1996) Predicting the distribution of tsetse flies in West Africa using temporal Fourier processed meteorological satellite data. Ann Trop Med Parasitol 90: 225–241.
44. Rogers DJ, Williams BG (1994) Tsetse distribution in Africa: seeing the wood and the trees. In: Edwards PJ, May RM, Webb NR, editors. Large-scale ecology and conservation biology. 35th symposium of the Britush Ecological Society with the Society for Conservation Biology. Chapter 11. pp. 249–273. Oxford, UK: Blackwell Scientific Publications.
45. Scharlemann JPW, Benz D, Hay SI, Purse BV, Tatem AJ, et al. (2008) Global data for ecology and epidemiology: A novel algorithm for temporal fourier processing MODIS data. PLoS ONE 3.
46. Zhang X, Friedl MA, Schaaf CB, Strahler AH, Hodges JCF, et al. (2003) Monitoring vegetation phenology using MODIS. Remote Sens Environ 84: 471–475.
47. Jones P (1987) Current availability and deficiencies in data relevant to agro-ecological studies in the geographic area covered by the IARCS. In: A.H. Bunting (Ed), Agricultural Environments. CAB International, Wallingford, UK, pp. 69–83.
48. Jones PG, Thornton PK (2009) Croppers to livestock keepers: livelihood transitions to 2050 in Africa due to climate change. Environ Sci Policy 12: 427–437.
49. Hijmans RJ, Cameron SE, Parra JL, Jones PG, Jarvis A (2005) Very high resolution interpolated climate surfaces for global land areas. International Journal of Climatology 25: 1965–1978.
50. CIESIN, IFPRI, World Bank and CIAT(2004) Global Rural Urban Mapping Project (GRUMP), Beta Version. New York, Center for Internation Earth Science Information Network (CIESIN), Columbia University; International Food Policy Research Institute (IFPRI); The World Bank & Centro Internacional de Agricultura Tropical (CIAT). Palisades, NY: Socioeconomic Data and Applications Center (SEDAC), Columbia University. Available: http://sedac.ciesin.columbia.edu/data/sets/browse. Accessed 2014 April 16.
51. Nelson A (2008) Travel time to major cities: A global map of Accessibility. Global Environment Monitoring Unit - Joint Research Centre of the European Commission, Ispra Italy. Available: http://gem.jrc.ec.europa.eu/. Accessed 2014 April 16.
52. USGS-EROS (1996) Global 30 Arc-Second Elevation Data Set. 1996. US Geological Survey (USGS) - Earth Resources Observation Systems (EROS). EROS Data Center (EDC) Distributed Active Archive Center (DAAC), Sioux Falls, South Dakota, USA. Available: http://eros.usgs.gov/#/Find_Data/Products_and_Data_Available/GTOPO30. Accessed 2014 April 16.
53. Griguolo S, Mazzanti M (1996) ADDAPIX: pixel-by-pixel classification for zoning and monitoring. Rome: FAO Technical Report SD:GCP/INt/578/NET. Revised May 2000. Rome, Italy. pp. 76.
54. Olson DM, Dinerstein E, Wikramanayake ED, Burgess ND, Powell GVN, et al. (2001) Terrestrial ecoregions of the world: A new map of life on Earth. BioScience 51: 933–938.
55. Zuur A, Ieno EN, Smith GM (2007) Analysing Ecological Data. XXVI, 672 p.
56. Gilbert M, Xiao X, Chaitaweesub P, Kalpravidh W, Premashthira S, et al. (2007) Avian influenza, domestic ducks and rice agriculture in Thailand. Agric Ecosyst Environ 119: 409–415.
57. Weimin M (2010) Distribution and characteristics of duck-fish farming systems in Eastern China. Smallholder Poultry Production. Rome: Food and Agriculture of the United Nations (FAO). pp. 28.
58. MacLeod M, Gerber P, Opio C, Henderson B, Dietze K, et al. (2013) Greenhouse gas emissions from pig and chicken supply chains – A global life cycle assessment Rome: Food and Agriculture Organization (FAO) of the United Nations. pp. 196.
59. Martin V, Pfeiffer DU, Zhou X, Xiao X, Prosser DJ, et al. (2011) Spatial distribution and risk factors of highly pathogenic avian influenza (HPAI) H5N1 in China. PLoS Pathogens 7.
60. Butler D (2013) Mapping the H7N9 avian flu outbreaks. Nature doi:101038/nature201312863.
61. Horby P, Tatem AJ, Huang Z, Gilbert M, Robinson TP, et al. (2013) H7N9 is a virus worth worrying about. Nature doi:101038/496399a 496(7446): 399.
62. Openshaw S (1983) The modifiable areal unit problem. Concepts and techniques in modern geography. Norwich, UK: Geo Books Vol. 38
63. Van Boeckel TP, Thanapongtharm W, Robinson T, D'Aietti L, Gilbert M (2012) Predicting the distribution of intensive poultry farming in Thailand. Agric Ecosyst Environ 149: 144–153.
64. Fritz S, McCallum I, Schill C, Perger C, Grillmayer R, et al. (2009) Geo-wiki.org: The use of crowdsourcing to improve global land cover. Remote Sens 1: 345–354.
65. Fritz S, McCallum I, Schill C, Perger C, See L, et al. (2012) Geo-Wiki: An online platform for improving global land cover. Environ Model Softw 31: 110–123.
66. Elith JH, Graham CP, Anderson R, Dudík M, Ferrier S, et al. (2006) Novel methods improve prediction of species' distributions from occurrence data. Ecography 29: 129–151.

2

Effects of Naturally Occurring Six- and Twelve-Nucleotide Inserts on Newcastle Disease Virus Replication and Pathogenesis

Anandan Paldurai[1], Sa Xiao[1], Shin-Hee Kim[1], Sachin Kumar[1], Baibaswata Nayak[1], Sweety Samal[1], Peter L. Collins[2], Siba K. Samal[1]*

1 Virginia-Maryland Regional College of Veterinary Medicine, University of Maryland, College Park, Maryland, United States of America, **2** Laboratory of Infectious Diseases, National Institute of Allergy and Infectious Diseases, Bethesda, Maryland, United States of America

Abstract

Newcastle disease virus (NDV) isolates contain genomes of 15,186, 15,192 or 15,198 nucleotides (nt). The length differences reflect a 6-nt insert in the 5′ (downstream) non-translated region (NTR) of the N gene (15,192-nt genome) or a 12-nt insert in the ORF encoding the P and V proteins (causing a 4-amino acid insert; 15,198-nt genome). We evaluated the role of these inserts in the N and P genes on viral replication and pathogenicity by inserting them into genomes of two NDV strains that have natural genome lengths of 15,186 nt and represent two different pathotypes, namely the mesogenic strain Beaudette C (BC) and the velogenic strain GB Texas (GBT). Our results showed that the 6-nt and 12-nt inserts did not detectably affect N gene expression or P protein function. The inserts had no effect on the replication or virulence of the highly virulent GBT strain but showed modest degree of attenuation in mesogenic strain BC. We also deleted a naturally-occurring 6-nt insertion in the N gene from a highly virulent 15,192-nt genome-length virus, strain Banjarmasin. This resulted in reduced replication *in vitro* and reduced virulence *in vivo*. Thus, although these inserts had no evident effect on gene expression, protein function, or replication *in vivo*, they did affect virulence in two of the three tested strains.

Editor: Toru Takimoto, University of Rochester Medical Center, United States of America

Funding: This research was supported by NIAID contract N01A060009 (85% support) and the NIAID NIH Intramural Research Program (15% support). The views expressed herein do not necessarily reflect the official policies of the Department of Health and Human Services, and the mention of trade names, commercial practices, or organizations does not imply endorsement by the U.S. Government. The funders had no role in study design, data collection and analysis, decision to publish, or preparation of the manuscript.

Competing Interests: The authors have declared that no competing interests exist.

* Email: ssamal@umd.edu

Introduction

Newcastle disease (ND) is one of the most important diseases of domesticated and wild birds [1,2]. The causative agent ND virus (NDV) causes a highly contagious and lethal disease that accounts for huge economic losses to the poultry industry worldwide [1–3]. NDV is a single stranded negative sense RNA virus in the genus *Avulavirus* under the family *Paramyxoviridae* [4,5]. The genome of NDV contains six genes encoding the nucleocapsid protein (N), phosphoprotein (P), matrix protein (M), fusion protein (F), hemagglutinin-neuraminidase protein (HN), and large polymerase protein (L). In addition, the P gene encodes an additional protein called V that is expressed by RNA editing.

Naturally occurring NDV strains exhibit a spectrum of virulence, with mortality in chickens ranging from 0 to 100% [1–3]. Based on the degree of virulence, NDV strains are classified as lentogenic (low virulence), mesogenic (moderate virulence) and velogenic (high virulence) pathotypes [1–3]. In addition, NDV strains are categorized into two phylogenetically divergent classes, namely class I and class II. Class I strains are typically isolated from healthy water fowl and are not associated with disease. Class II contains strains that cause infections ranging from inapparent to highly fatal. These two classes are further divided into genotypes based on partial or complete nucleotide sequence of the F gene. Currently, class I strains represent a single genotype and class II strains represent at least XVIII genotypes [6–9].

The complete genome sequence analysis of NDV strains reveal the existence of genome lengths of 15,186 nucleotides (nt) [2,4,10–12], 15,192 nt [13–15] or 15,198 nt [16–20]. All these genome lengths are divisible by six conforming to the 'rule of six' that is observed in all viruses of the subfamily *Paramyxovirinae* [4]. These sequence length variations in the NDV genome was identified in the nucleoprotein gene and in the phosphoprotein gene as a 6-nt and 12-nt insert sequences, respectively. Previous studies involving genome sequence analysis of NDV strains identified the presence of the N-gene and P-gene inserts and related them to the natural history of NDV as: the 15,186-nt genome-length viruses circulated between 1930 and 1960, and the 15,192-nt and 15,198-nt genome-length viruses emerged after 1960 [10–20]. The 15,186-nt and 15,192-nt genome-length viruses belong to the NDV genetic class II and the 15,198-nt genome-length viruses belong to NDV genetic class I. Currently, all three genome-length viruses are circulating in bird populations around the world. The sequence alignment and phylogenetic tree analysis revealed that NDV strains which belonged to a particular genome-length assignment clustered together (Fig. 1). The percent nt sequence identities of NDV genomes suggest a very close genetic relationship of a particular genome-length virus strains to others (Table S1). In addition, our laboratory recently identified a unique virus of the 15,198-nt genome-length containing a 6-nt insert in the N gene and another 6-nt insert in the intergenic sequence between HN and L genes [22]. This later HN-L insert will not be addressed in the present study.

All the 15,192-nt genome-length viruses contain a 6-nt insert (e.g., AGGGUG in strain ZJ1) in the 5′ (downstream) noncoding region of the N gene after genome position 1647 [13,14] (Fig. 1a), and all previously-analyzed 15,198-nt genome-length viruses contain a 12-nt insert (e.g., ACCCUCUGCCCC in strain Alaska 415) in the ORF encoding the P and V proteins after genome position 2381 [16–20]. The 12-nt insertion increases the lengths of the P and V proteins by four amino acids (aa) without affecting their reading frames. The aa sequence introduced in P and V proteins are WETG and VGDG, respectively, at aa position 166 to 169 (e.g., strain Alaska 415). The importance of these inserts in NDV biology is not known.

In this study, we investigated the biological significance of the 6-nt N and 12-nt P inserts by introducing them separately by reverse genetics into the genomes of two genetically cloned 15,186-nt genome-length viruses strain Beaudette C (BC) [11,23] and strain Texas GB (GBT) [24]. Reciprocally, we also evaluated the effect of deleting the 6-nt N insert from a naturally-occurring 15,192-nt genome-length strain Banjarmasin (Ban) [25,26]. The strains BC and GBT are genetically closely related and belong to genotype II, and the strain Ban belongs to genotype VII. All three strains belong to NDV phylogenetic class II and possess an identical sequence ^{112}RRQKR↓F^{117} at the proteolytic cleavage site of their fusion proteins but differ in virulence. BC is a mesogenic strain and GBT and Ban are velogenic strains.

Our results showed that the addition of the 6-nt N or the 12-nt P insert into the genome of 15,186-nt genome-length viruses or the deletion of the 6-nt insert from a 15,192-nt genome virus resulted in a decrease of virulence. These results suggest that the 6-nt and the 12-nt inserts found in the 15,192-nt and 15,198-nt genome-length viruses may not have any direct role in replication and virulence but they make up the optimal genome-length that is required for efficient virus replication and pathogenesis.

Materials and Methods

Cells and viruses

A chicken embryo fibroblast cell line (DF-1), a human epidermoid carcinoma cell line (HEp-2), and a human embryonic kidney cell line (293T) were obtained from the American Type Culture Collection (ATCC, Manassas, VA). The cell lines were grown in Dulbecco's minimal essential medium (DMEM) with 10% fetal bovine serum (FBS) and maintained in DMEM with 2% FBS. The modified vaccinia virus strain Ankara (MVA) expressing T7 RNA polymerase was kindly provided by Dr. Bernard Moss (NIH, Bethesda, MD). The recombinant (r) NDV strains BC (rBC), GBT (rGBT), Banjarmasin (rBan), and their mutant derivatives were grown in nine-day-old embryonated specific-pathogen-free (SPF) chicken eggs in an enhanced biosafety level 3 (BSL-3+) containment facility certified by the USDA following the guidelines of the IACUC, University of Maryland.

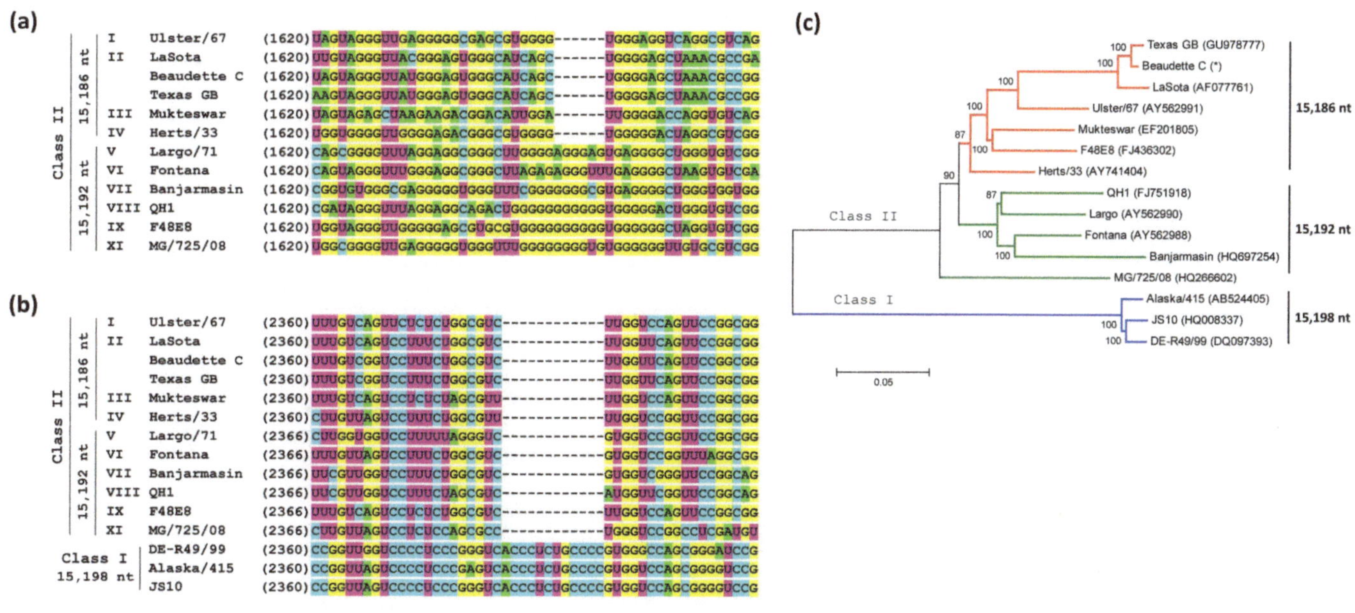

Figure 1. Nucleotide sequence alignment and phylogenetic tree analysis of NDV strains. (a) Nucleotide (nt) sequence alignment of part of the 5′ (downstream) non-translated region (NTR) of the Nucleocapsid protein (N) gene of NDV strains to illustrate the 6-nt insert that is characteristic of 15,192-nt size class viruses. (b) Nt sequence alignment of part of the ORF of the Phosphoprotein (P) gene NDV strains to illustrate the 12-nt insert that is found in many of the 15,198-nt size class viruses. All sequences shown are negative-sense and gaps indicate absence of the insert sequence. The nucleotide residues are color coded; U-violet, A-green, G-yellow and C-blue. (c) Phylogenetic tree analysis based on the nt sequences of complete genomes of NDV strains. Note the clustering of NDV strains with respect to their genome-length. Branches in each cluster is color coded: red-15,186 nt; green-15,192 nt; blue-15,198 nt. The tree was constructed by bootstrap analysis (1000 replications) using the neighbor-joining of the Kimura-2-parameter method for nt differences in the MEGA 4.0 phylogenetic analysis program [21]. Scale bar shows number of base substitutions per site. Bootstrap values are shown at the nodes. Note the clustering of unique genome-length viruses. Asterisk (*) indicate the reference for the sequence of strain BC [11]. The genetic class designations are indicated for NDV strains in all three panels.

Reverse genetic systems for NDV strains BC, GBT, and Ban

Full-length antigenome cDNA clones of NDV strains BC and GBT were constructed in the present study by sequential cloning into pBR322/HDr vector using a previously-described strategy [23]. First a 112 nt linker sequence containing 9 unique restriction enzyme (RE) sites in the order of AscI, PacI, PmeI, AsiSI, AgeI, SnaBI, BstBI, MluI and RsrII, was cloned between AscI and RsrII sites in the pBR322/HDr vector. Among these RE sites, AgeI site was a unique site present in the genomes of BC and GBT. The antigenomes of BC and GBT were constructed as 8 matching fragments using the 9 restriction enzyme sites noted above, which were spaced identically in each antigenome construct (Fig. 2a). The segments were synthesized by PCR from BC full length plasmid DNA [23] and from viral RNA using RT-PCR for GBT. PCR was performed with the high fidelity platinum *Pfx* polymerase, and the gel purified fragments were digested and sequentially cloned into the pBR322/HDr vector [23]. The sequential cloning of N, P, M, F and HN genes was performed as segments 1, 2, 3, 4 and 5. The L gene was cloned as three fragments, namely, 6, 7 and 8. In total, 16 nt changes were introduced in the antigenomes of strains BC and GBT to introduce the RE sites and to modify a naturally occurring RsrII site in the P gene. All of the RE sites were introduced into non-translated regions with the exception of the BstBI and MluI sites that were introduced into the L ORF. The nt changes in the L ORF were introduced in such a way that the aa sequence was not altered. The nt changes made are A(1768)T, C(1769)T, C(1773)T, A(3221)G, A(3222)T, T(3227)A, T(4452)G, T(4453)C, T(4457)C, A(4458)G, T(4459)C, A(8327)C, G(8330)A, G(10396)A, A(13537)G, and A(13537)G. Support plasmids expressing the N, P, and L proteins of strain GBT were constructed using the pGEM7Z (+) expression vector. Support plasmids for NDV strains BC and Ban were previously constructed in our laboratory [23,25].

Construction and rescue of mutant viruses of NDV strains BC, GBT, and Ban

A 6-nt (AGGGUG) or 12-nt (ACCCUCUGCCCC) insert conforming to the respective consensus sequence (see Results and Fig. 2a) was introduced separately into the N (after nt position 1647) or P (after nt position 2381) genes of strains BC and GBT using overlap PCR and cloned using RE sites AscI and PacI for N gene and PacI and PmeI for P gene, respectively. In addition, the existing 6-nt N insert that occurs naturally in strain Ban was deleted by the same method using RE sites AscI and PacI (Fig. 2b).

Virus growth kinetics and plaque morphology

The growth kinetics of rBC, rGBT, rBan, and their mutant viruses were determined under multi-cycle growth conditions in DF-1 cells. The virus was inoculated at a multiplicity of infection (MOI) of 0.01 PFU into DF-1 cells grown in DMEM with 10% FBS at 37°C. Aliquots from the medium supernatant were collected at 8-h intervals until 64 h post infection for rBC and rGBT viruses and their mutants (Fig. 3a, b). For rBan and its mutant, DF-1 cells were infected with an MOI of 0.01 PFU, and aliquots from the medium supernatant were collected at 12 h intervals for 48 h (Fig. 3c). Viral titers were assayed by limiting dilution in DF-1 cells, and titers were determined using the method of Reed and Muench [27] and expressed as 50%-tissue-culture-infectious-dose (TCID50) units. Plaque assays were performed to determine the plaque morphology: plaques were photographed and measured on day 5 in the case of the rBC and rGBT groups of viruses, and on day 7 for rBan and its mutant virus (Fig. 3d).

Production of N protein antiserum and immunoblot analysis

A 15-aa synthetic peptide was custom synthesized (GenScript) in which first aa was an added cysteine for conjugation and aa 2 to 15 corresponded to aa 191 to 204 of the N protein of NDV strain LaSota. One rabbit was injected with 1 mg of KLH-conjugated synthetic N protein peptide in Freund's complete adjuvant to raise anti-N protein antiserum. After 2 weeks, a booster immunization was given with 0.5 mg of the peptide in Freund's incomplete adjuvant, and the hyperimmune serum was collected 2 weeks later. Western blot analysis was performed using NDV-infected cell lysates to confirm the specificity of the antisera to NDV N protein (data not shown).

Expression of N protein in the recombinant viruses, rBC and rBC-N6 and rBan and rBan-ΔN6, were examined by immunoblot analysis. Briefly, DF-1 cells were infected at a MOI of 0.1 PFU. The cells were harvested at 24 h post infection, the lysed proteins were denatured, reduced, separated by NuPAGE 4–12% Bis-Tris gel (Life Technologies, Grand Island, New York), and analyzed by immunoblotting using a 1:100 dilution of anti-N peptide antibody described above. β-Tubulin was used as the loading control. The band density of N protein was quantitated and compared between rBC and rBC-N6 and between rBan and rBan-ΔN6 using ImageJ analysis [28] (Fig. 4a, b).

Minigenome system for NDV strain BC

We developed a minigenome system for strain BC. A cDNA was designed to encode a negative-sense mini-genome containing (Fig. 4c): the 3′-terminal 221 nt of the BC genome, including the 55-nt leader region and complete upstream non-translated region of N gene, followed by the 660-nt chloramphenicol acetyl transferase (CAT) reporter gene in negative sense, followed by the 5′-terminal 265 nt of the BC genome, including the last 152 nt of the L gene (containing the last 42 nt of the coding region and the complete downstream non translated region) and the 113-nt trailer region. In the mini-genome cDNA, the leader region was flanked by the hepatitis delta virus ribozyme and the trailer was flanked by a T7 promoter sequence, so that T7 transcription would yield a negative-sense mini-genome (Fig. 4c). The mini-genome cDNA was constructed from three fragments containing (i) the leader and upstream N sequence, (ii) the CAT sequence, and (iii) the downstream L and trailer sequence. These three fragments were joined sequentially by two rounds of overlapping PCR using high fidelity *Pfx* polymerase. The final product was cloned into pBR322/HDr between RE sites AscI and RsrII as shown in Figure 4c, and its sequence was confirmed.

Expression plasmids of BC N, P, L, and P with 12 nt insertion also were cloned separately in pCDNA3.1 (+) expression vector. 0.8 μg of minigenome plasmid and 0.8 μg of N, 0.6 μg of P or P with 12 nt insert (P12) and 0.5 μg of L plasmids were transfected using Lipofectamine 2000 reagent on to a 80% monolayer of 293T cells in 12-well cell culture plate. MVA-T7 was used to infect the monolayer at the same time. Media was changed after 3 h, and incubated for 48 h and samples for CAT-ELISA were processed following the manufacturer's protocol and the OD values were recorded at 405 nm (Fig. 4d). Plasmids N and P were used along with BC minigenome to serve as control.

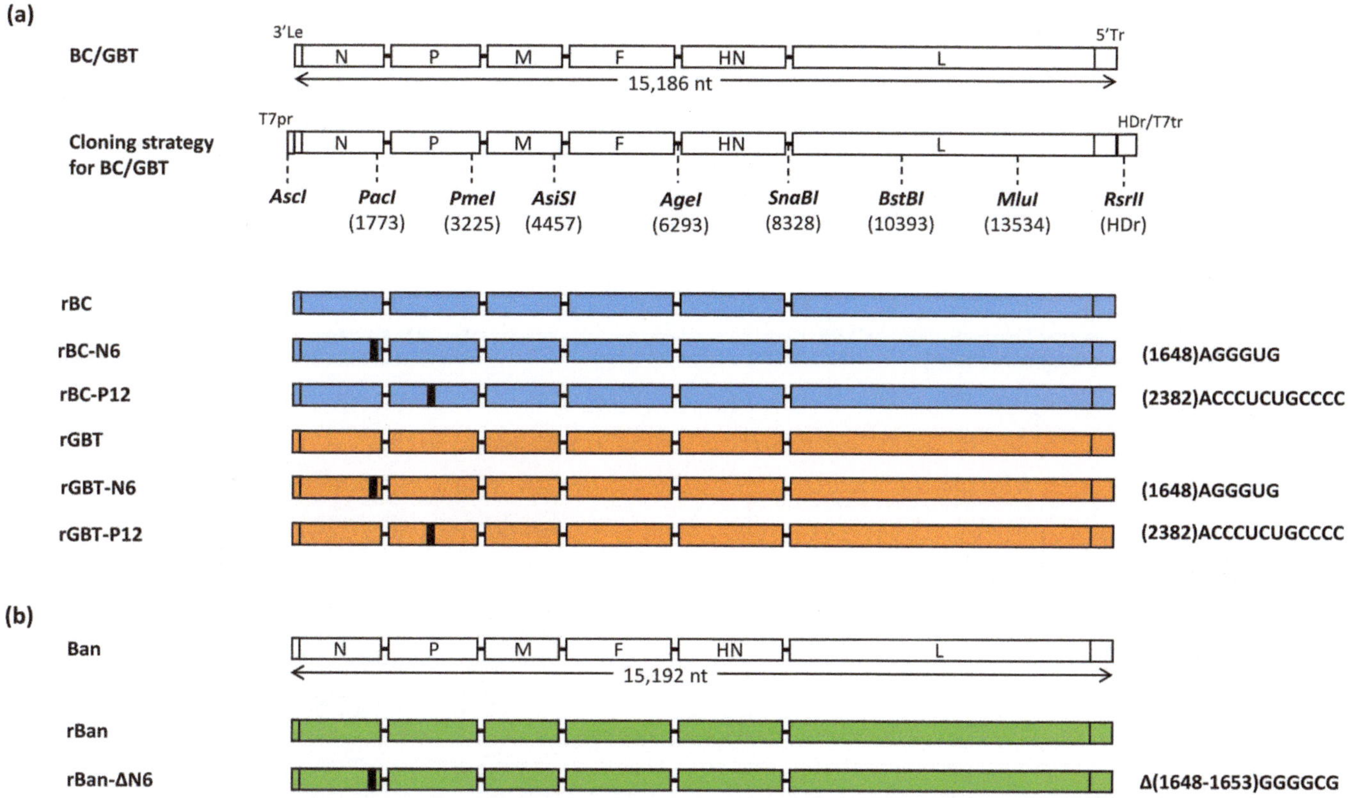

Figure 2. Gene map, reverse genetic cloning strategy for NDV strains Beaudette C, GB Texas and Banjarmasin. (a) Gene map and cloning strategy for NDV strains BC and GBT and their mutant viruses. Top two schematic gene maps show genetic structure, genome-length and cloning strategy for NDV strains BC and GBT. The location of RE sites in the antigenome cDNA clones of strains BC and GBT are shown. The numerals indicate genome nt position. AscI and RsrII sites are present before T7 promoter (T7pr) sequence and within hepatitis delta virus ribozyme/T7 terminator (HDr/T7tr) sequence, respectively, in the plasmid vector pBR322 (see Materials and Methods section). Bottom six gene maps illustrate the recombinant, 6-nt and 12-nt insert mutant viruses. The diagrams of N and P gene boxes show the position (indicated by a small box in black) of the 6-nt and 12-nt inserts in rBC and rGBT to generate mutant viruses rGBT-N6 and rBC-N6 (genome lengths of 15,192 nt) and rGBT-P12 and rBC-P12 (genome lengths of 15,198 nt). The nt position and sequence of the insert is given on the left. (b) Gene map of recombinant and 6-nt deletion mutant of NDV strain Ban. The recombinant and the 6-nt deleted viruses are indicated by rBan and rBan-ΔN6, respectively. The deleted 6-nt sequence and the nt position (indicated by a small box in black) in the 15,192-nt genome of Ban is provided on the left. Le and Tr indicate leader and trailer regions, respectively.

Pathogenicity studies

The pathogenicity of the parental and mutant viruses was quantified by the MDT test in nine-day-old embryonated chicken eggs and the ICPI test in one-day-old chicks [3]. To evaluate replication and pathogenicity of the rBC and rGBT viruses and their mutant derivatives in birds, two-week-old SPF chickens in groups of 13 were inoculated with 0.2 ml of 10^6 PFU of each virus by the oculonasal route. Three birds from each group were euthanized at 3 DPI and tissues from lung, trachea, spleen, brain and intestine were collected. For virus titration, the tissue samples were homogenized, and the supernatant was serially diluted and used to infect DF-1 cells, with duplicate wells per dilution. Infected wells were identified by HA assay of the supernatant, and the titer was calculated using the method of Reed and Muench [27] and expressed as TCID50/g of tissue (Fig. 5).

The remaining 10 chickens in each group were observed for clinical signs of disease until 14 days post infection (DPI). The birds were scored daily as follows: 0 for normal, 1 for sick, 2 for paralysis/twitching/wing drop, 3 for prostration, and 4 for death. A mean score per virus group per day was generated for comparison. The mortality pattern was observed daily for the entire 14 days to generate the survival pattern of chickens among the virus groups (See Results and Fig. 6).

For rBan and its mutant virus, chickens in groups of 10 were inoculated with 0.2 ml of 2×10^4 PFU of virus by the oculonasal route. This lower dose (compared to the BC and GBT groups) was used because of the greater virulence of rBan. The birds in each group were observed daily for 14 days and scored for disease as described for the rBC and rGBT groups (Fig. 6).

For *in vivo* experiments, nine-day-old embryonated chicken eggs (MDT assay), one-day-old White Leghorn chicks (ICPI assay), and two-week-old White Leghorn chickens (Pathogenesis study) were used. A New Zealand White rabbit was used for the immunization study. The chicken eggs and the animals were SPF and were procured from the Sunrise Farms Inc., Stuarts Draft, Virginia and from the Charles River Laboratories, Germantown, Maryland, respectively. The animals were housed and cared for in accordance with established guidelines, and the experimental procedures were performed with approval from Institutional Animal Care and Use Committee of the University of Maryland. The end point for all the *in vivo* experiments was death but chicks in ICPI assay and chickens in the pathogenesis study that showed terminal signs of disease. For example, chickens showing paralysis and movement restriction, were euthanized using a higher dose of gaseous anesthetic Isoflurane.

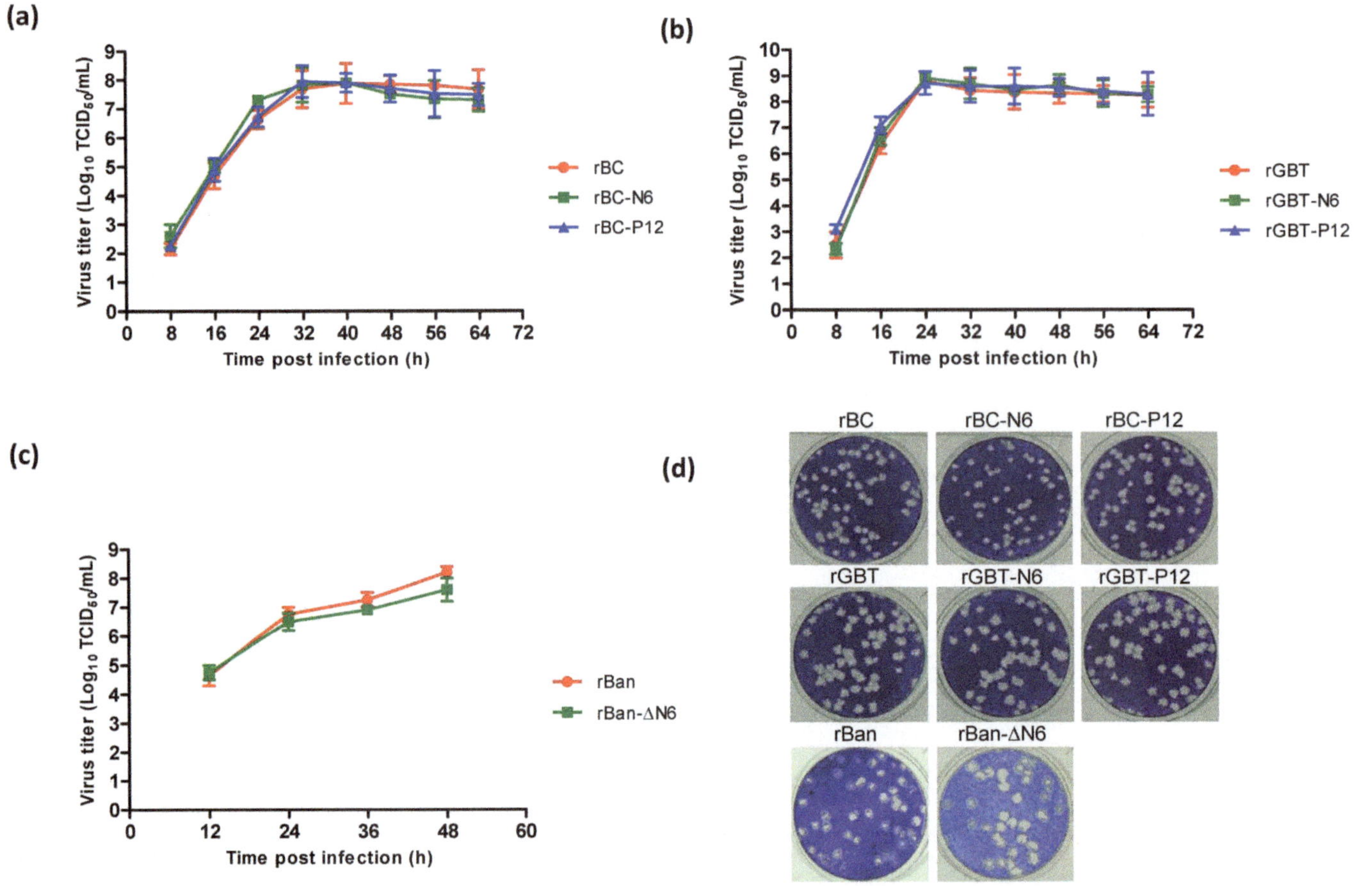

Figure 3. Growth kinetics and plaque morphology of recombinant NDV strains in chicken embryo fibroblast (DF-1) cells. The multi-cycle growth kinetics of recombinant BC (rBC) (a), GBT (rGBT) (b) and Ban (rBan) (c) in parallel with their mutant viruses in DF-1 cells. Values are the means of triplicate wells. Error bars indicate mean±SEM. (d) Plaque morphology of rBC, rGBT and rBan group viruses in DF-1 cells. Note the larger plaque size of GBT and Ban viruses compared to BC viruses, and the similarity between the mutant viruses and their parents.

Ethics Statement

All pathogenicity studies were conducted under biosafety level (BSL3)-enhanced conditions at the University of Maryland. Animals were cared for in accordance with established guidelines, and the experimental procedures were performed with approval from Institutional Animal Care and Use Committee of the University of Maryland, protocol number R-12-93.

Statistical analysis

Statistically significant differences in data from different recombinant virus groups were evaluated by one-way analysis of variance (ANOVA). Growth kinetics for various groups were analyzed using correlation of XY pairs (Pearson) and P value (two tailed). P values below 0.05 were regarded as being significant for all analyses. Experiments were repeated a minimum of three times. Statistical analysis for mean and standard deviation of data and one-way ANOVA was done by using Prism 5.0 computer software (GraphPad Software Inc., San Diego, CA).

Results

Design and rescue of recombinant wild type and mutant viruses

In the present study, we investigated the functional significance of the 6-nt insert in the N gene and the 12-nt insert in the P gene by introducing them separately by reverse genetics into the genomes of two 15,186-nt genome-length viruses representing two different NDV pathotypes, namely the moderately virulent strain BC and the highly virulent strain GBT. Consensus sequences for the 6- and 12-nt inserts were determined by aligning the sequences of the N and P genes of representative 15,192- and 15,198-nt genome-length NDV strains (Fig. 1a, b). This showed that the 6-nt insert had conserved residues at positions 2, 3 and 4 (−GGG−) (Fig. 1; sequences are negative sense), while the 12-nt insert was found conserved in the representative strains (ACCCU-CUGCCC) (Fig. 1b). We therefore chose the 6-nt sequence AGGGUG and the 12-nt sequence ACCCUCUGCCC for insertion into BC and GBT. We also performed deletion of a naturally occurring 6-nt insert (GGGGCG) from the N gene 5′NTR of a velogenic NDV strain Ban containing 15,192-nt genome-length [25].

We constructed and recovered the wild type (wt) viruses rBC and rGBT, which are recombinant versions of strains BC and GBT (Fig. 2a). We then constructed and recovered the mutant derivatives rBC-N6 and rGBT-N6, in which the 6-nt insert AGGGUG was inserted into the N gene after position 1647 (resulting in viral genomes of 15,192 nt) (Fig. 2a). We also constructed the mutant derivatives rBC-P12 and rGBT-P12, in which the 12-nt insert ACCCUCUGCCC was inserted into the P gene after position 2381 (resulting in viral genomes of 15,198 nt) (Fig. 2a). The parental recombinant and genome-length mutant

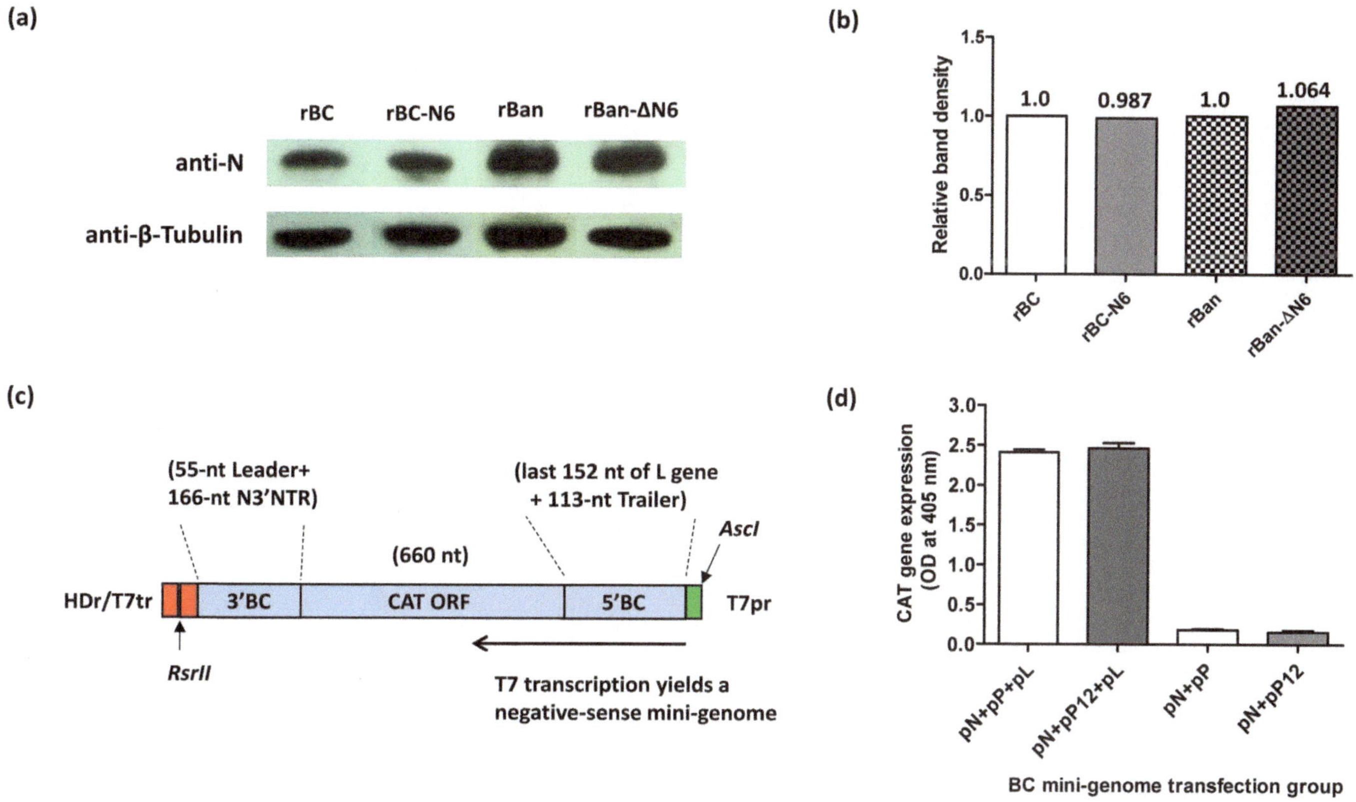

Figure 4. Comparative analysis of nucleocapsid protein expression and phosphoprotein function. (a) Nucleocapsid protein expression in DF-1 cells infected with rBC and rBC-N6 and rBan and rBan-ΔN6. Replicate cell monolayers were infected with rBC and rBC-N6 and rBan and rBan-ΔN6 at an MOI of 0.1, and were harvested at 24 h post-infection. Cell lysates were prepared and analyzed by polyacrylamide gel electrophoresis and immunoblotting with a polyclonal serum against a peptide prepared from the sequence of the N protein. β-Tubulin was used as the loading control. (b) The density of the N protein bands at 24 h was quantified to compare the N protein expression between parental viruses rBC and rBan to their respective N6 and ΔN6 mutant viruses using ImageJ program [28]. Note the similarity between the band densities of rBC and BC-N6 and rBan and rBan-ΔN6. (c) Map of the cDNA encoding the BC minigenome, which consisted of the first 166 nt from the leader end of the BC genome, followed by the CAT ORF, followed by the last 152 nt of the trailer end of the BC genome. (d) Analysis of mini-genome activity in lysates from transfected cells using an ELISA for the CAT protein to compare the activities of the wt and P12 versions of the P protein of strain BC. The N+P and N+P12 transfections are negative controls. CAT expression was expressed as absorbance at 405 nm.

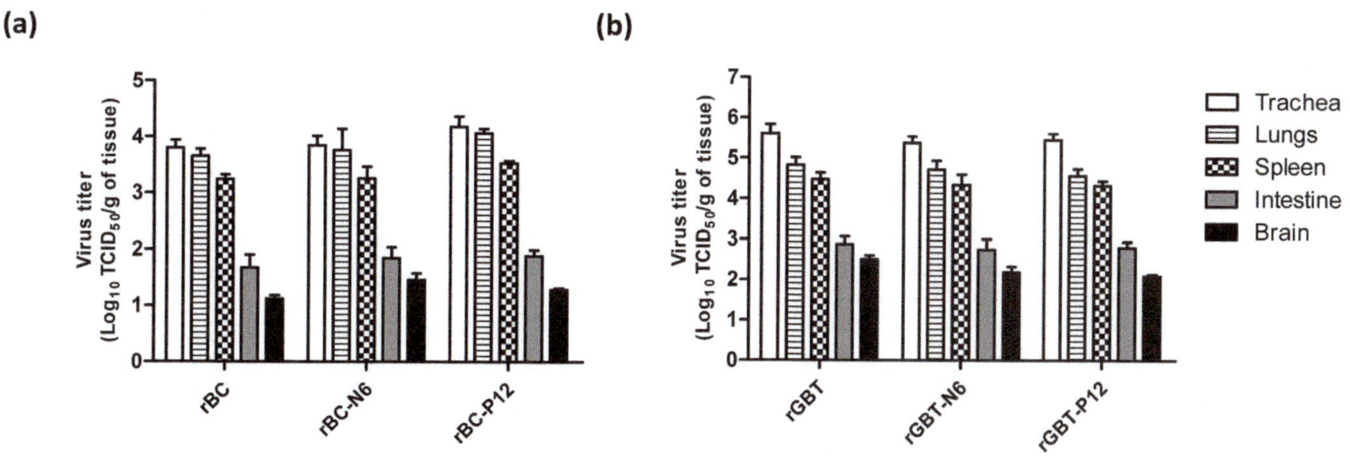

Figure 5. Virus titers of rBC and rGBT and their mutants in two-week-old chickens following oculonasal inoculation. Tissue samples from the trachea, lungs, spleen, intestine, and brain of 3 chickens (n = 3) from each indicated virus group were harvested on day 3 post infection, and virus titers were determined by limiting dilution assay [27]. The mean virus titer from 3 chickens per group was given for each tissue sample. Error bars indicate mean±SEM.

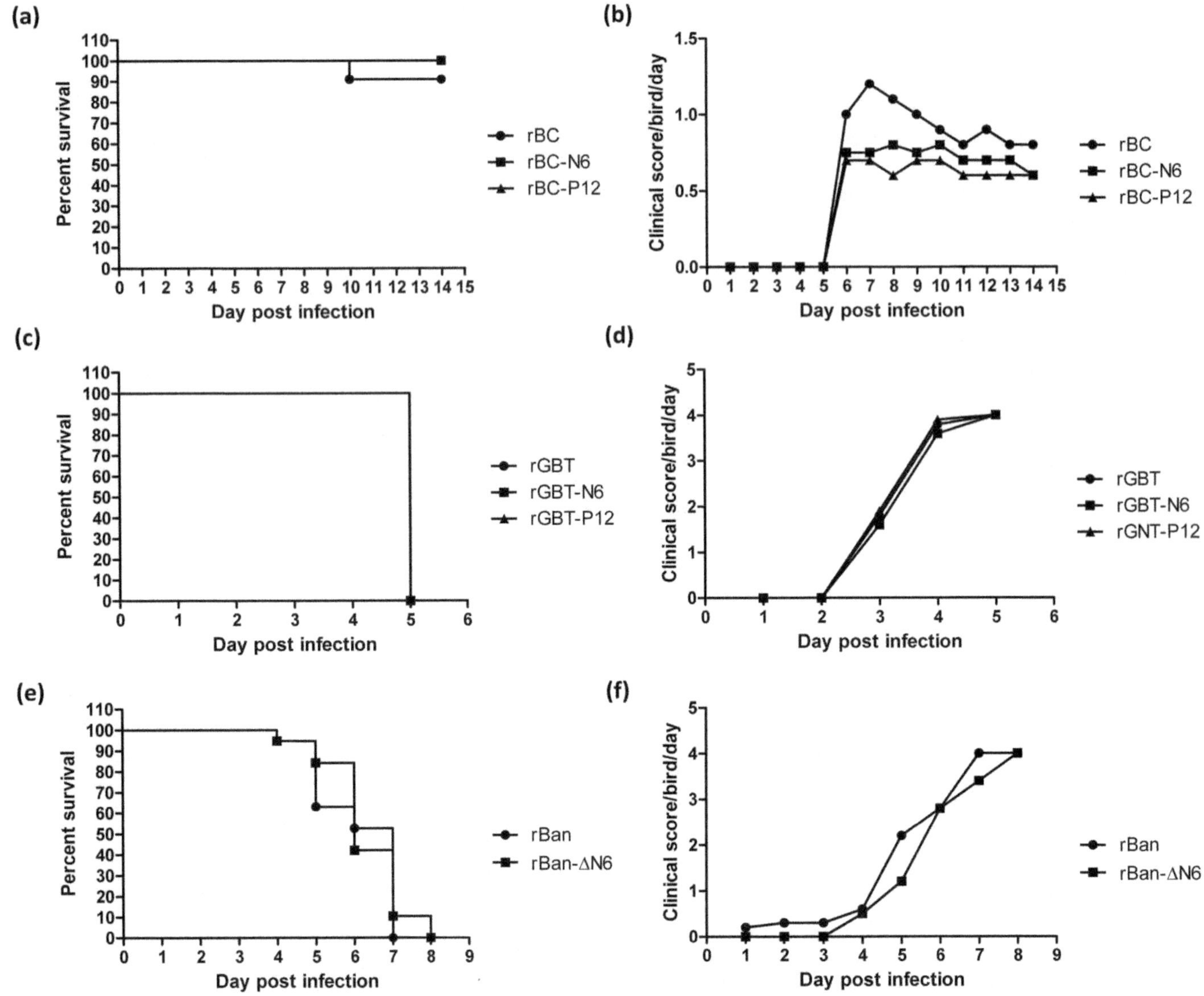

Figure 6. Percent survival and clinical score curves for recombinant and mutant viruses. Percent survival curve and clinical score curves for recombinant NDV strains BC (a, b), GBT (c, d) and Ban (e, f) in two-week-old chickens following oculonasal inoculation. The birds (10 per group) were clinically scored for 14 days using a scoring system for the clinical signs: 0, normal; 1, sick; 2, paralysis/twitching/wing drop; 3, prostration; and 4, death. The mean scores per group per day are plotted in the graph.

viruses were serially passaged 5 times in nine-day-old embryonated chicken eggs and 5 times in chicken embryo fibroblast DF-1 cells and the stability of the created restriction enzyme sites and insert sequences were confirmed by sequence analysis.

We previously developed a reverse genetic system for the virulent 15,192-nt genome-length strain Ban [25], which has a naturally-occurring 6-nt insert (GGGGCG from genome nt position 1648–1653) in the N gene. We used this system to delete the 6-nt sequence resulting in the virus rBan-ΔN6 (to generate a 15,186 nt genome) (Fig. 2b). This virus also was passaged 5 times in embryonated eggs and its sequence confirmed.

Multi-cycle growth kinetics and plaque morphology

The multi-cycle growth kinetics and plaque morphology of the N6 and P12 mutant viruses were evaluated *in vitro* in DF-1 cells using standard procedures [23]. The growth kinetics and titers of BC N6 and P12 derivatives were relatively similar compared to their parental biological and recombinant BC parents and reached their maximum titers at 32 h post infection (PI) (Fig. 3a). The biological and recombinant versions of the parental GBT strain (wt GBT and rGBT, respectively) had similar growth patterns and plaque morphologies (data not shown). Compared with the parental viruses, rGBT-N6 and rGBT-P12 had very similar growth kinetics throughout the course of 64 h PI and reached maximum titers at 24 h indicating a higher growth kinetics than BC viruses (Fig. 3b). The rBan and rBan-ΔN6 viruses had similar growth kinetics at 12 and 24 h, but at later times, i.e., in 36 and 48 h the mean titer ($\log_{10}$ TCID50/mL) of rBan was 7.25 and 8.2 compared to 6.9 and 7.6 of rBan-ΔN6, respectively (Fig. 3c). The plaque sizes of the various viruses were compared by measuring the diameters of 20 randomly picked plaques for each virus. The mean plaque diameters (in mm) were: 1.83±0.12, 1.76±0.1 and 1.87±0.15 for rBC, rBC-N6 and rBC-P12, respectively; and 2.82±0.16, 2.91±0.19 and 2.87±0.17 for rGBT, rGBT-N6, and rGBT-P12, respectively (Fig. 3d). Thus, there were no significant differences in plaque size between the mutant viruses and their respective parental recombinant viruses, although overall the plaque sizes of the BC viruses were substantially less than those of the GBT viruses. The plaques produced by the rBan and rBan-ΔN6 viruses were large and relatively similar in size with a diameter of 2.95±0.31 and 3.12±0.23 mm, respectively (Fig. 3d).

Immunoblot analysis for nucleocapsid protein expression

To investigate the influence of the 6-nt insert in the N gene (which occurred in the downstream non-translated sequence) on N protein expression, replicate DF-1 monolayers were infected with 0.1 MOI of the rBC and rBC-N6 and rBan and rBan-ΔN6 viruses, and cells were harvested at 24 h, and lysates were prepared and analyzed by gel electrophoresis (Fig. 4a). The relative band densities for rBC and rBC-N6 and rBan and rBan-ΔN6 were 1.0 and 0.987 and 1.0 and 1.064, respectively, suggesting no apparent difference in expression levels between the rBC and rBC-N6 viruses and between the rBan and rBan-ΔN6 viruses (Fig. 4b).

BC mini-genome CAT reporter gene assay for P protein function

To evaluate the effect of the 12-nt insertion in the P gene (which occurred within the ORF and added 4 aa to P and V), we developed a mini-genome system for strain BC. In this system, a mini-genome cDNA was constructed to encode a negative-sense genome analog that contained the 3′ leader and 5′ trailer regions of strain BC flanking a negative-sense copy of the CAT gene under the control of BC gene-start and gene-end transcription signals (Fig. 4c). This was transfected into 293T cells together with N, P, and L support plasmids (namely, pN, pP and pL) and MVA-T7 vaccinia virus, and at 48 h the cells were harvested and assayed for CAT expression by ELISA. The minigenome complemented with wt pN, pP and pL yielded a mean OD value of 2.412 and with pN, pP12 (12-nt in P gene ORF) and pL resulted in a mean OD value of 2.462 (Fig. 4d). Negative controls in which the BC minigenome was complemented with pN and pP or with pN and pP12 yielded mean OD values of 0.186 and 0.158, respectively. The close similarity between the transfections with wt P compared to mutant P12 indicated that the insertion of 4 aa within the P protein did not affect its function.

Mean death time (MDT) and intracerebral pathogenicity index (ICPI)

To determine the effect of the 6-nt and 12-nt inserts on the virulence of NDV, the parental and mutant viruses were evaluated for MDT in nine-day-old embryonated chicken eggs and for ICPI in one-day-old chicks (Table 1). The MDT and ICPI values of the biological wt versus the recombinant wt viruses of strains BC and GBT were similar, indicating that the recombinant viruses retained the pathogenicity phenotype of the biological parents. The mutant viruses (rBC-N6, rBC-P12, rGBT-N6, and GBT-P12) also had MDT values similar to those of their respective parental biological and recombinant viruses (Table 1). In contrast, the MDT value of the ΔN6 virus was higher than that of rBan, indicative of a decrease in virulence (Table 1).

In the ICPI test, highly virulent strains are defined as having values approaching 2.0. The ICPI values of wt BC, wt rBC, rBC-N6, and rBC-P12 were 1.6±0.02, 1.58±0.035, 1.54±0.01, and 1.52±0.045, respectively. The ICPI values of wt GBT, wt rGBT, rGBT-N6, and rGBT-P12 were 1.9±0.02, 1.88±0.035, 1.9±0.015, and 1.86±0.02, respectively (Table 1). These results indicate that the 6- and 12-nt inserts either had little effect or were slightly attenuating in the BC virus, and had little or no effect in the GBT virus. The ICPI values of rBan and rBan-ΔN6 were 1.81±0.025 and 1.68±0.135, respectively, suggesting attenuation of rBan-ΔN6 compared to its parental recombinant virus (Table 1).

Virus replication and pathogenesis in two-week-old chickens

To study the pathogenesis of these viruses under conditions modeling natural infection, two-week-old chickens in groups of 13 were infected by the oculonasal route with 200 μL of PBS containing 10^6 PFU of each recombinant virus per bird. Three days later, 3 birds from each group were sacrificed and virus titers in the trachea, lungs, spleen, intestine, and brain were determined (Fig. 5). Chickens infected with rBC, rBC-N6, or rBC-P12 had low virus titers in all 5 organs compared to the rGBT, rGBT-N6, and rGBT-P12 (Fig. 5). There were no consistent differences between the N6 and P12 mutants and their respective parents.

The remaining 10 chickens in each virus group were observed for clinical signs of disease until 14 days post infection (DPI). In the case of the BC virus groups, all of the chickens survived the 14-day experiment except for 1 chicken in the rBC group that died on day 10 (Fig. 6a). Chickens in the rBC group first showed mild clinical signs on 6 DPI, which increased in severity till 11 DPI and then decreased during recovery. The clinical signs included ruffled feathers, lethargy, somnolence, and self-isolation but there was no neurological signs observed. In the rBC group, chickens were severely sick, with scores substantially exceeding those of the rBC-N6 and rBC-P12 (Fig. 6b). In the rGBT, rGBT-N6, and rGBT-P12 groups, mild signs of paralysis were first observed on 3 DPI and the chickens displayed progressive neurological signs including tremors, wing drop, torticollis, opisthotonus and prostration on 4 DPI. All 10 chickens died on day 5 in rGBT, rGBT-N6, and rGBT-P12 groups (Fig. 6c, d).

In the rBan group, 1, 4, and 1 birds died on days 4, 5, and 6 DPI, respectively, and the remaining 4 birds died on 7 DPI (Fig. 6e). In the rBan-ΔN6 group, the time of death was delayed by approximately 1 day: specifically, 1, 1, 4, and 3 birds died on days 4, 5, 6, 7 DPI, respectively, and the remaining 1 bird died on 8 DPI (Fig. 6e). The disease signs include dyspnea, gasping, ruffled feathers, and self-isolation. In the clinical scoring, the scores of rBan was generally higher compared to rBan-ΔN6 except on day 6 (and 8, when all birds in each group were dead) (Fig. 6f). The mortality pattern and the clinical scores indicate a reduction in the virulence of rBan-ΔN6 compared to rBan.

Discussion

NDV strains have natural genome lengths of 15,186 nt, 15,192 nt, and 15,198 nt. The two longer genome lengths are due to the presence of naturally-occurring 6-nt and 12-nt inserts in, respectively, the 5′ (downstream) non-translated region of the N gene and in the coding sequence for the P and V proteins. We evaluated the effects of these inserts by introducing consensus 6- and 12-nt inserts into the NDV strains BC and GBT, which are genetically closely related but differ in pathotype. Specifically, BC is a moderately virulent strain whereas GBT is a highly virulent strain used as a standard challenge virus in the U.S. We also deleted the 6-nt insert from the naturally-occurring 15,192-nt genome-length virulent NDV strain Ban, to evaluate its effect on replication and pathogenicity.

We analyzed the parental and mutant viruses for a number of features. *In vitro* growth was analyzed by multi-cycle growth kinetics and plaque size. Possible effects on N gene expression due

Table 1. Mean death time (MDT) assay and intracerebral pathogenicity index (ICPI) assay scores of parental and N6 and P12 mutant viruses of NDV strains Beaudette C (BC), Texas GB (GBT) and Banjarmasin (Ban).

Virus	MDT (h)*	ICPI score[#]
wtBC	60±2.0	1.60±0.020
rBC	59±1.0	1.58±0.035
rBC-N6	58±1.5	1.54±0.010
rBC-P12	61±3.0	1.52±0.045
wtGBT	48±1.0	1.90±0.020
rGBT	47±1.5	1.88±0.035
rGBT-N6	46±0.5	1.90±0.015
rGBT-P12	47±1.0	1.86±0.020
rBan	52±2.0	1.81±0.025
rBan-ΔN6	56±1.0	1.68±0.135

*Pathotype definitions by MDT: >90 h, lentogenic; 60 to 90 h, mesogenic; <60 h, velogenic.
#Pathotype definitions by ICPI: velogenic strains approach the maximum score of 2.00, whereas lentogenic strains approach scores close to 0.
The values are the mean±SEM from three independent experiments.

to the presence of the N6 insert in the downstream non-translated region were evaluated by Western blot analysis of the N protein accumulation. Possible effects on P gene function due to the P12 insert, which adds four aa to P and V, were evaluated for the strain BC using a minigenome system. Virulence was scored by the standard MDT and ICPI tests with chicken eggs and one-day-old chicks, respectively. In addition, pathogenicity in two-week-old chickens was evaluated by replication, tropism, clinical disease, and mortality. Different results were obtained with the three different strains.

With the virulent strain GBT, the introduction of the 6-nt insert into the N gene, or the 12-nt insert into the P gene, had no discernible effect in any of the assays, including *in vitro* growth, N gene expression, P protein function, MDT, ICPI, and pathogenicity in two-week-old chickens. One possibility is that the very high level of virulence of the GBT strain obscured possible subtle effects of the inserts.

With the mesogenic strain BC, the introduction of these inserts did not significantly affect the growth kinetics in DF-1 cells. These results indicate that insertion of 6 nt or 12 nt into a 15,186-nt genome-length virus did not result in a growth advantage, but rather was neutral. The plaque sizes of the parental and mutant viruses were similar, suggesting that these inserts do not affect growth sufficient to result in observable difference in plaque size. No effects were observed in N gene expression or P protein function. There was no difference in MDT, but the presence of the inserts was associated with a somewhat reduced ICPI score, indicative of attenuation. Also, the inserts did not reduce BC replication in two-week-old birds but they did reduce clinical disease and mortality. Thus, the N6 and P12 inserts were associated with reduced virulence, and this effect did not appear to be due to a reduction in replication *in vivo*.

With the virulent strain Ban, deletion of the naturally-occurring 6-nt "insert" from the N gene slightly lowered replication *in vitro*, decreased virulence based on MDT, ICPI, and clinical disease and mortality in two-week-old birds, but no effect was observed in N gene expression.

Thus, while the inserts did not detectably affect strain GBT, they did affect the pathogenicity of strains BC and Ban. However, the effects were not consistent with regard to associating the presence of an insert with increased or decreased virulence. Specifically, whereas the insertion of N6 or P12 into the 15,186-nt genome of BC (to create a 15,192-nt or 15,198-nt genome, respectively) resulted in slight attenuation, the converse manipulation, namely the removal of the 6-nt "insert" from the 15,192-nt genome of strain Ban (to create a 15,186-nt genome) also resulted in attenuation. These results suggest that genome-length is a fitness controlling parameter. Any change in the naturally-occurring genomes – whether to add inserts or remove inserts – is somewhat detrimental to the virus. Thus, the naturally-occurring inserts presumably existed evolutionarily because they provide some selective advantage to that particular strain.

It was somewhat surprising that the insertion or removal of these short nt sequences would have a detectable effect on virulence, given the very small incremental change in genome-length conferred by the insertion or deletion of a 6-nt of 12-nt insert. It might have been expected that these inserts would affect expression of the respective gene or, in the case of the P12 insert that inserted 4 aa into P and V, the function of the respective proteins. Surprisingly, neither effect was observed. This is offered with the caveat that we did not directly evaluate V protein function. It appears that both proteins accommodate this aa insertion without much alteration in the phenotype of the virus. In addition, the effects were not specific to the N or P gene, and instead the effects were similar to N6 or P12. It may be that these inserts have some effect on genomic RNA folding, or on the hexamer organization of the nucleocapsid.

The origin of these inserts in nature is unknown, although they appear to have been introduced after 1960 [11,29], it is possible that NDV strains with genome lengths of 15,192 nt and 15,198 nt existed in nature before 1960 but were not identified due to lack of extensive nucleotide sequencing. The size of each insert conforms to the "rule of six" [4,30]. The nucleotide sequence of the inserts shows some variation among strains, indicating that the length of the insert is more important than the sequence. The likeliest mechanism of introduction of these inserts would be polymerase stuttering, with the rule of six placing a strong selective pressure for inserts to conform to the rule. There is evidence of genome-length variation in other APMVs. For example, APMV-2 strains Yucaipa and England have genome lengths of 14,904 nt, strain Kenya has a genome-length of 14,196 nt, and strain Bangor has a genome-length of 15,024 nt [31]. In APMV-3, strain Wisconsin has a genome-length of 16,182 nt compared to 16,272 nt for strain Netherlands [32]. In APMV-4, strain Delaware has a genome-length of 15,048 nt compared to 15,054 nt for strain Hong Kong [33]. In APMV-6, strain Hong Kong has a genome-length of 16,236 nt compared to 16,230 nt for strain IT4524-2 [34]. Thus, variations in genome lengths among members of genus *Avulavirus* was known, but the importance of this variation was not known.

The virus strains that naturally contain these inserts (namely, the 15,192-nt and 15,198-nt genome-length) differ substantially in nucleotide sequence from viruses that lack these inserts (the 15,186-nt genome-length) (Table S1). Strains BC and GBT (15,186-nt genome-length) share 99.1% nt sequence identity. Similarly, strains BC and GBT (both belong to genotype II of class II) share substantial identity with other 15,186-nt strains, including those of genotype I (e.g., Ulster; 90.4 and 90.7%, respectively), II (LaSota; 97.0 and 97.5%), III (Mukteswar, 87.9 and 88.1%), and IV (Herts 33, 88.0 and 88.3%). In contrast, strains BC and GBT share less identity with NDV class II strains that possess the additional 6 nt, such as: genotype V (Largo; 85.4 and 85.6%), VI (Fontana; 85.5 and 85.7%), VII (ZJ1; 83.4 and 83.6%), VIII (QH1; 84.5 and 84.6%), IX (F48E8; 87.9 and 88.1%), and XI (MG 725 08; 82.6 and 82.8%). Strains BC and GBT also share less nt identity with class I viruses, such as Alaska 415 (72.6 and 72.6%) and JS10 (72.5 and 72.5%). Thus, the 15,186-nt viruses of class II, genotypes I, II, III, and VI appear to form one relatively highly related group, with 88–99% nt identity, whereas viruses with longer genomes, of class II genotypes V, VI, VII, VIII, and IX, as well as class I, generally more divergent from strains BC and GBT, with only 72–85% identity (except for genotype IX, 88%).

The ecology and evolution of NDV is not well understood. Currently, the circulation of all three genome-length viruses (15,186-nt, 15,192-nt, and 15,198-nt) in bird populations indicate their successful establishment and survival. The NDV strains of genome-length 15,186-nt are a well-studied group that include well-defined lentogenic, mesogenic and velogenic pathotypes. Although the 15,192-nt genome-length NDV are isolated frequently from outbreaks in poultry in recent years, the spectrum of virulence within this group of viruses remains to be studied comprehensively. The viruses with genome-length 15,198-nt are lentogenic in nature and are frequently isolated from shorebirds and waterfowl [16–20]. However, the pigeon-origin NDV strains (pigeon paramyxoviruses) contain a genome-length of 15,192-nt and a polybasic fusion protein cleavage site sequence but are not pathogenic to chickens [35]. There are also cases in which NDV strains that phylogenetically cluster to 15,192-nt genome-length viruses, containing a polybasic fusion protein cleavage site sequence are isolated from apparently healthy chickens [36,37]. These natural infections in birds indicate that the host species may be playing a major role in the evolution of NDV. The wider phylogenetic distance among the 15,186-nt, 15,192-nt, and 15,198-nt genome-length NDV strains points to a possibility that these genome-length viruses might have originated independently. Future studies on extensive phylogenetic analyses of NDV genomes are necessary to determine the time of divergence of different genome-length viruses in evolution.

In summary, our results showed that the 6-nt and 12-nt inserts did not detectably affect N gene expression or P protein function. The inserts had no effect on the replication or virulence of the highly virulent GBT strain. They also had no significant effect on replication of strain BC *in vivo*, but resulted in a modest degree of attenuation. We also deleted a naturally-occurring 6-nt insertion in the N gene from a highly virulent 15,192-nt genome-length virus, strain Ban. This resulted in reduced replication *in vitro* and reduced virulence *in vivo*. Thus, although these inserts had no evident effect on gene expression, protein function, or replication *in vivo*, they did affect virulence in two of the three tested strains. These results suggest that NDV has evolved to produce different genome lengths which is optimal for the replication and pathogenesis of that strain in a particular host and environment.

Supporting Information

Table S1 Per cent nucleotide sequence identities among the genome sequences of representative Newcastle disease virus strains.

Acknowledgments

We thank Daniel D Rockemann, Girmay T Gebreluul, and all our laboratory members for their excellent technical assistance and help. We thank Andrea F Perez for BSL-3 coordination.

Author Contributions

Conceived and designed the experiments: AP SX SKS. Performed the experiments: AP SX SHK SK. Analyzed the data: AP SX SKS PLC. Contributed reagents/materials/analysis tools: SK BN SS. Contributed to the writing of the manuscript: AP SKS PLC.

References

1. Alexander DJ (2003) Newcastle disease, other avian paramyxoviruses, and pneumovirus infections, p. 63–99. *In* J.M. Saif, H.J. Barnes, J.R. Glisson, A.M. Fadly, L.R. McDougald, and D.E. Swayne (ed.), Diseases of Poultry, 11th ed. Iowa State University Press, Ames, Iowa.
2. Samal SK (2011) Newcastle disease and related avian paramyxoviruses. In The Biology of Paramyxoviruses, 69–114. Edited by Samal S. K. Norfolk: Caister Academic Press.
3. Alexander DJ (1989) Newcastle disease, p.114–120. *In* H. G. Purchase, L. H. Arp, C. H. Domermuth, and J. E. Pearson (ed.), A laboratory manual for the isolation and identification of avian pathogens, 3rd ed. American Association for Avian Pathologists, Inc., Kennett Square, PA.
4. Lamb RA, Parks GD (2007) Paramyxoviridae: the viruses and their replication, p. 1449–1496. *In* D. M. Knipe, and P. M. Howley (ed.), Fields virology, 5th ed. Wolters Kluwer-Lippincott Williams & Wilkins, Philadelphia, PA.
5. Mayo MA (2002) Virus Taxonomy-Houston. Arch Virol 147: 1071–1076.
6. Aldous EW, Mynn JK, Banks J, Alexander DJ (2003) A molecular epidemiological study of avian paramyxovirus type 1 (Newcastle disease virus) isolates by phylogenetic analysis of a partial nucleotide sequence of the fusion protein gene. Avian Pathol 32: 239–256.
7. Diel DG, da Silva LH, Liu H, Wang Z, Miller PJ, et al. (2012) Genetic diversity of avian paramyxovirus type 1: Proposal for a unified nomenclature and classification system of Newcastle disease virus genotypes. Infect Genet Evol 12: 1770–1779.
8. Snoeck CJ, Adeyanju AT, Owoade AA, Couacy-Hymann E, Alkali BR, et al. (2013) Genetic diversity of Newcastle disease virus in wild birds and pigeons in West Africa. Appl Environ Microbiol 79(24): 7867–7874.
9. Snoeck CJ, Owoade AA, Couacy-Hymann E, Alkali BR, Okwen MP, et al. (2013) High genetic diversity of Newcastle disease virus in poultry in West and Central Africa: co-circulation of genotype XIV and newly defined genotypes XVII and XVIII. J Clin Microbiol 51(7): 2250–2260.
10. de Leeuw O, Peeters B (1999) Complete nucleotide sequence of Newcastle disease virus: evidence for the existence of a new genus within the subfamily Paramyxovirinae. J Gen Virol 80: 131–136.
11. Krishnamurthy S, Samal SK (1998) Nucleotide sequences of the trailer, nucleocapsid protein gene and intergenic regions of Newcastle disease virus strain Beaudette C and completion of the entire genome sequence. J Gen Virol 79: 2419–2424.
12. Romer-Oberdorfer A, Mundt E, Mebatsion T, Buchholz UJ, Mettenleiter TC (1999) Generation of recombinant lentogenic Newcastle disease virus from cDNA. J Gen Virol 80: 2987–2995.
13. Huang Y, Wan HQ, Liu HQ, Wu YT, Liu XF (2004) Genomic sequence of an isolate of Newcastle disease virus isolated from an outbreak in geese: a novel six nucleotide insertion in the noncoding region of the nucleoprotein gene. Arch Virol 149(7): 1445–1457.
14. Ujvari D (2006) Complete nucleotide sequence of IT-227/82, an avian paramyxovirus type-1 strain of pigeons (*Columba livia*). Virus Genes 32: 49–57.

15. Miller PJ, Decanini EL, Afonso CL (2010) Newcastle disease: evolution of genotypes and the related diagnostic challenges. Infect Genet Evol 10(1): 26–35.
16. Czegledi A, Ujvari D, Somogyi E, Wehmann E, Werner O, et al. (2006) Third genome size category of avian paramyxovirus serotype 1 (Newcastle disease virus) and evolutionary implications. Virus Res 120(1–2): 36–48.
17. Kim LM, King DJ, Curry PE, Suarez DL, Swayne DE, et al. (2007a) Phylogenetic diversity among low virulence Newcastle disease viruses from waterfowl and shorebirds and comparison of genotype distributions to poultry-origin isolates. J Virol 81: 12641–12653.
18. Kim LM, King DJ, Suarez DL, Wong CW, Afonso CL (2007b) Characterization of class I Newcastle disease virus isolates from Hong Kong live bird markets and detection using real-time reverse transcription-PCR. J Clin Microbiol 45: 1310–1314.
19. Liu H, Chen F, Zhao Y, Zheng D, Li J, et al. (2010) Genomic characterization of the first class I Newcastle disease virus isolated from the mainland of china. Virus Genes 40(3): 365–371.
20. Seal BS, Wise MG, Pedersen JC, Senne DA, Alvarez R, et al. (2005) Genomic sequences of low-virulence avian paramyxovirus-1 (Newcastle disease virus) isolates obtained from live-bird markets in North America not related to commonly utilized commercial vaccine strains. Vet Microbiol 106: 7–16.
21. Kumar S, Dudley J, Nei M, Tamura K (2008) MEGA: a biologist centric software for evolutionary analysis of DNA and protein sequences. Brief Bioinformatics 9: 299–306.
22. Kim SH, Nayak S, Paldurai A, Nayak B, Samuel A, et al. (2012) Complete genome sequence of a novel Newcastle disease virus strain isolated from a chicken in West Africa. J Virol 86(20): 11394–5.
23. Krishnamurthy S, Huang Z, Samal SK (2000) Recovery of a virulent strain of Newcastle disease virus from cloned cDNA: expression of a foreign gene results in growth retardation and attenuation. Virology 278: 168–182.
24. Paldurai A, Kumar S, Nayak B, Samal SK (2010) Complete genome sequence of highly virulent neurotropic Newcastle disease virus strain Texas GB. Virus Genes 41(1): 67–72.
25. Xiao S, Nayak B, Samuel A, Paldurai A, Kanabagattebasavarajappa M, et al. (2012a) Generation by reverse genetics of an effective, stable, live-attenuated Newcastle disease virus vaccine based on a currently circulating, highly virulent Indonesian strain. PLoS One 7(12): e52751.
26. Xiao S, Paldurai A, Nayak B, Samuel A, Bharoto EE, et al. (2012b) Complete genome sequences of Newcastle disease virus strains circulating in chicken populations of Indonesia. J Virol 86(10): 5969–5970.
27. Reed LJ, Muench H (1938) A simple method of estimation of 50% end points. Am J Hyg 27: 493–497.
28. Schneider CA, Rasband WS, Eliceiri KW (2012) NIH Image to ImageJ: 25 years of image analysis. Nature Methods 9: 671–675.
29. Miller PJ, Kim LM, Afonso CL, Ip HS (2009) Evolutionary dynamics of Newcastle disease virus. Virology 391: 64–72.
30. Calain P, Roux L (1993) The rule of six, a basic feature for efficient replication of Sendai virus defective interfering RNA. J Virol 67: 4822–4830.
31. Subbiah M, Nayak S, Collins PL, Samal SK (2010) Complete genome sequences of avian paramyxovirus serotype 2 (APMV-2) strains Bangor, England and Kenya: evidence for the existence of subgroups within serotype 2. Virus Res 152(1–2): 85–95.
32. Kumar S, Nayak B, Samuel AS, Xiao S, Collins PL, et al. (2010) Complete genome sequence of avian paramyxovirus-3 strain Wisconsin: evidence for the existence of subgroups within the serotype. Virus Res 149(1): 78–85.
33. Parthiban M, Kaliyaperumal M, Xiao S, Nayak B, Paldurai A, et al. (2013) Complete genome sequence of an avian paramyxovirus type 4 from North America reveals a shorter genome and new genotype. Genome Announc 1(1): e00075–12.
34. Xiao S, Subbiah M, Kumar S, De Nardi R, Terregino C, et al. (2010) Complete genome sequences of avian paramyxovirus serotype 6 prototype strain Hong Kong and a recent novel strain from Italy: evidence for the existence of subgroups within the serotype. Virus Res 150(1–2): 61–72.
35. Dortmans JC, Koch G, Rottier PJ, Peeters BP (2009) Virulence of pigeon paramyxovirus type 1 does not always correlate with the cleavability of its fusion protein. J Gen Virol 90(11): 2746–50.
36. de Almeida RS, Maminiaina OF, Gil P, Hammoumi S, Molia S, et al. (2009) Africa, a reservoir of new virulent strains of Newcastle disease virus? Vaccine 27(24): 3127–3129.
37. de Almeida RS, Hammoumi S, Gil P, Briand FX, Molia S, et al. (2013) New avian paramyxoviruses type I strains identified in Africa provide new outcomes for phylogeny reconstruction and genotype classification. PLoS One 8(10): e76413.

3

Evolution of an Expanded Mannose Receptor Gene Family

Karen Staines, Lawrence G. Hunt, John R. Young, Colin Butter*

The Pirbright Institute, Compton, United Kingdom

Abstract

Sequences of peptides from a protein specifically immunoprecipitated by an antibody, KUL01, that recognises chicken macrophages, identified a homologue of the mammalian mannose receptor, MRC1, which we called MRC1L-B. Inspection of the genomic environment of the chicken gene revealed an array of five paralogous genes, *MRC1L-A* to *MRC1L-E*, located between conserved flanking genes found either side of the single *MRC1* gene in mammals. Transcripts of all five genes were detected in RNA from a macrophage cell line and other RNAs, whose sequences allowed the precise definition of spliced exons, confirming or correcting existing bioinformatic annotation. The confirmed gene structures were used to locate orthologues of all five genes in the genomes of two other avian species and of the painted turtle, all with intact coding sequences. The lizard genome had only three genes, one orthologue of *MRC1L-A* and two orthologues of *the MRC1L-B* antigen gene resulting from a recent duplication. The Xenopus genome, like that of most mammals, had only a single *MRC1*-like gene at the corresponding locus. *MRC1L-A* and *MRC1L-B* genes had similar cytoplasmic regions that may be indicative of similar subcellular migration and functions. Cytoplasmic regions of the other three genes were very divergent, possibly indicating the evolution of a new functional repertoire for this family of molecules, which might include novel interactions with pathogens.

Editor: Michelle L. Baker, CSIRO, Australia

Funding: This work was funded by the BBSRC (Biotechnology and Biological Sciences Research Council) under grant number BBS/E/I/00001423 as part of the Institute Strategic Programme Grant to the Avian Viral Diseases Programme at the Pirbright Institute. The funders had no role in study design, data collection and analysis, decision to publish, or preparation of the manuscript.

Competing Interests: The authors have declared that no competing interests exist.

* Email: colin.butter@avianimmunology.org

Introduction

Recent evolution of the repertoire of molecules involved in the function of the immune system has resulted in substantial divergence in the composition and functions of the gene families to which these molecules belong. Even among mammals, different families of molecules may carry out equivalent functions in different species [1]. While the functions of many molecules in immunity are well conserved between mammalian and avian species, in other cases there is extensive divergence in molecular repertoires, with cytokines and chemokines providing examples [2]. These differences often involve gene duplication followed by functional diversification [3]. Thus evolution has led to variety in molecular details in spite of more conserved underlying mechanisms in solutions to the problems of infection. Variation in molecular repertoires may underlie some of the differences between species in host-pathogen interactions. An understanding of these differences will be essential to optimise approaches to immune protection.

The mannose receptor C-type 1 gene (*MRC1, CD206*) is the eponymous member of the mannose receptor family. Their gene products are type I transmembrane glycoproteins containing arrays of C-type lectin domains (CTLDs). The family also includes DEC205 (CD205), MRC2 (Endo180, CD280) and Phospholipase A_2 receptor (PLA_2R), each having important functions in immunity [4]. These receptors all have an N-terminal cysteine-rich domain (CysR) followed by a single fibronectin type II domain (FNII), then either 8 (MRC1, MRC2 and PLA_2R) or 10 (DEC205) CTLDs separated by linker regions. They have a transmembrane domain and a short cytoplasmic tail containing motifs that signal endocytosis. In mammals, *DEC205* and *PLA_2R* genes are arranged in tandem on one chromosome, while the others are unlinked. In the three genes encoding 8 CTLDs, the 30 exon gene structure and the splicing phases of all introns are completely conserved. The CTLDs fall into two groups, one having an extra pair of cysteine residues at the N-terminal end of the domain (domains 2, 3, 4, 6, 8) [5]. While individual CTLDs generally have low affinities for carbohydrate ligands, the molecules can exhibit high affinities for complex carbohydrate by cooperative binding [6]. Only the fourth CTLD of human MRC1 retains strong enough binding to have lectin activity on its own [7].

The mannose receptor is a recycling endocytosis receptor, rapidly internalised via clathrin-coated vesicles and delivered to early endosomes, with the majority of the receptors in the intracellular location in the steady state [8]. Endocytosis of bound molecules underlies the primary function of the mannose receptor in the recognition of pathogen associated molecular patterns and their consequent uptake for engulfment and for antigen presentation [9]. A soluble form of the mammalian mannose receptor, produced by proteolytic cleavage [10], may also function in the delivery of antigens to lymphoid follicles [11]. Clearance by binding to the mannose receptor may also be involved in the regulation of levels of some hormones [12]. In chickens, the orthologue of mammalian PLA_2R acts as an Fc receptor (FcRY), the functional equivalent of mammalian FcRn, extending the range of its endocytic targets to immune complexes [13].

Binding of the mannose receptor by a virus may elicit immunomodulatory responses [14]. It may also facilitate viral entry in a cell either indirectly, as with HIV [15], or directly, as with Dengue [16]. In the mouse, binding of influenza virus by the mannose receptor, in addition to its more widespread binding to sialic acid, is important for virus entry into macrophages [17]. The virus replicates inside infected macropahges, but they do not release infective virus. Instead, the infection enhances the presentation of influenza virus antigens and stimulates the generation of pro-inflammatory cytokines. Thus the participation of the mannose receptor in allowing infection of macrophages contributes to innate and eventually to adaptive protection [18]. Reciprocally driven evolution of the virus and the mannose receptor in different species may thus be a significant contributor to differences in host-pathogen interactions.

Employing mass spectrometry of immunoprecipitated antigen, we identified a molecule recognised by a macrophage marker antibody, KUL01 [19], as a chicken homologue of MRC1. Inspection of neighbouring avian genome sequence revealed that the locus contained five tandemly repeated genes encoding similar molecules that are likely to have arisen through duplication, of a single ancestral MRC1 gene, in the avian lineage. Very different cytoplasmic sequences and differences in relative transcript levels in tissues indicate diversification of function among the duplicated genes.

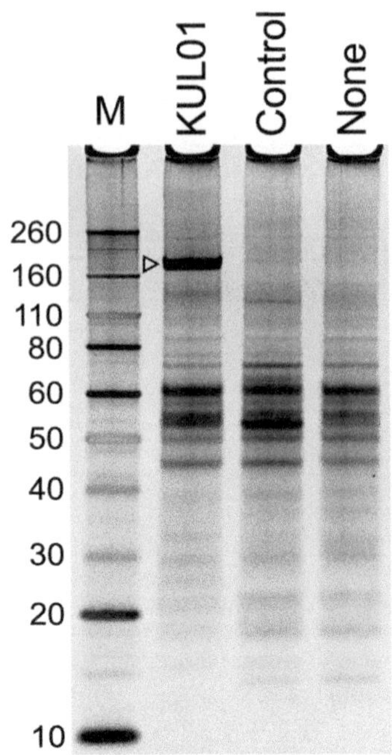

Figure 1. KUL01 specifically precipitates a molecule with apparent molecular weight 180 kDa. Track M contains molecular weight standards. The other tracks contain materials absorbed from a precleared lysate of the HD11 macrophage cell line, by agarose beads to which were attached either KUL01, an isotype matched control antibody, or no antibody, and eluted at low pH. The open arrowhead points to the band(s) specifically absorbed by the KUL01 antibody, which were analysed by mass spectroscopy.

Results

The KUL01 antibody recognises a homologue of the macrophage mannose receptor MRC1

KUL01 antibody bound to agarose beads was used to adsorb proteins from a lysate of the transformed chicken macrophage cell line HD11, which were analysed by SDS PAGE after elution at low pH. Specific bands, obtained from beads coated with KUL01 but not from those coated with control antibody, were excised, digested with trypsin and analysed my mass spectroscopy. The major specifically recognised molecule was a (doublet) band with an apparent molecular weight of 180 kDa (figure 1). By Mascot search of the NCBI non-redundant chicken proteins in the IPI database, a sufficient number of peptides from the tryptic digest of this band were identified as being derivable from the sequence IPI00814304 to unequivocally identify it as the source of antigen specifically adsorbed by KUL01 (figure S1 and table S1). It was annotated as being a chicken homologue of MRC1.

Genomic context of chicken MRC1 orthologues

The genomic context of the gene for the KUL01 antigen was inspected to see whether additional evidence from conserved gene order would support its identification as the orthologue of MRC1. Inspection of the region between orthologues of the highly conserved genes, *SLC39A12* and *STAM*, that flank *MRC1* in mammals, revealed multiple segments with similarity to the *MRC1* gene. Existing annotation and EST data, together with manual examination, allowed the definition of five potential *MRC1L* genes. For convenience, these were labelled *MRC1L-A to E* in sequence in the direction of their transcription (which is inverse to the genome map). Annotations of this gene array from different sources varied widely, in detailed exon composition, splicing sites and numbers of genes. To evaluate the predicted gene models, a series of PCR primers were designed for amplification of segments of the predicted transcripts from RNA. PCR products were amplified from RNA from the HD11 transformed macrophage cell line, and from a cDNA library from RPRL Line 0 chicken spleen.

All predicted exons were amplified from spliced transcripts from the Line 0 chicken cDNA. All the transcript sequences confirmed in this way contained intact reading frames for MRC1-like proteins. These were submitted to the ENA database and received accession numbers HF569039, HF566127, HF569040, HF569041, HF569042, in order *MRC1L-(A to E)* and are provided in figure S2, together with their genomic locations. The *MRC1L-B* and *–C* genes are now correctly annotated in the ENSEMBL database (ENSGALT00000043091, ENSGALT00000014059). Annotation of the other genes is currently inaccurate, with errors as described in file S1 and are liable to change in subsequent database versions. Differences from the corresponding red jungle fowl genomic sequences are enumerated in table S2. The exon structures of the genes and their coding content are compared in figure 2. All encoded eight CTLDs. All except D also contained the exons encoding CysR and FNII receptor domains. That exception apart, the 30-exon structures are identical to that of the mammalian MRC1 genes, with all splice phases conserved and very similar exon lengths for all except the terminal exons.

One alternative splice acceptor site, for exon 8 of the MRC1L-E gene, resulting in the insertion of six amino acids, was found in a minority of the sequenced clones from Line 0 cDNA. While that was the only variant transcript in the Line 0 cDNAs, in the HD11 RNA, more frequent alternatively spliced transcripts were detected for *MRC1L-E*, most of which resulted in interruption of the open reading frame, so that no intact open reading frame for *MRC1L-E* was found in the HD11 cDNA. Thus it is possible the alternative splicing seen in HD11 was an artefact of the transformation of

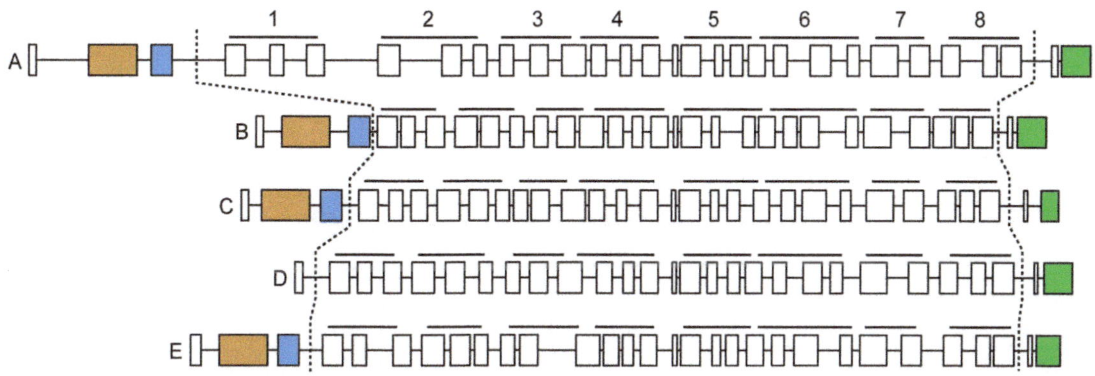

Figure 2. Structure of paralogous *MRC1* genes in the chicken genome. Exons are shown to scale as rectangles. Introns are drawn to 1/10 of the exon scale, except for the shortest which are expanded for visibility. Orange and blue exons are the CysR and FNII domains in all genes except D. The terminal green exon contains transmembrane and cytoplasmic regions. The central array of exons encodes the eight CTLDs indicated by the black bars above each gene.

these cells. The alternative spliced transcripts are illustrated in figure S3.

The locations of conserved features in the CTLDs of the chicken MRC1L genes are shown in figure 3. The tryptophan/hydrophobic/glycine/hydrophobic (WIGL) motif characteristic of the family [20] is present in all these domains of all genes, with minor variations. Four cysteine residues are also conserved in all these domains, an outer pair forming the disulphide bond spanning most of the domain, and an inner pair forming the disulphide bond stabilising the β3–β4 hairpin [21].

MRC1L genes in other species

The UCSC genome browser BLAT search [22,23] with individual and concatenated chicken genes was used to locate orthologous genes in genomes of other birds (turkey and zebrafinch), painted turtle, lizard and Xenopus (sequences in figure S4 and locations in figure S2). In all cases, the alignments with the highest scoring similarities were found between a pair of highly conserved orthologues of the same flanking genes, *SLC39A12* and *STAM*. Exons missing from these BLAT alignments were easily identified by manual inspection. The arrangements of these genes are compared with the orthologous region of the mouse genome in figure 4. The genes in the three birds are very similar, in structure and size of all five genes. The two gaps between the coding sequences of genes C, D and E are small compared with those between the upstream genes. The turtle appears to have a very similar set of five genes, although they occupy a segment of genome twice the length of that in the birds. The lizard genome contains only three genes, while the Xenopus genome, like the mammalian, contains only one *MRC1L* gene. The mouse genome, like that of other mammals, contains an additional gene, *TMEM236*, between the shared flanking genes.

Phylogenetic trees were constructed using a variety of sequence subsets and methods. The great majority of the results had similar topology to the tree depicted in figure 5. Several of the genes identified in other species were missing all or parts of exons in gaps in the genome assemblies. Some signal peptide exons were uncertain, and gene D lacked CysR and FNII domain exons. To avoid bias by these omissions, the tree shown was constructed using just those parts of the CTLDs that were available from all of the genes involved. All species had a single gene that was placed in the same clade as the mammalian *MRC1* gene in 100% of bootstrapped trees. For the avian and turtle genes, the same pattern of species was found for each gene, implying that these arose by duplication before the divergence of these species. In contrast, the lizard lacked orthologues of genes C, D and E, but appeared to have two relatively similar genes of the gene represented in chickens by the KUL01 antigen. Thus the simplest consistent history of this gene family would be an original duplication of the ancestral MRC1 gene, giving rise to the *MRC1L-B* gene, followed in the shared avian and turtle ancestor by further duplications producing genes *C*, *D* and *E*, and in the lizard lineage by a second duplication of the *MRC1L-B* gene. Trees constructed using all the separated CTLDs generally gave the same pattern of species within a clade representing each domain, providing no evidence for domain reassortment. The majority produced the same topology as the tree shown, although bootstrap values were lower. Where the topologies differed, the bootstrap values were insufficient to support any contrary implications. A minority of alternative tree construction methods failed to place the lizard genes 2 and 3 in the MRC1L-B clade.

The cytoplasmic regions of the *MRC1L* gene products are compared in figure 6. The pattern of similarities between sequences are consistent with the evolutionary history that was implied by phylogenetic analysis. This part of the protein is highly conserved between the single mammalian *MRC1* gene and the other genes assigned to the same clade by analysis of the CTLDs. In these molecules, it contains potential motifs involved in targeting to the endocytic pathway, φxNxxY [24,25] and (DE)xxxLZ [25,26]. These motifs are shared by the genes that fall into the MRC1L-B clade that includes the KUL01 antigen, except for the replacement of tyrosine by histidine in the second of the two lizard genes in this clade. The group of genes including mammalian MRC1 also has a di-aromatic motif (YF) that may be involved in endosome sorting [27]. Although the latter is absent from the MRC1L-B orthologues, there are several other residues conserved between these two groups of proteins. In contrast, the cytoplasmic regions of the three downstream genes, found only in the bird and turtle genomes, are highly divergent between paralogues, although well conserved among orthologues. The product of MRC1L-C has only very short cytoplasmic sequences beyond the positively charged region expected to lie immediately inside the plasma membrane. Products of genes D and E have cytoplasmic sequences quite different from each other as well as from those of the MRC1L-A and MRC1L-B molecules. None of the downstream genes contain the endocytosis motifs conserved in the two upstream genes, although the MRC1L-D genes do have a

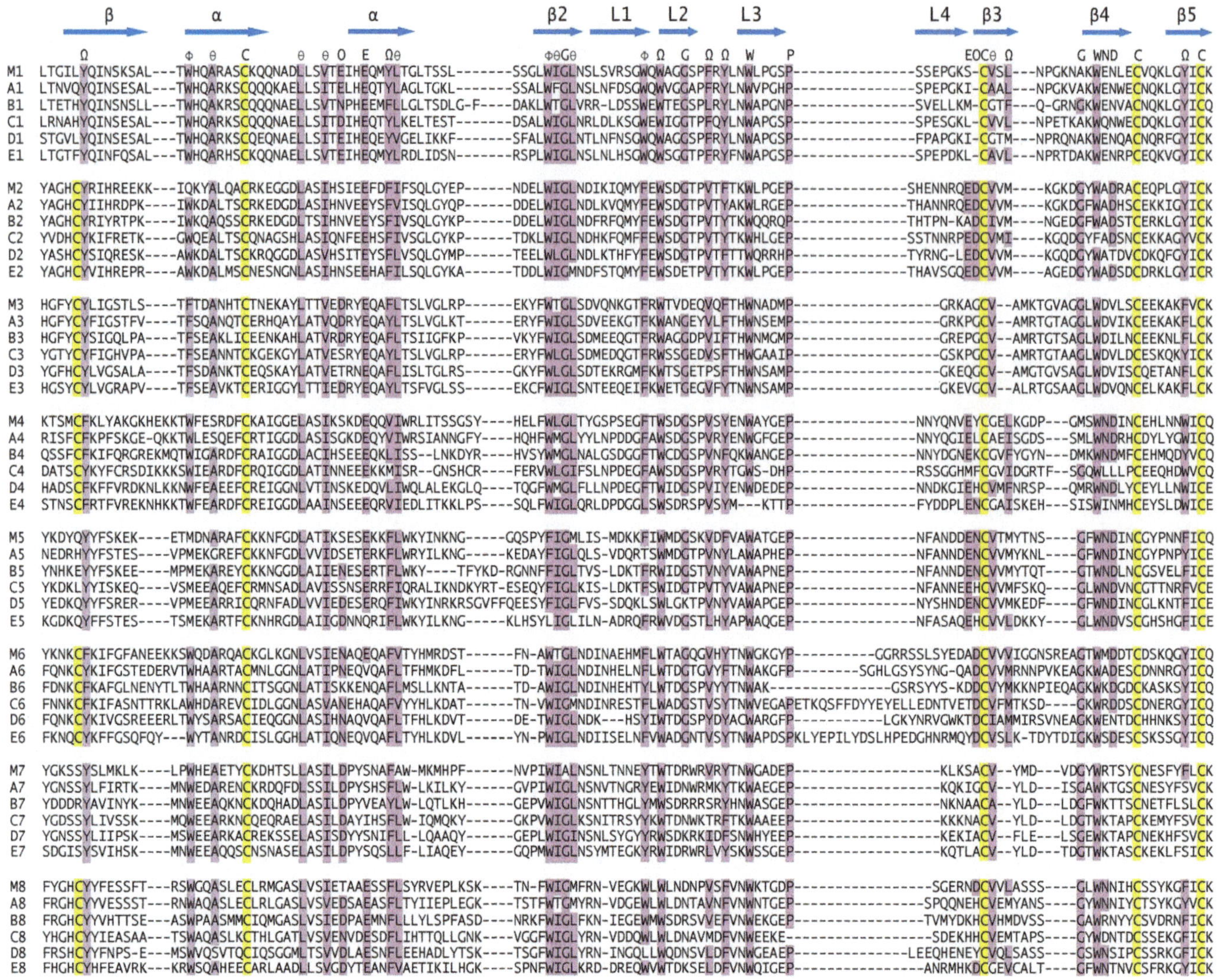

Figure 3. C type lectin domains of the avian MRC1 orthologue gene products. Sequences are labelled on the left, M being the mouse MRC1 sequence while the chicken genes are labelled A to E in genome order in the direction of their transcription, with sequential numbers to indicate the domains in order. Dashes indicate missing residues in the alignment. The short linker peptides between domains are omitted from this figure. Residues reported [20,51] to be conserved throughout the mannose receptor family are indicated above the sequences using the symbols Ω, aromatic or aliphatic; φ, aromatic; θ, aliphatic; C, E, G, P, W, N, D the standard amino acid codes; O, carbonyl oxygen containing (DNEQ). The corresponding residues in the sequences are shaded, yellow for cysteine and purple for the others. Additional cysteine residues in domains 2, 3, 4, 6 and 8 are also shaded. Likely locations of secondary structural features in the mouse sequence [52] are indicated by blue arrows above the sequence; β, beta strand; α alpha helix; L loop.

potential alternative endocytic pathway targeting motif YxxZ (FxxZ in the turtle) [28].

Transcription in tissues

Amplification of the spliced cDNAs for all five genes from the HD11 cell line suggested that all five genes might be transcribed in macrophages. PCR products were also obtained for all the genes from a spleen cDNA library. To obtain a more general picture of the pattern of transcript levels from these genes, quantitative PCR assays were developed for each and applied to compare levels of mRNA for each gene in different normal tissues. The mRNA levels, relative to 28S rRNA, found in various tissues from six Line 0 birds are shown in figure 7.

Exceptionally, the level of *MRC1L-A* transcript was highest in the liver whilst the level in the skin was highest for the other four genes, though only marginally so for *MRC1L-B*. Genes *C*, *D* and *E* had remarkably similar patterns of transcript levels in tissues, possibly indicating coordinated regulation. There was some variation between genes in the levels in different parts of the gut, although duodenum always had lower levels than distal regions of the digestive tract. Within the lymphoid tissues the highest level was always seen in the spleen. Relative transcript levels of all the genes were lowest in either kidney or liver. These assays are not calibrated to compare transcript levels between different genes.

The same assay was used to compare levels of expression, relative to 28S RNA, in several transformed cell lines (figure S5). Expression was clearly highest in the two macrophage cell lines, HD11 and MQ. Much lower levels of MRC1L-A were detected in some of the T cell derived cell lines.

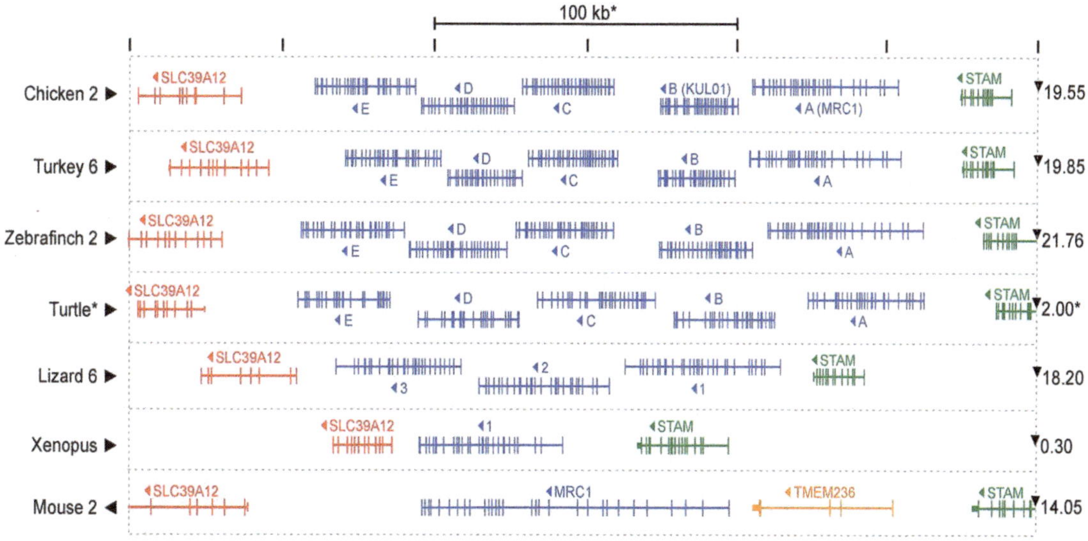

Figure 4. Arrangement the MRC1 orthologue locus in different species. Species are labelled at the left, with a numeral indicating the chromosome where that is known. Black arrowheads indicate the relative orientations of the reference genome maps. The conserved flanking genes SLC39A12 and STAM are indicated in red and green respectively. An additional gene TMEM236, found only in mammalian genomes, is coloured yellow. Predicted MRC1 paralogues are shown in blue. Vertical lines represent the exons of each gene. All the genomes are represented at the same scale, so that the region between vertical dotted lines is 300 kilobase pairs, except in the case of the Painted Turtle, where it represents 600 kilobase pairs. The location in megabase pairs of the right hand end of the map in the chromosome, or other map segment, is indicated at the right. The coding sequences of all genes shown run from right to left in this map, as indicated by arrowheads.

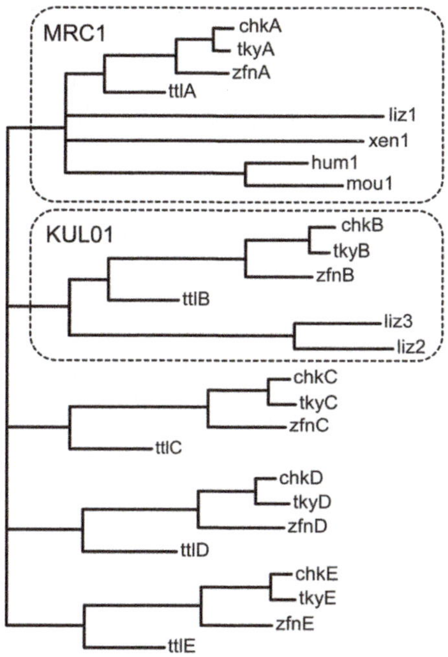

Figure 5. Evolutionary relationships of avian MRC1L genes. A maximum likelihood phylogenetic tree was constructed from predicted exons encoding all the CTLDs, using the Tamura-Nei model in the MEGA software, with 100 bootstrap datasets. All nodes with bootstrap values less than 100 were coalesced into multifurcations. Leaves are labelled with a three letter species code (chk, chicken (*Gallus gallus*); tky, turkey (*Maleagris gallopavo*); zfn, zebrafinch (*Taeniopygia guttata*); ttl, painted turtle (*Chrysemys picta bellii*); liz, lizard (*Anolis carolinensis*); xen, *Xenopus tropicalis*; hum, human (*Homo sapiens*); mou, mouse (*Mus musculus*); followed by either a letter or a number indicating the order of the genes in the direction of transcription. Clades representing orthologues of the MRC1 (human) and KUL01 (chicken) genes are surrounded by dotted lines.

```
hum1  KKRRVHLPQEG-AFENTLYFNSQSSPGTSDMKDLVGNIEQNEHSVI
mou1 KKRHALHIPQEA-TFENTLYFNSNLSPGTSDTKDLMGNIEQNEHAII
xen1  KRQKNKPPEDN-SFDNNLYFDGDRVPATHDTNILVENIEQNEHAIS
liz1  KKRNQHLVTEE-NFENSLYFNSNSAPGTSDTKDLVLNMEQNEHGAI
chkA  KRRKNRLATND-SFENNLYFNSD---GTGDTKDLVTNIERNEHATL
tkyA  KRRKNRLSTND-SFENNLYFNSD---GTGDTKDLVTNIERNEHATL
zfnA  KRRKNCLPTND-SFENNLYFNGDAVPGISDTKDLVTNIEQNEHATL
ttlA  RKRKNHMATND-SFENNLYFNTDAVPGTSDTKDLVDNIEQNEHAIL

liz2  RRRRGQPQTLG-GFDNSLYNKDRVVIPQKDPESLANNNEERLTSFRGNPS
liz3  KKQRKQQQNAA-GFNNSLHE-DNVIILQNDKELLVNNKAGD
chkB  KKRREQTTVTA-SFGNAIYCGTPDP-GTHESKCLVTNIEENEQAML
tkyB  KKRHEQTTVTA-SFGNAIYCGSPDP-GTHESKCLVTNIEENE
zfnB  KRRRDRQMFTA-GFDNAIYR-SDL--GTHESNCLVTNIEENE
ttlB  KKKRHNQLPTDVSFDNTLYCNRDAVPVASDSKYLVANIEQNEQAML

chkC  KRKRQNQLLRD
tkyC  KRKRQNQLSRD
zfnC  KRKRQNQLSTDSGNETLLR
ttlC  KKKRQNQL

chkD  KIKIQSEAERAVGQQSMLLEYSSALDRENDENDPASSKGGSERSDV
tkyD  KMKIQNEADQAAGQHSMLLEYSSAPARENNENNPASS
zfnD  KIKTGSGTGREVRRSSSQLEYSRALTAGDNGSGATNNKEKNEQSVV
ttlD  RKKRQNKLQTDASFNNVLLEHRDTVTGESDTKDSVDKKDQNEHTVI

chkE  RNKGQ-NQISISARMSGSEAALDIQEDDAHTNK
tkyE  RNKGQ-NQVSISARMSGSEAAVDIQGNDAHANK
zfnE  RRKRQ-NLPHISTRMSGSEATVDIQVKDTHSDM
ttlE  KRKNQDNFLPIVTRMSDTKESVDNQEQDEHAVA
```

Figure 6. Alignments of cytoplasmic regions of MRC-like genes from various species. Gene names are as described in the legend to figure 5. Shaded residues show the locations of peptide motifs that may be involved in targeting to the endocytic pathway; green for the φxNxxY, red and blue for the (DE)xxxLZ motif, and purple for YxxZ (φ indicating a bulky hydrophobic residue and Z indicating a hydophobic residue). Light green shading indicates an overlapping potential di-aromatic endosome sorting motif in the MRC1 and MRC1L-A sequences.

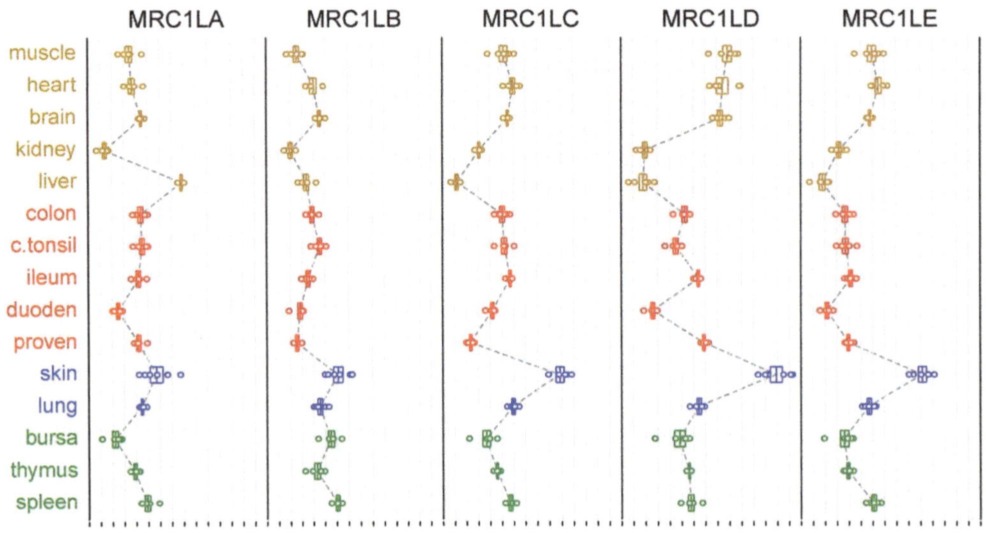

Figure 7. Relative levels of each MRC1 orthologue mRNA in different tissues, measured by quantitative PCR. Tissues, as labelled at the left, are grouped according to preponderance of immune function. For each gene, relative levels of mRNAs are plotted horizontally using a logarithmic scale with arbitrary origins. Circles are individual measurements from each of six birds. Boxes are centered on the means, and their ends indicate the standard errors of those means. All measurements were normalised relative to a constant level of 28S rRNA in each sample and adjusted to the log2 scale using the measured PCR efficiency of standard dilution series, before calculation of means and standard errors. Grey vertical lines and small scale bars at the bottom indicate two-fold differences in relative mRNA measurements.

Discussion

In the human genome, the region of chromosome 10 between the flanking markers *SLC39A12* and *STAM* is annotated as containing a tandemly repeated region, each repeat containing the genes *TMEM236* and *MRC1*. The repeated genes are part of a duplicated segment of about 200 kB with greater than 99% identity, separated by a large gap. There are only two BAC end pairs spanning the gap. In contrast all other mammals that we examined, including other primates, have only one copy of the *TMEM236* and *MRC1* genes between the same flanking marker orthologues, without the gap. While a very recent duplication in humans cannot be ruled out, it seems much more likely that this is a mis-assembled region in the human genome and thus that all mammals carry only a single *MRC1* gene. In species from other classes of terrestrial vertebrate, examination of the region of the genomes between the most highly similar homologues of the flanking markers revealed that some of these contained multiple, tandemly arranged diverged paralogues of *MRC1*. *Xenopus tropicalis* genomes contained only a single gene, the lizard *Anolis carolinensis* had three, while three birds and the painted turtle had five. This indicated duplication of the ancestral *MRC1* gene in the avian lineage and its precursors. The most likely sequence of events would have been an initial duplication producing the ancestors of chicken *MRC1L-A* and *MRC1L-B* genes, followed by a much more recent duplication of the latter in the lizard, and by further early duplications in the common ancestor of birds and turtles. In this context, it is of note that the phylogenetic position of the turtle has been the subject of much debate over a number of decades. Whilst a recent report based on an analysis of microRNAs suggested that turtles form a clade with lizards [29], subsequent reports place them in the archosaur lineage with birds and the crocodylia [30,31]. The more recent proposal is compatible with the simplest possible history of the MRC1 genes described in the present report.

Chicken orthologues of the adjacent *DEC205* [32] and *PLA$_2$R* genes, and of the *MRC2* gene, are found elsewhere in the genome. The additional genes in the *MRC1* locus are therefore not relocated orthologues of these genes.

All the identified genes in all the species examined had intact reading frames coding for proteins with the CTLD structure normally found in members of the mannose receptor family. All were found as spliced mRNAs in the chicken. Thus it is unlikely that any of the duplicated genes is a pseudogene, although differently spliced variants of the genes *D* and *E* transcripts were found in HD11 cDNA that had interrupted reading frames. The physical distances between the genes *C, D* and *E* were small, and the pattern of variation of their transcript levels in tissues was very similar. It may be that the transcription of these three genes is co-ordinately regulated by a shared set of upstream *cis*-acting elements. Indeed, the PCR amplifications used to confirm splice junctions would not have detected splicing between exons in different genes, so that the existence of splice variants that combine segments of the three genes, in a manner similar to the TWEPRIL transcripts from the TWEAK-APRIL genes in mouse [33], is not excluded.

The HD11 cell line contained mRNA for all five *MRC1L* genes, but peptides from protein immunoadsorbed by KUL01 included only those from MRC1L-B. This would be consistent with the KUL01 epitope being exclusive to MRC1L-B. However, the similarities between the MRC1L paralogues, while low, are sufficient that we could not exclude the possibility of recognition of the product of one or more of the other genes in the context where KUL01 is applied as a macrophage marker. To test this possibility we conducted two further experiments. As shown in figure S6, treatment of HD11 cells with transfection reagents including a small interfering RNA (siRNA) with 25/25 nucleotide identity to *MRC1L-B* cDNA sequence, caused 90% reduction in the median level of binding of fluorescently labelled KUL01 antibody, compared with the identical levels observed after the same treatment with either a control siRNA without or with no siRNA. The maximum similarity of the effective siRNA with the other *MRC1L* cDNA sequences, in either orientation, were 15/18 (A), 15/23 (C), 16/20 (D) and 17/22 (E). These are similar to the maximum similarity of the control siRNA with MRC1L-B cDNA (16/25), and would not generally be expected to be sufficient for cross-interference. However, since off-target interference effects have been reported with lower similarities, this observation does not completely exclude the possibility of cross reaction with the product of another MRC1L gene. In a second experiment, figure S7, we observed that that the KUL01 antibody only identified MRC1-B when expression plasmids coding for potential extracellular regions of all five MRCIL genes, as fusion proteins, were transfected into COS-7 cells. This provides compelling evidence that the KUL01 anybody binds the product of the MRC1L-B gene and not the remaining paralogues. Whilst the qRT-PCR analysis of MRC1L-B transcripts is consistent with the observed staining patterns reported with KUL01 across a number of immune-related tissues [19] it is not possible from the present data to infer the cellular distribution of the expression of the remaining MRC1L molecules, although, except for MRC1L-A in the liver, the similarity of the transcript profiles would be consistent with their predominant expression in the same cells as MRC1L-B.

In mammals, MRC1 is a multi-functional molecule. Being a pathogen-associated pattern recognition receptor, its involvements in uptake of antigen for presentation are important functions in innate and adaptive immune responses [9,34], but it also has roles in the clearance of hormones [12] and the regulation of circulating cytokine levels [35–37]. Cellular expression of the molecule is not restricted to macrophage alone but is also present on immature dendritic cells, reflecting its role in antigen capture [38].

The information presented here does not tell us whether a shared ancestor of birds and mammals had multiple *MRC1L* genes, with subsequent gene loss in the mammalian lineage, or whether it had a single gene that was subsequently duplicated only in the avian lineage. The former possibility would allow the hypothesis that the modern functions of mammalian MRC1 might have been distributed between the original paralogous genes. The latter model would have allowed the evolution of novel functional roles for the newly duplicated genes. The similarities between the cytoplasmic domains of MRC1L-A and MRC1L-B, especially with regard to trafficking signals, suggest biological functions similar to the mammalian MRC1, with the possibility of functional redundancy between these molecules. The very different cytoplasmic sequences of the other genes might reflect substantial functional divergence of these from the mammalian *MRC1* genes.

The immune functions of MRC1 in the macrophage have given it an important role in determining the effectiveness of the response to influenza virus infection, at least in the lungs of mice. This presents a single interaction that is likely to be an effective target for evolution of viral virulence. If the additional genes in birds have similar functions in avian macrophages, then there is scope for redundant interactions with the virus that might be harder to evade. Expression of all these genes in macrophages is suggestive of conservation of these interactions. It will therefore be important to investigate whether these molecules have suitable carbohydrate binding activities, whether they are involved in endocytosis and phagocytosis, and whether modulation of their expression affects the susceptibility and response to influenza infection of avian macrophages. We have observed abortive replication of influenza in an avian macrophage cell line (KS and CB, Unpublished observations), which would allow a similar protective role for the *MRC1L* genes to that of *MRC1* in the mouse, in generating effective responses. The involvement of multiple molecules, increasing redundancy in virus receptors, could increase the robustness of this immune mechanism in birds.

The known interaction of the mannose receptor with influenza virus in mice allows the hypothesis that a similar situation occurs in birds, facilitating infection of macrophages but leading to a protective innate immune response [18]. There are other enveloped avian viruses, including Marek's Disease Virus, Infectious Bronchitis Virus and Newcastle Disease Virus, that might be supposed to induce IFN-α by interaction with the mannose receptor [14].

Examples in which the mannose receptor acts as an innate pattern recognition molecule include the internalization of the yeast cell-wall particle zymosan [39], the phagocytosis of Pneumocystis by human alveolar macrophages [40] and Mycobacterium tuberculosis by the monocytic human cell line THP-1 [41]. The mannose receptor also appears to play a role in modulating the adaptive immune response through a role in myeloid plasticity [42]. However, the full repertoire of host-pathogen interactions allowed by the mannose receptor, and particularly the relevance of an expanded Mannose Receptor gene family, remains to be elucidated.

Materials and Methods

Ethics statement

All animal procedures were performed in accordance with the UK Animals (Scientific Procedures) Act 1986 [43]. This study was approved by the Pirbright Institute Ethical Review Panel and the UK Home Office under project licence 30/2683.

Experimental animals

RPRL (Regional Poultry Research Laboratory, East Lansing, MI.) Line O birds were obtained from the Compton specific pathogen free breeding facility, from parents negative for antibodies to specified pathogens, and were kept in controlled-environment isolation rooms with food and water provided *ad libitum*. For RNA preparations, tissue sections (approximately 500 mg), from birds between 4 and 5 weeks old, were collected into RNA Later stabilization fluid (Ambion, UK).

Antibodies, cells and cell lines

KUL01 is a monoclonal IgG1 antibody that recognises an antigen present on the surface of at least a subset of macrophages in chickens [19]. Purified antibody was purchased from Southern Biotech (Alabama).

The retrovirus-transformed macrophage-like cell line HD11 [44] was cultured in RPMI 1640 medium (Invitrogen), 10% FCS. Lines used in figure S5 are described in the figure legend.

Immunoprecipitation

Five to seven million HD11 cells pelleted at 200×g for 5 min were washed 3 times in PBS and resuspended in 500 µl of ice cold lysis buffer consisting of 20 mM TrisHCl, 100 mM NaCl, 0.5% v/v NP40 pH 7.6 to which 10 µl/ml HALT protease inhibitor cocktail and 10 µl/ml EDTA (Pierce Thermo product 87786) had been added. After vigorous mixing and incubation on ice for 30 minutes, Cell debris was then removed by centrifugation at 17,000×g for 15 minutes at 4°C and the lysate was stored at −80C.

Immunoprecipitations were carried out using a Thermo Scientific Pierce Immunoprecipitation kit (product number 1859011), following the manufacturer's instructions. Three hundred µg of antibody (Southern Biotech) was coupled to 100 µl AminoLink Plus Coupling Resin. Lysates were pre-cleared by two overnight incubations, mixing end over end at 4°C with agarose resin (Thermo Scientific) previously washed in lysis buffer, and then incubated for 2.5 hours with the immobilized antibody. After washing three times with 400 µl lysis buffer, bound proteins were eluted using five 100 µl aliquots of 0.1 M glycine. HCl, pH 2.8 including 0.5% (v/v) NP-40. Proteins were recovered from the pooled eluates by addition of trichloroacetic acid to 10% (w/v) and incubated on ice over night before pelleting in a microfuge at 17,000×g for 20 min at 4°C. Pellets were washed with 1 ml of ice cold 90% (v/v) acetone in water, then dried in a speed vac before resuspension and heating to ≥80°C in PAGE sample buffer including DTT for 10 min. PAGE was performed using 4–12% polyacrylamide Tris-Tricine gels in MES buffer and proteins visualised by rinsing the gels in water then incubating for 1–2 hours in Imperial stain (Thermo Scientific) followed by de-staining in water.

Peptide analysis

Bands of interest were excised from PAGE gels, cut into 1 mm cubes and individually placed in a covex 96 well microtitre plate. Reduction with DTT, alkylation with iodoacetamide and digestion using trypsin (Promega V511A) were all performed using a Hewlett Packard MassPREP robot. Digested extracts were transferred into low volume glass sample vials (Chromocol), dried in a speedvac then resuspended in 10 µl of 3% acetonitrile with 0.1% TFA. Liquid chromatography was carried out using a Waters NanoAquity UPLC system which supplied solvents A (0.1% formic acid in water) and B (0.1% formic acid in acetonitrile) to a 1.7 µm, 75 µm ×250 mm, BEH 130 C18 column (Waters) (HPLC solvents were all LC-MS grade from Fisher Scientific). Sample was concentrated onto a 180 µm ×20 mm, 5 µm Symmetry C18 trap (Waters) for 3 minutes at 15 µl/min, and separated at 250 nl/min using a gradient which ramped initially from 3–10% B over 1 minute then to 50% B over 41 minutes and to 85% B in 3 minutes followed by a wash step at this concentration for 2 minutes before re-equilibration at 3% B. Ionised peptides were analysed by a quadrupole time of flight (Q-ToF) Premier mass spectrometer (Waters) in data-dependent acquisition mode where a MS survey scan was used to automatically select multicharged peptides for further MS/MS fragmentation. From each survey scan up to four peptides were selected for fragmentation. MS/MS collision energy was dependent on precursor ions mass and charge state. A reference spectrum was collected every 10 seconds from Glu-fibrinopeptide B(785.8426 m/z), introduced *via* a reference sprayer. Raw MS/MS specta were processed using ProtenLynx Global Server (Waters) and were searched against the NCBInr database using the Mascot search algorithm.

RNA and quantitative PCR

RNA was extracted from 100 mg samples, of fifteen tissues from six birds of the same inbred line, using the Trizol Plus RNA Purification kit (Life Technologies), according to the manufacturer's instructions. Homogenisation was performed using a Mixer Mill MM300 (Retsch) and 3 mm stainless steel cone balls (Retsch). An on-column DNase digestion step was included (Purelink DNAse, Life Technologies). The majority of samples were diluted to have A_{260} approximately 1.0. Some samples with low RNA yields were used at up to ten-fold lower A_{260}.

Primers and probes for real-time quantitative PCR assay of 28S rRNA [45] and of the five predicted chicken macrophage mannose receptor mRNAs are detailed in table S3. The *MRC1L* cDNA primers and probes were designed so that the primers were entirely in different exons and the probe was approximately centred on an intron-exon boundary. *MRC1L* gene primers and probes were designed using Genscript primer design software (https://www.genscript.com/ssl-bin/app/primer) and Primer Express (Applied Biosystems, Foster City, California, USA). These primers gave no detectable signal after 40 cycles with 2.5 ng chicken genomic DNA in the standard assay conditions.

Probes incorporated 5-carboxyfluorescein (FAM) at the 5′ end and N,N,N,N′ tetramethyl-6-carboxyrhodamine (TAMRA) at the 3′ end. Assays were carried out using the Superscript III platinum one-step qRT-PCR kit (Invitrogen). Amplification and detection of specific products were carried out with the 7500 Fast Real Time System (Taqman; Applied Biosystems) with the following cycle profile: 50°C for 5 min, 95°C for 2 min and then 40 cycles of 95°C for 3 sec and 60°C for 30sec.

To measure the PCR efficiencies, six 10-fold dilutions, of the highest expressing tissue for each MRC1-L assay, and of HD11 RNA for the 28S assay, were used in triplicate measurements. All *MRC1L* gene mRNA measurements were normalised to the levels of 28S ribosomal RNA in the samples using the equation $Xt = Ct - s(Ct' - Q)/s'$ where Ct is the gene-specific threshold cycle, Ct′ is the threshold cycle for the 28S ribosomal RNA assay (on a constant dilution of the sample), s and s′ are slopes of linear regressions of threshold cycles (C_T) against $\log_{10}$(RNA) for target gene and 28S assays respectively. All sample Ct values were within the range of the standard plots. Details of the normalisation calculations and of statistical analyses confirming differential expression between tissues are provided in document S1 and document S2.

Sequencing and bioinformatics

Primers listed in table S4 were designed to amplify overlapping segments of the five predicted transcripts. Preparative PCR amplifications were carried out using methods described elsewhere [32], using templates of a line 0 chicken spleen cDNA library [46], freshly prepared total RNA from line 0 chicken spleen and total RNA from the cell line HD11. Amplified products excised from agarose gels were cloned into the pGEM-T-Easy vector (Promega). DNA prepared using the Qiagen QIAprep spin miniprep kit were used for sequencing. Sequencing reactions were performed by GATC Biotech. Sequence data were analysed using STADEN [47]. Multiple clones of PCR products were sequenced from each amplification to obtain the consensus sequence and to identify clones free from PCR errors.

Extensive use was made of the ClustalW [48]. The UCSC genome browser (http://genome.ucsc.edu; [49]) during the manual refinement of gene structures and in the preparation of figure 4. Assembly versions used were chicken, WUGSC 2.1/galGal3; turkey, TGC Turkey_2.01/melGal1; zebra finch, WUGSC 3.2.4/taeGut1; lizard, Broad AnoCar2.0/anoCar2; painted turtle, v3.0.1/chrPic1; Xenopus tropicalis, JGI 4.2/xenTro3; mouse, GRCm38/mm10; human, GRCh/hq19. Phylogenetic analyses were carried out using the MEGA package [50].

Supporting Information

Figure S1 Peptide sequences from MRC1L-B found in trypic digest of KUL01-adsorbed material.

Figure S2 Chicken MRC1L cDNA sequences and genomic locations of orthologues.

Figure S3 Alternative splicing in MRC1L-E cDNA.

Figure S4 Predicted sequences of MRC1L orthologues in other species.

Figure S5 Relative mRNA levels of MRC1L genes in chicken cell lines.

Figure S6 Suppression of KUL01 antigen expression by MRC1L-B specic siRNA.

Figure S7 KUL01 specifically recognises the MRC1L-B gene product in transfected COS cells.

Table S1 List of peptides from tryptyic digest of KUL01-adsorbed material.

Table S2 Differences between Line 0 cDNA sequence and genomic jungle fowl sequence.

Table S3 Primers and probes for TaqMan quantitative PCR.

Table S4 Primers used in amplifying chicken MRC1L cDNAs.

Document S1 Statistical analysis of qPCR data for MRC1L genes in different tissues.

Document S2 Statistical test for differences in MRC1L transcripts between tissues.

File S1 Chicken MRC1L genes: Links to ENSEMBL identifiers & Errors in release 75.

Acknowledgments

The authors would like to thank Dr John Hammond, for advice pertaining to phylogenetic analysis, and the dedicated staff of the Institute's animal services.

Author Contributions

Conceived and designed the experiments: KS LGH JRY CB. Performed the experiments: KS LGH JRY CB. Analyzed the data: KS LGH JRY CB. Contributed reagents/materials/analysis tools: JRY. Wrote the paper: KS LGH JRY CB.

References

1. Barten R, Torkar M, Haude A, Trowsdale J, Wilson MJ (2001) Divergent and convergent evolution of NK-cell receptors. Trends in Immunology 22: 52–57.
2. Kaiser P, Poh TY, Rothwell L, Avery S, Balu S, et al. (2005) A genomic analysis of chicken cytokines and chemokines. Journal of Interferon and Cytokine Research 25: 467–484.
3. Hughes AL (1994) The Evolution of Functionally Novel Proteins after Gene Duplication. Proceedings of the Royal Society B-Biological Sciences 256: 119–124.
4. Weis WI, Taylor ME, Drickamer K (1998) The C-type lectin superfamily in the immune system. Immunological Reviews 163: 19–34.
5. Taylor ME, Conary JT, Lennartz MR, Stahl PD, Drickamer K (1990) Primary Structure of the Mannose Receptor Contains Multiple Motifs Resembling Carbohydrate-Recognition Domains. Journal of Biological Chemistry 265: 12156–12162.
6. Taylor ME, Drickamer K (1993) Structural Requirements for High-Affinity Binding of Complex Ligands by the Macrophage Mannose Receptor. Journal of Biological Chemistry 268: 399–404.
7. Taylor ME, Bezouska K, Drickamer K (1992) Contribution to Ligand-Binding by Multiple Carbohydrate-Recognition Domains in the Macrophage Mannose Receptor. Journal of Biological Chemistry 267: 1719–1726.
8. Tietze C, Schlesinger P, Stahl P (1982) Mannose-Specific Endocytosis Receptor of Alveolar Macrophages - Demonstration of 2 Functionally Distinct Intracellular Pools of Receptor and Their Roles in Receptor Recycling. Journal of Cell Biology 92: 417–424.
9. Stahl PD, Ezekowitz RAB (1998) The mannose receptor is a pattern recognition receptor involved in host defense. Current Opinion in Immunology 10: 50–55.
10. Martinez-Pomares L, Mahoney JA, Kaposzta R, Linehan SA, Stahl PD, et al. (1998) A functional soluble form of the murine mannose receptor is produced by macrophages in vitro and is present in mouse serum. Journal of Biological Chemistry 273: 23376–23380.
11. Martinez-Pomares L, Gordon S (1999) Potential role of the mannose receptor in antigen transport. Immunology Letters 65: 9–13.
12. Fiete DJ, Beranek MC, Baenziger JU (1998) A cysteine-rich domain of the "mannose" receptor mediates GalNAc-4-SO4 binding. Proceedings of the National Academy of Sciences of the United States of America 95: 2089–2093.
13. Tesar DB, Cheung EJ, Bjorkman PJ (2008) The chicken yolk sac IgY receptor, a mammalian mannose receptor family member, transcytoses IgY across polarized epithelial cells. Molecular Biology of the Cell 19: 1587–1593.
14. Milone MC, Fitzgerald-Bocarsly P (1998) The mannose receptor mediates induction of IFN-alpha in peripheral blood dendritic cells by enveloped RNA and DNA viruses. Journal of Immunology 161: 2391–2399.
15. Nguyen DG, Hildreth JEK (2003) Involvement of macrophage mannose receptor in the binding and transmission of HIV by macrophages. European Journal of Immunology 33: 483–493.
16. Miller JL, Dewet BJM, Martinez-Pomares L, Radcliffe CM, Dwek RA, et al. (2008) The mannose receptor mediates dengue virus infection of macrophages. Plos Pathogens 4.
17. Reading PC, Miller JL, Anders EM (2000) Involvement of the mannose receptor in infection of macrophages by influenza virus. J Virol 74: 5190–5197.
18. Upham JP, Pickett D, Irimura T, Anders EM, Reading PC (2010) Macrophage Receptors for Influenza A Virus: Role of the Macrophage Galactose-Type Lectin and Mannose Receptor in Viral Entry. Journal of Virology 84: 3730–3737.
19. Mast J, Goddeeris BM, Peeters K, Vandesande F, Berghman LR (1998) Characterisation of chicken monocytes, macrophages and interdigitating cells by the monoclonal antibody KUL01. Veterinary Immunology and Immunopathology 61: 343–357.
20. Weis WI, Kahn R, Fourme R, Drickamer K, Hendrickson WA (1991) Structure of the Calcium-Dependent Lectin Domain from a Rat Mannose-Binding Protein Determined by Mad Phasing. Science 254: 1608–1615.
21. Zelensky AN, Gready JE (2003) Comparative analysis of structural properties of the C-type-lectin-like domain (CTLD). Proteins-Structure Function and Genetics 52: 466–477.
22. Kent WJ (2002) BLAT - The BLAST-like alignment tool. Genome Research 12: 656–664.
23. Kent WJ, Sugnet CW, Furey TS, Roskin KM, Pringle TH, et al. (2002) The human genome browser at UCSC. Genome Research 12: 996–1006.
24. East L, Isacke CM (2002) The mannose receptor family. Biochimica Et Biophysica Acta-General Subjects 1572: 364–386.
25. Mellman I (1996) Endocytosis and molecular sorting. Annual Review of Cell and Developmental Biology 12: 575–625.
26. Pond L, Kuhn LA, Teyton L, Schutze MP, Tainer JA, et al. (1995) A Role for Acidic Residues in Di-Leucine Motif-Based Targeting to the Endocytic Pathway. Journal of Biological Chemistry 270: 19989–19997.
27. Schweizer A, Stahl PD, Rohrer J (2000) A di-aromatic motif in the cytosolic tail of the mannose receptor mediates endosomal sorting. Journal of Biological Chemistry 275: 29694–29700.
28. Sandoval IV, Bakke O (1994) Targeting of membrane proteins to endosomes and lysosomes. Trends Cell Biol 4: 292–297.
29. Hedges SB (2012) Amniote phylogeny and the position of turtles. Bmc Biology 10.
30. Chiari Y, Cahais V, Galtier N, Delsuc F (2012) Phylogenomic analyses support the position of turtles as the sister group of birds and crocodiles (Archosauria). Bmc Biology 10.
31. Crawford NG, Faircloth BC, McCormack JE, Brumfield RT, Winker K, et al. (2012) More than 1000 ultraconserved elements provide evidence that turtles are the sister group of archosaurs. Biology Letters 8: 783–786.
32. Staines K, Young JR, Butter C (2013) Expression of Chicken DEC205 Reflects the Unique Structure and Function of the Avian Immune System. PLoS One 8: e51799.
33. Pradet-Balade B, Medema JP, Lopez-Fraga M, Lozano JC, Kolfschoten GM, et al. (2002) An endogenous hybrid mRNA encodes TWE-PRIL, a functional cell surface TWEAK-APRIL fusion protein. Embo Journal 21: 5711–5720.
34. Prigozy TI, Sieling PA, Clemens D, Stewart PL, Behar SM, et al. (1997) The mannose receptor delivers lipoglycan antigens to endosomes for presentation to T cells by CD1b molecules. Immunity 6: 187–197.
35. Shibata Y, Metzger WJ, Myrvik QN (1997) Chitin particle-induced cell-mediated immunity is inhibited by soluble mannan - Mannose receptor-mediated phagocytosis initiates IL-12 production. Journal of Immunology 159: 2462–2467.
36. Vautier S, MacCallum DM, Brown GD (2012) C-type lectin receptors and cytokines in fungal immunity. Cytokine 58: 89–99.

37. Yamamoto Y, Klein TW, Friedman H (1997) Involvement of mannose receptor in cytokine interleukin-1 beta (IL-1 beta), IL-6, and granulocyte-macrophage colony-stimulating factor responses, but not in chemokine macrophage inflammatory protein 1 beta (MIP-1 beta), MIP-2, and KC responses, caused by attachment of Candida albicans to macrophages. Infection and Immunity 65: 1077–1082.
38. Sallusto F, Cella M, Danieli C, Lanzavecchia A (1995) Dendritic cells use macropinocytosis and the mannose receptor to concentrate macromolecules in the major histocompatibility complex class II compartment: downregulation by cytokines and bacterial products. J Exp Med 182: 389–400.
39. Underhill DM, Ozinsky A, Hajjar AM, Stevens A, Wilson CB, et al. (1999) The Toll-like receptor 2 is recruited to macrophage phagosomes and discriminates between pathogens. Nature 401: 811–815.
40. Zhang JM, Zhu JP, Bu X, Cushion M, Kinane TB, et al. (2005) Cdc42 and RhoB activation are required for mannose receptor-mediated phagocytosis by human alveolar macrophages. Molecular Biology of the Cell 16: 824–834.
41. Diaz-Silvestre H, Espinosa-Cueto P, Sanchez-Gonzalez A, Esparza-Ceron MA, Pereira-Suarez AL, et al. (2005) The 19-kDa antigen of Mycobacterium tuberculosis is a major adhesin that binds the mannose receptor of THP-1 monocytic cells and promotes phagocytosis of mycobacteria. Microbial Pathogenesis 39: 97–107.
42. Mishra PK, Morris EG, Garcia JA, Cardona AE, Teale JM (2013) Increased Accumulation of Regulatory Granulocytic Myeloid Cells in Mannose Receptor C Type 1-Deficient Mice Correlates with Protection in a Mouse Model of Neurocysticercosis. Infection and Immunity 81: 1052–1063.
43. UK Home Office (1986) Guidance on the Operation of the Animals (Scientific Procedures) Act.
44. Beug H vKA, Doderlein G, Conscience J-F, Graf T (1979) Chicken hematopoietic cells transformed by seven strains of defective avian leukemia viruses display three distinct phenotypes of differentiation. Cell 18: 375–390.
45. Moody A, Sellers S, Bumstead N (2000) Measuring infectious bursal disease virus RNA in blood by multiplex real-time quantitative RT-PCR. J Virol Methods 85: 55–64.
46. Tregaskes CA, Bumstead N, Davison TF, Young JR (1996) Chicken B-cell marker chB6 (Bu-1) is a highly glycosylated protein of unique structure. Immunogenetics 44: 212–217.
47. Staden R (1996) The Staden sequence analysis package. Molecular Biotechnology 5: 233–241.
48. Larkin MA, Blackshields G, Brown NP, Chenna R, McGettigan PA, et al. (2007) Clustal W and clustal X version 2.0. Bioinformatics 23: 2947–2948.
49. Meyer LR ZA, Hinrichs AS, Karolchik D, Kuhn RM, Wong M, et al. (2012) The UCSC Genome Browser database: extensions and updates 2013. Nucleic Acids Res Nov 15.
50. Tamura K, Peterson D, Peterson N, Stecher G, Nei M, et al. (2011) MEGA5: Molecular Evolutionary Genetics Analysis Using Maximum Likelihood, Evolutionary Distance, and Maximum Parsimony Methods. Molecular Biology and Evolution 28: 2731–2739.
51. Kim SJ, Ruiz N, Bezouska K, Drickamer K (1992) Organization of the Gene Encoding the Human Macrophage Mannose Receptor (Mrc1). Genomics 14: 721–727.
52. Harris N, Super M, Rits M, Chang G, Ezekowitz RAB (1992) Characterization of the Murine Macrophage Mannose Receptor - Demonstration That the down-Regulation of Receptor Expression Mediated by Interferon-Gamma Occurs at the Level of Transcription. Blood 80: 2363–2373.

Histone Deacetylase Inhibitors Selectively Target Homology Dependent DNA Repair Defective Cells and Elevate Non-Homologous Endjoining Activity

Stephanie Smith[1], Jennifer Fox[1], Marco Mejia[2], Wanvipa Ruangpradit[2], Alihossein Saberi[3], Sunmi Kim[1,3,4], Yongjun Choi[1], Sehyun Oh[8], Yucai Wang[5,7], Kyungho Choi[4], Lei Li[5,6], Eric A. Hendrickson[8], Shunichi Takeda[3], Mark Muller[2], Kyungjae Myung[1]*

1 Genome Instability Section, Genetics and Molecular Biology Branch, National Human Genome Research Institute, National Institutes of Health, Bethesda, Maryland, United States of America, **2** Department of Molecular Biology and Microbiology, College of Medicine, University of Central Florida, Orlando, Florida, United States of America, **3** Department of Radiation Genetics Kyoto University, Medical School, Kyoto, 606-8501 Japan, **4** Department of Environmental Health School of Public Hearth, Seoul National University, Seoul, Korea, **5** Department of Experimental Radiation Oncology, The University of Texas MD Anderson Cancer Center, Houston, Texas, United States of America, **6** Department of Genetics, The University of Texas MD Anderson Cancer Center, Houston, Texas, United States of America, **7** The University of Texas Graduate School of Biomedical Sciences at Houston, Houston Texas, United States of America, **8** Department of Biochemistry, Molecular Biology and Biophysics, University of Minnesota Medical School, Minneapolis, Minnesota, United States of America

Abstract

Background: We have previously used the ATAD5-luciferase high-throughput screening assay to identify genotoxic compounds with potential chemotherapeutic capabilities. The successful identification of known genotoxic agents, including the histone deacetylase inhibitor (HDACi) trichostatin A (TSA), confirmed the specificity of the screen since TSA has been widely studied for its ability to cause apoptosis in cancer cells. Because many cancers have acquired mutations in DNA damage checkpoints or repair pathways, we hypothesized that these cancers may be susceptible to treatments that target compensatory pathways. Here, we used a panel of isogenic chicken DT40 B lymphocyte mutant and human cell lines to investigate the ability of TSA to define selective pathways that promote HDACi toxicity.

Results: HDACi induced a DNA damage response and reduced viability in all repair deficient DT40 mutants although *ATM*-nulls were least affected. The most dramatic sensitivity was observed in mutants lacking the homology dependent repair (HDR) factor *BLM* or the non-homologous end-joining (NHEJ) and HDR factors, *KU/RAD54*, suggesting an involvement of either HDR or NHEJ in HDACi-induced cell death. To extend these findings, we measured the frequencies of HDR and NHEJ after HDACi treatment and monitored viability in human cell lines comparably deficient in HDR or NHEJ. Although no difference in HDR frequency was observed between HDACi treated and untreated cells, HDR-defective human cell lines were clearly more sensitive than wild type. Unexpectedly, cells treated with HDACis showed a significantly elevated NHEJ frequency.

Conclusions: HDACi targeting drugs induced significant increases in NHEJ activity in human cell lines but did not alter HDR frequency. Moreover, HDR is required for cellular resistance to HDACi therapy; therefore, NHEJ does not appear to be a critical axis for HDACi resistance. Rather, HDACi compounds induced DNA damage, most likely double strand breaks (DSBs), and HDR proficiency is correlated with cell survival.

Editor: Sebastian D. Fugmann, Chang Gung University, Taiwan

Funding: This research was supported by the NIH grants GM088351, CA154461 to EAH, the NIH grants CA127945, CA097175 to LL, the UCF College of Medicine to MTM, a grant-in-aid from the Ministry of Education, Culture, Sports, Science and Technology of the Japanese Government (MEXT, number 20241012) to ST, the National Research Foundation of Korea (NRF) funded by the Ministry of Education, Science and Technology (357-2011-D00133), the intramural Research Programs of the National Human Genome Research Institute and NIH R03 MH092164-01 to KM. The funders had no role in study design, data collection and analysis, decision to publish, or preparation of the manuscript.

Competing Interests: The authors have declared that no competing interests exist.

* E-mail: kmyung@mail.nih.gov

Introduction

DNA double strand breaks (DSBs) are toxic lesions that represent a major threat to cell survival. Homologous recombination (HR), also known as homology dependent repair (HDR) and non-homologous end joining (NHEJ) are two major pathways that repair DNA DSBs [1,2,3]. The HDR pathway, which is largely considered an error free process, functions mainly in the S and G2 phases of the cell cycle when a sister chromatid is available for use as a template [4]. In eukaryotes, the RAD51 strand exchange protein is a central player in HDR and mediates the process of synapse from a wild type allele {for review see [2]}. Other HDR proteins generally function as positive or negative regulators of RAD51. Positive regulators include BRCA1 and

BRCA2. BRCA1 binds directly to the DSB, participates in the processing of the DSB by promoting 5′-end resection, and is required for the recruitment of RAD51 [4]. BRCA2 promotes RAD51-mediated strand exchange, thus controlling the assembly of the nucleofilament required for synapse [4]. Negative regulators of HDR such as BLM and FANCM have evolved to prevent uncontrolled or unscheduled HDR [5], which could ultimately lead to genomic DNA rearrangements [2]. BLM [2], RecQ5 [6], and FANCJ [7] helicases were reported to destabilize RAD51-coated single-stranded DNA (ssDNA) and FANCM is a translocase that disrupts intermediate RAD51-coated D-loops [2]. Recently, PARI [8] and RTEL [9] have been suggested as putative homologs to the yeast anti-recombination protein, Srs2. Given the importance of HDR in genome stability, it is not surprising that many of the proteins involved in HDR have been found to increase cancer susceptibility when mutated. Mutations in BRCA2 and/or BRCA1 increase predisposition to breast and ovarian cancers [4], while mutations in BLM or FANCM are associated with syndromes showing elevated genomic instability and cancer susceptibility in general [2,10].

NHEJ is an error-prone pathway whereby the two broken ends of the DSB are conjoined by direct ligation without regard to sequence homology, but generally involve microhomology of a few bases. Whereas HDR is the major repair mechanism in the S and G2 phases of the cell cycle, the NHEJ pathway is primarily active in G1 in part because the repair protein 53BP1 binds to the broken ends and prevents resection, thereby repressing an early key step in HDR [3]. During NHEJ, the KU70-KU80 heterodimer (Ku) holds the broken ends in direct proximity and recruits other NHEJ proteins including the DNA-dependent protein kinase catalytic subunit (DNA-PKcs), Artemis, and DNA Ligase IV (LIGIV). DNA-PKcs, Ku and the DNA at the site of the DSB together form an active kinase complex (DNA-PK). Ku, Artemis, XRCC4 and LIGIV are all targets of DNA-PK, although phosphorylation of these proteins is, surprisingly, dispensable for NHEJ *in vivo* [11,12,13]. In contrast, autophosphorylation of DNA-PKcs is required for proper NHEJ [14]. Artemis and Ku participate in the processing of the DSB, and then the heterodimeric complex of XRCC4 and LIGIV ligate the broken DNA ends [15]. As with HDR, inappropriate NHEJ is detrimental to the cell and results in chromosomal deletions, insertions or translocations, especially when more than one DSB is available for repair [16]. Because Ku spatially stabilizes DSB ends, its loss can also lead to inappropriate joining outcomes [16]. Mutations in *ARTEMIS* are associated with severe combined immunodeficiency and predisposition to lymphomas [16]. Germ-line mutations in *LIGIV* result in LIG4 syndrome and predispose individuals to lymphoid malignancies [16]. Lastly, mutations of *DNA-PKcs* cause severe combined immunodeficiency in mice [17,18,19,20]. In animals, NHEJ appears to be the major pathway for DSB repair while HDR, a high fidelity process, is much more limited. Recent evidence has suggested that the DNA synthesis associated with HDR can also reprogram DNA methylation signatures in the repaired segment, thereby leading to silencing of tumor suppressor genes or activation of oncogenes in daughter cells [21,22,23].

We recently developed a robust ATAD5-luciferase high-throughput screening (HTS) assay based on the stabilization of the DNA damage response protein ATAD5 to identify genotoxic compounds and potential chemotherapeutic agents that act by inducing DNA damage [24,25]. The ATAD5-luciferase HTS is a tractable cell based screen that identified histone deacetylase inhibitors (HDACis) as potent DNA damaging agents [25]. There is significant general interest in epigenetic therapeutics and these agents are currently under intense investigation for potential use as anti-cancer drugs [26]. HDACi therapeutics increase histone acetylation levels by inhibiting deacetylation of histones thus modifying the chromatin structure and regulating gene expression [27]. HDACis are highly pleiotropic and have numerous non-histone targets including p53, NF-kB and Rb/E2F showing widespread effects [26]. In the case of p53, this tumor suppressor protein is stabilized and transcriptionally activated by hyperacetylation, which in turn activates DNA repair or pro-apoptotic proteins [28]. Induction of cell cycle arrest, apoptosis and differentiation, coupled with inhibition of metastasis and angiogenesis, all combine to give HDACis a diverse set of anti-cancer abilities [27,28]. TSA has been widely studied and shown to increase apoptosis in a variety of cancer types. TSA also increases the effectiveness of platinum-based therapies in human bladder cancer cells [29]. Another HDACi suberoylanilide hydroxamic acid (SAHA), has been extensively researched and was approved by the FDA in 2006 for use in the treatment of cutaneous T cell lymphoma [28]. Currently HDACis are being chemically modified to form new compounds combining the properties of the HDACis and other anti-cancer agents [27].

Because DNA repair pathways are well conserved evolutionarily we employed a panel of isogenic chicken DT40 B lymphocyte cell lines to investigate whether HDACis specifically kill DNA repair-deficient cells. Ease of target integration, a short doubling time and an unusually long S phase are all characteristics that make DT40 cells ideal for studying DNA repair and genotoxicity [30]. Here, we further examine the role that DNA repair pathways play in HDR, a pivotal pathway in defining resistance to HDACi; however, two different HDACi drugs strongly stimulate the process of NHEJ. Thus, elevation of an error prone pathway may aid in cytotoxicity of HDACi in cancer.

Results and Discussion

Previously we developed a high-throughput screen that used ATAD5 as a biomarker to detect genotoxic compounds, and described a preliminary screen of small chemical libraries [25]. In this screen, we found that HDACis, including TSA, increased the protein level of ATAD5 {Figure 1a and [25]} and activated DNA damage responses (Figure 1b). In addition to an increased level of γH2AX protein, pulsed-field gel electrophoresis (PFGE) confirmed a slight increase in DNA DSBs after treatment with TSA indicated by shorter DNA fragments. Many transformed cells are defective in repairing certain types of DNA damage due to deficiencies in DNA repair pathways. Transformed cells are usually highly susceptible to HDACi drugs such as TSA or SAHA [31] which also induce DNA damage (Figure 1b); thus, we reasoned that DNA repair pathways such as HDR and NHEJ are likely important in defining drug sensitivity in tumors. To test this, a panel of isogenic chicken DT40 B lymphocyte cell lines, each of which is defective in a different DNA repair pathway (Table 1), was screened for viability after treatment with increasing concentrations of TSA. The viability of the DT40 cells was assessed 48 hr after treatment, using the CellTiter-Glo luminescent cell viability assay to detect ATPase activity. Compared to wild-type, all mutant DT40 cell lines tested displayed some degree of sensitivity to TSA (Figure 2a and Table 2). *ATM*-deficient cells were not as strongly affected as other nulls but were still sensitized to TSA (Figure 2a and Table 2). To determine if the effect was specific to TSA, we also measured the viability of DT40 cell lines treated with increasing concentrations of another HDACi, SAHA (Figure 2b). The toxicity profiles of cells treated with either TSA or SAHA fell into three groups. *XPA*-, *SHPRH*-, *BLM*-, and *KU70/RAD54*-null cells fell into the first group of cells sensitive to both TSA and SAHA. *POLβ*-,

REV3-, *FEN1*-, *UBC13*- and *FANCC*-null cells fell into the second group and only exhibited sensitivity to TSA. Finally, *ATM*-null cells were in a group by themselves and exhibited sensitivity similar to wild-type in the presence of both TSA and SAHA (Figure 2a and b and Table 2). It appeared that DNA damage caused by TSA requires all of the DNA repair pathways with the possible exception of the ATM-dependent DNA damage response, which is not thought to be required in HDR in normal mouse cells [32]. Also, base excision repair, the fanconi anemia pathway, and translesion synthesis polymerases appeared to be dispensable for the repair of SAHA-induced DNA damage.

KU70/RAD54- and *BLM*-null DT40 cells were the most sensitive to both TSA and SAHA treatment compared to the other mutant cell lines. *KU70/RAD54*-null cells are NHEJ and HDR defective (NHEJ, due to the absence of *KU70* and HDR due to the loss of *RAD54*) [2,3]. In contrast, *BLM*-null cells exhibit a hyper-recombination phenotype [33]. To test the possibility that HDACi treatment causes promiscuous HDR, we measured the frequency of sister chromatid exchange (SCE) in human retinal pigment epithelial (RPE) cells after TSA treatment. The frequency of SCE events for both treated and control-treated cells was not significantly different (Figures 3a and b). We also performed a single DSB-induced HDR assay using DR-GFP as a reporter in human U2OS cells [34] and found that there was no difference in HDR frequency between TSA-treated and control-treated cells (Figures 3c and d). A similar and complementary approach was performed using a HeLa cell line (iHO4.5GFP) containing twin DR-GFP reporter cassettes [35] that undergo HDR following I-SceI-induced DSB formation in the 5′ cassette [23]. In iHO4.5GFP cells, the I-SceI gene is under the control of the tet-on promoter which activates upon exposure to doxycycline (Figure 3e). Using this assay, we found that there was no significant difference in the HDR frequency of TSA or SAHA-treated cells compared to control-treated cells (Figures 3f and Figure S1a). It is possible that the decrease in HDR frequency and clear toxicity observed at higher doses of TSA (data not shown) resulted from a suppression of HDR [36,37]. Taken together, these data indicate that treatment with TSA or SAHA does not increase the frequency of HDR. Indirect evidence that HDACi drugs do not induce promiscuous HDR repair comes from iHO4.5GFP uninduced (minus Dox) cells treated with TSA. If TSA or SAHA directly or indirectly caused genome wide DNA damage and HDR in the DR-GFP reporter, we would expect to see an increase in the percent GFP readout in the absence of I-SceI as some DNA damage and HDR should be randomly directed to the DR-GFP locus. As shown in Figure 3f and Figure S1a, there was no obvious increase in the percentage of GFP positive cells in uninduced iHO4.5GFP cells treated with HDACi alone.

The protein 53BP1 is recruited to DSBs and inhibits the 5′ to 3′ single-strand resection that initiates HDR [38]. ATM and DNAPKcs, which are both required for NHEJ, phosphorylate

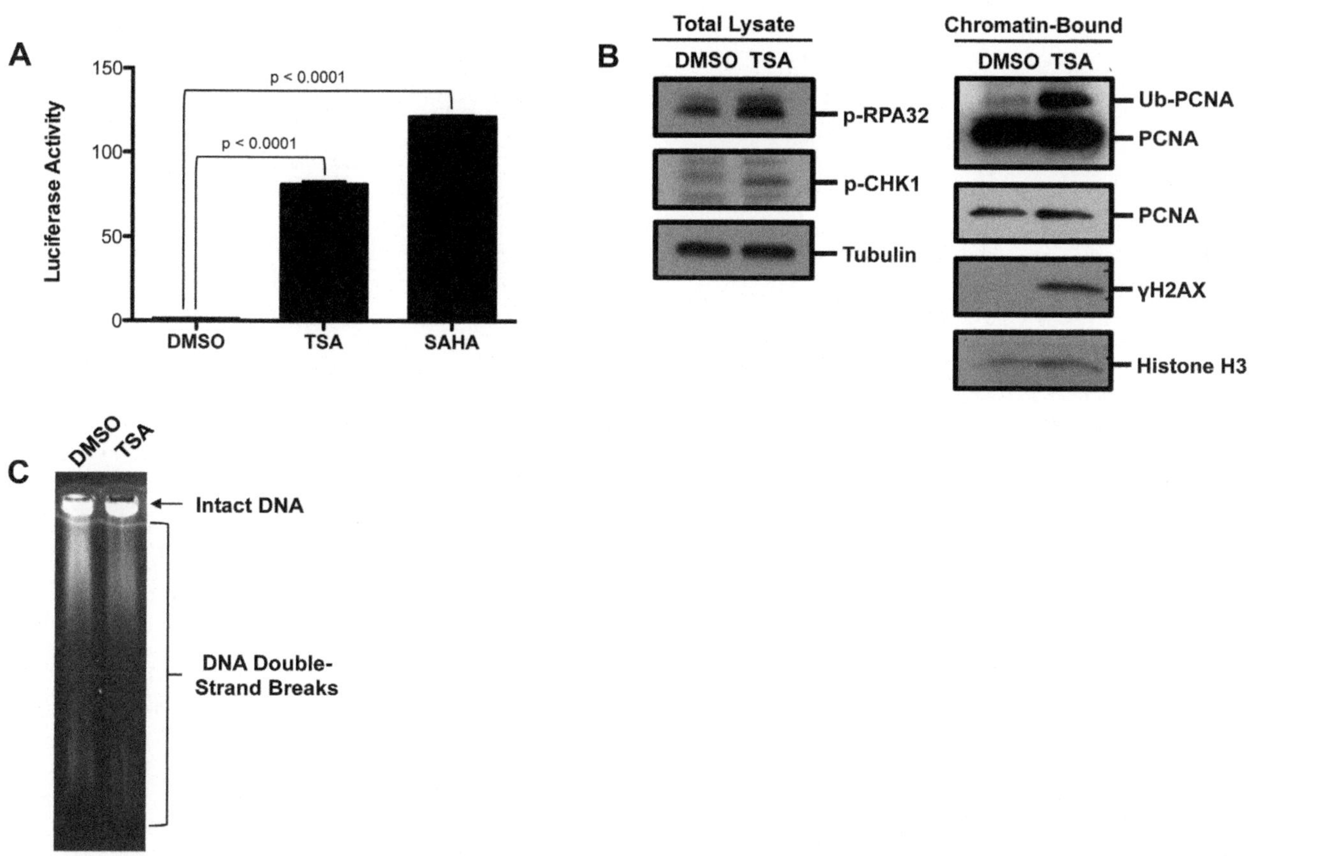

Figure 1. Trichostatin A induces DNA damage. (A) HEK293T ELG1-LUC cells were treated with 0.75 μM TSA or 50 μM SAHA for 48 hr. LUC activity was measured using One-Glo. The graph represents average LUC activity ± SD. Significance was calculated using a two-tailed t-test. (B) HEK293T cells were treated with 50 μM TSA for 24 hr. Using the indicated antibodies proteins levels were visualized by Western blot analysis from either the chromatin-bound fraction or total cell lysate. (C) HEK293T cells were treated with 100 uM TSA for 24 hours and then Pulsed-field gel electrophoresis was performed.

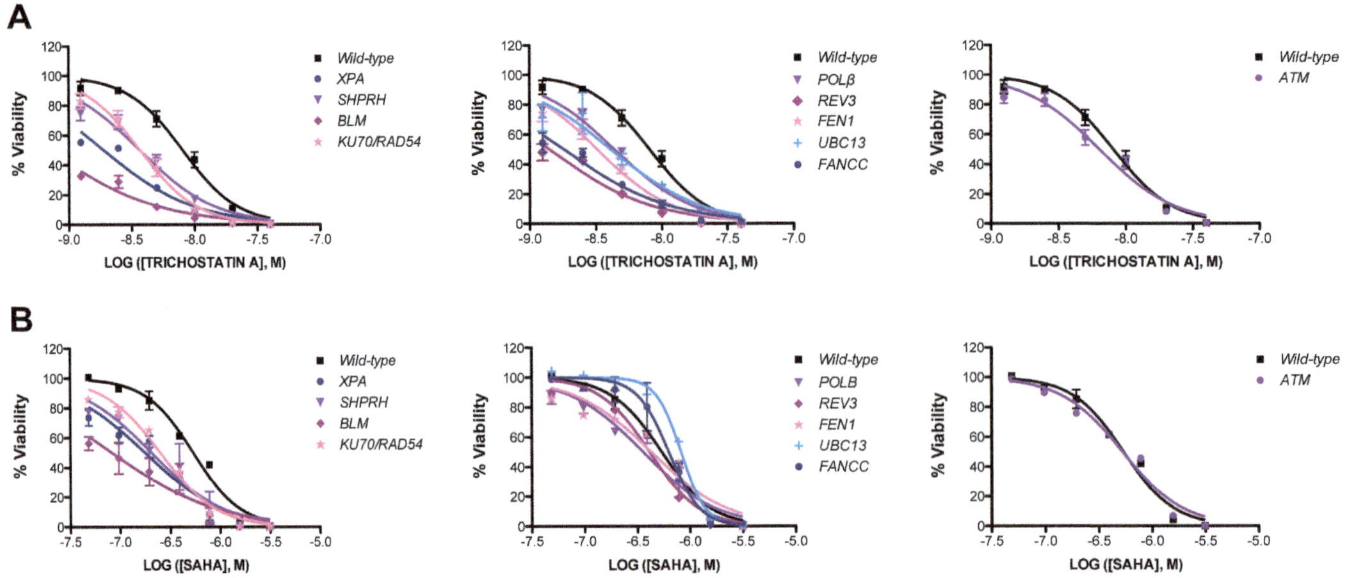

Figure 2. Viability of isogenic chicken DT40 B lymphocyte cell lines following 48 hr treatment with (A) 0 to 0.04 μM TSA and (B) 0 to 3.125 μM SAHA. Viability was determined using CellTiter-Glo. The data represent the average of 3 independent experiments ± SD.

53BP1 and p-53BP1 is a good marker for NHEJ initiation and suppression of HDR. Human RPE cells were treated with TSA, SAHA, DMSO as a negative control or hydroxyurea (HU) as a positive control and the formation of p-53BP1 foci was monitored by fluorescence microscopy. After a 1-hr treatment, there was no difference in the number of p-53BP1 foci per cell in cells treated with TSA, SAHA or DMSO (Figures 4a and b). Even after a 24-hr treatment, we did not observe any difference in p-53BP1 foci in TSA- or SAHA-treated cells compared to DMSO (data not shown). In contrast, the majority of HU-treated cells had more than 20 p-53BP1 foci (Figures 4a and b). We also used a HeLa cell-based assay to measure the frequency of NHEJ with a dedicated GFP reporter that cannot repair I-SceI DSBs by HDR (Figure 4c). IHN20.22 cells contain a single copy of a GFP cassette under the control of a CMV promoter that has been disrupted by an internal adenoviral exon. Flanking the adenoviral exon are twin I-SceI sites placed in an inverted orientation. Digestion with I-SceI results in incompatible ends that must be repaired by NHEJ [39]. These cells also have one stable copy of a cassette that encodes for doxycycline-induced I-SceI expression. Using this assay we found NHEJ to be significantly increased in cells treated with higher concentrations of TSA or SAHA compared to non-treated cells (Figures 4d and e and Figure S2a). We performed an additional NHEJ assay using the U2OS cell line EJ2-GFP [40]. Unlike the previous NHEJ assay, digestion with I-SceI in this cell line generates compatible ends that are repaired by NHEJ. Using this assay, we found that treatment with 100 nM TSA increased NHEJ frequency although not at a statistically significant level (Figure S2b). Reduction of 53BP1 by siRNA did not increase end joining of compatible ends (Figure S2c and d). Finally, we note that SAHA treated IHN20.22 cells in the absence of I-SceI cleavages (no Dox treatment) display rather large increases in NHEJ frequency as determined by increases in the percentage of GFP positive cells (Figure S2e). From this result we infer that HDACi induced DNA damage involves the generation of DSBs that are sensed and acted upon by the NHEJ pathway. Based on independent and complementary approaches, we conclude that HDACi treatment increased the frequency of NHEJ at the DSB sites; however, we did not observe enhanced 53BP1 recruitment to chromatin as noted (Figures 4a and b). The recruitment of p-53BP1 into sites of DNA damage, in particular at DSBs, involves histone H4 acetylation [41] and others have shown that HDACi treatment can suppress 53PB1 focus formation [42].

Differences between avian and human cells could account for our inability to detect an increase in HDR frequency; therefore, we analyzed viability profiles in mammalian cell models. Logistically, this is difficult since many of the comparable human cell lines are not available. Nonetheless, to determine if human cells defective in NHEJ were sensitive to HDACi, we knocked down *KU80* expression in HeLa cells with siRNA, and then treated the cells with increasing concentrations of TSA, SAHA or, as a positive control, MMS for 48 hr. Whereas *KU86*-knockdown cells exhibited a reduced viability after treatment with MMS compared to control knockdown cells ($p = 0.03$ for EC50s), there was no difference in viability between control and *KU80*-knockdown cells after treatment with TSA or SAHA even though we achieved an almost complete reduction in KU80 protein level (Figure 5a and Figure S1d). In addition, we treated *LIG4*-null HCT116 cells, which are severely defective in NHEJ [43,44], with increasing concentrations of TSA, SAHA or MMS and monitored viability. *LIG4*-null cells are sensitive to a wide range of DNA damaging agents [44] and they were therefore slightly more sensitive to MMS treatment compared to wild type although not at a statistically significant level (Figure 5b). However, we did not observe any reduction in viability of *LIG4*-null cells compared to HCT116 after treatment with either TSA or SAHA (Figure 5b). TSA can therefore enhance NHEJ frequency at DSBs, but NHEJ is dispensable for cell survival after TSA-induced DNA damage. Likewise, HCC1937 cells, which lack a functional *BRCA1* gene and are therefore defective in HDR [45], were treated with TSA, SAHA or MMS and viability was assessed after 48 hr. Compared to the control cells that were complemented by *BRCA1* cDNA expression (wild-type), *BRCA1* deficient HCC1937 cells exhibited sensitivity to TSA and SAHA that was similar to that of MMS (Figure 6a). To determine if HDR is indeed necessary to repair HDACi induced damage, we knocked down *RAD51* expression

Table 1. Cell lines used in this study.

Cell Type	Mutation/Name	Pathway or Description	Origin
Chicken DT40	Wild-type		Evans *et al.* 2010
Chicken DT40	*XPA*	Nucleotide Excision Repair	Evans *et al.* 2010
Chicken DT40	*SHPRH*	DNA Post-replication Repair	This study
Chicken DT40	*BLM*	DNA Replication and Repair	Evans *et al.* 2010
Chicken DT40	*FANCC*	Interstrand crosslink Repair	Evans *et al.* 2010
Chicken DT40	*KU70/RAD54*	Non-homologous End Joining/Homologous Recombination	Evans *et al.* 2010
Chicken DT40	*POLβ*	Base Excision Repair	Evans *et al.* 2010
Chicken DT40	*REV3*	Translesion DNA Synthesis	Evans *et al.* 2010
Chicken DT40	*FEN1*	Base Excision Repair, Nucleotide Excision Repair, DNA Replication	Evans *et al.* 2010
Chicken DT40	*UBC13*	DNA Post-replication Repair	Evans *et al.* 2010
Chicken DT40	*ATM*	Cell Cycle Checkpoint	Evans *et al.* 2010
Human Lymphoblast	Wild-type		Candotti *et al.* 1997
Human Lymphoblast	*BLM*	DNA Replication and Repair	Coriell
Human Lymphoblast	*XPA*	Nucleotide Excision Repair	Coriell
Mouse Embryonic Fibroblast	Wild-type		Krijger *et al.* 2011
Mouse Embryonic Fibroblast	*SHPRH*	DNA Post-replication Repair	Krijger *et al.* 2011
Human Embryonic Kidney	HEK293T		ATCC
Human Embryonic Kidney	HEK293T ELG1-LUC		Fox *et al.* 2012
Human Cervical Adenocarcinoma	HeLa		ATCC
Human Cervical Adenocarcinoma	HeLa IHN20.22	Non-homologous End Joining Assay Cell Line	This study
Human Cervical Adenocarcinoma	HeLa IHN20.41	Non-homologous End Joining Assay Cell Line	This study
Human Cervical Adenocarcinoma	HeLa iHO4.5GFP	Homologous Recombination Assay Cell Line	This study
Human Colorectal Cancer	HCT116		ATCC
Human Colorectal Cancer	HCT116 *FANCM*	Interstrand Crosslink Repair	Wang *et al.* 2013
Human Colorectal Cancer	HCT116 *LIG4*	Non-homologous End Joining	Fattah *et al.* 2010 Oh *et al.* 2013
Human Ductal Carcinoma	*BRCA1* Corrected		Yu *et al.* 2006
Human Ductal Carcinoma	*BRCA1*	Homologous Recombination	Yu *et al.* 2006
Human Osteosarcoma	U2OS DR-GFP	Homologous Recombination Assay Cell Line	Xia *et al.* 2006
Human Osteosarcoma	U2OS EJ2-GFP	Alternative End Joining Assay Cell Line	Gunn *et al.* 2012
Human Retinal Pigmented Epithelium	RPE		ATCC

Table 2. EC50 values for isogenic chicken DT40 B lymphocyte cell lines following 48 hour treatment with TSA and SAHA.

	EC50	
	TSA nM	SAHA μM
Wild-type	8.1	0.54
ATM	6.4	0.53
POLβ	4.4	0.36
UBC13	4.1	0.82
KU70/RAD54	3.7	0.25
SHPRH	3.7	0.21
FEN1	3.2	0.82
XPA	1.9	0.18
FANCC	1.8	0.63
REV3	1.4	0.41
BLM	0.7	0.08

with siRNA in HeLa cells and then treated with increasing concentrations of TSA, SAHA or MMS and measured viability after 24 hours. Compared to the control knockdown cells, cells with a reduced expression of *RAD51* were more sensitive to both TSA and SAHA (Figure 6b and Figure S1e). RAD51 protein levels were only reduced by one-third, compared to control knockdown cells, which may have resulted in a decreased sensitivity to TSA and SAHA. Although we did not observe the large reduction in viability that was seen in DT40 cells, the sensitivity of *BRCA1*-deficient cells and *RAD51* deficient cells to HDACi and MMS is mutually consistent with the notion that HDR is required to repair HDACi-induced damage.

Because the results of our experiments with *KU70/RAD54*-null avian cells were also slightly different from what we observed using mammalian cell lines, we repeated viability assays using mammalian cell lines lacking *XPA*, *BLM*, *SHPRH*, *or FANCM* [46]. We chose to test these cell lines because the *XPA*-, *BLM*- *SHPRH*- and *FANCC*-null avian cells were some of the most sensitive to either TSA, SAHA or both. After a 48-hr treatment, *XPA*- and *BLM*-mutant human lymphocytes displayed a mild sensitivity to TSA (Figures 7a and b). EC50 values for *XPA*- and *BLM*-mutants were

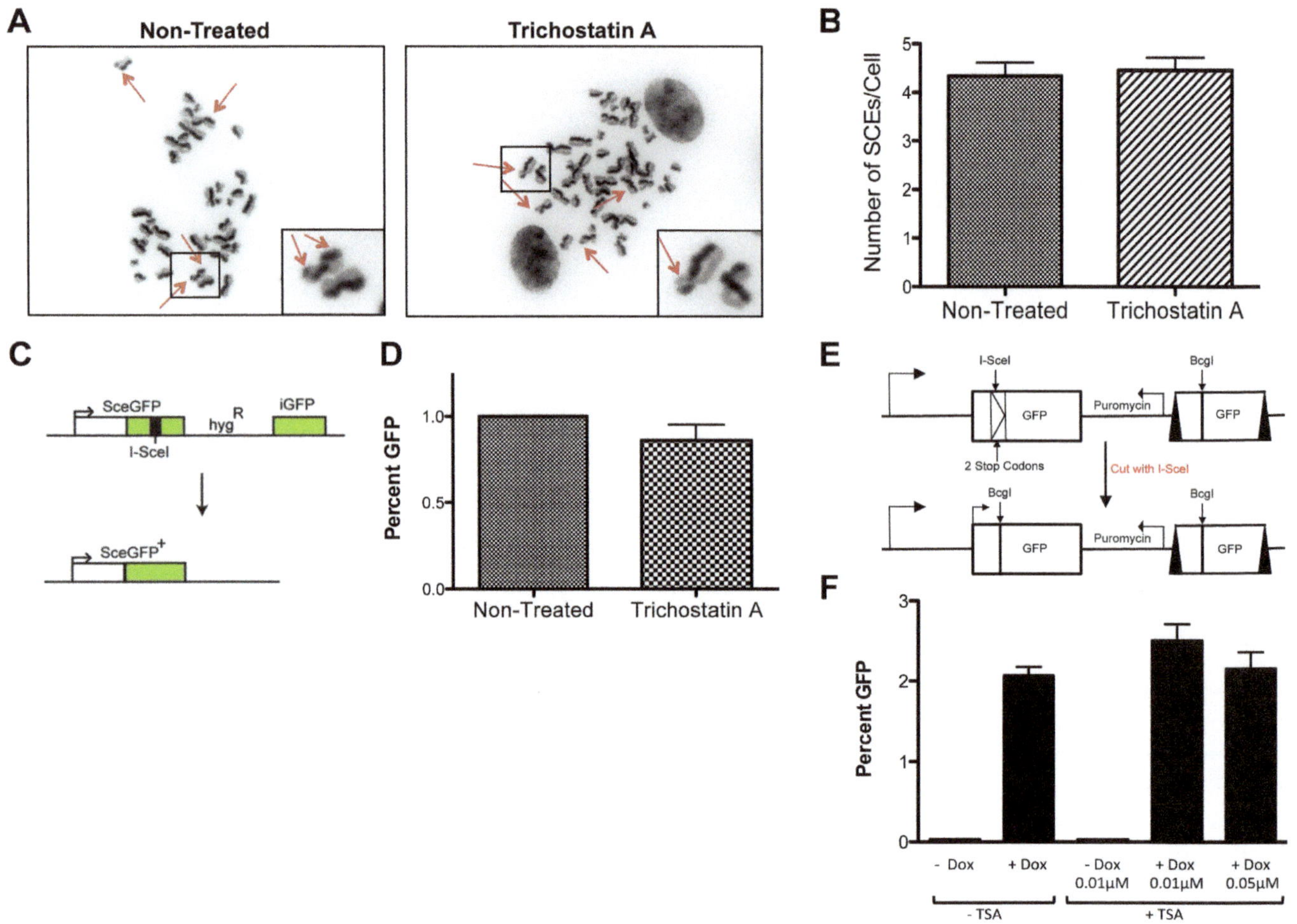

Figure 3. The effect of HDACis on SCE and HR Frequency. (A) RPE cells were treated with 0.2 μM TSA for 48 hr. Representative images of metaphase spreads with arrows indicating SCEs (Magnification: 100×). (Inset) Magnification of the boxed region. (B) The graph represents the average number of SCEs per cell ± SD following treatment. Non-significance was determined using a two-tailed t-test. (C) Schematic of DR-GFP HR frequency assay. (D) U2OS DR-GFP cells were transfected with pCGA-I-SCEI and then treated with 0.25 μM TSA for 48 hr. The graph represents the average HR frequency ± SD following treatment determined by FACS analysis. Non-significance was determined using a two-tailed t-test. (E) Schematic of twin reporter DR-GFP HR assay. (F) HeLa iHO4.5GFP cells were pulsed for 24 hr with Dox, washed and chased in the presence of the indicated amounts of TSA. The percentage of GFP-positive cells was determined by FACS analysis. The graph represents the average percent GFP ± SD. The difference between +Dox/−TSA and +Dox/+TSA not significant and was determined using a two-tailed t-test.

significantly different than wild-type ($p = 0.009$ and $p = 0.02$, respectively). Although the EC50 values for SAHA treated *XPA*- and *BLM*-mutants were not significantly different, there was a clear sensitivity of the mutants at lower survival percentages (Figures 7a and b). *XPA*- and *BLM*-mutants were both more sensitive to MMS compared to wild-type (Figure S1b). This result was similar to that observed in *BRCA1*-deficient cells (Figure 6a) with the sensitivity differences between wild-type and mutant reduced compared to what was observed in DT40 cells. *SHPRH*-null MEFs did not show any sensitivity to either TSA or SAHA when compared to wild-type MEFs (Figure 7c) and likewise, we did not observe any difference in viability between *FANCM*-deficient HCT116 cells compared to the control (Figure 7d) following treatment with TSA or SAHA. As expected *FANCM*-null cells were highly sensitive to treatment with MMS (Figure S1c). We concluded that there are slight differences in the sensitivity of avian and mammalian cells to HDACi therapeutics, but reaction to HDACi treatment also varies widely between human tumors [47] and the differences we observed might not be species specific. Collectively, however, our data also indicate that TSA and SAHA can be used to enhance the killing of cancer cells defective in specific DNA repair pathways including those dependent on BRCA1 or Rad51 (HDR), XPA (NER), or BLM.

The fact that NHEJ repair events are significantly enhanced by HDACi strategies suggests that an error prone pathway of break repair may contribute to toxicity by this class of drugs. In fact, it has been shown that high doses of TSA induce aneuploidy in lymphoblasts [48]. In marked contrast, the HDR pathway may reconcile HDACi induced genotoxicity and provide a mechanism that promotes survival of those cells that have this pathway intact. The potential for HDACi drugs to target cells with HDR defects and stimulate NHEJ events is significant. Our findings predict that combining epigenetic drugs with traditional genotoxic therapies represents a rational strategy to target cancer cells, which frequently display HDR repair defects. In addition, activation of NHEJ, which is a prominent, error prone path in human cells, also contributes to the cytotoxic activity of HDACi in cancer cells. Future studies will be required to fully understand the contribution of NHEJ and HDR in directing tumor cell death by epigenetic agents; however, we have powerful genetic and cell based

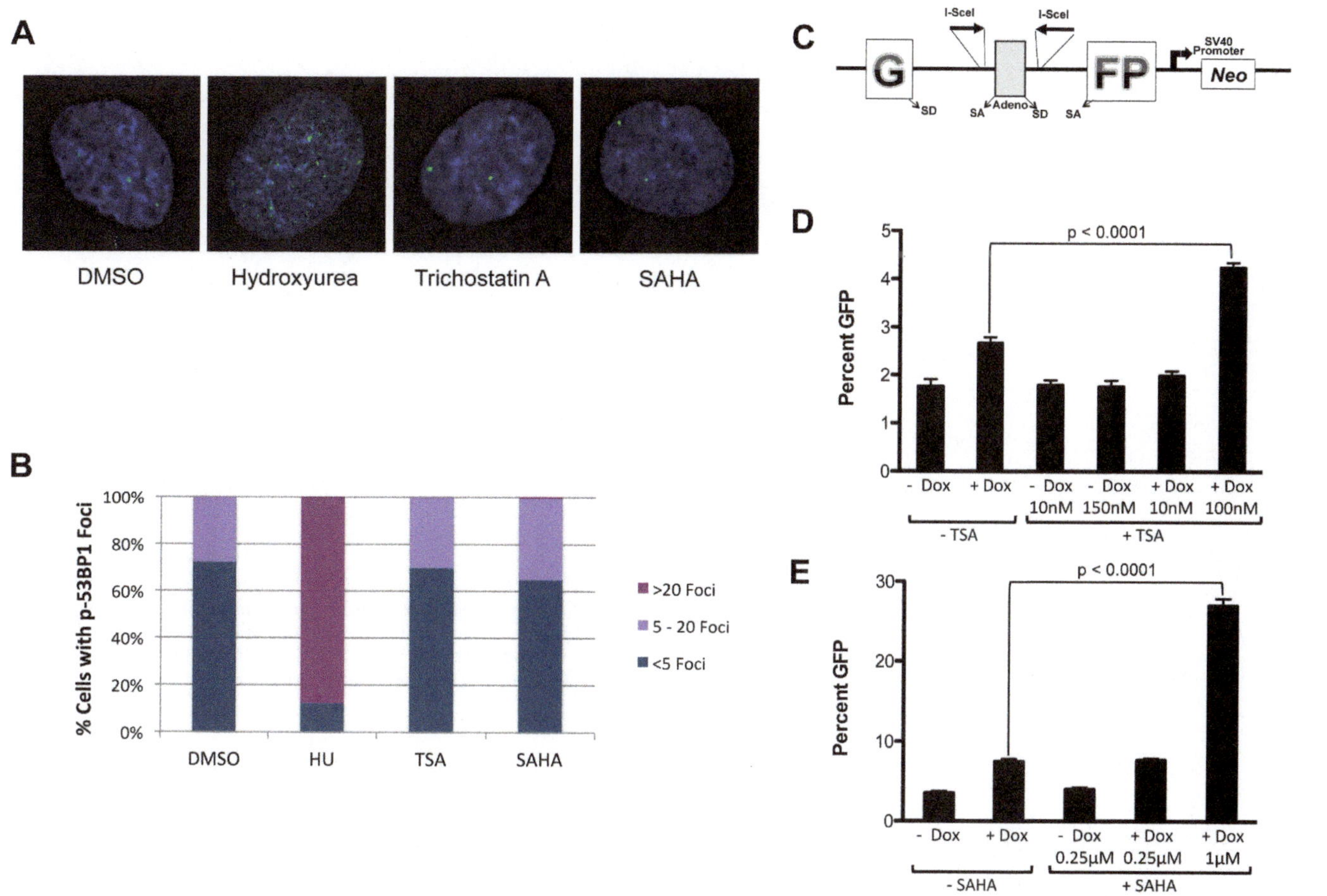

Figure 4. The effect of HDACi on NHEJ. (A) Representative images of RPE nuclei (blue) with p-53BP1 foci (green) after a 24 hr treatment with 2 mM HU or 1 hr treatment with either 0.5 μM TSA or 32 μM SAHA. (B) The percentage of RPE cells containing the indicated number of p-53BP1 foci following treatment as described in A was determined from at least 145 cells per treatment. (C) Schematic of NHEJ assay. HeLa IHN20.22 cells were pulsed for 24 hr with Dox, washed and chased in the presence of the indicated amounts of TSA (D) or SAHA (E) for 3 days. The graphs represent the average percent GFP ± SD. Significance between +Dox/−TSA or SAHA and +Dox/+TSA or SAHA was calculated using a two-tailed t-test. The percentage of GFP-positive cells was determined by FACS analysis.

reporting tools to enhance our understanding of each repair pathway.

Materials and Methods

Chicken *RAD5* (human SHPRH homolog) Cloning and Gene Targeting Vectors

Two *RAD5* disruption constructs, RAD5-puro and RAD-bsr, were generated from genomic PCR products combined with puromycin and blasticidin selection marker cassettes. Genomic DNA sequences were amplified using SalI primer 5′-TATAA-GTCGA- CAGGTTGGAATCTACCTTCTGGAAGCAGG-3′ and BamHI primer 5′-TATAAGGATCCTAGA- TTTTCAC-TCCATCCAGAGTAATGACC-3′ (for the left arm of the KO construct); and NotI primer 5′-TATAAGCGGCCGCTTTGC-TACAACACTTATTTGTTGCAACAGG-3′ and BamHI primer 5′-TATAAGGATCCGAAATAGACGGCTTCTCAAAAGAA-CGCTGG3′ (for the right arm primer of the KO construct). Amplified PCR products were cloned into pBluescript II K. The BamHI site was used to clone marker gene cassettes. 0.4 kb of fragment from the genomic DNA amplified using the primers 5′-CAAAAAGATGACAGTCGTTCAAATCTAAATC- TGGG-3′ and 5′-CTTTAGAGCTTGACCCTCTCCAGG-3′ was used as a probe for Southern blot analysis.

Human *FANCM* and *LIGIV* Targeting

The mutants were generated in the HCT116 cell background. The construction and phenotypes of *LIGIV*-null cells [43,44] and *FANCM*-null cells [46] have been described.

Cell Culture

Isogenic DT40 cell lines [30], each defective in a different DNA repair pathway (Table 1), were cultured in RPMI (Life Technologies) supplemented with 10% fetal bovine serum (FBS, Hyclone), 1% chicken serum (Life Technologies), 50 μM 2-mercaptoethanol (Sigma), 1 mM L-glutamine (Life Technologies) and 1% penicillin-streptomycin (Life Technologies). *BLM*- and *XPA*-defective lymphocytes (Coriell) were cultured in RPMI supplemented with 15% FBS and 2 mM L-glutamine. Wild-type human lymphocytes [49] were cultured in RPMI supplemented with 10% FBS, 1 mM L-glutamine, 1 mM sodium pyruvate (Life Technologies), 1% non-essential amino acids (Life Technologies), 50 μM 2-mercaptoethanol and 50 μg/ml gentamycin sulfate (Life Technologies). Wild-type and *SHPRH* mouse embryonic fibroblasts (MEFs) [50], RPE (ATCC), HEK293T (human embryonic kidney) (ATCC), HeLa

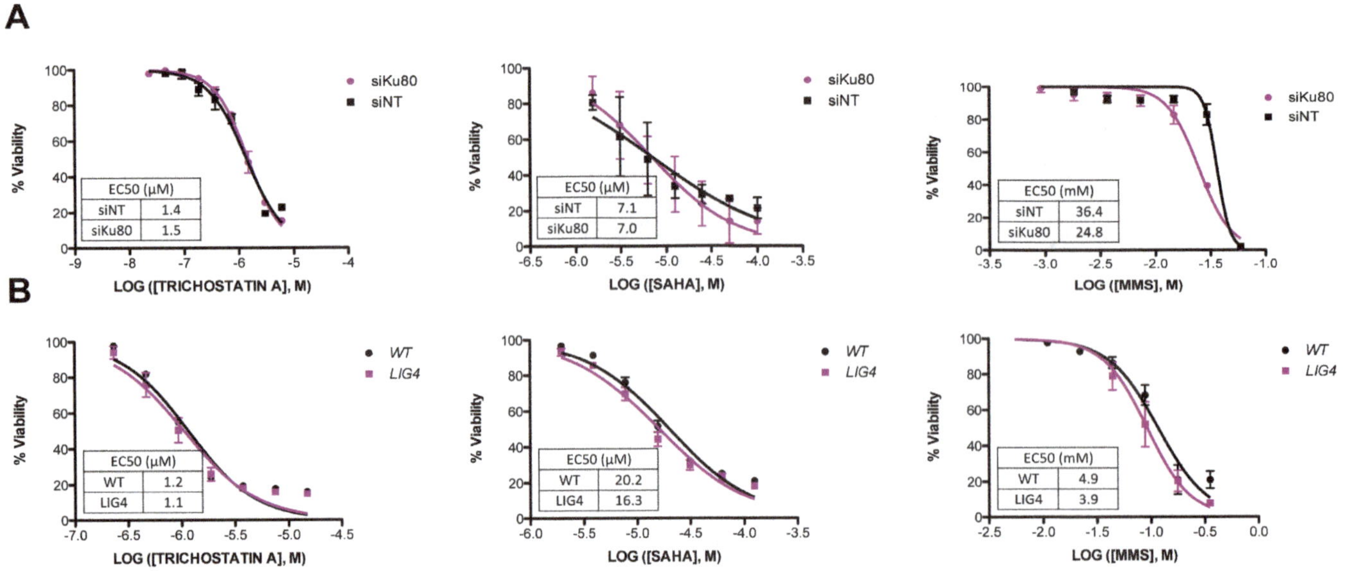

Figure 5. Viability of NHEJ deficient cells after treatment with HDACis. The indicated cells were treated for 48 hr with 0 to 1.5 μM TSA, 0 to 100 μM SAHA or 0 to 118 mM MMS. Viability was determined using CellTiter-Glo. The data represent the average of 3 independent experiments ± SD. (A) Hela cells after 24 hr transfection with either non-targeting siRNA or siRNA against *KU80*. (B) HCT116 *LIG4*-null or wild-type HCT116 cells. (C) HCC1937 cells, lacking a functional *BRCA1* gene, or HC1937 cells complimented by *BRCA1* cDNA expression (wild-type).

(human cervical adenocarcinoma) (ATCC), HCT116 (human colorectal cancer cell) (ATCC), U2OS EJ2-GFP [40], isogenic HCT116 *FANCM*- [43,46] and *LIG4*- [43,44] null cells, HCC1937 cells complimented with a *BRCA1* cDNA and HCC1937 [45] were cultured in DMEM with Glutamax (Life Technologies) supplemented with 10% FBS and 1% penicillin- streptomycin. U2OS DR-GFP [34,51] cells were cultured in McCoys modified 5A (Life Technologies) supplemented with 10% FBS, 2 mM L-glutamine and 1% penicillin-streptomycin. All cell lines were maintained in a humidified environment of 5% CO_2 and 95% air at 37°C.

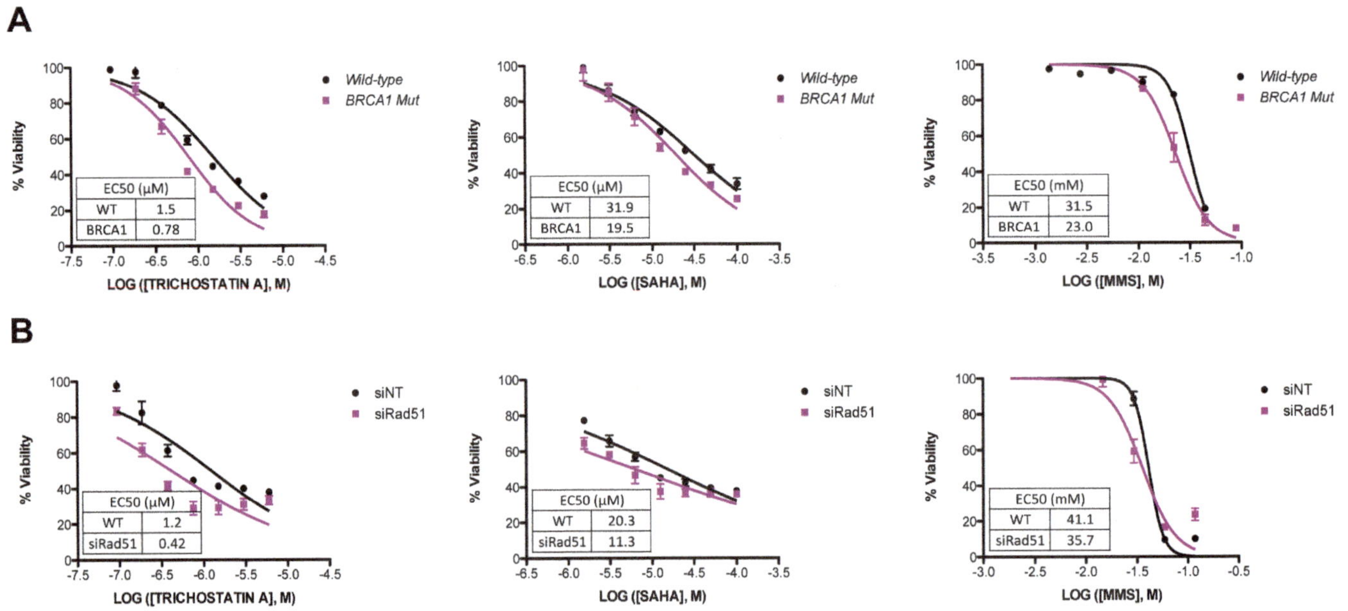

Figure 6. Viability of HDR deficient cells after treatment with HDACis. The indicated cells were treated for 48 hr with 0 to 1.5 μM TSA, 0 to 100 μM SAHA or 0 to 118 mM MMS. Viability was determined using CellTiter-Glo. The data represent the average of 3 independent experiments ± SD. (A) HCC1937 cells, lacking a functional *BRCA1* gene, or HC1937 cells complimented by *BRCA1* cDNA expression (wild-type). EC50 differences between wild-type and *BRCA1* after treatment with TSA and SAHA were significant at $p = 0.0009$ and $p = 0.02$ respectively. EC50 differences between wild-type and *BRCA1* after MMS treatment were not significant $p = 0.07$. (B) Hela cells after 2×24 hr transfection with either non-targeting siRNA or siRNA against *RAD51*. EC50 differences between siNT and siRAD51 after treatment with TSA and SAHA were significant at $p < 0.0001$ and $p = 0.03$ respectively. EC50 differences between siNT and siRAD51 after MMS treatment were not significant $p = 0.07$.

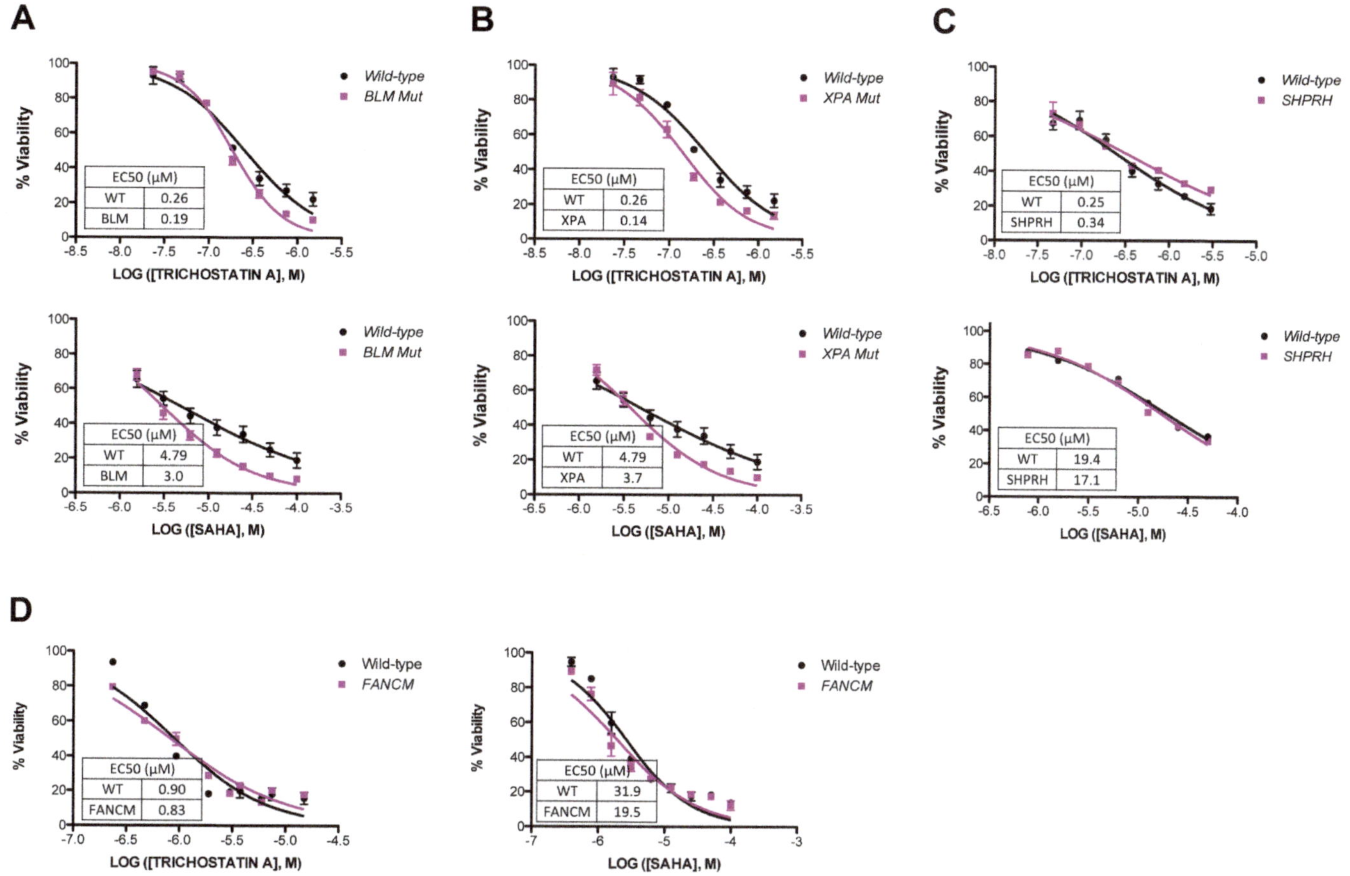

Figure 7. Effect of HDACi on the viability of mammalian cell lines. (A) *BLM* and (B) *XPA* human lymphocytes were treated with 0 to 1.5 μM TSA or 0 to 100 μM SAHA for 48 hours. (C) *SHPRH* MEFs were treated with 0 to 1.5 μM TSA or 0 to 100 μM SAHA for 48 hours. (D) *FANCM* human colorectal cancer cells were treated with 0 to 1.5 μM TSA or 0 to 100 μM SAHA for 48 hr. Viability was determined using CellTiter-Glo. The data represent the average of 3 independent experiments ± SD.

Luciferase Assay

HEK293T ELG1-LUC cells [25] were plated at a density of 10,000 cells per well in a 96-well white, assay plate (Costar). 24 hr after seeding, cells were treated with 0.75 μM TSA or 50 μM SAHA and then incubated for an additional 48 hr. Either One-Glo luciferase reagent (Promega) to quantify luciferase activity or Cell-Titre Glo to quantify cell viability was added to each well. Luminescence intensity was measured using a Fluoroskan Ascent Luminometer (Thermo Scientific). Luciferase levels were normalized to cell viability.

Protein Analysis

HEK293T cells were grown in 10-cm tissue-culture plates to ~90% confluence and treated with 0.75 μM TSA, or DMSO (negative control) for 24 hr. To obtain total lysate, the cells were resuspended in lysis buffer [50 mM Tris, pH 7.5, 150 mM NaCl, 1% Nonidet P-40, 5 mM EDTA, protease inhibitors (Roche)] and lysed on ice for 30 min. Chromatin-bound fractions were isolated as described [52]. Proteins in the total lysate or the chromatin-bound fraction were separated by SDS-PAGE using a 4–15% tris-glycine gel (Bio-Rad) and transferred to a polyvinylidene difluoride membrane. Proteins in the membrane were detected by the ECL Western Blotting Detection System (GE Healthcare). HRP-conjugated anti-PCNA was purchased from Santa Cruz Biotechnology. Rabbit antiphospho-RPA32 (S4/S8), and rabbit antiphospho-CHK1 (S317) antibodies were purchased from Bethyl Laboratories. HRP-conjugated anti–β-tubulin antibody was purchased from Abcam. Rabbit antihistone H3 antibody was purchased from Upstate. Mouse antiphospho-histone H2AX (S140, 3F2) antibody was purchased from GeneTex.

Pulsed-Field Gel Electrophoresis

HEK293T cells were treated with 100 uM TSA for 24 hours and then Pulsed-field gel electrophoresis was performed as described [25].

siRNA Knockdown of *KU80* or *RAD51*

HeLa cells were transfected once with ON-TARGETplus NON-targeting siRNA or siRNA targeting *KU80* (Dharmacon) or twice with siRNA targeting *RAD51* (Dharmacon) using Lipofectamine RNAi Max (Life Technologies). 24 hr post-transfection, cells were treated with TSA (final concentration = 0 μM to 0.04 μM, Sigma) or SAHA (final concentration = 0 μM to 3.125 μM, Cayman Chemical Company). 48 hr following treatment, cell viability was determined using Cell Titer-Glo (Promega) according to the manufacturer's protocol. Viability was quantified on a Fluoroskan Ascent Luminometer (Thermo Scientific). Dose-response curves were generated using GraphPad Prism. Protein levels were visualized using antibodies against KU80 or RAD51 using whole cell extract prepared 72 hr after transfection.

Viability Assays

All cells were cultured in 96-well white, assay plates (Costar). DT40 cells were plated at a density of 1,000 cells per well. TSA (final concentration = 0 μM to 0.04 μM, Sigma) or SAHA (final concentration = 0 μM to 3.125 μM, Cayman Chemical Company) were added immediately after plating and cells were treated for 48 hr. Human lymphoblasts were plated at a density of 20,000 cells per well. TSA (final concentration = 0 μM to 1.5 μM) or SAHA (final concentration = 0 μM to 100 μM) were added immediately after plating and cells were treated for 48 hr. MEFs and fibroblasts were plated at a density of 5,000 cells per well. TSA (final concentration = 0 μM to 1.5 μM) or SAHA (final concentration = 0 μM to 100 μM) were added 24 hr after plating and cells were treated for 48 hr. Following treatment, cell viability was determined using Cell Titer-Glo (Promega) according to the manufacturer's protocol. Viability was quantified on a Fluoroskan Ascent Luminometer (Thermo Scientific). Dose-response curves were generated using GraphPad Prism.

Sister Chromatid Exchange (SCE) Assay

SCE was carried out as described [25]. Briefly, RPE cells were treated with 0.2 μM TSA for 48 hr. Cells were washed with PBS and then cultured in the presence 5 μg/ml BrdU for an additional 48 hours. Colcemid (0.05 μg) was added 3 hr prior to preparation of metaphase spreads. Metaphase spreads on slides were prepared by standard hypotonic treatment and fixation with methanol and glacial acetic acid and incubated at 45°C for 18 hr before staining with 2 mg/ml Hoechst 33258 in 2x SSC solution. The slides, mounted with Sorensen's phosphate buffer pH 7.0, were then treated by UV light for 30 min and subsequently incubated at 65°C for 1 hr in 2x SSC. Chromosomes on slides were stained with 4% Giemsa in Sorenson's buffer pH 6.8 for 30 min and monitored under microscope. Images of 50 metaphase spreads for each cell line were captured from 2 independent experiments.

Immunofluorescence and Microscopy

5×10^4 RPE cells were plated in each well of a 4-well chamber slide (Nunc). 24 hr after plating, cells were treated for an additional 24 hr with 2 mM HU or 1 hr with either 0.5 μM TSA or 32 μM SAHA. Following treatment, slides were washed with PBS then fixed with 4% paraformaldehyde/0.2% Triton X-100 in PBS for 20 min. After a brief wash with PBS, slides were permeabilized with 0.5% NP40 in PBS for 10 min and then washed with 0.5% BSA/0.175% Tween-20 in PBS. Slides were blocked for 1 hr in 1% donkey serum/2% BSA in PBS and then incubated in rabbit antiphospho-53BP1-Ser1778 (Cell Signaling) diluted 1:1000 in 3% BSA in PBS for 2 hr. After extensive washes with 0.5% BSA/0.175% Tween-20 in PBS, slides were incubated for 1 hr in Alexa-Fluor 488-conjugated goat anti-rabbit IgG secondary antibody (Invitrogen) diluted 1:250 in 3% BSA in PBS. Following washes in 0.5% BSA/0.175% Tween-20 in PBS, slides were mounted with ProLong Gold Antifade Reagent with DAPI (Life Technologies). Wide-field images were collected using a Personal DeltaVision system (Applied Precision Inc., Issaquah, WA, USA) mounted on an inverted Olympus IX71 microscope with an oil immersion UPlanSApo 100×/1.40 objective lens. All images were acquired using a CoolSNAP ES2 camera with 1×1 binning. Excitation filters 390/18 and 490/20 with corresponding emission filters 435/48 and 528/38 were used to collect the DAPI and Alexa-Fluor 488. All images were collected using the same settings and all were deconvolved using an iterative constrained method with 10 cycles, medium noise filtering in SoftWoRx version 4.0.0. At least 145 cells were imaged from each treatment.

Recombination Reporter Assays

A U2OS cell line stably transfected with a single copy of an intact DR-GFP reporter gene (gift from Dr. M. Jasin at the Memorial Sloan-Kettering Institute) was used to measure the HDR frequency [34,51]. A single DSB was introduced by expressing the I-SceI endonuclease. Cells were treated with 0.25 μM TSA at 24 hr after transfection. After a 48 hr treatment, cells were analyzed on a BDFACSCalibur with a 15 mW 488 nm argon laser. GFP emission was detected with a 530/30 band-pass filter and DsRed was detected with a 670LP filter. Data was analyzed using FlowJo. The HDR frequency was determined by the number of cells expressing GFP divided by the number of cells expressing DsRed (as an indicator for transfection). Experiments were repeated at least 3 times, and the average values are reported.

The Hela cell line iHO4.5GFP was used to measure the HDR frequency. This cell line contains the DR-GFP reporter twin cassettes (GFP-I, GFP-II) that are mutated and GFP minus. Adjacent to the Cassette I, a unique I-SceI site was engineered and the I-SceI gene introduced and placed under control of the Tet-on promoter. Cells were either continuously exposed to doxycycline (Dox) for 7 days, (new Dox added each day with medium change) or pulsed with Dox for 24 hr and then washed and chased in Dox-free medium for 7 days. HDR frequency was measured by FACS analysis and reported as the percentage of GFP cells. The percent GFP readout reveals the HDR frequency, based on Q-PCR analyses, as shown previously [23].

Non-Homologous End Joining Reporter Assays

Two different clones of NHEJ reporter cells were constructed and tested (IHN20.22 and IHN20.41 with similar results using other clones, not shown). The NHEJ based reporter is based on the construct from Mao et al. [39] and consists of a single GFP cassette disrupted by an internal adenoviral exon and a Neomycin selectable marker. The cassette also includes the CMV promoter; however, due to the exon insertion, the cells are GFP minus. Flanking the adenoviral exon are twin I-Sce1 sites that were placed in an inverted orientation. Digestion with the homing endonuclease I-Sce1, creates a DS DNA break with incompatible ends, which are repaired by NHEJ. To create an inducible I-SceI system, a stably transfected HeLa cell lines were made containing a single integrated copy of the NHEJ (GFP) cassette. The construct was validated by sequencing and qPCR to confirm copy number. Two lentiviruses (pLV-TetO-HA-Sce1 and rtTA) were used to co-infect this stable line. A number of clones were screened to identify a single copy GFP cassette line that was induced by doxycycline addition in a Tet-on format and two clones were selected for this study. Following induction of I-SceI by addition of doxycycline, DS DNA breaks are produced that flank the adenoviral exon. The breaks can only be repaired by the NHEJ pathway (not HDR) and in some repair products WT GFP is produced [53,54]. The percent GFP was determined by FACS analysis as previously described [22,23]. For this analysis, 2×10^5 IHN20.22 or IHN20.41 cells were plated in 35 mm dishes, plus or minus Dox (or DMSO negative controls). Cells were pulsed with 0.5 ug Doxycycline/mL for 24 hours to induce a detectable and synchronous wave of NHEJ repair. At this time, TSA at the indicated concentrations was added and the GFP measured as a time course over 3 days by FACS analysis. Induction of I-SceI gene expression was not affected by HDACi treatment, using this approach. NHEJ was also analyzed using a complementary approach with a U2OS cell line carrying an End Joining (EJ-5) reporter in genome [40]. To measure NHEJ, 1×10^5 U2OS EJ2-GFP cells were plated in each well of a 6-well plate, and transfected the next day with 3 μg of I-SceI expression vector (pCGA-I-SCE) and 10 μl of Lipofectamine LTX (Life Technologies) in culture medium without antibiotics. 24 hr after transfection, cells were treated with either DMSO as a negative control, or with 100 nM TSA. NHEJ frequencies were measured by FACS analysis (48 hr post-treatment) to reveal the total percent GFP. siRNA knockdown was performed one time 24 hours prior to transfection of I-SceI with ON-TARGETplus NON-targeting siRNA, siRNA targeting *KU80* (Dharmacon) or siRNA targeting *53BP1* (Dharmacon) using Lipofectamine RNAi Max (Life Technologies). Protein levels were visualized using antibodies against KU80 or 53BP1 using whole cell extract prepared 72 hr after transfection.

Statistical Analyses

The Graphpad Prism 5 (Graphpad Prism®) software package was used to perform statistical analyses.

Densitometry Analyses

AlphaView SA (Cell Biosciences) software was used to perform densitometry analyses.

Supporting Information

Figure S1 (A) HeLa iHO4.5GFP cells were pulsed for 24 hr with Dox, washed and then chased in the presence of the indicated amounts of SAHA. The graph represents the average percent GFP ± SD. The difference between +Dox/−SAHA and +Dox/+SAHA not significant and was determined using a two-tailed t-test. (B) *BLM* and *XPA* human lymphocytes were treated with 0 to 118 mM MMS for 48 hr. Viability was determined using CellTiter-Glo. (C) *FANCM* human colorectal cancer cells were treated with 0 to 118 mM MMS for 48 hr. Viability was determined using CellTiter-Glo. (D) 72 hr after transfection with either non-targeting siRNA or siRNA against KU86, protein levels were visualized using antibodies against KU86. Relative densitometry is shown on right. (E) 72 hr after transfection with either non-targeting siRNA or siRNA against RAD51, protein levels were visualized using antibodies against RAD51. Relative densitometry is shown on right.

Figure S2 (A) HeLa IHN20.41 cells were pulsed for 24 hr with Dox, washed and chased in the presence of the indicated amounts of SAHA for 3 days. The percentage of GFP-positive cells was determined by FACS analysis. The graph represents the average percent GFP ± SD. Significance between +Dox/−SAHA and +Dox/+SAHA was calculated using a two-tailed t-test. (B) U2OS EJ2-GFP cells were transfected with pCGA-I-SCEI and then treated with 100 nM TSA for 48 hr. The graph represents the average NHEJ frequency ± SD following treatment determined by FACS analysis. The difference between non-treated and TSA treated was not significant and was determined using a one-tailed t-test. (C) U2OS EJ2-GFP cells were transfected with non-targeting siRNA or siRNA targeting *KU80* or *53BP1*. 24 hr after knockdown, the cells were transfected with pCGA-I-SCEI and then treated 24 hr later with 100 nM TSA for 48 hr. The graph represents the average NHEJ frequency ± SD following treatment determined by FACS analysis. The difference between non-targeting and *KU80* knockdown was significant and was determined using a two-tailed t-test. The difference between non-targeting and *53BP1* knockdown was not significant and was determined using a two-tailed t-test. (D) 72 hr after transfection with either non-targeting siRNA, siRNA against Ku80 or siRNA against 53BP1, protein levels were visualized using antibodies against indicated proteins. Relative densitometry is shown on right. (E) Analysis of SAHA induced NHEJ in iHN20.22 cells. The NHEJ reporter cells were not treated with Doxycycline in order to assess direct genotoxicity and NHEJ recovery in the absence of directed DSBs at the I-Sce1 site. Cells were incubated for 24 hr. in the indicted concentrations of SAHA and percent GFP was determined by FACS ± SD.

Acknowledgments

We thank Drs. C. Austin (NCATS), M. Xia (NCATS), and R. Huang (NCATS) for initial screening; Dr. J. Chen and Dr. M. Jasin for providing cells; and members in the Myung laboratory for helpful discussions and comments on the manuscript; and K.M. especially thanks E. Cho.

Author Contributions

Conceived and designed the experiments: SS JF M. Meija M. Muller KM. Performed the experiments: SS JF M. Meija WR AS SK YC. Analyzed the data: SS JF M. Muller KM. Contributed reagents/materials/analysis tools: SS M. Meija SO YW KC LL EAH ST M. Muller KM. Wrote the paper: SS M. Muller KM.

References

1. Smith S, Sikdar N, Liaw H, Lee K, Myung K (2009) Pathways for suppressing and promoting gross chromosomal rearrangements in Saccharomyces cerevesiae. In: Witt SN, editor. Yeast as a Model for Human Disease. Kerala, India: Transworld Research Network. pp. 249–276.
2. Krejci L, Altmannova V, Spirek M, Zhao X (2012) Homologous recombination and its regulation. Nucleic Acids Research 40: 5795–5818.
3. Chapman JR, Taylor MRG, Boulton SJ (2012) Playing the End Game: DNA Double-Strand Break Repair Pathway Choice. Molecular Cell 47: 497–510.
4. Roy R, Chun J, Powell SN (2012) BRCA1 and BRCA2: different roles in a common pathway of genome protection. Nat Rev Cancer 12: 68–78.
5. Chu WK, Hickson ID (2009) RecQ helicases: multifunctional genome caretakers. Nat Rev Cancer 9: 644–654.
6. Hu Y, Raynard S, Sehorn MG, Lu X, Bussen W, et al. (2007) RECQL5/Recql5 helicase regulates homologous recombination and suppresses tumor formation via disruption of Rad51 presynaptic filaments. Genes & Development 21: 3073–3084.
7. Sommers JA, Rawtani N, Gupta R, Bugreev DV, Mazin AV, et al. (2009) FANCJ Uses Its Motor ATPase to Destabilize Protein-DNA Complexes, Unwind Triplexes, and Inhibit RAD51 Strand Exchange. Journal of Biological Chemistry 284: 7505–7517.
8. Moldovan G-L, Dejsuphong D, Petalcorin MIR, Hofmann K, Takeda S, et al. (2012) Inhibition of Homologous Recombination by the PCNA-Interacting Protein PARI. Molecular Cell 45: 75–86.
9. Barber LJ, Youds JL, Ward JD, McIlwraith MJ, O'Neil NJ, et al. (2008) RTEL1 Maintains Genomic Stability by Suppressing Homologous Recombination. Cell 135: 261–271.
10. Mathew CG (2006) Fanconi anaemia genes and susceptibility to cancer. Oncogene 25: 5875–5884.
11. Douglas P, Gupta S, Morrice N, Meek K, Lees-Miller SP (2005) DNA-PK-dependent phosphorylation of Ku70/80 is not required for non-homologous end joining. DNA Repair 4: 1006–1018.
12. Wang Y-G, Nnakwe C, Lane WS, Modesti M, Frank KM (2004) Phosphorylation and Regulation of DNA Ligase IV Stability by DNA-dependent Protein Kinase. Journal of Biological Chemistry 279: 37282–37290.
13. Yu Y, Wang W, Ding Q, Ye R, Chen D, et al. (2003) DNA-PK phosphorylation sites in XRCC4 are not required for survival after radiation or for V(D)J recombination. DNA Repair 2: 1239–1252.
14. Goodarzi AA, Yu Y, Riballo E, Douglas P, Walker SA, et al. (2006) DNA-PK autophosphorylation facilitates Artemis endonuclease activity.
15. Lieber MR (2010) The Mechanism of Double-Strand DNA Break Repair by the Nonhomologous DNA End-Joining Pathway. Annual Review of Biochemistry 79: 181–211.
16. Kasparek TR, Humphrey TC (2011) DNA double-strand break repair pathways, chromosomal rearrangements and cancer. Seminars in Cell & Developmental Biology 22: 886–897.
17. Kirchgessner C, Patil C, Evans J, Cuomo C, Fried L, et al. (1995) DNA-dependent kinase (p350) as a candidate gene for the murine SCID defect. Science 24: 1178–1183.

18. Blunt T, Finnie NJ, Taccioli GE, Smith GCM, Demengeot J, et al. (1995) Defective DNA-dependent protein kinase activity is linked to V(D)J recombination and DNA repair defects associated with the murine scid mutation. Cell 80: 813–823.
19. Peterson SR, Kurimasa A, Oshimura M, Dynan WS, Bradbury EM, et al. (1995) Loss of the catalytic subunit of the DNA-dependent protein kinase in DNA double-strand-break-repair mutant mammalian cells. Proceedings of the National Academy of Sciences 92: 3171–3174.
20. Miller RD, Hogg J, Ozaki JH, Gell D, Jackson SP, et al. (1995) Gene for the catalytic subunit of mouse DNA-dependent protein kinase maps to the scid locus. Proceedings of the National Academy of Sciences 92: 10792–10795.
21. Lee GE, Kim JH, Taylor M, Muller MT (2010) DNA Methyltransferase 1-associated Protein (DMAP1) Is a Co-repressor That Stimulates DNA Methylation Globally and Locally at Sites of Double Strand Break Repair. Journal of Biological Chemistry 285: 37630–37640.
22. Lee B, Morano A, Porcellini A, Muller MT (2012) GADD45alpha inhibition of DNMT1 dependent DNA methylation during homology directed DNA repair. Nucleic Acids Research 40: 2481–2493.
23. Cuozzo C, Porcellini A, Angrisano T, Morano A, Lee B, et al. (2007) DNA Damage, Homology-Directed Repair, and DNA Methylation. PLoS Genet 3: e110.
24. Sikdar N, Banerjee S, Lee K-y, Wincovitch S, Pak E, et al. (2009) DNA damage responses by human ELG1 in S phase are important to maintain genomic integrity. Cell Cycle 8: 3199–3207.
25. Fox JT, Sakamuru S, Huang R, Teneva N, Simmons SO, et al. (2012) High-throughput genotoxicity assay identifies antioxidants as inducers of DNA damage response and cell death. Proceedings of the National Academy of Sciences 109: 5423–5428.
26. Ho AS, Turcan S, Chan TA (2013) Epigenetic therapy: use of agents targeting deacetylation and methylation in cancer management.
27. Ai T, Cui H, Chen L (2012) Multi-targeted histone deacetylase inhibitors in cancer therapy. Curr Med Chem 19: 475–487.
28. Li D, Marchenko ND, Moll UM (2011) SAHA shows preferential cytotoxicity in mutant p53 cancer cells by destabilizing mutant p53 through inhibition of the HDAC6-Hsp90 chaperone axis. Cell Death Differ 18: 1904–1913.
29. Jasek E, Lis GJ, Jasinska M, Jurkowska H, Litwin JA (2012) Effect of Histone Deacetylase Inhibitors Trichostatin A and Valproic Acid on Etoposide-induced Apoptosis in Leukemia Cells. Anticancer Research 32: 2791–2799.
30. Evans TJ, Yamamoto KN, Hirota K, Takeda S (2010) Mutant cells defective in DNA repair pathways provide a sensitive high-throughput assay for genotoxicity. DNA Repair 9: 1292–1298.
31. Lee J-H, Choy ML, Ngo L, Foster SS, Marks PA (2010) Histone deacetylase inhibitor induces DNA damage, which normal but not transformed cells can repair. Proceedings of the National Academy of Sciences 107: 14639–14644.
32. Kass EM, Helgadottir HR, Chen C-C, Barbera M, Wang R, et al. (2013) Double-strand break repair by homologous recombination in primary mouse somatic cells requires BRCA1 but not the ATM kinase. Proceedings of the National Academy of Sciences 110: 5564–5569.
33. Tikoo S, Sengupta S (2010) Time to Bloom. Genome Integrity 1: 14.
34. Xia B, Sheng Q, Nakanishi K, Ohashi A, Wu J, et al. (2006) Control of BRCA2 Cellular and Clinical Functions by a Nuclear Partner, PALB2. Molecular Cell 22: 719–729.
35. Pierce AJ, Johnson RD, Thompson LH, Jasin M (1999) XRCC3 promotes homology-directed repair of DNA damage in mammalian cells. Genes & Development 13: 2633–2638.
36. Kotian S, Liyanarachchi S, Zelent A, Parvin JD (2011) Histone Deacetylases 9 and 10 Are Required for Homologous Recombination. Journal of Biological Chemistry 286: 7722–7726.
37. Adimoolam S, Sirisawad M, Chen J, Thiemann P, Ford JM, et al. (2007) HDAC inhibitor PCI-24781 decreases RAD51 expression and inhibits homologous recombination. Proceedings of the National Academy of Sciences 104: 19482–19487.
38. Bunting SF, Callen E, Wong N, Chen H-T, Polato F, et al. (2010) 53BP1 Inhibits Homologous Recombination in Brca1-Deficient Cells by Blocking Resection of DNA Breaks. Cell 141: 243–254.
39. Mao Z, Bozzella M, Seluanov A, Gorbunova V (2008) Comparison of nonhomologous end joining and homologous recombination in human cells. DNA Repair 7: 1765–1771.
40. Gunn A, Stark JM (2012) I-SceI-Based Assays to Examine Distinct Repair Outcomes of Mammalian Chromosomal Double Strand Breaks. In: Bjergb√¶k L, editor. DNA Repair Protocols: Humana Press. pp. 379–391.
41. Murr R, Loizou J, Yang Y, Cuenin C, Li H, et al. (2006) Histone acetylation by Trrap-Tip60 modulates loading of repair proteins and repair of DNA double-strand breaks.
42. Hsiao K-Y, Mizzen CA (2013) Histone H4 deacetylation facilitates 53BP1 DNA damage signaling and double-strand break repair. Journal of Molecular Cell Biology.
43. Fattah F, Lee EH, Weisensel N, Wang Y, Lichter N, et al. (2010) Ku Regulates the Non-Homologous End Joining Pathway Choice of DNA Double-Strand Break Repair in Human Somatic Cells. PLoS Genet 6: e1000855.
44. Oh S, Wang Y, Zimbric J, Hendrickson EA (2013) Human LIGIV is synthetically lethal with the loss of Rad54B-dependent recombination and is required for certain chromosome fusion events induced by telomere dysfunction. Nucleic Acids Research 41: 1734–1749.
45. Yu X, Fu S, Lai M, Baer R, Chen J (2006) BRCA1 ubiquitinates its phosphorylation-dependent binding partner CtIP. Genes & Development 20: 1721–1726.
46. Wang Y, Leung JW, Jiang Y, Lowery MG, Do H, et al. (2013) FANCM and FAAP24 Maintain Genome Stability via Cooperative as Well as Unique Functions. Molecular Cell 49: 997–1009.
47. Nalabothula N, Carrier F (2011) Cancer cells' epigenetic composition and predisposition to histone deacetylase inhibitor sensitization. Epigenomics 3: 145–155.
48. Olaharski AJ, Ji Z, Woo J-Y, Lim S, Hubbard AE, et al. (2006) The Histone Deacetylase Inhibitor Trichostatin A Has Genotoxic Effects in Human Lymphoblasts In Vitro. Toxicological Sciences 93: 341–347.
49. Candotti F, Oakes SA, Johnston JA, Giliani S, Schumacher RF, et al. (1997) Structural and functional basis for JAK3-deficient severe combined immunodeficiency. Blood 90: 3996–4003.
50. Krijger PHL, Lee K-Y, Wit N, van den Berk PCM, Wu X, et al. (2011) HLTF and SHPRH are not essential for PCNA polyubiquitination, survival and somatic hypermutation: Existence of an alternative E3 ligase. DNA Repair 10: 438–444.
51. Nakanishi K, Yang Y-G, Pierce AJ, Taniguchi T, Digweed M, et al. (2005) Human Fanconi anemia monoubiquitination pathway promotes homologous DNA repair. Proceedings of the National Academy of Sciences of the United States of America 102: 1110–1115.
52. Lee K-y, Yang K, Cohn MA, Sikdar N, D'Andrea AD, et al. (2010) Human ELG1 Regulates the Level of Ubiquitinated Proliferating Cell Nuclear Antigen (PCNA) through Its Interactions with PCNA and USP1. Journal of Biological Chemistry 285: 10362–10369.
53. Kuchma M, Kim J, Muller M, Arlen P (2012) Prostate Cancer Cell Surface-Associated Keratin 8 and Its Implications for Enhanced Plasmin Activity. The Protein Journal 31: 195–205.
54. Merolla F, Luise C, Muller MT, Pacelli R, Fusco A, et al. (2012) Loss of CCDC6, the First Identified RET Partner Gene, Affects pH2AX S139 Levels and Accelerates Mitotic Entry upon DNA Damage. PLoS ONE 7: e36177.

5

Extensive Microbial and Functional Diversity within the Chicken Cecal Microbiome

Martin J. Sergeant[1], Chrystala Constantinidou[1], Tristan A. Cogan[2], Michael R. Bedford[3], Charles W. Penn[4], Mark J. Pallen[1]*

1 Division of Microbiology and Infection, Warwick Medical School, University of Warwick, Coventry, United Kingdom, **2** School of Clinical Veterinary Science, Bristol, United Kingdom, **3** AB Vista Feed Ingredients, Marlborough, United Kingdom, **4** Institute of Microbiology and Infection, University of Birmingham, Birmingham, United Kingdom

Abstract

Chickens are major source of food and protein worldwide. Feed conversion and the health of chickens relies on the largely unexplored complex microbial community that inhabits the chicken gut, including the ceca. We have carried out deep microbial community profiling of the microbiota in twenty cecal samples via 16S rRNA gene sequences and an in-depth metagenomics analysis of a single cecal microbiota. We recovered 699 phylotypes, over half of which appear to represent previously unknown species. We obtained 648,251 environmental gene tags (EGTs), the majority of which represent new species. These were binned into over two-dozen draft genomes, which included *Campylobacter jejuni* and *Helicobacter pullorum*. We found numerous polysaccharide- and oligosaccharide-degrading enzymes encoding within the metagenome, some of which appeared to be part of polysaccharide utilization systems with genetic evidence for the co-ordination of polysaccharide degradation with sugar transport and utilization. The cecal metagenome encodes several fermentation pathways leading to the production of short-chain fatty acids, including some with novel features. We found a dozen uptake hydrogenases encoded in the metagenome and speculate that these provide major hydrogen sinks within this microbial community and might explain the high abundance of several genera within this microbiome, including *Campylobacter*, *Helicobacter* and *Megamonas*.

Editor: John Parkinson, Hospital for Sick Children, Canada

Funding: The work was funded by the BBSRC. The funders had no role in study design, data collection and analysis, decision to publish, or preparation of the manuscript.

Competing Interests: Mike Bedford is employed by AB Vista Feed Ingredients. There are no patents, products in development or marketed products to declare.

* E-mail: m.pallen@warwick.ac.uk

Introduction

The domestic chicken occupies a special place in science and society. It is the most common domesticated animal, the most important food production animal and the most abundant and widely distributed bird in the world, scattered across islands and continents from the Arctic to the Falklands. Chickens provide a case study in domestication, a process began >7,000 years ago in South-East Asia [1]. Chickens have also played a key role in the history of science, from Aristotle's description of a chick embryo [2] to Darwin's account of their domestication [3]. The chicken has been adopted as a laboratory organism for research in genetics, embryology, development, immunology, virology and cancer [4]. The completion of the chicken genome sequence was a landmark in basic and applied biology [5]. However, the nuclear and mitochondrial genomes of the chicken represent just a small part of the gene pool associated with this bird.

Chickens, like other birds, have proportionally smaller intestines and shorter transit digestion times than mammals, but do not appear to any less efficient at digestion than their mammalian counterparts [6]. This may be explained, in part, by the fact that the chicken gastrointestinal tract is home to a complex microbial community, the chicken gut microbiota, which underpins the links between diet and health in this bird. The healthy chicken gut microbiota plays important roles in assimilating nutrients from food, in producing vitamins and essential amino acids and in preventing harmful pathogens from gaining a foothold [7]. The chicken gut microbiota also acts as source of human infections and as a reservoir of antibiotic-resistance determinants [8]. An optimal gut microbiota can increase agricultural productivity, as evidenced by the ability of antibiotics to promote growth in chicks [9]. This microbiota is also home to a rich collection of genes, the chicken gut microbiome, likely to include many sequences of scientific interest and biotechnological potential.

The chicken gastrointestinal tract consists of a crop, where food can be stored, followed by a proventriculous or true stomach which leads to the muscular gizzard, where digesta are ground, before entering the small and finally large intestine. The most densely populated microbial community within the chicken gut is found in the ceca, a pair of blind-ended sacs that open off the large intestine [10]. At the entrance to each cecum, long intertwining villi sieve out coarse particulate material, allowing only soluble or fine particulate digesta to enter the lumen. Whereas the transit time through the upper intestine is only 2.5 hours, digesta dwell in the ceca for 12–20 hours, potentially allowing a longer time for digestion and absorption of nutrients. Various roles have been assigned to the cecal microbiota in wild birds [10] but its function in the modern commercial broiler is unclear and, in some experiments, the caeca have been removed without impairing the chicken's development [10]. However, this microbiota has been implicated in many processes; nitrogen recycling by breakdown of uric acid [11], supplying B vitamins to their hosts [12] and producing essential amino acids required by their host [13]. Particularly relevant to the intensive farming of chickens is the cecum's role in digestion of non-starch polysaccharides NSPs [14], which are found in the grains used in commercial chicken feed. Some authors suggest as much as 10% of energy needs is recovered from a well-functioning cecum [14,15], with chicken fed high fiber showing a dramatic increase in the size of this organ [16]. The fermentation of breakdown products of NSPs produces short chain volatile fatty acids (SCFA), which are absorbed across the mucosa and catabolised by the host [6]. Such SCFA not only contribute to the nutrition of the chicken, they also lower pH which can inhibit acid-sensitive pathogens and improve mineral absorption [7]. In particular, butyrate has been shown to reduce *Salmonella* infection [17] and it is also able to stimulate epithelial cell growth [18]. Molecular hydrogen produced during the fermentation process [16] if allowed to accumulate can lead to inhibition of this process. Therefore, for efficient fermentation this gas needs to be removed by hydrogen-consuming bacteria [19]. These interactions are poorly understood and therefore the current study used metagenomics to identify pathways in the chicken ceca microbiome for NSP breakdown, SCFA production and hydrogen consumption.

Previous culture-based studies have established that, as in other vertebrates, the phylums *Bacteroidetes* and *Firmicutes* predominated in the chicken cecal microbiota [20–22]. Attempts at culture-independent phylogenetic profiling using 16S rRNA gene sequences have yielded insights into the composition of the chicken cecal microbiome [23–27] and more recent studies have shown the domination by *Fimicutes*, especially of the *Clostridiales* order [28]. Similarly, studies using metagenomics, the whole-scale sequencing of DNA extracted from a microbial community without target-specific amplification or culture, have provided glimpses into the function of this complex microbial community [29,30]. However, most previous studies have examined pooled samples, thus ignoring variation in individual chickens, and have not achieved sufficient depth of coverage to provide a global picture of the taxonomic diversity and functional repertoire of the whole microbiome. This study aimed to address these points and analyzed cecal contents from 10 broiler chickens from the same flock on a commercial farm to an unprecedented depth, and on one sample produced the largest metagenomic analysis to date in order to illuminate the function of the cecal microbiota in chickens.

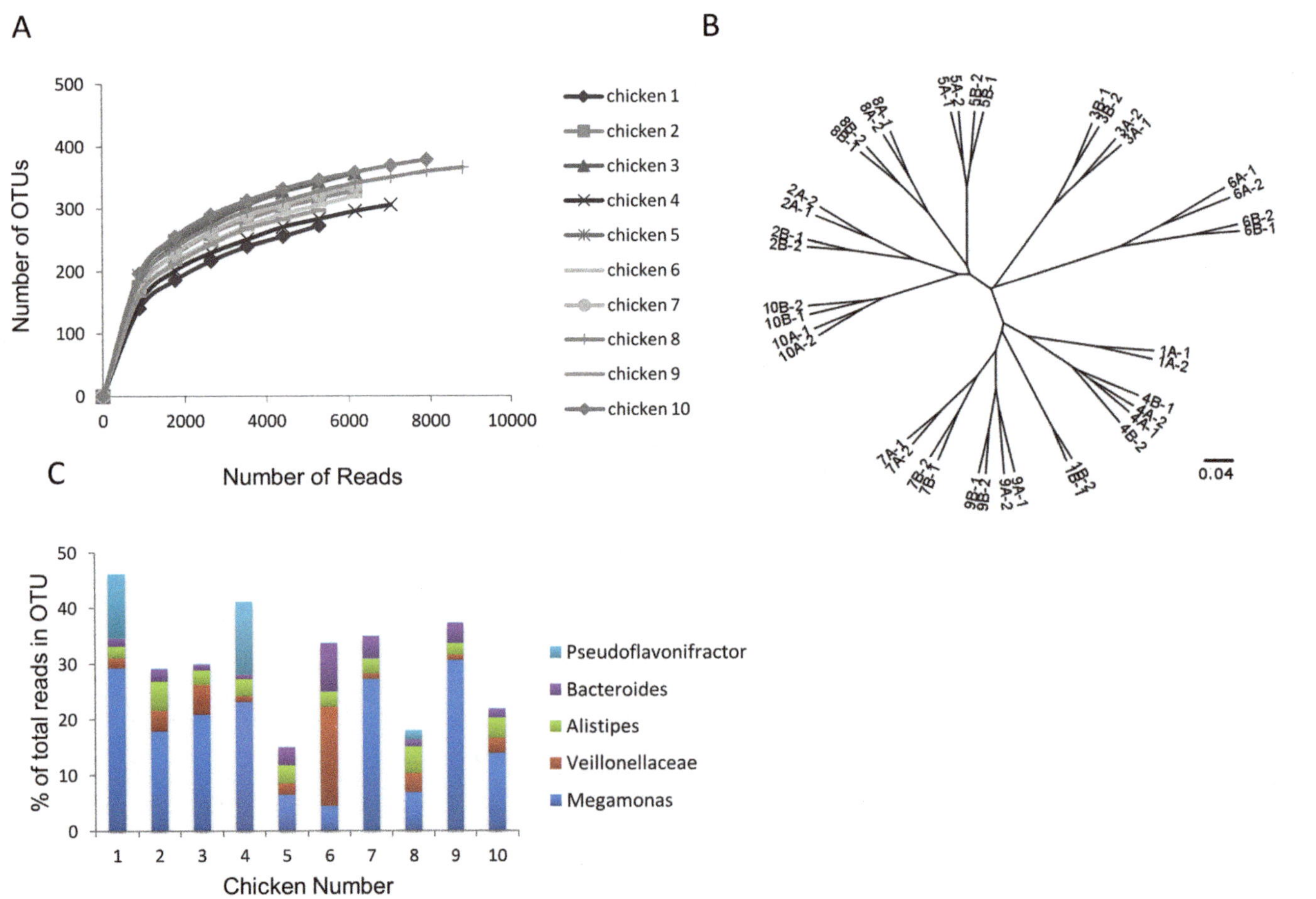

Figure 1. Summary of 16S analysis. (A) Rarefaction curves of the OTUs clustered at 97% sequence identity for each chicken, based on the averages of the four replicates per bird. (B) Hierarchical clustering visualizing similarities among cecal samples. The number in each label indicates each individual chicken and the letter each individual ceca (either A or B). Technical replicates of each ceca were carried out. (C) Bar chart showing the proportion of reads assigned to the top 5 most abundant OTUs in each chicken.

Table 1. Draft genome sequences recovered from the chicken cecal metagenome.

Draft Genome ID	# of contigs	Size (Mbp)	G+C %	Depth of Coverage	Taxonomic Assignment	Closest Genome	Similarity to closest genome[a]	Size of closest genome	Completeness by closest genome[b]	Completeness by core genes[c]
4	555	5.49	44	21	*Bacteroides*	*Bacteroides dorei 5_1_36/D4*	100%	5.53	99%	86%
1	761	3.30	50	23	*Enterobacteriaceae*	*Escherichia albertii TW07627 a*	100%	4.70	70%	24%
3	570	3.01	58	31	*Firmicutes*	*Clostridium cellulovorans 743B*	58%	5.26	57%	81%
29	91	2.80	49	67	*Clostridiales*	*Subdoligranulum sp. 4_3_54A2FAA*	90%	4.21	67%	93%
36	63	2.71	52	39	*Bacteroidales*	*Tannerella sp. 6_1_58FAA_CT1*	92%	3.84	70%	91%
2	636	2.59	53	19	*Lachnospiraceae 3_1_57FAA_CT1*	*Lachnospiraceae bacterium 3_1_57FAA_CT1*	94%	7.69	34%	27%
7	448	2.53	61	38	*Subdoligranulum variabile*	*Subdoligranulum variabile DSM 15176*	88%	3.24	78%	62%
34	77	2.51	42	254	*Veillonellaceae*	*Megamonas hypermegale ART12/1*	94%	2.56	98%	95%
45	37	2.44	62	942	*Alistipes*	*Alistipes sp. HGB5*	95%	3.46	71%	88%
16	218	2.31	58	27	*Bacteroidales*	*Alistipes indistinctus YIT 12060*	93%	3.09	75%	90%
5	521	2.30	56	14	*Victivallis vadensis*	*Victivallis vadensis ATCC BAA-548*	75%	4.58	50%	53%
38	56	2.25	54	79	*Clostridiales*	*Clostridium sp. MSTE9*	77%	3.51	64%	92%
14	257	2.20	61	39	*Bacteroidales*	*Alistipes sp. HGB5*	94%	3.46	64%	89%
6	508	1.93	63	40	*Ruminococcaceae bacterium D16*	*Lachnospiraceae bacterium 7_1_58FAA*	96%	3.21	60%	68%
23	129	1.81	56	57	*Bacteroidetes*	*Flavobacterium columnare ATCC 49512*	83%	3.16	57%	93%
30	89	1.80	57	41	*Dialister*	*Dialister succinatiphilus YIT 11850*	79%	2.46	73%	95%
44	38	1.73	29	47	*Campylobacter jejuni*	*Campylobacter jejuni 81-176*	99%	1.62	107%	89%
11	274	1.72	68	53	*Coriobacteriaceae*	*Atopobium parvulum DSM 20469*	86%	1.54	111%	88%
17	212	1.68	51	70	*Clostridiales*	*Ruminococcus torques L2-14*	94%	3.34	50%	89%
43	42	1.67	34	92	*Helicobacter pullorum*	*Helicobacter pullorum MIT 98-5489*	99%	1.92	87%	89%
8	364	1.50	45	13	*Bacteroides*	*Bacteroides thetaiotaomicron VPI-5482*	99%	6.29	24%	7%
12	297	1.48	64	94	*Bifidobacterium*	*Bifidobacterium gallicum DSM 20093*	93%	2.02	73%	79%
18	188	1.43	47	46	*Clostridiales*	*Clostridium leptum DSM 753*	74%	3.27	44%	86%
10	286	1.34	62	19	*Coriobacteriaceae*	*Coriobacterium glomerans PW2*	88%	2.12	63%	78%

Table 1. Cont.

Draft Genome ID	# of contigs	Size (Mbp)	G+C %	Depth of Coverage	Taxonomic Assignment	Closest Genome	Similarity to closest genome[a]	Size of closest genome	Completeness by closest genome[b]	Completeness by core genes[c]
15	222	1.30	50	15	*Clostridiales*	*Ruminococcus albus 8*	79%	3.69	35%	70%

[a]Closest genome was identified based on blastp of the translated *rpoB* gene from the draft genome against the ncbi nr database [b] Completeness based on the sum size of total contigs compared to the size of the closest genome [c] Completeness based on the % of core genes present (see methods).

Experimental Procedures

Ethics statement

In accordance with the United Kingdom Animal (Scientific Procedures) Act of 1986, this study did not require a Home Office project license because no regulated procedures were carried out. Chickens were humanely killed at a designated establishment by cervical dislocation, which is an appropriate method under Schedule 1 of the Act.

Samples collection, DNA extraction and PCR amplification

Cecal samples were collected from Ross broilers at 42 days, housed indoors under standard commercial conditions. They had been fed on a wheat based diet with 5% maize which contained ionophores but no antibiotics. The feed conversion ratio was standard for the breed and there was no feed withdrawal period before the birds were sacrificed. The cecal contents were a typical brown colour and like toothpaste in constituency. Birds were euthanized by cervical dislocation and the ceca removed and transported to the laboratory on ice. The cecal surface was sterilized with 70% ethanol, a longitudinal incision was made with a scalpel and the edges pulled back. Contents were removed into a sterile tube and flash frozen in liquid nitrogen and stored at −70°C. DNA was extracted and PCR amplification of 16S rRNA sequences was performed as described previously [31] using primers F20 and R19 flanking the variable regions V1–V3 and an annealing temperature of 55°C. Sequencing of amplicons was carried out on the Roche FLX Titanium instrument as described previously [31].

Phylogenetic analysis of 16S rRNA gene sequences

Reads were truncated where flow signals were less than 0.7 and all sequences were trimmed to 600 flows (around 350 bp in length). Clustering of the reads into Operation Taxonomic Units (OTUs) which share 97% identity was achieved using Uparse [32]. Other methods were also attempted (Text S1 and Figure S5). The following modifications to the standard Uparse pipeline were carried out. Pre-clustering (-cluster_smallmem) was included, which clustered sequences exhibiting two or less nucleotide difference. In addition, an extra chimera checking step (-uchime_ref) against the default reference database was performed. The resulting sequences were taken as defining putative operational taxonomic unites (OTUs) or phylotypes. OTU sequences were assigned to a taxonomic lineage using QIIME (assign_taxonomy.py) [33]. In addition, all OTU sequences were BLAST-searched against the NCBI nr database.

The resultant sequences, frequencies and taxonomic assignments were formatted into an OTU table that was compatible with the QIIME pipeline [33]. QIIME was used to calculate Simpsons' index and construct rarefaction curves. Dendograms depicting the similarity of bacterial communities were constructed via the jackknifed_beta_diversity script from QIIME, exploiting the Bray Curtis method to compute a similarity matrix and then the un-weighted pair-group method with arithmetic mean (UGPMA) to cluster the results. Jacknifed support was included to account for the different sampling depths. A hundred rarefied tables were generated at sample size that corresponded to the number of reads in the smallest sample to produce bootstrap values.

Metagenome sequencing and analysis

DNA extracted from cecum 1A was used for metagenome sequencing. Library preparation and sequencing on one channel

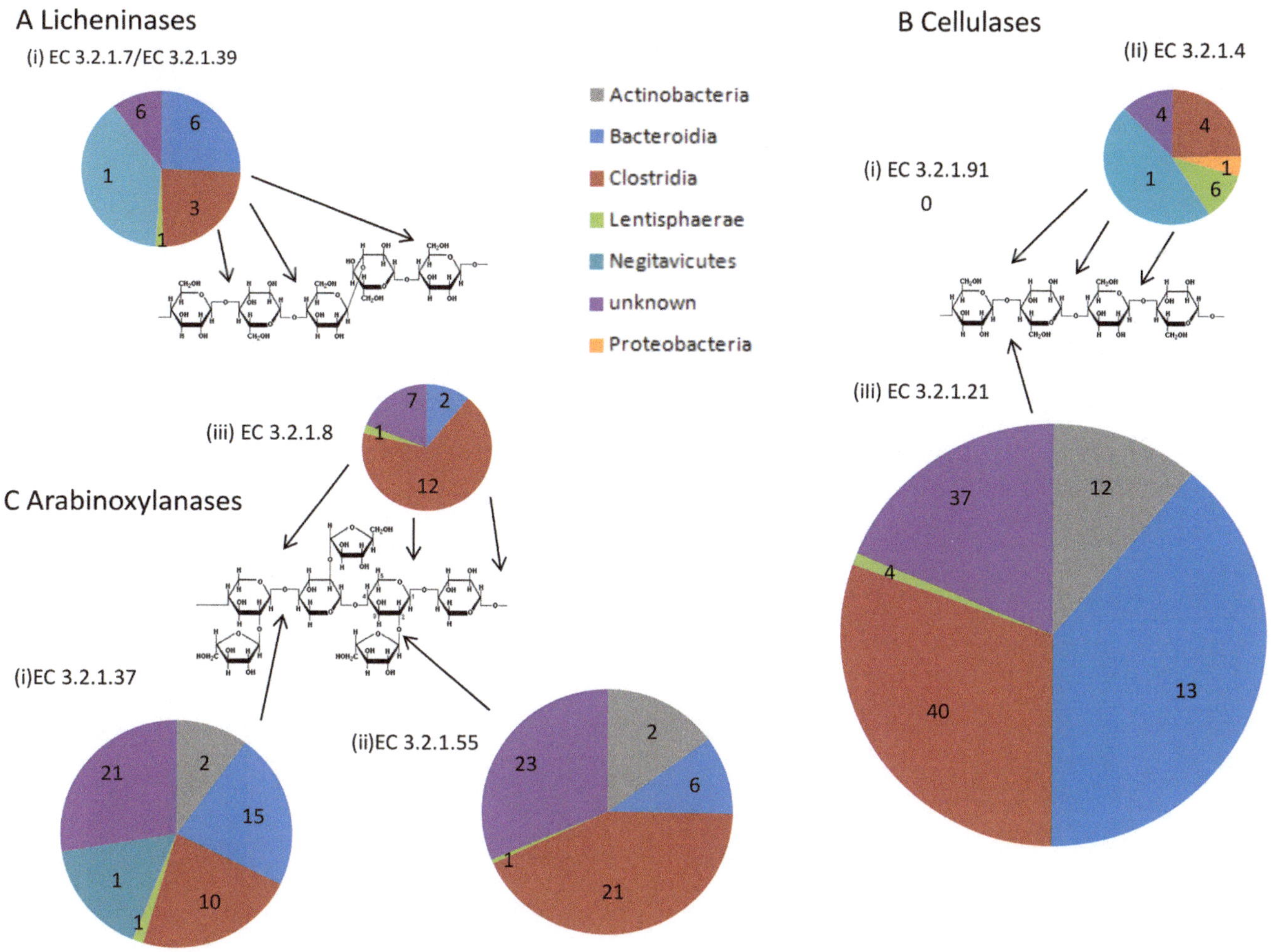

Figure 2. Polysaccharide-degrading enzymes in the chicken cecal metagenome. The figure shows each class of enzyme as judged by SEED/KEGG annotation and GH (see methods) for three types of NSP. The size of pie chart reflects abundance of the enzyme class; numbers indicate quantity of genes assigned to each bacterial Taxon at the class level.

of the Illumina MiSeq 2000 were performed according to the manufacturer's instructions by Source BioScience, Nottingham UK.

Preliminary analysis of the data involved blasting 260 000 reads against the NCBI nr database and obtaining taxonomic from the output using MEGAN(45). A comprehensive analysis was then carried out and is summarized in Figure S4a. Initially, the reads were filtered and trimmed with CLC workbench (CLC bio, Denmark) using the default settings and reads below 60 bases were removed. The 81,772,788 reads that remained were assembled into contigs (environmental gene tags) using CLC work bench under the default settings. Coding sequences (CDSs) were predicted using MetaGene [34] and translated into protein sequences which were searched against the NCBI NR database using BLASTP. BLAST results were fed into MEGAN [35], which provided KEGG and SEED annotations as well as assigning a taxonomic origin using the software's LCA algorithm. Coverage of each environmental gene tag (EGT) was assessed by mapping reads to the EGT using BWA [36].

A taxonomic assignment was made for each EGT whenever > 50% of the CDSs from the EGT had been assigned by MEGAN to the same taxon, otherwise the EGT's taxonomic assignment was scored as unknown. Functional domains were assigned to each predicted protein using Hidden Markov Models (HMMs). This was achieved using hmmsearch from HMMER [37] against the PFAM [38] and TIGRFAMS databases. Signal sequences were predicted using SignalP [39] and antibiotic resistance assigned using the ARDB package [40]. Known patterns were identified in the data using stand alone tool from the PROSITE web site [41]. All the information was stored in a MySQL database (Figure S4A) for easy retrieval and linking of the different threads of information.

Binning of EGTs

Z scores for the 256 tetra-nucleotides in each EGT were calculated as described previously [42]. Pairwise comparisons of EGT Z scores were performed using the Pearson correlation coefficient and the results assembled into a matrix. The matrix was then used to cluster EGTs at various identity levels using the cluster.classic command from MOTHUR [43]. Initial seed clusters were obtained at 0.25 identity. Clusters were merged into putative genomes if they had similar depth-of-coverage and an identical taxonomic assignment at the family level. The validity of putative genomes was assessed by determining whether the house-keeping genes, *rpo*B, *rec*A, *gro*EL and *gyr*B were single copy. Taxonomic status confirmed by when bacterial 'core' genes from

Table 2. Number of genes containing GH domains in different metagenomes.

	Macropod[a]	Termite[b]	Bovine[c]	Panda[d]	chicken
Cellulases					
GH5	10	56	1451	3	151
GH6	0	0	0	0	0
GH7	0	0	1	0	0
GH9	0	9	795	0	14
GH44	0	6	?	0	41
GH45	0	4	115	0	0
GH48	0	0	0	0	0
Total	10(2)	74(11)	2365(9)	3(1)	206(2)
Endohemicellulases					
GH8	1	5	329	2	21
GH10	11	46	1025	2	60
GH11	0	14	165	0	0
GH12	0	0	0	0	0
GH26	5	15	369	0	18
GH28	2	6	472	1	93
GH53	9	12	?	0	21
Total	28(5)	98(14)	2360(9)	13(3)	213(2)
Debranching Enzymes					
GH51	12	18	?	5	84
GH54	0	0	?	0	0
GH62	0	0	1	0	0
GH67	5	10	120	2	12
GH78	25	0	1260	2	425
Total	42(8)	18(3)	1381(5)	9(2)	521(5)
Oligosaccharide-degrading enzymes					
GH1	61	22	253	101	263
GH2	24	23	1436	1	998
GH3	72	69	2844	18	1275
GH29	2	0	939	1	232
GH35	3	3	158	4	54
GH38	3	11	272	10	73
GH39	1	3	315	9	45
GH42	8	24	374	18	367
GH43	10	16	?	0	340
GH52	0	3	0	0	0
Total	184(33)	174(24)	6591(23)	162(36)	3647(38)
Sum	557	704	27755	448	9033
CDS	78896	82789	2547270	49844	595178
%GH	0.71	0.85	1.09	0.90	1.52

Data are grouped according to Allgier *et al* [68]. The numbers in parenthesis are relative to total number of GH containing genes. The data is take from [a]wallaby [55] [b]termite [44], [c]panda [69] and [d]bovine rumen [70].

the human microbiome project (http://hmpdacc.org/tools_protocols/tools_protocols.php) were blasted against putative genomes with a cut off value of $1e^{-10}$. Completeness of putative genomes was assessed by comparing the size of the genome with that of the closest relative in the GenBank.

Functional domain analysis

Most glucosyl Hyrdrolase (GH) domains were detected using PFAM HMMs as described previously [44]. To detect GH domains without an HMM, metagenomic protein sequences were blasted against a set of GH domains described previously [44] with an e-value cut off 10^{-6}. Xylanase, licheninase and cellulase sequences were detected using predictions of enzyme activities

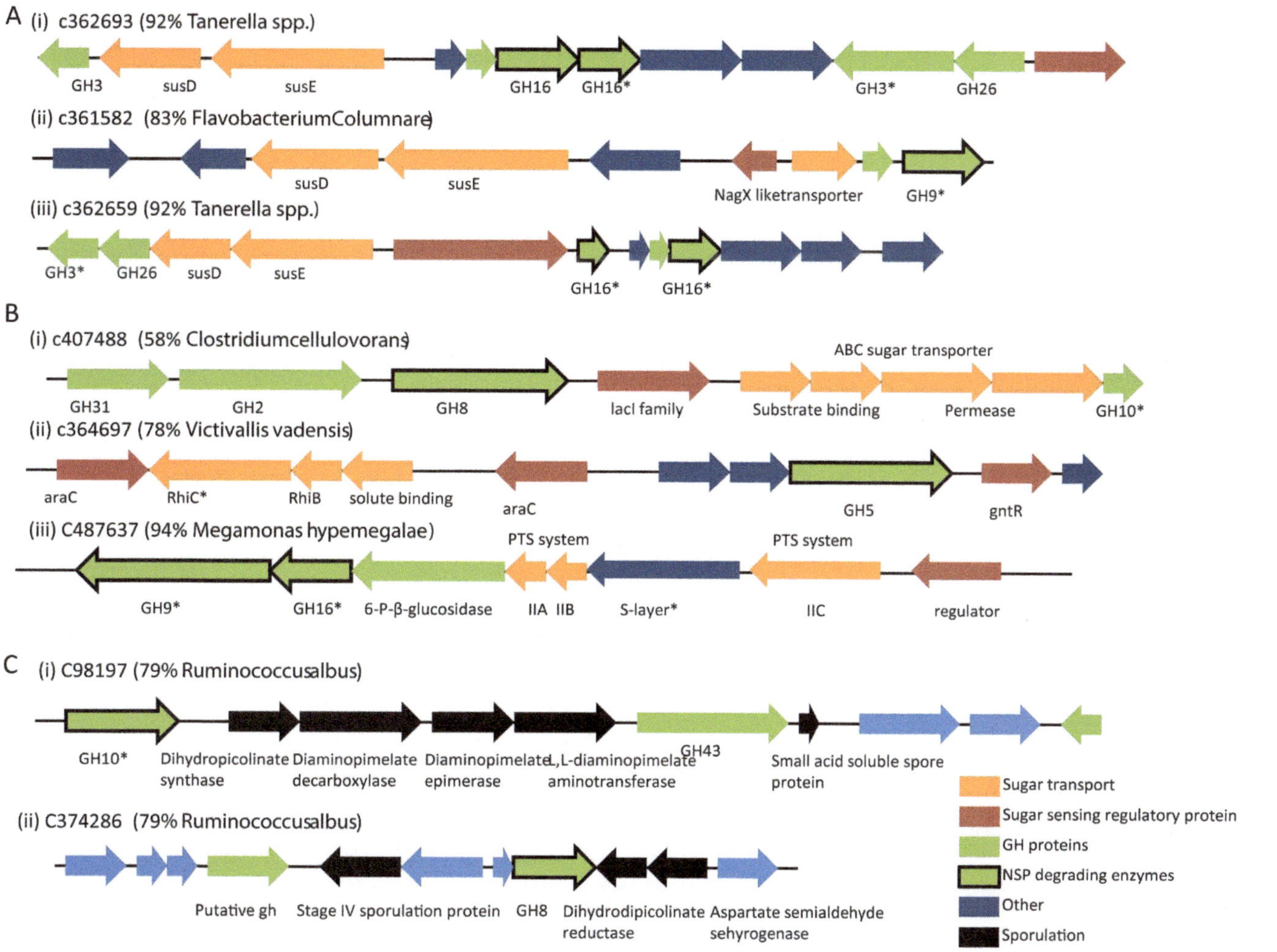

Figure 3. Gene clusters associated with polysaccharide degradation and utilization. NSP degrading genes were identified by SEED/KEGG annotation and GH domain (see methods). (A) Gene clusters encoding putative PUL systems from various *Bacteroidetes*. (B) Gene cluster encoding putative integrated polysaccharide degradation and utilization systems from various *Firmicutes*. (C) NSP degrading enzymes associated with sporulation genes * indicates predicted signal peptide.

from the SEED and KEGG annotations, combined with the appropriate GH domains as specified by the Cazy Website [45] (Table S6). Gene contexts were visualised in Artemis.

Fermentation to acetate was examined by looking for putative acetate kinase (TIGR0016) and phosphate acetyltransferase (TIGR00651) that were adjacent to each other in EGTs. To investigate fermentation to butyrate, 3-hydroxybuturyl-CoA dehydrogenase (BCD), models were constructed using HMM, based on 10 BCD proteins from divergent prokaryotes. Putative BCD genes were indentified using this model and were further verified by looking for an adjacent Electron Transfer Flavoprotein (PF01021). Putative butyryl-CoA:acetate Coa transferase genes was found by using the conserved sequence AFVDIAKAG [46]. The alternative pathway was identified by adjacent transbutyrylase (TIGR02706) and butyrate kinase (TIGR02707) genes. Fermentation to propionoate was investigated by searching for the methyl-Malonyl-CoA:pyruvate transcarboxylase gene using as a SEED/KEGG annotation of EC 2.1.3.1 and the epimerase gene was putatively identified using a SEED annotation of EC 5.1.99.1 and TIGR03081. Methylmalonyl decarboxylase genes were identified by a SEED/KEGG annotation of EC4.1.1.41 and TIGR01117.

Putative uptake hydrogenases were identified with the patterns [EGMQS]RXC[GR][IV]CXXX[HT]XXX[AGS]X(0,4)[VANQD] or [AFGIKLMV][HMR]XX[HR][AS][AFLY][DN]PC[FILMV]X-C[AGS]XH [47]. The dissimilatory 5′ phophosulfate resuctase (APS) present in suphate reducers was putatively identified if genes with TIGR02064 and TIG02066 models were adjacent to each other. The AcetylCoa Synthase beta subunit responsible for the CO dehydrogenase reaction in acetogens was identified by the conserved sequences LCGAVSW and PMTSCGC [48]. A search for the methyl-coenzyme M reductase present in methanogens was performed by looking for adjacent genes containing TIGR03256 and TIG03257 domains.

Results and Discussion

Microbial diversity in the chicken cecum

From the ten chickens, we recovered 414,070 16S sequences, which were classified into 699 phylotypes using a 97% sequence identity threshold. Rarefaction curves suggest that sampling has reached saturation and that the number of phylotypes in individual chickens ranges from ~200 to ~350 (Figure 1A). Sequences from 232 phylotypes showed less than 97% identity to

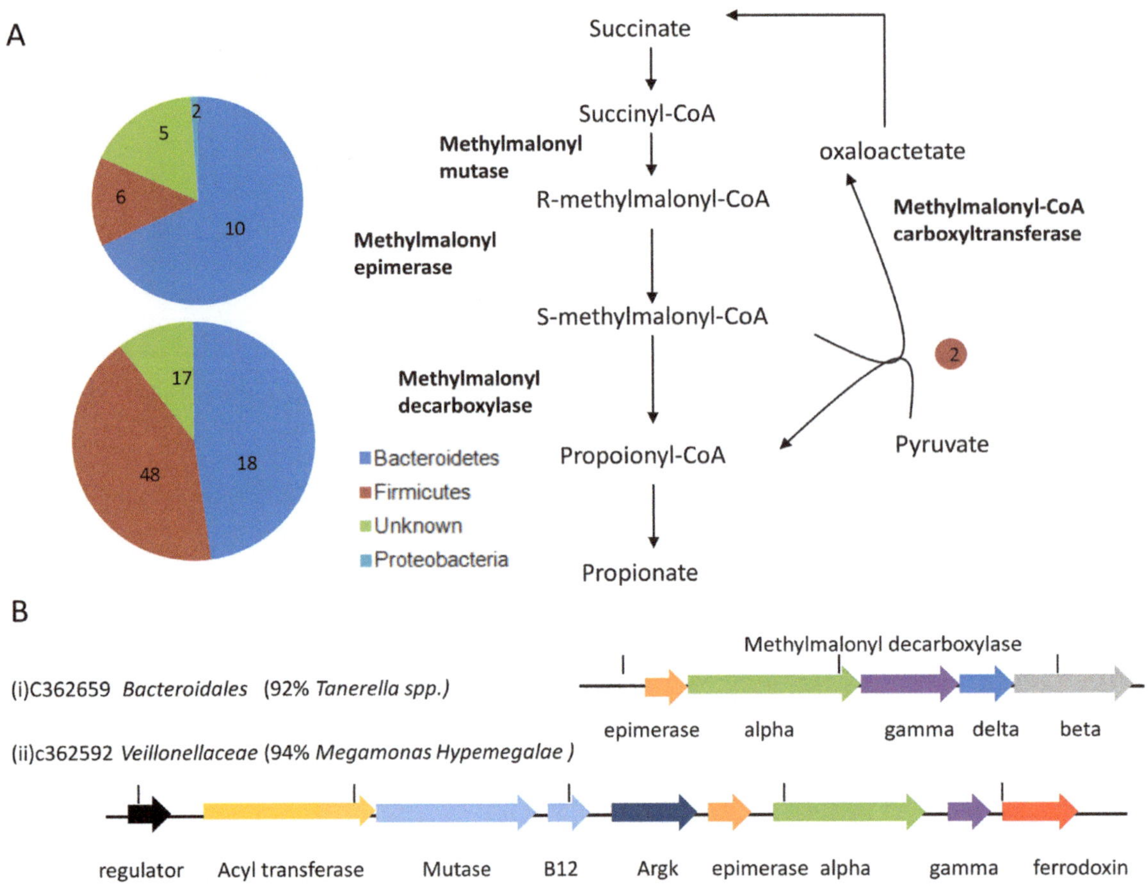

Figure 4. Pathways and gene clusters associated with propionoate production in the chicken cecal metagenome. (A) Pathways involved in propionoate production showing the putative genes identified coding for the enzymes involved. Size of pie chart reflects abundance of the gene class; numbers indicate quantity of genes assigned to each taxon. (B) Operon structure of two Methylmalonyl decarboxylase loci.

any sequence in GenBank (Data Set S1) and therefore potentially represent new species. The majority of these OTUs contained large numbers of reads and hence are unlikely to be due to sequencing or PCR errors (Figure S1).

Previous studies have shown large inter-chick variation of microbiota community structure with both T-RLFP [49] and quantitative PCR [50], so we were curious to determine how much variation occurs within the same region of the gut. We analysed biological replicates from each bird (two ceca) and technical replicates for each sample and found that samples from the same bird clustered together, with the exception of bird 1(Figure 1B). Furthermore, in all but one case (bird 4), individual ceca from the same chicken could be differentiated with technical replicates clustering together. Simpson's diversity index varied between ceca and birds, with the highest value (i.e. least evenness) in bird 1 (Table S1), which was dominated by *Megamonas* and *Alistipes* (Figure 1C).

Curiously, in our samples, *Lachnospriceae*, *Ruminococcaceae* and *Bacteroides* appear to be less abundant than might be expected from previous studies (Figure S2). This can largely be explained by the unprecedented numerical dominance of the class *Negativicutes* (over 20% of all sequences) and in particular, by the high prevalence of a single novel species of *Megamonas*, which accounts for nearly a third of the reads in one of the birds, chicken 9 (Figure 1C).

The chicken cecal metagenome

We obtained a hundred and twenty million 110-base reads from the contents of a single cecal sample (cecum 1A). A taxonomic analysis of a subset of reads (Table S2) showed that, of the reads that could be assigned to a taxon, >98% were bacterial, with < 1% assigned to the chicken and fewer than one in a thousand assigned to archaea, other eukaryotes (e.g. the cereal fungus *Magnaporthe orazae* and the alga *Chlamydomonas reinharrdii*) or to viruses (bacteriophages and Fowl Adenovirus).

Reads were incorporated into a 337-Mbp assembly, with an N_{50} of 647 bp and consisting of 648,251 environmental gene tags (EGTs). From this assembly, we predicted 108,103 complete coding sequences (CDS) and 595,178 partial CDSs. Of the EGTs greater than 2 kb about 13% could be assigned to a known species (Figure S3A), suggesting that the majority of EGTs that we have recovered represent new species. Seven percent of EGTs could not even be assigned to a known domain (Figure S3A). The majority of these showed, on homology searching, just a few weak matches to phage genes. Since phages largely contain genes with unknown functions [51] these EGTs probably represent phages.

When the taxonomic distribution predicted from the 16S analysis is compared with that from the metagenomics data, there is a discrepancy in the ratio of *Firmicutes* to *Bacteroidetes* (Figure S3b). This is largely due to differences in the ratio of reads from the genus *Alistipes*, which belongs to the *Bacteroidetes*, to those from *Megamonas*, which belongs to the *Firmicutes*, (19.9 and

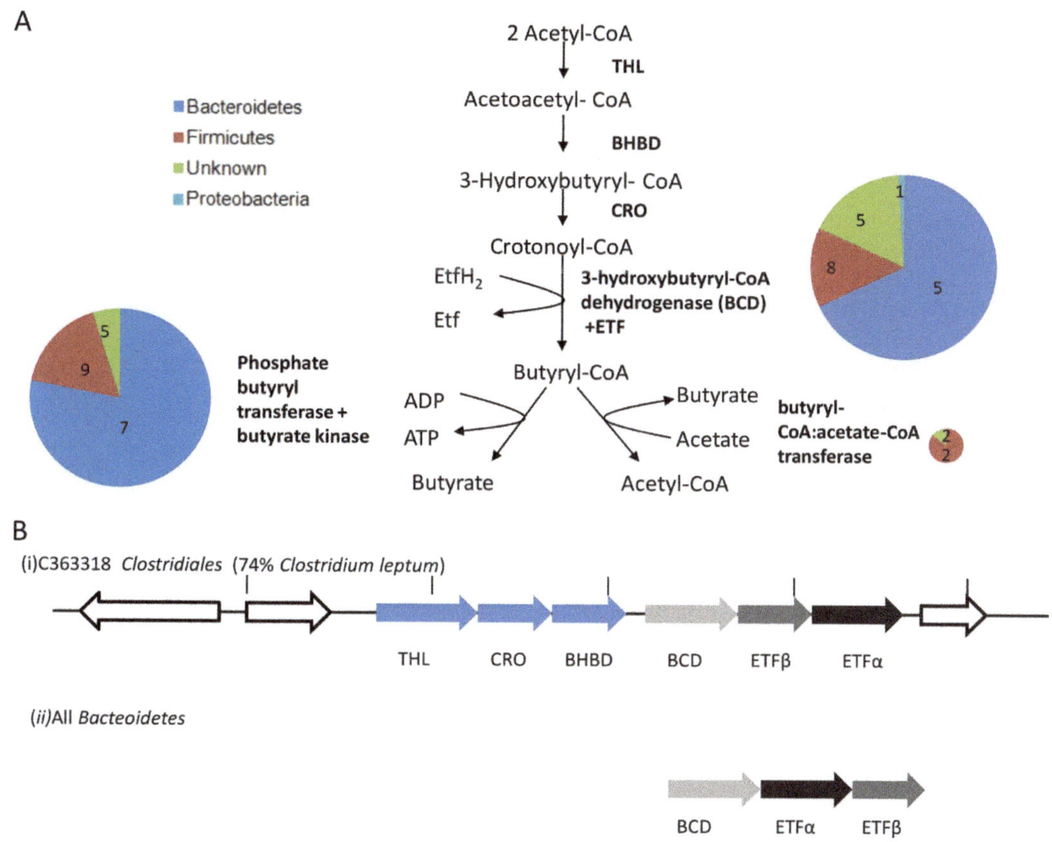

Figure 5. Pathways and gene clusters associated with butyrate production in the chicken cecal metagenome. (A) Pathways involved in butyrate production showing the putative genes identified coding for the enzymes involved. Size of pie chart reflects abundance of the gene class; numbers indicate quantity of genes assigned to each taxon. (B) Operon structure of two butyryl-CoA:acetate-CoA transferase (BCD) loci.

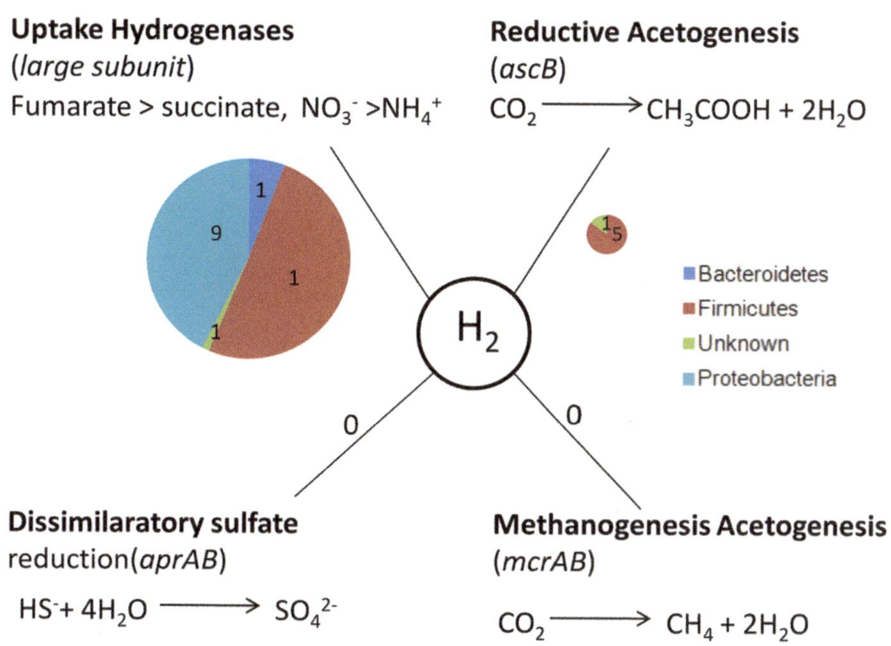

Figure 6. Potential Hydrogen sinks in the Chicken cecal metagenome. The key genes involved in each pathway that could potentially use hydrogen are shown. The size of pie chart reflects abundance of the gene class; numbers indicate quantity of genes assigned to each taxon.

16.3% in the 16S data set; 32% of and 9% in the metagenome), probably reflecting differential amplification in the 16S PCR.

EGTs were binned according to Z-score, coverage and taxonomic assignment, allowing us to reconstruct two-dozen genomes larger than 1Mbp (Table 1). Only five genomes showed a ≥99% match within the rpoB gene to sequences in GenBank; suggesting most of the draft genomes we have recovered represent new species.

Antibiotic resistance genes were investigated using the ARDB database pipeline [40] and the results are shown in data S2. The most common predicted resistance was against tetracycline and bacitracin. In addition a vancomycin resistance operon in *Enterococcus* was detected.

Polysaccharide-degrading enzymes

The grain that forms the basis of most commercial chicken diets is rich in non-starch polysaccharides, with β-glucans, including cellulose, predominating in barley and oats and arabinoxylans abundant in wheat, maize and rye. In comparison to a set of other known metagenomes, the chicken cecal microbiome contains the largest proportion of sequences (1.5%) representing glycosyl-hydrolase (GH) domains (Table 2). Within this microbiome, we found sequences from over two hundred different non-starch polysaccharide-degrading enzymes (Figure 2).

In line with the expectation that less soluble, larger polymers are excluded from the cecum, we found that, in comparison to other microbial communities, the chicken cecal microbiome (along with the panda microbiome) harbored the lowest proportion of cellulases and endohemicellulases (4%), but the largest proportion of oligosaccharide degrading enzymes (38%) within GH-contiaing genes (Table 2). In particular, glucanases acting on oligosaccharides (E.C. 3.2.1.4 and E.C. 3.2.1.1) predominate over endoglucanases (EC 3.2.1.4 and E.C 3.2.1.8) acting on full-length polymers of cellulose and xylan (Figure 2). We found no evidence of any sequences representing the exo-acting cellobiohydralase activity (E.C. 3.2.1.91) associated with the degradation of crystalline cellulose [52]. We found a greater abundance of sequences involved in degradation of xylans than for degradation of β-glucans in the ceca, which contrasts with the relative dominance of β glucanase activity over xylanase in the small intestine [53].

Enzymes involved in xylan and cellobiose degradation are similarly distributed across three main bacterial classes, *Actinobacteria*, *Clostridia* and *Bacteroidia* (Figure 2). However, among endoglucanases, there appears to be a relative under-representation of the *Actinobacteria*, with greater contributions from the *Negativicutes* and *Lentisphaerae* (in particular the species *Victivallis vadensis*).

In order to reap the benefits of extracellular non-starch polysaccharides (NSP) degradation, bacteria exploit multi-protein cellulosomes, characterized by dockerin motifs, or isolated cellulases which use carbohydrate binding modules (CBM) to attach to the substrate [52,54]. However, in our dataset, only 51 of 9498 GH domains were attached to binding modules and only two were attached to dockerin motifs (Table S3), again suggesting an absence or paucity of conventional cellulase activity.

Another complex enabling bacteria to exploit NSP degredation, which are present in *Bacteroides*, are polysaccharide utilization systems (PUL), which digest and import the products of polysaccharide degradation [55]. We found evidence of over 500 such systems in the *Bacteriodetes* from the chicken cecum, including representatives of a novel class of PUL recently identified in the Tammar Wallaby foregut that incorporates β-1,4 endoglucanases and β-1,4 endoxylanases [55] (Figure 3A).

We found additional genetic evidence of co-ordination of polysaccharide degradation with sugar transport and utilization (Figure 3B) – for example, in *Megamonas*, we found a gene cluster encoding secreted endo-glucanases, a cellobiose phosphotransferase system and a 6-phospho-beta-glucocidase, which together probably form an extracellular complex capable of degrading NSPs to cellobiose, which is then imported and cleaved to give D-glucose.

Some endoglucanases were not associated with regulatory genes or sugar transporters and therefore may not be involved in the exploitation of NSP for energy. For example, it has been suggested that some cellulase genes might be involved in biosynthesis of cellulose [56], as evidenced by their association in operons with cellulose synthesis genes. We found no evidence of biosynthetic cellulose activity in the chicken microbiome. However, we found two endoglucanase genes in a *Clostridiales* genome that were associated with sporulation genes (Figure 3C), which leads us to speculate that such endoglucanase genes may be implicated in breakdown of the cell wall or formation of the spore cortex.

Production of short-chain volatile fatty acids

Short-chain volatile fatty acids (SCFAs), such as acetic acid, propionic acid and butyric acid, are produced by microbial fermentation of the sugars released from non-starch polysaccharides and are found in the chicken ceca [57]. SCFAs elicit several beneficial effects. Absorption of SCFAs across the gut mucosa contributes to the nutrition of the chicken (6). In addition, SCFAs can inhibit the growth of pathogens and improve mineral absorption [17].

We found abundant evidence of acetate fermentation in the chicken cecal metagenome, with over 30 acetate kinase/phosphotransferase sequences (Table S4). One of pathways to propionate fermentation, the Wood-Werkman cycle, is poorly represented, with two methylmalonyl-CoA carboxytransferase genes found at low coverage (Figure 4A). However, an alternative propionate fermentation pathway, which exploits methylmalonyl-CoA decarboxylase and methylmalonyl-CoA epimerase appears to be well represented in this microbial community, with many genes encoding these enzymes (Figure 4A). As expected, we found that gene clusters from the *Bacteroidetes* that encode the alpha subunit also encode the beta, gamma and delta subunits of methylmalonyl-CoA decarboxylase together with methylmalonyl epimerase (Figure 4B). However, similar gene clusters from *Megamonas* and *Dialister* appear to lack genes for the beta subunit, which couples decarboxylation to export of Na^+ across the membrane, and the delta subunit, which holds the complex together [58]. Instead these clusters encode a ferredoxin gene, which, we speculate, may be involved in coupling decarboxylation to electron transport in a novel propionate fermentation pathway.

The first committed step in butyrate production is the conversion of crotonoyl-CoA to butyryl-CoA by 3-hydroxybutyryl-CoA dehydrogenase (BCD) [59]. Assignment of this enzyme to KEGG or SEED categories is hampered by similarities of this enzyme to acyl-CoA dehydrogenases involved in lipid metabolism. In butyrate-producing bacteria the BCD gene is found in an operon adjacent to electron transferring flavoproteins (ETF). The BCD:ETF complex conserves the energy of the reaction, which is believed to be used to generate proton-motive force [60].

We searched the chicken cecal microbiome for BCD sequences, using a protein-sequence-based hidden Markov model, twinned with evidence from genetic context (co-occurrence with adjacent ETF genes). This approach yielded nineteen sequences, mostly from *Bacteroidetes* and *Firmicutes*, but also a single sequence from

Escherichia spp (Figure 5A). In one *Firmicutes* EGT, there was enough adjacent sequence to reveal genomic context, which included the classic BDH operon structure [61] (Figure 5B). However in *Bacteroidetes* and *Escherichia*, the order of the BCD and ETF genes differed and they were not adjacent to other genes in the butyrate fermentation pathway.

After the formation of butyryl–CoA, butyrate fermentation can proceed either by butyryl-CoA:acetate:CoA transferase or via the enzymes phosphotransbutyrylase and butyrate kinase (Figure 5A). The former pathway is by far the most commonly used by butyrate-producing bacteria isolated from the human gut [61]. We detected only four sequences encoding butyryl-CoA:acetate:CoA transferase in our chicken cecal metagenome. This is in line with results from a recent study of butyrate-producing bacteria cultured from chicken ceca [62], where fewer than half the isolates contained the butyryl-CoA:aceate: CoA transferase gene, leading to speculation that another as yet unidentified acyl transferase might substitute for the canonical butyryl-CoA: acetate CoA transferase in some butyrate fermentation pathways. We found nineteen sequences corresponding to phosphotransbutylase and butyrate kinase, including seven from the *Bacteroidetes*. As *Bacteroidetes* appear to contain an energy conserving BCD/ETF complex and phosphotransbutylase/butyrate kinase genes, we speculate that they might have the potential to produce butyrate. In this context, it is worth noting that, although butyrate production is not generally associated with *Bacteroidetes* grown in culture, butyrate has been shown to be produced by *Bacteroides* spp, in colonized germ free mice [63].

Hydrogen sinks within the cecal microbiota

One of the goals of metagenomics, and of microbial ecology in general, is to explain why some taxa are so much more abundant than others in a given microbiology community. We speculated that high species abundance might be explained in the chicken cecal microbiome by the need for hydrogen sinks within this ecosystem.

During fermentation, NADH formed through glycolysis needs to be recycled to NAD^+. This can be achieved through reduction of pyruvate or acetyl CoA to SCFAs. Fermentation to acetate produces the most ATP by substrate level phosphorylation, but this route allows little NADH to be recycled. Hydrogenases provide an alternative route for NADH recycling, but one that leads to the production of molecular hydrogen [47]. Hydrogenases are inhibited by high levels of their own product, so without a sink for hydrogen within an ecosystem, accumulation of hydrogen leads to reduced fermentation and/or less energy-efficient fermentation to substances such as ethanol, butyrate and propionate [19,64]. The presence of bacteria that can act as a hydrogen sink not only results in a switch to the more productive fermentation to acetate, but also increased production of SCFAs which bring benefits to the host.

In some enteric microbiotas, methanogens act as major consumers of hydrogen. However, in our dataset, we found no evidence of potential methanogens (members of the *Euryarchaeota*), even though they have been reported in chicken cecal samples in other studies [65]. Sulfate reducers are also potential hydrogen consumer, but we found no evidence of *Desulfovibrio* spp. in our 16S and metagenomic data. Acetogenesis, the reduction of CO_2 to acetyl-CoA, provides another potential hydrogen sink, but we detected only six acetyl CoA synthase genes, (from the *Ruminococcae* and *Lachnospiraceae*) in our dataset (table S5 and Fig. 6).

Bacterial uptake NiFe hydrogenases link the oxidation of H_2 to the reduction of anaerobic electron acceptors such as NO_3^-, SO_4^-, fumarate or CO_2 [47]. Bacteria that possess these enzymes (such as *Wollinella* and *Campylobacter*) could potentially provide a significant hydrogen sink capable of facilitating acetate production in microbial ecosystems [66,67]. We found sequences for twelve uptake hydrogenases in our chicken cecal metagenome (Figure 6 and table S5), in several of the most abundant genera in this ecosystem (*Megamonas*, *Helicobacter*, *Campylobacter*). We speculate that the high abundance of these genera in the chicken cecum might, at least in part, be explained by their potential to remove hydrogen, which is likely to benefit not only the other members of the microbial community, but also, indirectly, the host, by improving recovery of energy from food.

Supporting Information

Figure S1 Relationship Between Size of OTU and Percentage Identity to Genbank Sequences. Graph showing relationship between the number of reads in an OTU and its percentage identity to the closest match in the NCBI nr database. Those OTUs showing limited homology still were comprised of many reads hence increasing the validity of the OTU.

Figure S2 Summary of Previous Studies on the Chicken Metagenome. Graph showing the relative amounts of different taxa within the chicken ceca from a number of different studies using different techniques (1). J.H.A. Apajalahti and A. Kettunen p. 124–126 in G. Perry, ed. *Avian Gut Function in Health and Disease*,2006. (2). W.E. Holben, K.P. Feris, A. Kettunen and J.H.A Apajalahti Appl. Envron. Microb, 70:2263–2270, 2004. (3). J.R. Lu, U. Idris, B. Harmon, C. Hofacre, J.J. Maurer and M.D. Lee. App. Environ. Microb. 69:6186–6823, 2003. ().G.R. Siragusa and M.G. Wise J. Appl. Microb. 102:1138–1149, 2007. (5). M.D. Cressman, Z. Yu, M.C. Nelson, S.J. Moeller, M.S. Liburn and H.N. Zerby. Appl Environ Microbiol 76:6572–6582 2010. (6). J.L. Danzeisen, H.B. Kim, R.E. Isaacson, Z.J. Tu and T.J. Johnson. Plos One 6:e27949. 2011 (7). This study.

Figure S3 Taxonomic Assignment of Metagenomic data. (A) The percentage of each EGT that could be assigned to a given taxonomic level. EGTs were assigned taxonomy based on the protein coding sequences they contained (see methods). (B) Comparison of phylogenetic assignment from pyrosequenced 16S amplicons and EGTs. (i) 260 000 110 bp reads assigned by MEGAN using the Least Common Ancestor algorithm. (ii) Taxonomic assignment of protein sequences from the assembled metagenomic data, abundance corrected by coverage. (iii) Taxonomic distribution of the genomes, abundance corrected by coverage and size of genome. (iv). Taxonomy of 16S, assigned using the rdp database project taxonomy.

Figure S4 Organization of the Metagenomic Data. (A) Flow diagram of the procedures used to analyse the metagenomic data. Grey boxes show the programs that were used for each step (B) Database scheama showing the structure of the MySQL database holding the metagenomic information.

Figure S5 Comparison of OTU pipelines. (A) Rareaction curves for each OTU picking method. The four reps for each chicken were merged (i) Mothur (ii) Custom (iii) Uparse. (B) PCA plots showing differences in OTU composition of each chicken (colour) when analysed by different pipelines (circle Uparse, triangle custom method and square Mothur). OTUs were merged according to taxonomic assignment by the RDP classifier at the family level. The axes represent the two principal components which are responsible for the most variation in the samples.

Table S1 Summary of the reads obtained for each of the 10 chickens.

Table S2 Broad Taxonomic assignment of a subset of reads from the chicken metagenome.

Table S3 Genes which contain both GH motifs and carbohydrate binding motifs (CBMs) or dockerin motifs.

Table S4 Predicted acetate kinase/phosphotransferase loci present in the chicken metagenome.

Table S5 Predicted Acetyl CoA synthase genes and the large subunit of uptake hydrogenases present in the Chicken metagenome.

Table S6 The assignment of putative NSP degrading enzymes based on SEED/KEGG annotation and GH domains.

Text S1 Comparisons of different techniques to cluster reads into OTUs from raw reads.

Data S1 List of all OTUs showing assigned taxonomy and their relative abundance in each sample.

Data S2 Table of antibiotic resistance genes present in the metagenome.

Acknowledgments

We thank Jan Kreft for suggestions that we should investigate the hydrogen metabolism of the chicken cecal microbiota.

Data deposition: The sequence reads reported in this paper have been deposited in the Sequence Read Archive (Accession no SRP019776). The EGTs are deposited the WGS database at NCBI (Accession no. SUB195828). Annotated EGTs and OTU information can also be accessed at the chicken microbiome project website (http://chickenmicrobiome.xbase.ac.uk/).

Author Contributions

Conceived and designed the experiments: MJP CWP. Performed the experiments: MJS CC. Analyzed the data: MJS. Contributed reagents/materials/analysis tools: TAC. Wrote the paper: MJS CWP MRB MJP.

References

1. Fumihito A, Miyake T, Takada M, Shingu R, Endo T, et al. (1996) Monophyletic origin and unique dispersal patterns of domestic fowls. Proc Natl Acad Sci U S A 93: 6792–6795.
2. Harre R (1981) Aristotle: the embryology of the chick. Great scientific experiments Oxford: Phaidon. 31–38.
3. Darwin C (1868) The variation of animals and plants under domestication. London: Murray.
4. Burt DW (2007) Emergence of the chicken as a model organism: implications for agriculture and biology. Poult Sci 86: 1460–1471.
5. Hillier LW, Miller W, Birney E, Warren W, Hardison RC, et al. (2004) Sequence and comparative analysis of the chicken genome provide unique perspectives on vertebrate evolution. Nature 432: 695–716.
6. McWhorter TJ, Caviedes-Vidal E, Karasov WH (2009) The integration of digestion and osmoregulation in the avian gut. Biol Rev 84: 533–565.
7. Apajalahti J (2005) Comparative gut microflora, metabolic challenges, and potential opportunities. J Appl Poultry Res 14: 444–453.
8. Zhou W, Wang Y, Lin J (2012) Functional Cloning and Characterization of Antibiotic Resistance Genes from the Chicken Gut Microbiome. Appl Environ Microb 78: 3028–3032.
9. Huyghebaert G, Ducatelle R, Van Immerseel F (2011) An update on alternatives to antimicrobial growth promoters for broilers. Vet J 187: 182–188.
10. Clench MH, Mathias JR (1995) The Avian Cecum – a Review. Wilson Bull 107: 93–121.
11. Karasawa Y (1999) Significant role of the nitrogen recycling system through the ceca occurs in protein-depleted chickens. J Exp Zool 283: 418–425.
12. Mcnab JM (1973) Avian Ceca – Review. World Poultry Sci J 29: 251–263.
13. Obst BS, Diamond JM (1989) Interspecific Variation in Sugar and Amino-Acid-Transport by the Avian Cecum. J Exp Zool: 117–126.
14. Jozefiak D, Rutkowski A, Martin SA (2004) Carbohydrate fermentation in the avian ceca: a review. Animal Feed Science and Technology 113: 1–15.
15. Hegde SN, Rolls BA, Coates ME (1982) THe effects of the gut microflora and dietary fibre on energy utilization by the chick. Br J Nutr 48: 73–80.
16. Jorgensen H, Zhao XQ, Knudsen KE, Eggum BO (1996) The influence of dietary fibre source and level on the development of the gastrointestinal tract, digestibility and energy metabolism in broiler chickens. Br J Nutr 75: 379–395.
17. Van Immerseel F, Boyen F, Gantois I, Timbermont L, Bohez L, et al. (2005) Supplementation of coated butyric acid in the feed reduces colonization and shedding of Salmonella in poultry. Poultry Sci 84: 1851–1856.
18. Kien CL, Blauwiekel R, Bunn JY, Jetton TL, Frankel WL, et al. (2007) Cecal infusion of butyrate increases intestinal cell proliferation in piglets. J Nutr 137: 916–922.
19. Stams AJM (1994) Metabolic Interactions between Anaerobic-Bacteria in Methanogenic Environments. Anton Leeuw Int J G 66: 271–294.
20. Salanitr JP, Blake IG, Muirhead PA (1974) Studies on Cecal Microflora of Commercial Broiler Chickens. Appl Microbiol 28: 439–447.
21. Salanitro JP, Blake IG, Muirhead PA, Maglio M, Goodman JR (1978) Bacteria Isolated from Duodenum, Ileum, and Cecum of Young Chicks. Appl Environ Microb 35: 782–790.
22. Mead GC (1989) Microbes of the Avian Cecum – Types Present and Substrates Utilized. J Exp Zool: 48–54.
23. Zhu XY, Zhong TY, Pandya Y, Joerger RD (2002) 16S rRNA-based analysis of microbiota from the cecum of broiler chickens. Appl Environ Microb 68: 124–137.
24. Lan PT, Hayashi H, Sakamoto M, Benno Y (2002) Phylogenetic analysis of cecal microbiota in chicken by the use of 16S rDNA clone libraries. Microbiology and Immunology 46: 371–382.
25. Lu JR, Idris U, Harmon B, Hofacre C, Maurer JJ, et al. (2003) Diversity and succession of the intestinal bacterial community of the maturing broiler chicken. Appl Environ Microb 69: 6816–6824.
26. Amit-Romach E, Sklan D, Uni Z (2004) Microflora ecology of the chicken intestine using 16S ribosomal DNA primers. Poultry Sci 83: 1093–1098.
27. Wei S, Morrison M, Yu Z (2013) Bacterial census of poultry intestinal microbiome. Poult Sci 92: 671–683.
28. Danzeisen JL, Kim HB, Isaacson RE, Tu ZJ, Johnson TJ (2011) Modulations of the Chicken Cecal Microbiome and Metagenome in Response to Anticoccidial and Growth Promoter Treatment. Plos One 6: e27949.
29. Qu A, Brulc JM, Wilson MK, Law BF, Theoret JR, et al. (2008) Comparative Metagenomics Reveals Host Specific Metavirulomes and Horizontal Gene Transfer Elements in the Chicken Cecum Microbiome. Plos One 3.
30. Kim T, Mundt E (2011) Metagenomic analysis of intestinal microbiomes in chickens. Methods Mol Biol 733: 185–194.
31. Sergeant MJ, Constantinidou C, Cogan T, Penn CW, Pallen MJ (2012) High-Throughput Sequencing of 16S rRNA Gene Amplicons: Effects of Extraction Procedure, Primer Length and Annealing Temperature. Plos One 7: e38094.
32. Edgar RC (2013) UPARSE: highly accurate OTU sequences from microbial amplicon reads. Nat Methods 10: 996–998.
33. Caporaso JG, Kuczynski J, Stombaugh J, Bittinger K, Bushman FD, et al. (2010) QIIME allows analysis of high-throughput community sequencing data. Nat Methods 7: 335–336.
34. Noguchi H, Park J, Takagi T (2006) MetaGene: prokaryotic gene finding from environmental genome shotgun sequences. Nucleic Acids Res 34: 5623–5630.
35. Huson DH, Auch AF, Qi J, Schuster SC (2007) MEGAN analysis of metagenomic data. Genome Res 17: 377–386.
36. Li H, Durbin R (2009) Fast and accurate short read alignment with Burrows-Wheeler transform. Bioinformatics 25: 1754–1760.
37. Eddy SR (1998) Hidden Markov models and genome sequence analysis. Faseb J 12: A1327–A1327.
38. Punta M, Coggill PC, Eberhardt RY, Mistry J, Tate J, et al. (2012) The Pfam protein families database. Nucleic Acids Res 40: D290–D301.

39. Petersen TN, Brunak S, von Heijne G, Nielsen H (2011) SignalP 4.0: discriminating signal peptides from transmembrane regions. Nat Methods 8: 785–786.
40. Liu B, Pop M (2009) ARDB-Antibiotic Resistance Genes Database. Nucleic Acids Res 37: D443–D447.
41. de Castro E, Sigrist CJA, Gattiker A, Bulliard V, Langendijk-Genevaux PS, et al. (2006) ScanProsite: detection of PROSITE signature matches and ProRule-associated functional and structural residues in proteins. Nucleic Acids Res 34: W362–W365.
42. Teeling H, Meyerdierks A, Bauer M, Amann R, Glockner FO (2004) Application of tetranucleotide frequencies for the assignment of genomic fragments. Environ Microbiol 6: 938–947.
43. Schloss PD, Westcott SL, Ryabin T, Hall JR, Hartmann M, et al. (2009) Introducing mothur: Open-Source, Platform-Independent, Community-Supported Software for Describing and Comparing Microbial Communities. Appl Environ Microb 75: 7537–7541.
44. Warnecke F, Luginbuhl P, Ivanova N, Ghassemian M, Richardson TH, et al. (2007) Metagenomic and functional analysis of hindgut microbiota of a wood-feeding higher termite. Nature 450: 560–U517.
45. Cantarel BL, Coutinho PM, Rancurel C, Bernard T, Lombard V, et al. (2009) The Carbohydrate-Active EnZymes database (CAZy): an expert resource for Glycogenomics. Nucleic Acids Res 37: D233–D238.
46. Louis P, Flint HJ (2007) Development of a semiquantitative degenerate real-time PCR-based assay for estimation of numbers of butyryl-coenzyme A (CoA) CoA transferase genes in complex bacterial samples. Appl Environ Microb 73: 2009–2012.
47. Vignais PM, Billoud B (2007) Occurrence, classification, and biological function of hydrogenases: An overview. Chem Rev 107: 4206–4272.
48. Gagen EJ, Denman SE, Padmanabha J, Zadbuke S, Al Jassim R, et al. (2010) Functional Gene Analysis Suggests Different Acetogen Populations in the Bovine Rumen and Tammar Wallaby Forestomach. Appl Environ Microb 76: 7785–7795.
49. Torok VA, Allison GE, Percy NJ, Ophel-Keller K, Hughes RJ (2011) Influence of antimicrobial feed additives on broiler commensal posthatch gut microbiota development and performance. Appl Environ Microbiol 77: 3380–3390.
50. Siragusa GR, Wise MG (2007) Quantitative analysis of the intestinal bacterial community in one- to three-week-old commercially reared broiler chickens fed conventional or antibiotic-free vegetable-based diets. J Appl Microbiol 102: 1138–1149.
51. Clokie MR, Millard AD, Letarov AV, Heaphy S (2011) Phages in nature. Bacteriophage 1: 31–45.
52. Warren RAJ (1996) Microbial hydrolysis of polysaccharides. Annu Rev Microbiol 50: 183–212.
53. Hubener K, Vahjen W, Simon O (2002) Bacterial responses to different dietary cereal types and xylanase supplementation in the intestine of broiler chicken. Arch Anim Nutr 56: 167–187.
54. Bayer EA, Belaich JP, Shoham Y, Lamed R (2004) The cellulosomes: Multienzyme machines for degradation of plant cell wall polysaccharides. Annu Rev Microbiol 58: 521–554.
55. Pope PB, Denman SE, Jones M, Tringe SG, Barry K, et al. (2010) Adaptation to herbivory by the Tammar wallaby includes bacterial and glycoside hydrolase profiles different from other herbivores. P Natl Acad Sci USA 107: 14793–14798.
56. Medie FM, Davies GJ, Drancourt M, Henrissat B (2012) Genome analyses highlight the different biological roles of cellulases. Nat Rev Microbiol 10: 227–U.
57. Meimandipour A, Soleimanifarjam A, Azhar K, Hair-Bejo M, Shuhaimi M, et al. (2011) Age effects on short chain fatty acids concentrations and pH values in the gastrointestinal tract of broiler chickens. Arch Geflugelkd 75: 164–168.
58. Bott M, Pfister K, Burda P, Kalbermatter O, Woehlke G, et al. (1997) Methylmalonyl-CoA decarboxylase from Propionigenium modestum cloning and sequencing of the structural genes and purification of the enzyme complex. Eur J Biochem 250: 590–599.
59. Colby GD, Chen JS (1992) Purification and Properties of 3-Hydroxybutyryl-Coenzyme-a Dehydrogenase from Clostridium-Beijerinckii (Clostridium Butylicum) Nrrl-B593. Appl Environ Microb 58: 3297–3302.
60. Louis P, Flint HJ (2009) Diversity, metabolism and microbial ecology of butyrate-producing bacteria from the human large intestine. Fems Microbiol Lett 294: 1–8.
61. Louis P, McCrae SI, Charrier C, Flint HJ (2007) Organization of butyrate synthetic genes in human colonic bacteria: phylogenetic conservation and horizontal gene transfer. Fems Microbiol Lett 269: 240–247.
62. Eeckhaut V, Van Immerseel F, Croubels S, De Baere S, Haesebrouck F, et al. (2011) Butyrate production in phylogenetically diverse Firmicutes isolated from the chicken caecum. Microb Biotechnol 4: 503–512.
63. Eastwood M (1995) Dietary fibre: mechanisms of action in human physiology and metabolism.
64. Macfarlane S, Macfarlane GT (2003) Regulation of short-chain fatty acid production. P Nutr Soc 62: 67–72.
65. Saengkerdsub S, Anderson RC, Wilkinson HH, Kim W-K, Nisbet DJ, et al. (2007) Identification and quantification of methanogenic archaea in adult chicken ceca. Appl Environ Microb 73: 353–356.
66. Howlett RM, Hughes BM, Hitchcock A, Kelly DJ (2012) Hydrogenase activity in the foodborne pathogen Campylobacter jejuni depends upon a novel ABC-type nickel transporter (NikZYXWV) and is SlyD-independent. Microbiology 158: 1645–1655.
67. Gross R, Simon J (2003) The hydE gene is essential for the formation of Wolinella succinogenes NiFe-hydrogenase. Fems Microbiol Lett 227: 197–202.
68. Allgaier M, Reddy A, Park JI, Ivanova N, D'Haeseleer P, et al. (2010) Targeted discovery of glycoside hydrolases from a switchgrass-adapted compost community. Plos One 5: e8812.
69. Zhu LF, Wu Q, Dai JY, Zhang SN, Wei FW (2011) Evidence of cellulose metabolism by the giant panda gut microbiome. P Natl Acad Sci USA 108: 17714–17719.
70. Hess M, Sczyrba A, Egan R, Kim TW, Chokhawala H, et al. (2011) Metagenomic Discovery of Biomass-Degrading Genes and Genomes from Cow Rumen. Science 331: 463–467.

6

Inhibition of Lipolysis in the Novel Transgenic Quail Model Overexpressing G_0/G_1 Switch Gene 2 in the Adipose Tissue during Feed Restriction

Sangsu Shin[1], Young Min Choi[1], Jae Yong Han[2], Kichoon Lee[1]*

1 Department of Animal Sciences, The Ohio State University, Columbus, Ohio, United States of America, **2** World Class University Biomodulation Major, Department of Agricultural Biotechnology, Research Institute for Agriculture and Life Sciences, College of Agriculture and Life Sciences, Seoul National University, Seoul, Korea

Abstract

In addition to the issue of obesity in humans, the production of low-fat meat from domestic animals is important in the agricultural industry to satisfy consumer demand. Understanding the regulation of lipolysis in adipose tissue could advance our knowledge to potentially solve both issues. Although the G_0/G_1 switch gene 2 (G0S2) was recently identified as an inhibitor of adipose triglyceride lipase (ATGL) *in vitro*, its role *in vivo* has not been fully clarified. This study was conducted to investigate the role of G0S2 gene *in vivo* by using two independent transgenic quail lines during different energy conditions. Unexpectedly, G0S2 overexpression had a negligible effect on plasma NEFA concentration, fat cell size and fat pad weight under *ad libitum* feeding condition when adipose lipolytic activity is minimal. A two-week feed restriction in non-transgenic quail expectedly caused increased plasma NEFA concentration and dramatically reduced fat cell size and fat pad weight. Contrary, G0S2 overexpression under a feed restriction resulted in a significantly less elevation of plasma NEFA concentration and smaller reductions in fat pad weights and fat cell size compared to non-transgenic quail, demonstrating inhibition of lipolysis and resistance to loss of fat by G0S2. Excessive G0S2 inhibits lipolysis *in vivo* during active lipolytic conditions, such as food restriction and fasting, suggesting G0S2 as a potential target for treatment of obesity. In addition, transgenic quail are novel models for studying lipid metabolism and mechanisms of obesity.

Editor: Raul M. Luque, University of Cordoba, Spain

Funding: This work was supported by Korea Research Foundation (KRF-2009-220-F00006), Next-Generation BioGreen 21 Program (No. PJ008142012013) funded by Rural Development Administration of Republic of Korea and by Agriculture and Food Research Initiative Competitive Grant no. 2010-65206-20716 from the USDA National Institute of Food and Agriculture. The funders had no role in study design, data collection and analysis, decision to publish, or preparation of the manuscript.

Competing Interests: The authors have declared that no competing interests exist.

* Email: lee.2626@osu.edu

Introduction

Obesity is considered a major health problem in an increasing number of countries and is underscored by adiposity. Adiposity collectively refers to fat cell numbers and sizes in the body and is regulated by developmental, nutritional, and hormonal signals. Major health issues closely associated with obesity include diabetes, hypertension, and cardiovascular diseases. In adult animals, including humans, changes in adipose tissue mass mainly result from plasticity of adipocyte sizes rather than from changes in cell numbers. Mature adipocytes are composed of 70 - 90% triacylglycerides (TAG) that are synthesized and hydrolyzed in response to energy status, regulating adipocyte size and consequently affecting fat mass. In addition, it is important to produce low-fat meat in the agricultural industry as providing a high-quality meat is a possible approach to reducing obesity.

Recent discoveries in the initial process of lipolysis to hydrolyze TAG into a fatty acid and diacylglycerol (DAG) revealed a complicated regulation of adipocyte size [1–3]. Adipose triglyceride lipase (ATGL, also named patatin-like phospholipase domain containing protein 2) is a recently discovered TAG hydrolase, which is considered a major initiator of lipolysis in adipose tissues [1,4–7]. ATGL is mainly expressed in adipose tissues, and a deficiency of ATGL in mice causes excessive accumulation of fat [8]. ATGL is composed of a patatin domain, which has an active site for its enzyme activity, and a hydrophobic domain for binding to lipid droplets (LD) required for ATGL enzyme activity [2,9–11]. There are two major regulators of ATGL activity identified to date. Activation of ATGL requires comparative gene identification-58 (CGI-58), which recruits ATGL to the LD by binding directly to the amino acid sequence within the patatin domain of ATGL [2,11,12]. Another regulator of ATGL is the G_0/G_1 switch gene 2 (G0S2), which was recently identified as an inhibitor of ATGL in 3T3-L1 adipocytes [3]. Comparative analysis of G0S2 amino acid sequences among animals and humans revealed a conservation of the hydrophobic domain, which is required for binding directly to the patatin domain of ATGL [3,13,14]. Similar to ATGL, G0S2 expression is mainly found in adipose tissues and is greatly up-regulated during preadipocyte differentiation in humans, mice, pigs, and avian species [3,13–17]. In adipose tissues, G0S2 is more highly expressed in mature fat cells containing TAG than in preadipocytes, which suggests that G0S2 is closely related to fat metabolism. The expression of G0S2 in adipose tissues is also regulated by feeding conditions. Feeding conditions promote up-regulation while down-regulation occurs during fasting, further supporting the inhibitory role of

G0S2 in ATGL-mediated lipolysis [13,14,17]. Nutrition-dependent expression pattern of G0S2 usually displays an inverse relationship to ATGL expression; however, these findings need to be further validated to provide direct evidence for the inhibitory function of G0S2 *in vivo*.

Herein, we produced transgenic quail that overexpressed the G0S2 gene in adipose tissues to investigate the role of G0S2 *in vivo*. To test whether the exogenous G0S2 could affect fat metabolism depending on the energy conditions, quail were subjected to an *ad libitum* feeding condition, when the amounts of ATGL expression are very low and endogenous G0S2 expression is very high, as well as a feed restriction condition, when the amounts of ATGL expression are very high and G0S2 expression is low.

Materials and Methods

Experimental quail and ethics statement

Japanese quail (*Coturnix coturnix japonica*) used in this study were maintained in the poultry center at The Ohio State University (OSU). The quail were always allowed to access feed *ad libitum*, except in the feed restriction study. For feed restriction that ran in parallel with *ad libitum* feeding, each quail was fed *ad libitum* until 6 weeks of age and then restricted to 12 g (about 60% of daily normal intake) of feed per day for 2 weeks. To investigate the role of G0S2 under the various feeding conditions, five to eight male quail hatched from the same parents were used for each non-transgenic or transgenic group for both lines. For the fasting experiment, all four groups of quail were fasted for 4 or 12 hours at 7 weeks of age. All of the experimental procedures were conducted in accordance with protocols approved by the Institutional Animal Care and Use Committee (IACUC) of OSU and the Prevention of Cruelty to Animals Act (1986).

Vector construction

The chicken G0S2 gene was amplified from cDNA of chicken adipose tissue by PCR with forward, 5′- GCCTCAGAACG-GAGCTCTTCCT -3′, and reverse, 5′- GCAGCA-GAGCCGTGTGCT -3′, primers and cloned into the pCR2.1 (Invitrogen, Carlsbad, CA, USA) cloning vector [14]. For the adipose tissue-specific promoter, the 2 kb upstream promoter region of the chicken fatty acid binding protein 4 (cFABP4) gene was amplified from chicken genomic DNA by PCR with forward, 5′-CAGGTGCTTCAACTCTCTCCCAA-3′, and reverse, 5′-CAGGCCAGGTAGCAGTCTTTCAC-3′, primers and cloned into the pCR2.1 vector. To generate the pLT-cFABP4-cG0S2 lentiviral vector, cFABP4 promoter and cG0S2 gene were replaced to sites of the RSV promoter and green fluorescence protein gene, respectively, of pLTReGW vector described in our previous report [18].

Production and concentration of lentivirus

The lentivirus was produced by the methods used by Shin et al. [18]. Briefly, one third of the 95% confluent 293FT cells (Invitrogen) in a 100 mm culture dish were seeded one day before transfection, fed with fresh medium two hours before transfection, and co-transfected with 10 µg of transfer vector (pLT-cFABP4-cG0S2) and 10 µg of packaging mixture (pLP1, pLP2, and pLP/VSVG; Invitrogen) using calcium-phosphate co-precipitation for 6 hours. The medium was replaced with 5 ml fresh culture medium. After 2 days of transfection, the medium containing the virus was harvested, filtrated, and concentrated to 100 X by ultracentrifugation (Beckman Coulter, Inc., Brea, CA, USA) at 26,000 rpm for 2 hours.

Production of the founder quails

Fresh eggs of wild-type Japanese quail were cleaned and sanitized with 70% ethanol and placed laterally on a tray for 4 hours. After sanitizing the eggs again with 70% ethanol, a small window about 5 mm in diameter was made on the lateral apex of the eggshell using fine-tip tweezers. Then, 1 to 2 µl of concentrated virus was injected into the subgerminal cavity by using the microinjection system (Tritech Research, Inc., Los Angeles, CA, USA) under a stereomicroscope (Olympus America Inc., Center Valley, PA, USA). After sealing the window with paraffin film, the eggs were incubated for 14 days at 37.5°C and 60% relative humidity and then transferred to a hatching tray. The hatched chicks were grown until sexually mature.

Testcross and selection of transgenic offspring

The mature individual founder was mated with wild-type quail by placing a male founder with two female wild-type quail or one female founder with one male wild-type quail in a cage. The eggs were numbered, collected daily for one week, and stored in a cold room (13°C) until incubating. The hatched chicks were tagged and reared for 10 days to collect the feather pulp for extracting genomic DNA. The pulp from 1 to 2 feathers was incubated in 300 µl of the cell lysis buffer (200 mM NaCl, 50 mM Tris-Cl, 10 mM EDTA, 1% SDS, pH 8.0) containing proteinase K (0.1 mg/ml, Invitrogen) at 55°C for more than 3 hours. To remove the protein, 100 µl of 7.5 M ammonium acetate was added to the tube, mixed vigorously and then centrifuged at 13,000×*g* for 10 min. The supernatant was transferred to a new tube, and genomic DNA was precipitated by centrifuging after adding and mixing 300 µl of isopropanol. The pellet was washed with 70% ethanol followed by drying and dissolving in TE buffer containing RNase A (10 µg/ml, Qiagen, Valencia, CA, USA). Genomic DNA was used for genotyping PCR with a primer set, LTG0S2-F: 5′- GAGAAGAGACCGAGCCCATC -3′ for forward primer and LT-R: 5′- CGGGCCACAACTCCTCATAA -3′ for reverse primer. The positive offspring were chosen and reconfirmed by PCR with primers, LTG0S2-F and WPRE-R: 5′-AAGGGAGATCCGACTCGTCT -3′for reverse primer. Integration sites of transgene were identified by using the SiteFinding PCR [19]. The SiteFinding PCR was conducted with the primer of SiteFinder-1 and, then, the primary nested PCR was followed by adding the primer mixture of SFP1 and LT-TSP1 (5′-ACTGACAATTCCGTGGTGTT -3′). The PCR product was diluted into 100 µl of distilled water and used as a template for the secondary PCR. The secondary PCR was conducted with primer sets of SFP2 and LT-TSP2: 5′- ACGAGTCGGATCT-CCCTTTG -3′ or LT-TSP3: 5′- TGTGCCCGTCTGTT-GTGTGA -3′. The bands showing a different size of about 0.3 kb, which is caused by the different position of LT-TSP2 and LT-TSP3, were selected and analyzed to identify the sequences. Nucleotide sequences from each transgenic quail were used to compare the genomic location and sequence homology with chicken at the UCSC Genome Bioinformatics Site (http://genome.ucsc.edu/).

Tissue collection and weighing

After analyzing exogenous G0S2 expression levels of transgenic lines, two lines, FG1 and FG3, were selected for further study. Five F1 transgenic quail were selected and mated with wild-type quail to produce F2 offspring. Transgenic and non-transgenic male quail were selected by PCR using the primers LTG0S2-F, LT-R, and WPRE-R to detect the transgene, and USP1 and 3 to detect the W-specific DNA fragment [20]. Body weight was measured weekly from hatch until sacrifice at 8 weeks of age. After sacrifice, abdominal fat, subcutaneous fat (Figure S1), left pectoralis muscle, thigh muscle, heart, liver, lung, and kidney tissues were obtained and weighed. Blood samples for the short-term fasting condition were collected after fasting for 4 hours at 7 weeks of age. Other blood samples were collected before sacrifice at 8 weeks of age. After clotting, serum was separated by centrifuging at 1,500×*g* for 15 min. All tissue and serum samples were stored in a -80°C freezer until further study.

Antibody production and Western blotting

Protein samples were prepared from tissues by grinding with radioimmunoprecipitation assay buffer and centrifuging at 15,000×*g* for 10 min. The G0S2 protein on the membrane was probed with an rabbit anti-chicken G0S2 antibody, which was developed in our laboratory, and an anti-rabbit IgG antibody conjugated with horseradish peroxidase (HRP; Jackson ImmunoResearch, West Grove, PA, USA) was used for detection with an enhanced chemiluminescence system (ECL plus; Amersham, Pittsburgh, PA, USA) and Hyperfilm (Amersham). The specificities of antibodies for quail ATGL and FABP4 proteins were previously demonstrated [21,22]. After probing the membranes with these ATGL and FABP antibodies, the membranes were incubated with proper secondary antibodies conjugated with HRP. The amount of alpha-tubulin for reference was determined with an anti-alpha-tubulin antibody (12G10; Developmental Studies Hybridoma Bank, Iowa City, IA, USA) and an anti-mouse IgG antibody conjugated with HRP (Cell Signaling Technology, Danvers, MA, USA). The density of the band was determined by using the ImageJ program (NIH, Bethesda, MD, USA).

Histochemistry and cell size determination

Subcutaneous fat tissues from the non-transgenic and transgenic quail were fixed in 10% neutral buffered formalin (Sigma-Aldrich, St. Louis, MO, USA) for sectioning. All procedures, dehydration, embedding, sectioning, and staining with hematoxylin and eosin were conducted by the Comparative Pathology and Mouse Phenotyping Shared Resource at OSU. Images were taken randomly from sample slides using an AXIO-Vert.A1 optical microscope (Carl Zeiss Microscopy, Thornwood, NY, USA) equipped with an AxioCam MRc5 camera (Carl Zeiss Microscopy) and analyzed by using the ImageJ program to measure the area and cell numbers.

NEFA assay

The concentration of NEFA in serum was determined by using the NEFA-HR (2) kit that relies on the ACS-ACOD enzymatic method (Wako Diagnostics, Richmond, VA, USA). All procedures were conducted as the manufacturer's protocol. After transferring 5 µl of sera, standards, and deionized water to a 96-well plate, 200 µl of Color Reagent Solution A was added to each well, followed by mixing and incubation at 37°C for 5 min. Then, the first absorbance of each sample was measured at 550 nm for each well. After adding and mixing 100 µl of Color Reagent Solution B to each well, the plate was incubated again at 37°C for 5 min, and the second absorbance was measured at 550 nm for each well. The final absorbance of each sample was obtained by difference. A linear standard curve was generated using the Microsoft Excel program (Microsoft, Redmond, WA, USA), and the NEFA concentration of each sample was calculated based on the standard curve.

Statistical analysis

Data were presented as mean and standard error of means. Statistical analyses were performed using Student's t-test or analysis of variance. *P* values under 0.05 were considered significant.

Results

Generation of transgenic quail expressing exogenous G0S2 in adipose tissue

The 2 kb promoter of the chicken FABP4 gene and the chicken G0S2 gene were cloned and inserted into a lentiviral vector to express the exogenous G0S2 gene specifically in adipose tissue (Figure 1A). The recombinant lentivirus was injected into 238 quail eggs; 51 founder chicks hatched, and 39 founder quail sexually matured and were crossed with wild-type quail or founders. A total of six transgenic quail lines [FABP4 promoter-G0S2 (FG), FG1 to FG6 lines] were generated from four founders, and the transgene was confirmed by PCR (Figure S2, Table S1). Integration sites of the transgene were analyzed by SiteFinding-PCR (Table S2). Transgenic quail possessed only one copy of the transgene that was located in various integration sites, except for FG3 and FG5 lines, which were generated from the same founder.

Adipose-specific expression of exogenous G0S2 in transgenic quail lines was verified and quantified by western blot analysis using an anti-chicken G0S2 antibody that was recently developed in our laboratory. In wild-type chicken and quail, the G0S2 protein was highly expressed in adipose tissues and negligible in other tissues and organs (Figure S3A), verifying the specificity of the G0S2 antibody in chicken and quail. Among transgenic quail lines, both FG1 and FG3 transgenic quail at embryonic and adult ages expressed 2- to 3-fold more G0S2 proteins in adipose tissues than did non-transgenic quail (Figure 1B and C, and S3C and D). These two transgenic quail lines were used for further investigation of tissue distribution of the G0S2 protein. This abundant expression of G0S2 proteins in adipose tissues in both lines of transgenic quail indicates adipose-specific expression of the exogenous G0S2 protein under the control of the cFABP4 promoter (Figure S3B). Female quail were excluded because of confounding effects caused by their gradual increase in adipose lipolysis to support egg yolk production [23].

Overexpressed G0S2 has no effect on growth and fat mass *in vivo* under *ad libitum* feeding conditions

In *ad libitum* feeding conditions, there was no difference ($P>0.05$) in body weight between transgenic and non-transgenic quail in either line (Figure 2A and B). The percentages of fat tissue and organ weights relative to body weights were not different between transgenic and non-transgenic quail in both lines (Figure 2C–F). Consequently, overexpressed G0S2 did not affect growth and fat pad weights when sufficient energy was supplied from the diet.

G0S2 expression prevents loss of fat under feed restriction

Feed restriction was applied to quail to investigate the effect of G0S2 overexpression under induced lipolytic conditions. The rates of body weight loss by feed restriction were different between transgenic and non-transgenic quail; non-transgenic quail lost about 10 g, whereas FG1 lost only 1g and FG3 lost 5g (Figure 3A). Comparison of adipose tissue weights among these quail revealed that FG1 and FG3 transgenic lines had about 3.6-fold ($P<0.001$) and 2.0-fold ($P<0.001$) more subcutaneous fat around the neck and 5.0-fold ($P<0.01$) and 2.0-fold ($P<0.05$) more abdominal fat,

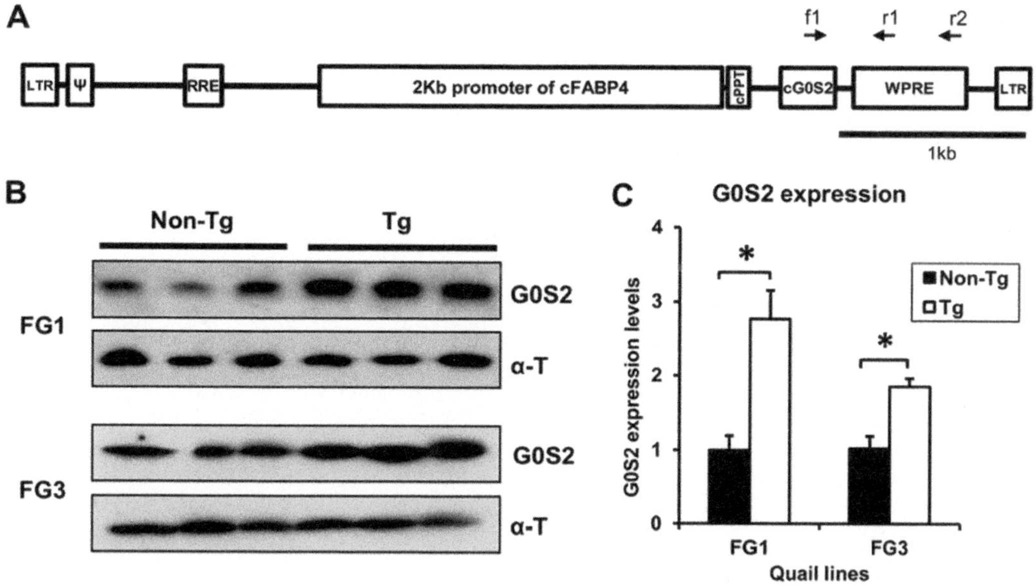

Figure 1. Lentiviral vector construct and its expression in adipose tissues of transgenic quail. (A) Diagram of lentiviral vector used for producing transgenic quail. The vector contains 2 kb promoter of chicken fatty acid binding protein and chicken G0S2 coding DNA sequences. The primers for detecting the transgene are presented as f1 for forward primer (LTG0S2-F) and r1 and r2 for reverse primers (LT-R and WPRE-R, respectively). (B) and (**C**) The expression level of G0S2 protein in adipose tissues of adult transgenic (Tg) and non-transgenic (Non-Tg) quail. Values are represented as mean ± SEM (n = 3). * indicates significance level of $P<0.05$.

respectively, than non-transgenic quail (Figure 3B and C). Compared with the fat pad weights in the *ad libitum* feeding condition, fat pad weights in non-transgenic quail were reduced 83% and 92% in subcutaneous and abdominal fat tissues, respectively, whereas in FG1 transgenic quail, they were reduced only 39% and 61% in the feed restriction condition. In the FG3 line, fat pad weights in non-transgenic quail were reduced 57% and 63% in subcutaneous and abdominal fat tissues, respectively, but in transgenic quail, they were reduced only 15% and 21%. These results clearly show that all transgenic lines have greater fat pads than non-transgenic quail under feed restriction, indicating that loss of fat during the feed restriction condition was significantly blocked by G0S2 expression in transgenic quail. There was no difference in other organ weights between transgenic and non-transgenic quail (Figure 3D and E), suggesting the effect of G0S2 overexpression could be limited to adipose tissue and not to other tissues in transgenic quail.

G0S2 prevents adipocyte hypotrophy caused by feed restriction

To investigate whether the differences in fat mass between transgenic quail and non-transgenic quail resulted from changes in fat cell size, the adipose tissues were sectioned, and the size of fat cells was determined. There was no difference in fat cell size between transgenic and non-transgenic quail fed *ad libitum*, as expected, because of the similar fat pad weights. However, the fat cell size of non-transgenic quail was less than that of the transgenic quail in a feed restriction condition (Figure 4A and B). In FG1, the fat cell size of non-transgenic quail was reduced ($P<0.001$) about 4-fold compared to transgenic quail after feed restriction for 2 weeks (Figure 4C). In FG3, the fat cell size of non-transgenic quail was also reduced ($P<0.05$) about 2-fold compared to the transgenic quail after feed restriction (Figure 4D). The rate of reduction in fat cell size in FG1 lines was more severe than in FG3 lines in both transgenic and non-transgenic quail after feed restriction. Therefore, overexpressed G0S2 prevented the adipocyte hypotrophy caused by feed restriction.

G0S2 inhibits lipolysis in adipose tissue *in vivo*

There was no difference in serum NEFA concentration during *ad libitum* feeding between transgenic and non-transgenic quail; however, it was significantly reduced in transgenic quail after short-term fasting and long-term feed restriction, which are considered to induce lipolysis (Figure 5A and B). Transgenic quail of both lines had lower ($P<0.05$) NEFA concentrations in blood than did non-transgenic quail at lipolytic conditions. Analysis of G0S2 and ATGL expression in adipose tissue revealed that G0S2 was expressed higher in transgenic quail than non-transgenic quail during *ad libitum* and 12 hours fasting while the ATGL was up-regulated by 12 hour fasting in both transgenic and non-transgenic quail (Figure 5C and D). Therefore, the ratio of ATGL to G0S2 was higher in non-transgenic quail than transgenic quail, and the ratio was increased more in non-transgenic quail during the fasting condition. The expression of FABP4 was not affected by feeding condition in transgenic and non-transgenic quail of both lines. These data suggest that overexpressed G0S2 in adipose tissues of transgenic quail decreased lipolysis by inhibiting the ATGL during a limited feeding condition.

Discussion

Recently, Japanese quail have been the focus of many biological studies because of their relatively small size, fast sexual maturation, abundant egg production, and domestication [24-28]. In addition, avian transgenesis has a powerful potential in the fields of biology, biomedicine, and agriculture to study embryo development and gene function, to produce therapeutic proteins in the egg, and to generate high-performing and disease-resistant poultry [29–31]. Importantly, based on conservation of the metabolic pathways in adipose tissue and similarity to regulation of gene expression in

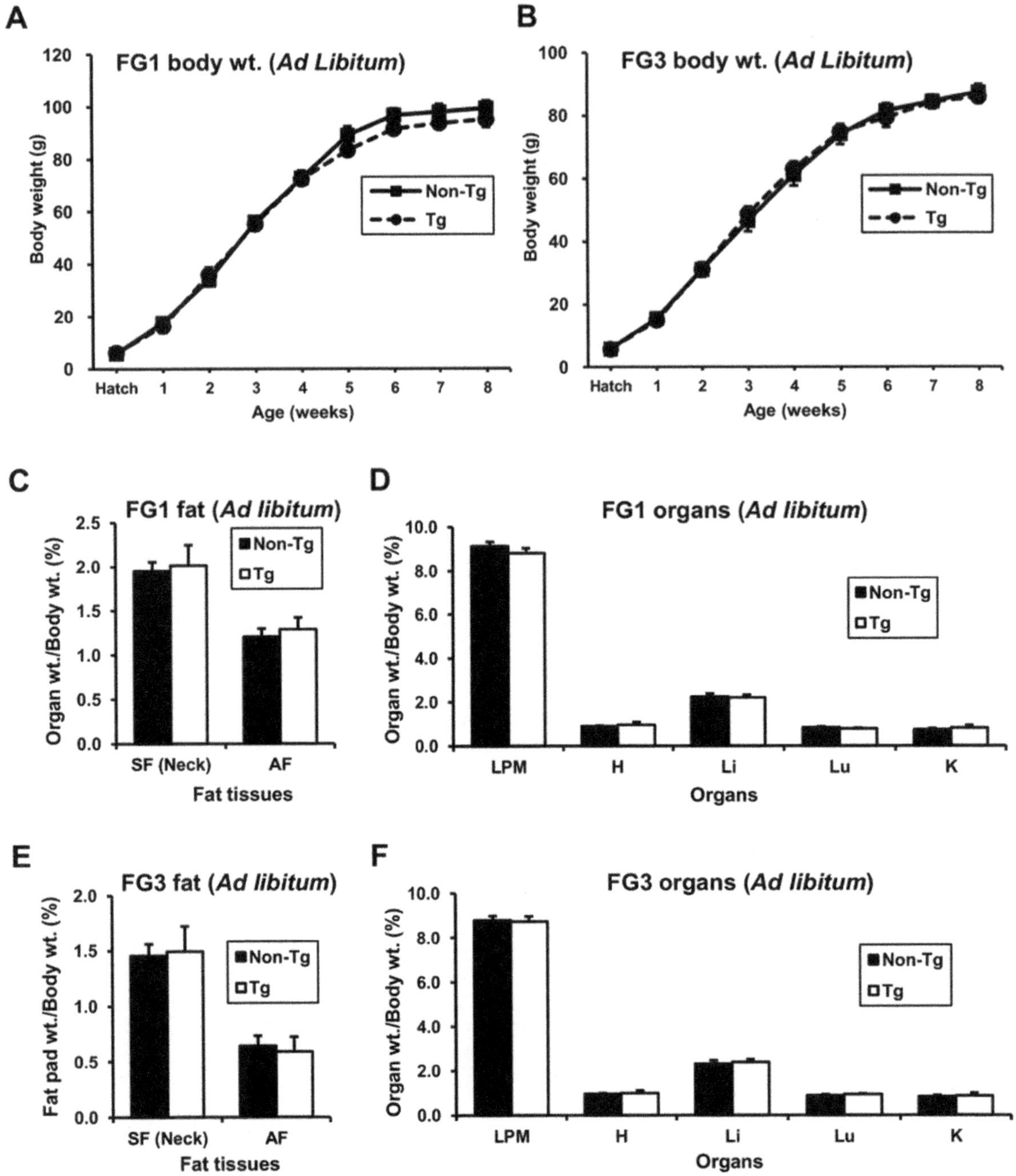

Figure 2. Analysis of growth and organ weights of transgenic and non-transgenic quail fed *ad libitum*. (A and B) Growth curve of FG1 and FG3 lines of transgenic and non-transgenic quail fed *ad libitum*. Body weights of male transgenic and non-transgenic quail were measured every week from hatch to 8 weeks of age. (C and D) Organ weights of FG1 quail fed *ad libitum*. Organ weights were measured and calculated to the percentage of total body weight. There was no difference between transgenic and non-transgenic quail in the tissue and organ weights ($n = 5$). SF: subcutaneous fat, AF: abdominal fat, LPM: left pectoralis muscle, H; heart, Li: liver, Lu: lung, and K: kidney. (E and F) Organ weights of FG3 quail fed *ad libitum*. FG3 did not show a difference in organ weight between transgenic ($n = 6$) and non-transgenic ($n = 8$) quail under the *ad libitum* feeding. Values are represented as mean ± SEM.

animals, quail were considered a particularly relevant avian model to study functions of target genes in adipose tissue [14,23,32].

Although the inhibitory function of G0S2 on ATGL proteins has been recently demonstrated *in vitro*, the anti-lipolytic role of G0S2 in adipose tissue and consequent effect on regulation of fat mass of animals in response to different energy statuses have not been extensively studied *in vivo*. In this study, we generated transgenic quail lines overexpressing the chicken G0S2 gene in adipose tissues under the control of the chicken FABP4 promoter to investigate its role *in vivo*. Adipose-specific expression of transgenes has successfully been achieved using the mouse FABP4 promoter in numerous transgenic mouse models, including ours [33]. Our comparative analysis of FABP4 promoters in mammals revealed conservation of important *cis*-acting elements for the

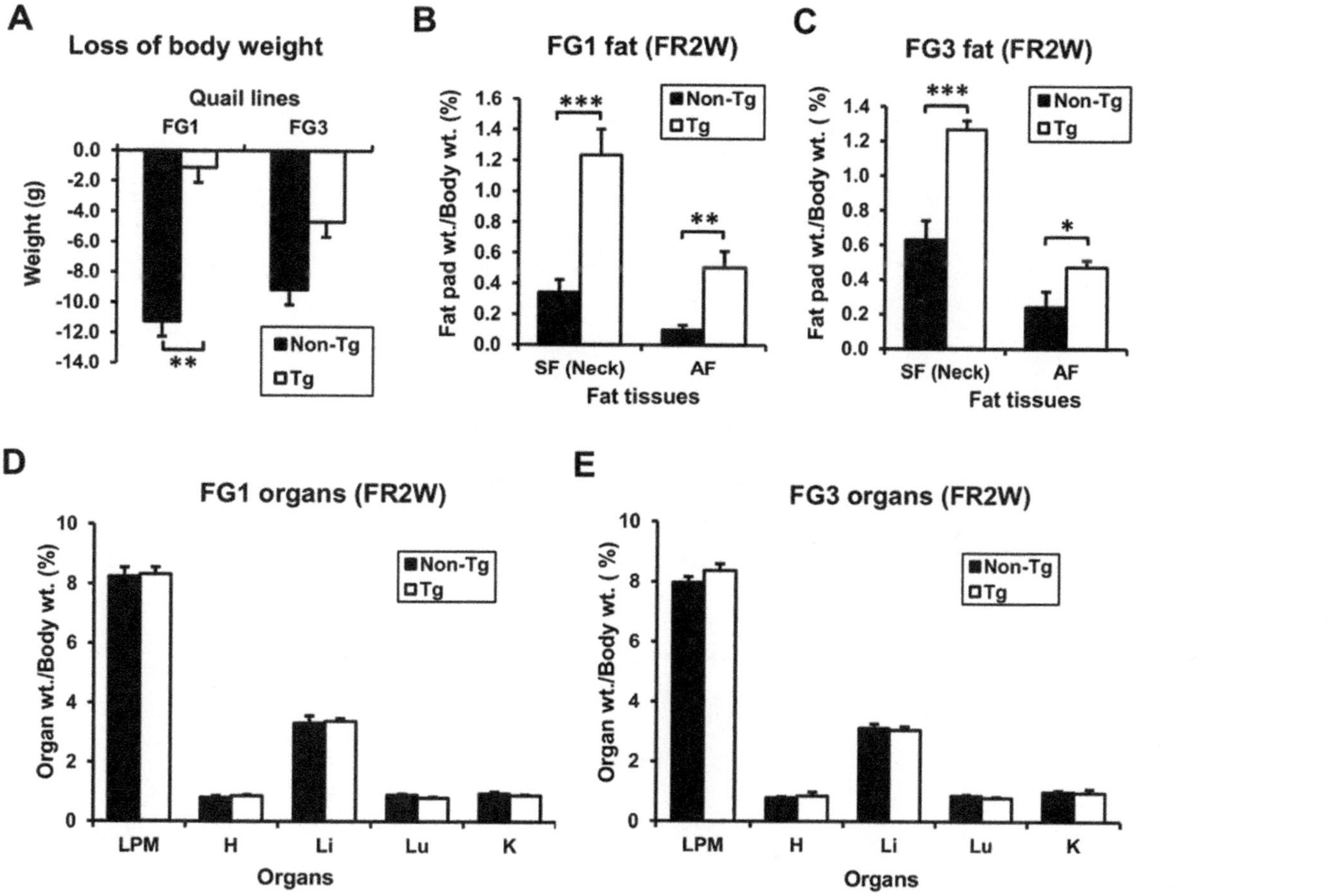

Figure 3. Analysis of body and organ weights of transgenic and non-transgenic quail that underwent feed restriction. (A) Changes of body weights after feed restriction for two weeks. Non-transgenic quail lost more body weight than transgenic quail in both lines. (B and C) Weights of fat pads after feed restriction. Both transgenic quail of FG1 and FG3 had significantly greater fat pads than non-transgenic quail after feed restriction. FR2W: feed restriction for 2 weeks. (D and E) Organ weights after feed restriction. There was no difference in non-adipose organ weights between transgenic and non-transgenic quail after feed restriction. $n = 6$ for each. Values are represented as mean ± SEM. *, **, and *** indicate significance levels of $P<0.05$, $P<0.01$, and $P<0.001$, respectively.

CAAT/enhancer binding protein α (C/EBPα) and peroxisome proliferator-activated receptor γ (PPARγ) binding sites [34]. In the current study, the chicken FABP4 promoter containing two putative C/EBPα and seven PPARγ binding sites successfully expressed the G0S2 protein about 2- to 3-fold greater in adipose tissues of transgenic quail than of non-transgenic quail. The expression of endogenous FABP4 was not affected by feeding conditions and it suggests that the exogenous G0S2 could be expressed stably regardless of feeding conditions.

In chickens, quail, pigs, and humans, expressions of ATGL and G0S2 genes in adipose tissue are dynamically regulated in an inverse relationship at different nutritional conditions such as normal feeding, fasting, and refeeding. Low levels of ATGL and high levels of G0S2 expression at normal feeding and refeeding conditions, and induction of ATGL and reduction of G0S2 expression during the fasting condition are tightly correlated with adipose lipolytic activities and blood levels of NEFA [13,14,17]. Under the *ad libitum* feeding condition, overexpression of G0S2 in adipose tissue did not change fat pad weights and fat cell sizes in either line of transgenic quail compared to the control non-transgenic quail. In addition, concentrations of blood NEFA were not different between transgenic and non-transgenic quail, suggesting that lipolytic activities were not affected by overexpression of G0S2 under the *ad libitum* condition. This is different from the result that basal lipolytic activity is reduced by 30 to 40% in fat extracts resulting in about a 2-fold increased fat mass in transgenic mice overexpressing G0S2 compared to wild-type mice [35].The absence of phenotypic responses to overexpression of G0S2 in the transgenic quail could be due to the *ad libitum* feeding condition; a sufficient energy supply from the diet could maintain low ATGL activity during which the inhibitory function of exogenous G0S2 would be minimal. Another plausible explanation based on our previous finding in normal chickens and quail is that high expression of endogenous G0S2 is sufficient to inhibit low amounts of ATGL during the *ad libitum* feeding condition, resulting in blood NEFA maintained at basal levels [14]. Therefore, exogenous G0S2 expression that would be metabolically redundant with high amounts of endogenous G0S2 in the adipose tissue of transgenic quail may not have any additional inhibitory effect on ATGL in an *ad libitum* feeding condition. This hypothesis could explain why G0S2 shows an inhibitory effect on lipolysis under the feed restriction condition while not increasing the fat mass during the *ad libitum* feeding condition.

The above results led us to hypothesize that enhanced ATGL-mediated lipolysis by low energy conditions, such as fasting or feed restriction, is inhibited by overexpression of G0S2. The inhibitory

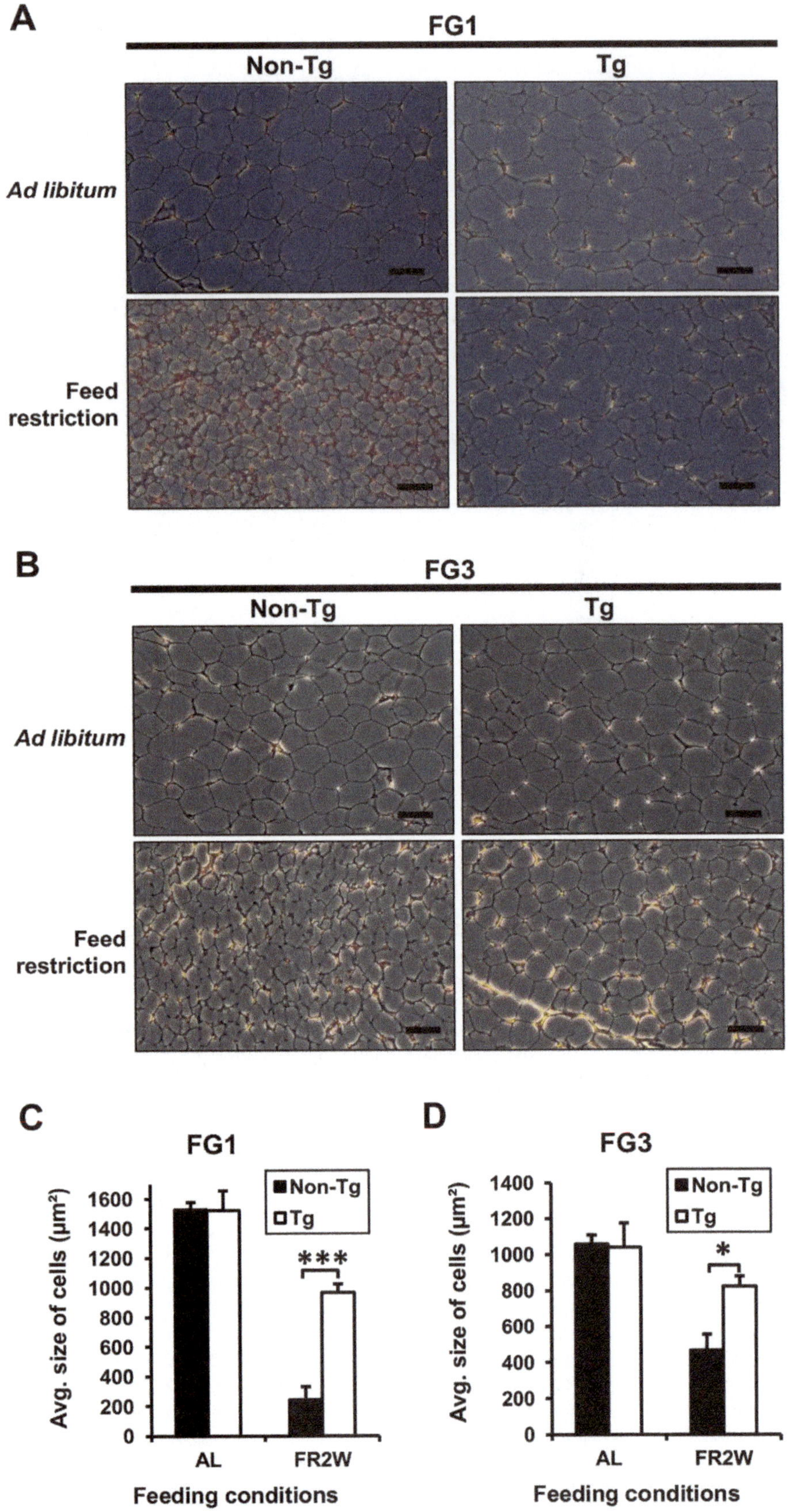

Figure 4. Comparison of fat cell size under the different feeding conditions. (A and B) Histology of fat tissues from transgenic and non-transgenic quail of FG1 and FG3. Fat cell size was almost the same between transgenic and non-transgenic quail in both lines fed *ad libitum*, while it shrank to different levels between them after feed restriction. All scale bars: 50 μm. (C and D) Numerical data of average fat cell size in different

feeding conditions. The average fat cell size of non-transgenic quail was significantly smaller than that of transgenic quail only after feed restriction ($n=3$). AL: *ad libitum* and FR2W: feed restriction for 2 weeks. Values are represented as mean ± SEM. * and *** indicate significance levels of $P<0.05$ and $P<0.001$, respectively.

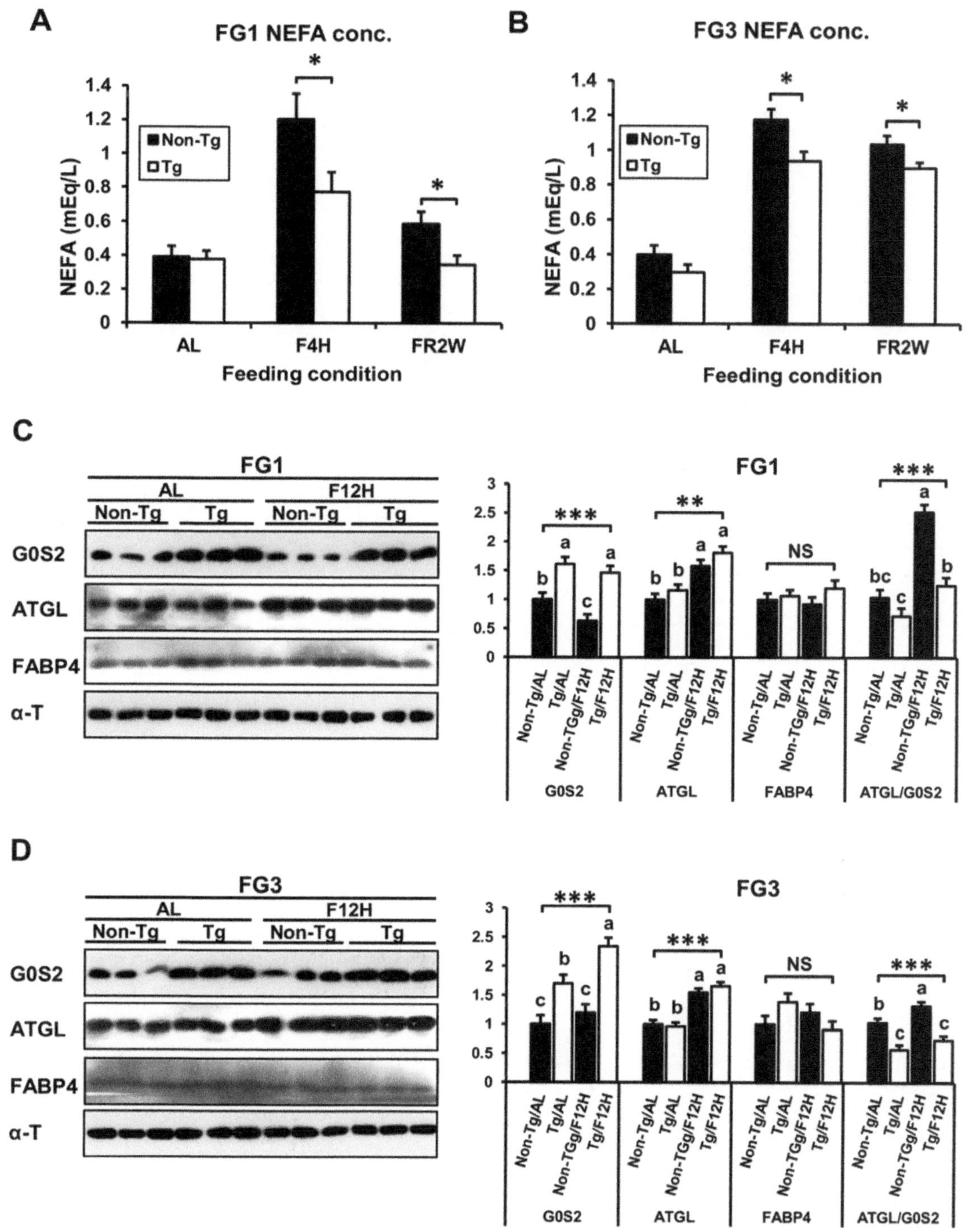

Figure 5. Blood NEFA levels and the expression of G0S2 and ATGL in fat tissues in different feeding conditions. (**A**) and (B) The levels of NEFA in serum were significantly lower in transgenic quail than in non-transgenic quail under the short-term fasting and feed restriction conditions ($n \geq 5$). AL: *ad libitum*, F4H: fasting for 4 hours, and FR2W: feed restriction for 2 weeks. (C) and (D) The expression of G0S2, ATGL, and FABP4 in fat tissues depending on feeding conditions, *ad libitum* (AL) vs. fasting for 12 hours (F12H). G0S2 was continuously higher in transgenic quail than non-transgenic quail. The expression of ATGL was higher in fasting condition in both transgenic and non-transgenic quail. The ratio of ATGL to G0S2 was highest in non-transgenic quail under the fasting condition. The expression of FABP4 was not significantly variable regardless of feeding condition. Values are represented as mean ± SEM. *, **, and *** indicate significance levels of $P<0.05$, 0.01, and 0.001, respectively. NS means non-significant.

effect of G0S2 on lipolysis *in vivo* was monitored by measuring sequential changes in NEFA release from adipose tissue into blood, in fat cell size, and in adipose tissue weights. In non-transgenic quail, feed restriction for two weeks significantly decreased adipose tissue mass, which is evidently caused by shrinking fat cell size when compared with the cell size before feed restriction. However, greater fat pad weights and fat cell sizes of all transgenic quail lines under the feed restriction status resulted from comparably lower levels of blood NEFA compared with non-transgenic quail lines. In addition, the expression of G0S2 was maintained higher in the adipose tissue of transgenic quail than non-transgenic quail while the ATGL expression was up-regulated, further suggesting the overexpressed G0S2 has the inhibitory role in ATGL activity during the lipolytic conditions. These data clearly indicate that G0S2 overexpression inhibits lipolysis in fat cells resulting in lower release of NEFA to the blood, consequently preventing the loss of TAG stored in lipid droplets that normally occurs by feed restriction. These findings are further supported by the *in vitro* studies showing that overexpression of G0S2 in HeLa cells has an inhibitory effect on lipolysis only under nutrient starvation [3]. Taken together, G0S2 has a significant inhibitory effect mainly on activated ATGL during lipolytic conditions to regulate the rate of TAG hydrolysis.

ATGL-mediated lipolysis could be tightly and inversely regulated by two major modulators: the up-regulation of CGI-58, which is required to activate ATGL in response to the negative energy status, and the induction of G0S2, which is needed to inhibit the activated ATGL during the transition from negative to positive energy status. In the current transgenic quail model, overexpression of G0S2 caused a resistance to loss of fat in a negative energy condition by disrupting the normal temporal regulation of ATGL. Considering the elevated expression of CGI-58 in adipose tissue during the negative energy condition [36], relatively low levels of blood NEFA in the transgenic quail under feed restriction suggest overexpression of G0S2 could dominate the regulation of ATGL by possibly ameliorating or overriding CGI-58 function. This is further supported by the finding that overexpression of G0S2 reduced the lipolytic activity of adipocytes overexpressing ATGL and CGI-58 *in vitro* [3]. Therefore, the treatment to regulate the G0S2 expression could be an ideal approach to change the adiposity in humans and other animals. In addition, it will be interesting to further investigate in the human population whether or not failure of fat loss under a diet program with reduced calorie intake could be related to the G0S2 gene. If so, it would be valuable to determine whether a low release of blood NEFA is attributed to increased G0S2 activity, possibly caused by elevated G0S2 expression or gain-of-function mutations on the G0S2 gene. It is reasonable that fasting or food restriction should be challenged to identify those relations, as the phenotype of G0S2 could not be detected with human individuals who normally access the diet *ad libitum*.

In conclusion, we successfully generated transgenic quail lines overexpressing exogenous G0S2. The excessive G0S2 had an inhibitory effect on lipolysis under feed restriction conditions, but did not enhance fat accumulation under the *ad libitum* feeding condition. Therefore, the G0S2 is a reasonable target gene to treat the adiposity in animals. To our knowledge, this is the first report that investigates gene function by using a transgenic bird and transgenic quail may be a useful animal model in the area of adipocyte biology and obesity research.

Supporting Information

Figure S1 Fat pads of quail. Quail has lots of subcutaneous fats around the neck (a), breast muscle (b and f), and legs (c and e). A big fat pad is located in the abdomen (d). Two major fat pads, subcutaneous fat around the neck (a) and abdominal fat (d), were used for measuring the parameters.

Figure S2 Detection of transgene in the transgenic quail genome and transgene expression levels. All transgenic quail were selected by PCR using two primer sets, ^{f1} + ^{r1} (412 bp) and ^{f1} + ^{r2} (798 bp), described in Figure 1A. 1–6: FG1-6 transgenic quail, 7: non-transgenic quail for negative control, and 8: plasmid for positive control.

Figure S3 Tissue distribution of G0S2 protein in wild-type chicken and quail and in transgenic quail lines. (A) The level of G0S2 protein in wild-type chicken and quail was investigated in various tissues including subcutaneous fat (SF), abdominal fat (AF), pectoralis muscle (PM), heart (H), liver (Li), lung (Lu), and kidney (K). G0S2 was mainly detectable in fat tissues and barely expressed in heart, liver, and lung. (B) The level of G0S2 protein in various tissues of transgenic quail lines was determined by using Western blot. Total G0S2 protein was mainly detected in adipose tissues. (C) and (D) The relative amounts of G0S2 protein in adipose tissues of transgenic and non-transgenic quail embryos. Two transgenic lines, FG1 and FG3, were selected and investigated to determine the expression level of G0S2 in adipose tissues of embryos at the age of 15 days. Values are represented as mean ± SEM. * and ** indicate significance levels of $P<0.05$ and $P<0.01$, respectively.

Table S1 The results of testcross for generating transgenic quail.

Table S2 Analysis of integration site of transgene on the transgenic quail genome.

Author Contributions

Conceived and designed the experiments: SS KL. Performed the experiments: SS YMC. Analyzed the data: SS KL. Contributed reagents/materials/analysis tools: JH. Wrote the paper: SS KL.

References

1. Zimmermann R, Strauss JG, Haemmerle G, Schoiswohl G, Birner-Gruenberger R, et al. (2004) Fat mobilization in adipose tissue is promoted by adipose triglyceride lipase. Science 306: 1383–1386.
2. Lass A, Zimmermann R, Haemmerle G, Riederer M, Schoiswohl G, et al. (2006) Adipose triglyceride lipase-mediated lipolysis of cellular fat stores is activated by CGI-58 and defective in Chanarin-Dorfman Syndrome. Cell Metab 3: 309–319.
3. Yang X, Lu X, Lombes M, Rha GB, Chi YI, et al. (2010) The G(0)/G(1) switch gene 2 regulates adipose lipolysis through association with adipose triglyceride lipase. Cell Metab 11: 194–205.
4. Jenkins CM, Mancuso DJ, Yan W, Sims HF, Gibson B, et al. (2004) Identification, cloning, expression, and purification of three novel human calcium-independent phospholipase A2 family members possessing triacylglycerol lipase and acylglycerol transacylase activities. J Biol Chem 279: 48968–48975.
5. Villena JA, Roy S, Sarkadi-Nagy E, Kim KH, Sul HS (2004) Desnutrin, an adipocyte gene encoding a novel patatin domain-containing protein, is induced by fasting and glucocorticoids: ectopic expression of desnutrin increases triglyceride hydrolysis. J Biol Chem 279: 47066–47075.

6. Schweiger M, Schreiber R, Haemmerle G, Lass A, Fledelius C, et al. (2006) Adipose triglyceride lipase and hormone-sensitive lipase are the major enzymes in adipose tissue triacylglycerol catabolism. J Biol Chem 281: 40236–40241.
7. Bezaire V, Mairal A, Ribet C, Lefort C, Girousse A, et al. (2009) Contribution of adipose triglyceride lipase and hormone-sensitive lipase to lipolysis in hMADS adipocytes. J Biol Chem 284: 18282–18291.
8. Haemmerle G, Lass A, Zimmermann R, Gorkiewicz G, Meyer C, et al. (2006) Defective lipolysis and altered energy metabolism in mice lacking adipose triglyceride lipase. Science 312: 734–737.
9. Duncan RE, Wang Y, Ahmadian M, Lu J, Sarkadi-Nagy E, et al. (2010) Characterization of desnutrin functional domains: critical residues for triacylglycerol hydrolysis in cultured cells. J Lipid Res 51: 309–317.
10. Kobayashi K, Inoguchi T, Maeda Y, Nakashima N, Kuwano A, et al. (2008) The lack of the C-terminal domain of adipose triglyceride lipase causes neutral lipid storage disease through impaired interactions with lipid droplets. J Clin Endocrinol Metab 93: 2877–2884.
11. Schweiger M, Schoiswohl G, Lass A, Radner FP, Haemmerle G, et al. (2008) The C-terminal region of human adipose triglyceride lipase affects enzyme activity and lipid droplet binding. J Biol Chem 283: 17211–17220.
12. Gruber A, Cornaciu I, Lass A, Schweiger M, Poeschl M, et al. (2010) The N-terminal region of comparative gene identification-58 (CGI-58) is important for lipid droplet binding and activation of adipose triglyceride lipase. J Biol Chem 285: 12289–12298.
13. Ahn J, Oh SA, Suh Y, Moeller SJ, Lee K (2013) Porcine G(0)/G(1) switch gene 2 (G0S2) expression is regulated during adipogenesis and short-term in-vivo nutritional interventions. Lipids 48: 209–218.
14. Oh SA, Suh Y, Pang MG, Lee K (2011) Cloning of avian G(0)/G(1) switch gene 2 genes and developmental and nutritional regulation of G(0)/G(1) switch gene 2 in chicken adipose tissue. J Anim Sci 89: 367–375.
15. Zandbergen F, Mandard S, Escher P, Tan NS, Patsouris D, et al. (2005) The G0/G1 switch gene 2 is a novel PPAR target gene. Biochem J 392: 313–324.
16. Schweiger M, Paar M, Eder C, Brandis J, Moser E, et al. (2012) G0/G1 switch gene-2 regulates human adipocyte lipolysis by affecting activity and localization of adipose triglyceride lipase. J Lipid Res 53: 2307–2317.
17. Nielsen TS, Vendelbo MH, Jessen N, Pedersen SB, Jorgensen JO, et al. (2011) Fasting, but not exercise, increases adipose triglyceride lipase (ATGL) protein and reduces G(0)/G(1) switch gene 2 (G0S2) protein and mRNA content in human adipose tissue. J Clin Endocrinol Metab 96: E1293–1297.
18. Shin SS, Kim TM, Kim SY, Kim TW, Seo HW, et al. (2008) Generation of transgenic quail through germ cell-mediated germline transmission. Faseb J 22: 2435–2444.
19. Tan G, Gao Y, Shi M, Zhang X, He S, et al. (2005) SiteFinding-PCR: a simple and efficient PCR method for chromosome walking. Nucleic Acids Res 33: e122.
20. Ogawa A, Solovei I, Hutchison N, Saitoh Y, Ikeda JE, et al. (1997) Molecular characterization and cytological mapping of a non-repetitive DNA sequence region from the W chromosome of chicken and its use as a universal probe for sexing carinatae birds. Chromosome Res 5: 93–101.
21. Lee K, Shin J, Latshaw JD, Suh Y, Serr J (2009) Cloning of adipose triglyceride lipase complementary deoxyribonucleic acid in poultry and expression of adipose triglyceride lipase during development of adipose in chickens. Poult Sci 88: 620–630.
22. Chen P, Suh Y, Choi YM, Shin S, Lee K (2014) Developmental regulation of adipose tissue growth through hyperplasia and hypertrophy in the embryonic Leghorn and broiler. Poult Sci doi.org/10.3382/ps.2013–03816.
23. Yang S, Suh Y, Choi YM, Shin S, Han JY, et al. (2013) Loss of fat with increased adipose triglyceride lipase-mediated lipolysis in adipose tissue during laying stages in quail. Lipids 48: 13–21.
24. Ottinger MA, Abdelnabi M, Li Q, Chen K, Thompson N, et al. (2004) The Japanese quail: a model for studying reproductive aging of hypothalamic systems. Exp Gerontol 39: 1679–1693.
25. Ball GF, Balthazart J (2010) Japanese quail as a model system for studying the neuroendocrine control of reproductive and social behaviors. Ilar J 51: 310–325.
26. Koksal F, Domjan M, Kurt A, Sertel O, Orung S, et al. (2004) An animal model of fetishism. Behav Res Ther 42: 1421–1434.
27. Seidl AH, Sanchez JT, Schecterson L, Tabor KM, Wang Y, et al. (2013) Transgenic quail as a model for research in the avian nervous system: a comparative study of the auditory brainstem. J Comp Neurol 521: 5–23.
28. Poynter G, Huss D, Lansford R (2009) Japanese quail: an efficient animal model for the production of transgenic avians. Cold Spring Harb Protoc 2009: pdb emo112.
29. Sang H (1994) Transgenic chickens—methods and potential applications. Trends Biotechnol 12: 415–420.
30. Scott BB, Velho TA, Sim S, Lois C (2010) Applications of avian transgenesis. Ilar J 51: 353–361.
31. Han JY (2009) Germ cells and transgenesis in chickens. Comp Immunol Microbiol Infect Dis 32: 61–80.
32. Serr J, Suh Y, Lee K (2009) Regulation of adipose triglyceride lipase by fasting and refeeding in avian species. Poult Sci 88: 2585–2591.
33. Lee K, Villena JA, Moon YS, Kim KH, Lee S, et al. (2003) Inhibition of adipogenesis and development of glucose intolerance by soluble preadipocyte factor-1 (Pref-1). J Clin Invest 111: 453–461.
34. Shin J, Li B, Davis ME, Suh Y, Lee K (2009) Comparative analysis of fatty acid-binding protein 4 promoters: conservation of peroxisome proliferator-activated receptor binding sites. J Anim Sci 87: 3923–3934.
35. Wueest S, Yang X, Liu J, Schoenle EJ, Konrad D (2012) Inverse regulation of basal lipolysis in perigonadal and mesenteric fat depots in mice. Am J Physiol Endocrinol Metab 302: E153–160.
36. Serr J, Suh Y, Lee K (2011) Cloning of comparative gene identification-58 gene in avian species and investigation of its developmental and nutritional regulation in chicken adipose tissue. J Anim Sci 89: 3490–3500.

7

Differential Responses of Cecal Microbiota to Fishmeal, *Eimeria* and *Clostridium perfringens* in a Necrotic Enteritis Challenge Model in Chickens

Dragana Stanley[1,2,3]⁹, Shu-Biao Wu[3,4]⁹, Nicholas Rodgers[3,4], Robert A. Swick[3,4], Robert J. Moore[2,3]*

1 Central Queensland University, School of Medical and Applied Sciences, Rockhampton, Queensland, Australia, 2 Australian Animal Health Laboratory, CSIRO Biosecurity Flagship, Geelong, Victoria, Australia, 3 Poultry Cooperative Research Centre, University of New England, Armidale, New South Wales, Australia, 4 School of Environmental and Rural Science, University of New England, Armidale, New South Wales, Australia

Abstract

Clostridium perfringens causes enteric diseases in animals and humans. In poultry, avian-specific *C. perfringens* strains cause necrotic enteritis, an economically significant poultry disease that costs the global industry over $2 billion annually in losses and control measures. With removal of antibiotic growth promoters in some countries this disease appears to be on the rise. In experimental conditions used to study disease pathogenesis and potential control measures, reproduction of the disease relies on the use of predisposing factors such as *Eimeria* infection and the use of high protein diets, indicating complex mechanisms involved in the onset of necrotic enteritis. The mechanisms by which the predisposing factors contribute to disease progression are not well understood but it has been suggested that they may cause perturbations in the microbiota within the gastrointestinal tract. We inspected changes in cecal microbiota and short chain fatty acids (SCFA) induced by *Eimeria* and fishmeal, in birds challenged or not challenged with *C. perfringens*. *C. perfringens* challenge in the absence of predisposing factors did not cause significant changes in either the alpha or beta diversity of the microbiota nor in concentrations of SCFA. Moreover, there was no *C. perfringens* detected in the cecal microbiota 2 days post-challenge without the presence of predisposing factors. In contrast, both fishmeal and *Eimeria* caused significant changes in microbiota, seen in both alpha and beta diversity and also enabled *C. perfringens* to establish itself post challenge. *Eimeria* had its strongest influence on intestinal microbiota and SCFA when combined with fishmeal. Out of 6 SCFAs measured, including butyric acid, none were significantly influenced by *C. perfringens*, but their levels were strongly modified following the use of both predisposing factors. There was little overlap in the changes caused following *Eimeria* and fishmeal treatments, possibly indicating multiple routes for progressing towards clinical symptoms of necrotic enteritis.

Editor: Gayatri Vedantam, University of Arizona, United States of America

Funding: This research was conducted within the Poultry CRC, established and supported under the Australian Government's Cooperative Research Centres Program, Contract 2.1.5. The funders had no role in study design, data collection and analysis, decision to publish, or preparation of the manuscript.

* Email: Rob.Moore@csiro.au

⁹ These authors contributed equally to this work.

Introduction

It has been more than half a century since necrotic enteritis (NE) was first reported in chickens by Parish *et al.* [1]. Despite decades of research, NE remains one of the major challenges in the poultry industry and is associated with extensive production losses worldwide [2]. Although *Clostridium perfringens* is clearly the pathogen responsible for NE, both field experience and efforts to experimentally reproduce the disease have shown that onset of NE is a complex process requiring one or a number of predisposing factors rather than just the presence of pathogenic *C. perfringens* strains [3,4].

In experimental disease challenge trials it is necessary to introduce predisposing factors, such as *Eimeria* co-infection, high protein feed (including fishmeal), indigestible non-starch polysaccharides, controlled immunosuppression or deliberate stressing of birds, to produce clinical symptoms in a substantial proportion of challenged birds [4]. Moreover, healthy birds often carry strains of *C. perfringens* without showing any clinical symptoms of NE. It is now clear that most of the *C. perfringens* strains colonizing healthy birds are non-pathogenic strains incapable of inducing NE. It has also been suggested that other bacteria may play a role in disease onset: for instance a significant reduction in *Weissella confusa* has been noted in *C. perfringens* challenged birds while uncultured mollicutes associated with human intestinal problems increased by 3.7 fold in NE birds [5]. Reduction of *Lactobacillus johnsonii* by NE [5] and independently by fishmeal [6] has also been reported.

The ban on the use of antibiotics as growth promoters in Europe has highlighted the growing need for alternatives to antibiotic supplementation as a way of controlling NE in poultry. It has been reported that addition of some short chain fatty acids (SCFAs) to chicken diets has the potential to help birds resist NE

[7,8]. It has also been noted that butyrate producing bacterial phylotypes are reduced in the intestinal microbiota during the onset of NE [5]. Interestingly SCFAs, especially butyrate, are also reduced in human colitis patients [9,10]. Butyrate aids mucosal immunity and differentiation of colonic regulatory T cells [11] and it has the ability to attenuate symptoms of colitis [12].

It has been recently shown that *Eimeria* co-infection and high fishmeal diets induce very significant changes in cecal microflora [6]. The present study was undertaken to further investigate the impact of fishmeal and *Eimera* on cecal microflora and SCFA changes in birds challenged and unchallenged with pathogenic *C. perfringens*. A 2 × 2 × 2 factorial arrangement of treatments was employed with fishmeal (− or +), *Eimeria* (− or +) and *C. perfringens (− or +)* as factors. Cecal microbial abundance in all treatment groups was correlated with concentrations of short chain fatty acids. The results produced in the present study suggest that, by itself, the pathogenic *C. perfringens* strain was unable to cause any significant changes in the cecal microbiota, and furthermore it demonstrated a total inability to establish itself and remain in the microbial community 2 days post-challenge, without the help of predisposing factors. We also found butyrate levels as well as other SCFAs were not significantly influenced by *C. perfringens* but were strongly influenced by the predisposing factors. This study identified microbiota and SCFA changes that correlated with the use of predisposing factors, which may be important in the successful induction of NE in the experimental systems. A deeper understanding of the factors affecting disease progression in experimental systems is likely to assist in the development of alternative control strategies for implementation in the field.

Materials and Methods

Animal trial

The animal trial was performed using day-old Cobb 500 male broiler chickens obtained from Baiada Country Road Hatchery, Tamworth, NSW, Australia. Chickens were vaccinated and initially handled as previously described [6]. Briefly, birds were raised in floor pens in a temperature controlled room. Water and food were provided ad libitum. The treatment groups were as follows: control (CTRL), high (25% w/w) fishmeal (Skretting, Tasmania) feed (FM), *Eimeria* (E) challenge group and a group with both fishmeal and *Eimeria* (E+FM). For *Eimeria* challenge chicks were gavaged *per os*, with a suspension of 5,000 oocysts of *E. acervulina* and *E. maxima*, and 2,500 oocysts of *E. brunetti* (Bioproperties Pty., Glenorie, NSW, Australia) in 1 mL PBS with unchallenged birds just receiving PBS. Each of the four main groups were divided into 6 pens of unchallenged and 6 pens of birds challenged with *C. perfringens* (strain EHE-NE18). At 14 and 15 days birds to be challenged were inoculated *per os* with 1 mL of *C. perfringens* suspension at a concentration of 10^8–10^9 CFU/mL. Birds in unchallenged groups received 1 mL of sterile thioglycollate broth (Oxoid). Two birds per pen were euthanized and the cecal digesta sampled on 16 d for subsequent microbiota analysis. Collected cecal digesta from two birds pooled to represent each pen was snap-frozen in liquid nitrogen and then stored at −20°C until required for DNA extraction. The NE lesion score was determined according to Prescott, *et al.* [13]. The fact that each predisposing factor had unchallenged control and challenged group of birds allowed us to compare, for the first time, the success of challenge to concomitant changes in microbiota and SCFAs induced in each of treatment groups. The graphical presentation of the design is given in Figure 1.

Animal ethics statement

All the birds were raised and handled humanely, and the animal trial was approved by the Animal Ethics Committee of the University of New England (AEC10/129). All procedures were according to "Australian code of practice for the care and use of animals for scientific purposes" (Australian Agricultural Council, 1997) and the "Australian model code of practice for the welfare of animals, Domestic Poultry" (Standing Committee on Agriculture and Resource Management, 1995).

Analysis of short chain fatty acids and enumeration of bacteria by culturing

The analysis of SCFAs and enumeration of bacteria followed the methods used by Wu *et al.* [14]. Briefly, SCFAs and lactate concentrations were measured in a 2.0 g cecal sample by gas chromatography using 2-ethylbutyric acid as an internal standard. The concentrations of organic acids were determined using a Varian CP3800 gas chromatograph (Varian Analytical Instruments, Palo Alto, CA). Varian Star 5.52 chromatography workstation (integration system) software (Varian Analytical Instruments) was used to process all the data. Total SCFA concentration was calculated by the sum of all the short chain organic acids including lactate measured in a sample, expressed as μmol/g digesta, and individual organic concentration was expressed as the level relative to the total SCFA (%). For the enumeration of the bacteria, approximately 1 g of cecal digesta sample was collected in reduced salt solution, and then homogenized for 2 min in CO_2-flushed plastic bags using a MiniMixH bag mixer (Interscience, St. Nora, France). The homogenized sample was serially diluted in six 10-fold steps. Aliquots (100 μL) from appropriate dilutions were plated on the following media to culture the respective bacteria; total anaerobic bacteria on Wilkins-Chalgren anaerobic agar (Oxoid, UK); coliform bacteria and lactose-negative enterobacteria on MacConkey agar (Oxoid, UK); lactic acid bacteria on de Man, Rogosa, and Sharpe agar (Oxoid, UK); and lactobacilli on Rogosa agar (Oxoid, UK). Bacterial numbers were expressed as $\log_{10}$ CFU/g digesta. Significant changes in SCFA profiles and cultured bacteria CFU were identified using ANOVA followed by Tukeys HSE test in R software.

Microbiota analysis

Cecal DNA was extracted as previously described [15] with QIAamp DNA stool kit (Qiagen). The DNA amplification procedure was carried out as previously described [16]. The primers used (forward primer [17], 5′ AGAGTTTGATCCTGG 3′; reverse primer a truncated version of W31 [18], 5′ TTACCGCGGCTGCT 3′) were selected to amplify the V1 to V3 region of the 16S rRNA gene. Sequencing was performed on a Roche/454 FLX+ Genome Sequencer according to manufacturer's instructions. The data pre-processing was done using PyroBayes [19] followed by further analysis in Qiime v1.6.0 [20] using usearch, uchime and uclust algorithms [21] at sequence similarity threshold of 97% and Blast taxonomy assignments. Sequences were trimmed using the parameters: minimum average quality score of 25, sequence lengths of 300–600 bases, no ambiguous sequences, and a maximum run of 6 bases in homopolymers. Low abundance operational taxonomic units (OTUs) were removed if they had less than 5 sequences and presence in less than 3 samples. The OTU abundance table was normalised using the average values from 100 rarefactions. Phylogenetic analysis was carried out using a variety of tools including the EzTaxon database [22], GreenGenes database

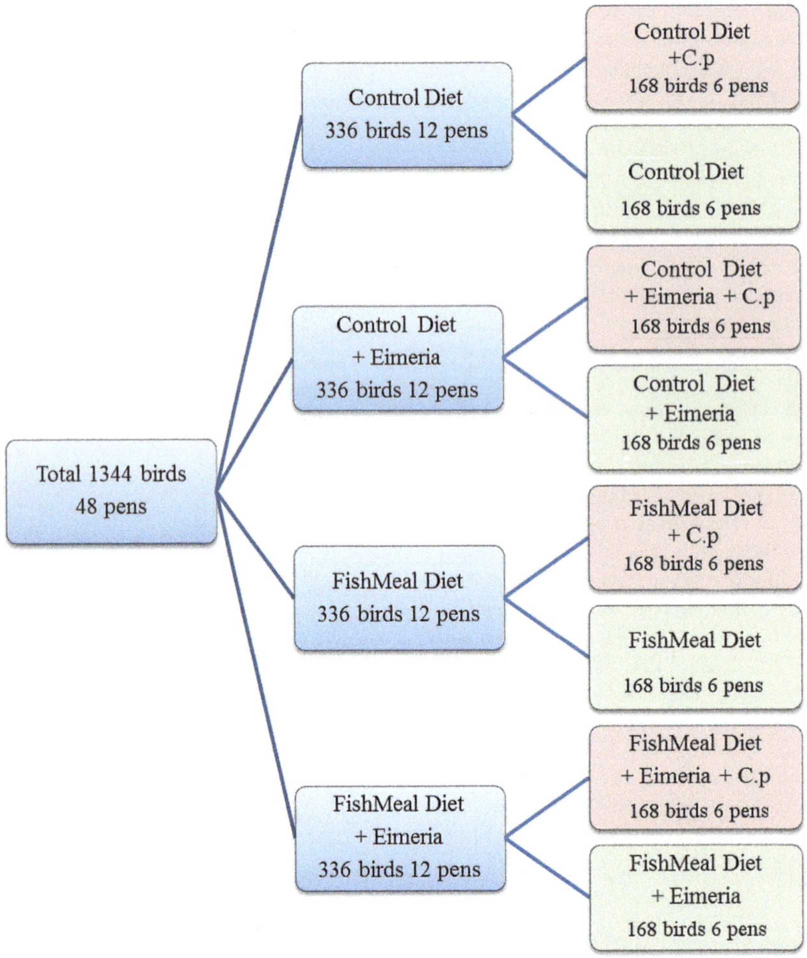

Figure 1. Diagram of the experimental design used in the animal trial. "C.p" was used to abbreviate *C. perfringens*.

(http://greengenes.lbl.gov/), BlastN 2.2.20 [23] and an R phylogenetic package, Ade4 (Analysis of Data functions for Ecological and Environmental data in the framework of Euclidean Exploratory) [24].

Results

Necrotic enteritis induction

Necrotic enteritis lesion scores in the small intestine of birds and NE induced mortalities observed in the different treatment groups are shown in Figure 2. In all sections of the GIT inspected, the highest NE lesion scores and mortality were recorded in the group challenged in the presence of both fishmeal and *Eimeria* (E+FM+Cp). The *Eimeria* challenge group also had high lesion scores. Lesions were detected in the challenged birds fed fishmeal, however, the NE induced mortality rate for this group was very low. Both lesion score and mortality data showed that challenge with *C. perfringens* without the presence of predisposing factors was not capable of producing clinical symptoms of NE. Other aspects of this trial, in particular the effects of different treatments on bird productivity before *C. perfringens* challenge, have been reported in a separate publication [6]. The NE lesion scores have been important to consider both in the current work with regard to microbiota changes and in the other publication in the context of productivity and hence different presentations of the lesion and mortality data are given.

Impact of treatments on microbiota diversity

The experimental design (Figure 1) allowed us to investigate the interaction of predisposing factors and *C. perfringens* infection on the overall microbiota composition within the ceca of treated birds. To inspect the effect of *Eimeria*, fishmeal and *C. perfringens,* individually and in combinations, on diversity and structure of cecal microbial communities, we have inspected alpha diversity measures (sample OTU richness) including chao1, dominance, Shannon, equitability, observed species and phylogenetic diversity using Qiime. Across all samples and groups the inspected alpha metrics were not significantly ($P<0.05$) influenced by the presence vs. absence of *C. perfringens* challenge. The influence of presence vs. absence of fishmeal was detected only in phylogenetic diversity metrics ($P=0.006$) while other metrics fell short of the threshold P-value for statistical significance. The greatest influence on alpha diversity was observed with the presence vs. absence of *Eimeria* with the reduction in diversity in the *Eimeria* groups giving P-values ranging from 0.001 for phylogenetic diversity to 0.008 for the equitability metric (Tables S1 and S2 in File S1). We have further dissected this finding to demonstrate that this difference is caused by a sample group containing both *Eimeria* and *C. perfringens* rather than other

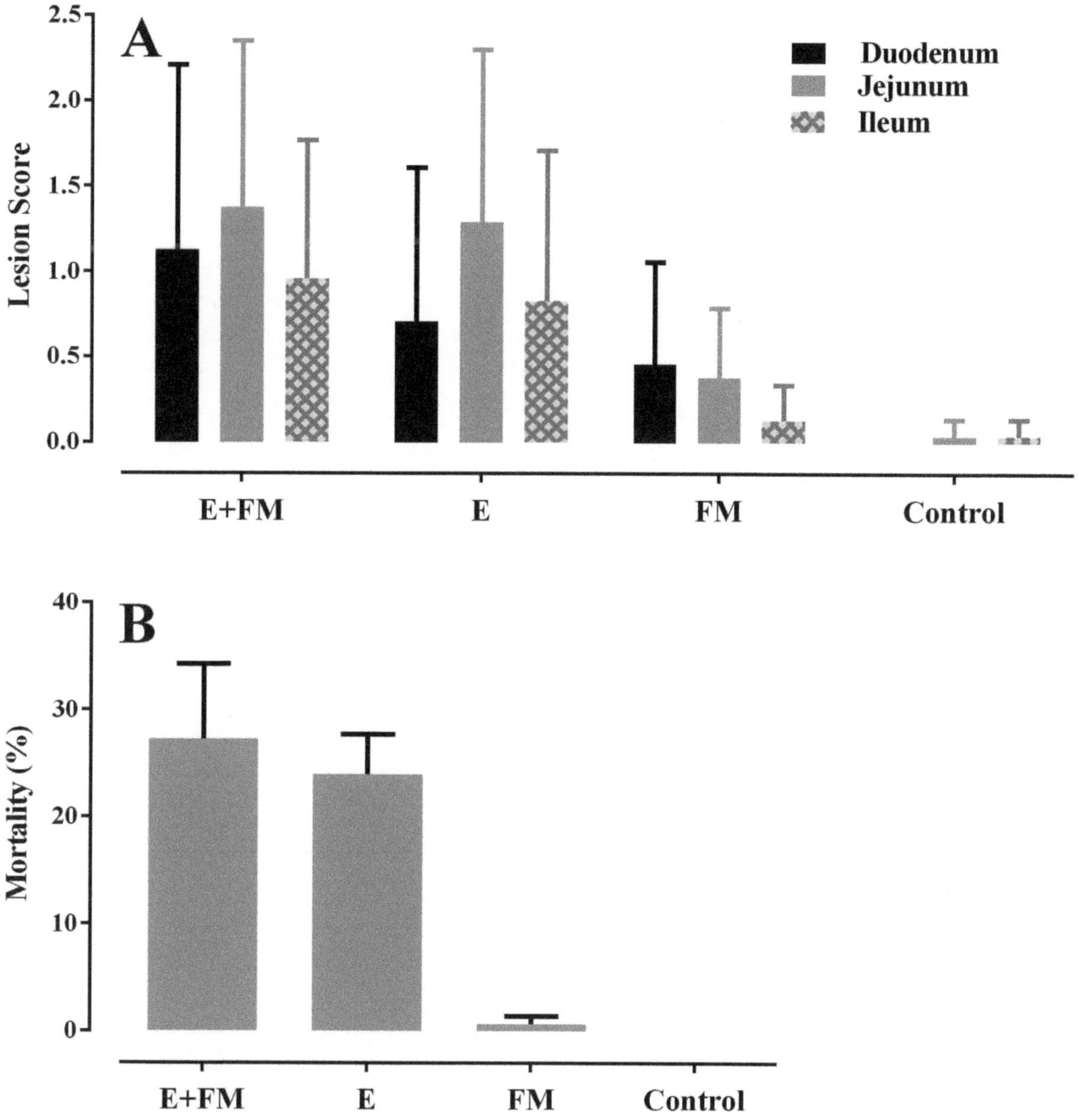

Figure 2. Barcharts showing lesion scores (A) and mortality (B) in groups challenged with *C. perfringens*. The groups not challenged with *C.perfringens* had no notable lesions or mortality. Lesions were scored as described in [13]. The bars show the standard errors. Missing bars indicate no lesions or mortality.

groups of samples containing *Eimeria* (E, E+FM or E+FM+Cp) (Figure S1 in File S1). The highest difference in alpha diversity between any two treatment groups was between control (no *Eimeria*, no fishmeal, no *C. perfringens*) vs. E+C groups. This comparison significantly affected all inspected alpha diversity measures with P-values ranging from 0.036 to 0.006. A bar-chart of species abundance (Figure S2 in File S1) demonstrates that the effect of combined *Eimeria* and *C. perfringens* on cecal microbiota composition was very pronounced.

Observing beta diversity (between sample OTU difference) using weighted and unweighted UniFrac and ADONIS statistics at 999 permutations, more differences between groups were observed in presence and absence (unweighted UniFrac) than in abundance (weighted UniFrac) of OTUs. Unweighted UniFrac demonstrated significant differences in OTUs within the cecal microbiota correlating with the presence vs. absence of *Eimeria* ($p<0.001$) and also by the presence vs. absence of fishmeal ($P<0.001$), while *C. perfringens* presence/absence produced insignificant ($P=0.058$) changes to the microbiota (Figure 3). Based on weighted UniFrac, *Eimeria* had the strongest influence ($P<0.001$) followed by fishmeal ($P=0.036$) with again insignificant influence of presence of *C. perfringens* ($P=0.168$). Finally, multivariate phylogenetic analysis (Ade4-generated PCA plot) visualised the differences between the groups using between class analyses, confirming the above results (Figure 4). The pyrosequencing data files used for this study have been deposited in the MGRAST metagenomics database (http://metagenomics.anl.gov/) with accession numbers 4567980.3 to 4568025.3.

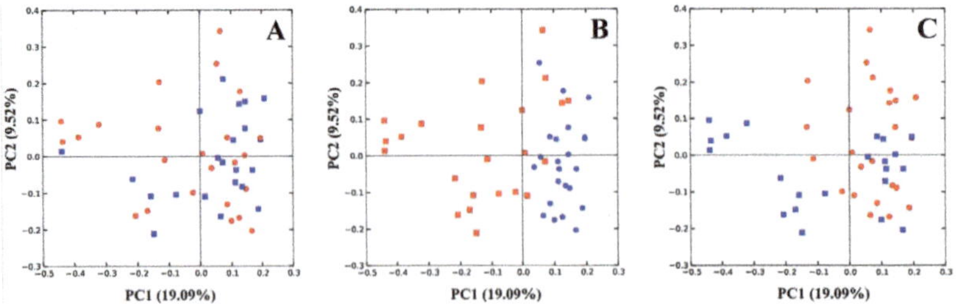

Figure 3. UnweightedUniFracPCA plot. Panel A is coloured by presence (red) and absence (blue) of *C. perfringens* in samples; in panel B samples are coloured according to presence (red) or absence (blue) of *Eimeria* and in panel C the same samples are coloured by presence (red) or absence (blue) of fishmeal diet.

Phylogeny of bacteria altered by predisposing factors and NE challenge

We used Ade4 between group multivariate phylogenetic analysis to identify the differences between treatment groups and to identify OTUs that most strongly influence between group differences at a confidence level cut-off of 95%. Figure 5 is a graphical representation of this analysis in the form of a 3D PCA plot (Figure 5A) and boxplots showing 3 selected OTUs across the treatment groups (Figure 5B–D). The 3D PCA plot presented in Figure 5A shows the relative relationship of treatment groups to OTUs. Based on the results of Ade4 analysis, the most affected phylotypes were related to the major chicken intestinal genera *Clostridium*, *Lactobacillus*, *Eubacterium* and *Ruminococcus*. OTU146 has 100% sequence similarity with the type strain of *Candidatus* Arthromitus, later renamed *Candidatus* Savagella [25], and was present at much higher frequency within the microbiota of *C. perfringens* challenged birds on the control diet than in all other groups (Figure 5B). Figure 5B also shows the presence of this OTU in three fishmeal containing groups and absence in three groups containing *Eimeria*. Among differentially abundant OTUs were OTU2877 and OTU655 with 98.5% and 99.58% similarity respectively to *C. perfringens* type strain (EzTaxon) (Figure 5C and 5D). *C. perfringens* was present in the challenged groups with predisposing factors, either used separately or together, but surprisingly was completely absent in all challenged birds that were not treated with predisposing factors (Figure 5C–D). All other OTUs marked as significantly different between groups in Ade4 analysis are provided in the form of bar-chart in a supplementary figure (Figure S3 in File S1) and their representative sequences are publically available on EMBL database under accession numbers HG810792 to HG810850.

SCFA production is altered during the challenge

Significant changes in SCFA profiles were produced by combinations of *C. perfringens* challenge and predisposing factors (Figure 6). The challenge with *C. perfringens* caused significant

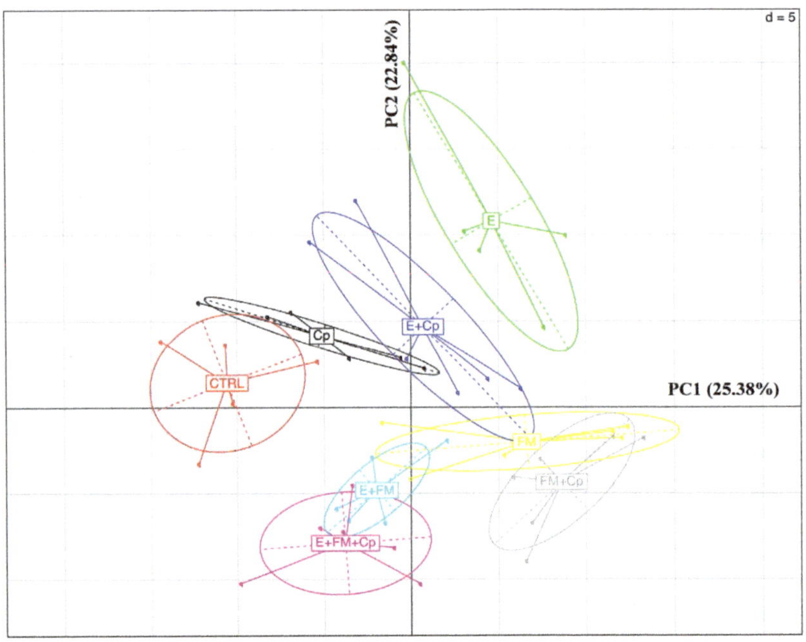

Figure 4. PCA plot generated using the Ade4 R phylogenetic package [24]. Principal Component Analysis combined with duality diagram functions (dudi) [32] was used to perform Between-Class Analysis (bca) with respect to sample assignment to treatment groups. Monte Carlo test based on 999 permutations demonstrates that groups are significantly (Monte Carlo P-value = 0.003) different. The graph shows sample and group relationship with respect to microbiota structure. The OTU table used for the analysis was 100 times rarefied (normalised) and OTUs with abundance lower than 0.001 were removed.

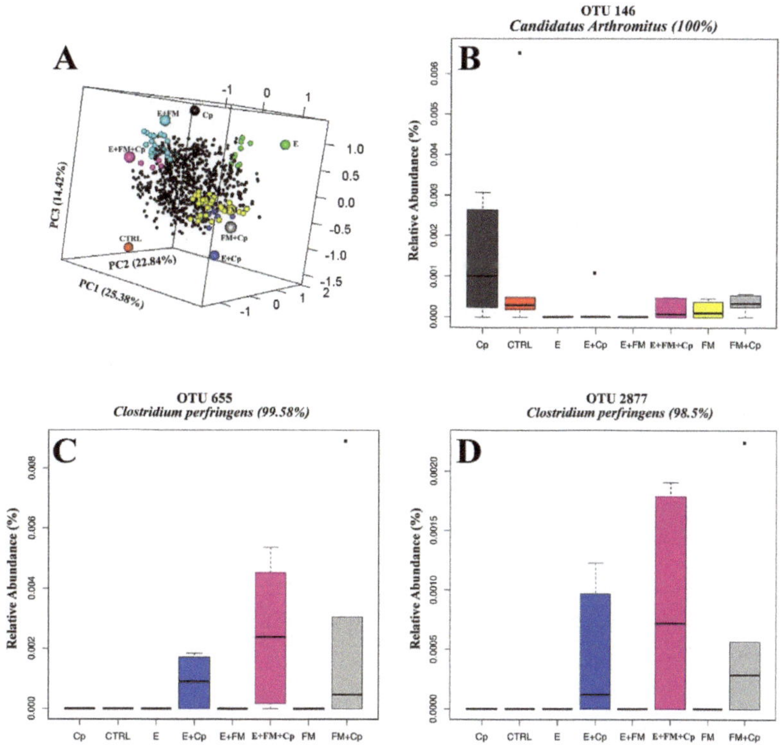

Figure 5. Duality diagram function and between class analyses presented in the form of a 3D PCA plot and selected significant OTUs in form of boxplots. The 3D graph (A) shows the relationship between sample groups and OTUs driving the sample differences. OTUs significantly different between groups were selected in Ade4 using the relative abundance table and confidence level of 95%; only OTUs with total abundance higher than 0.001 were retained in the analysis. The large circles represent treatment groups while small black circles represent OTUs. Only OTUs that are significantly associated with differences between groups are enlarged and coloured in the same colour as the sample they are distinguishing from others. Some of the significant OTUs are given in views B, C and D while all OTUs selected by Ade4 analysis are given in Figure S3. The boxes represent the limits of the second and third quartiles; the whiskers indicate the data within 1.5 times the interquartile range and the dots are outliers.

changes only in pH ($P = 0.0178$) with no significant changes in any of the SCFA inspected (P-values ranging from 0.97 to 1). Figure 6 shows that the majority of significant differences were observed in concentrations of isobutyric, isovaleric and propionic acid (lower right corner heat spot in Figure 6); in all of these comparisons at least one group of the 2 groups compared was challenged with *C. perfringens* and at least one group of the pair with *Eimeria*. There are no comparisons in this "hot spot" that did not contain at least one predisposing factor. Bar-charts showing concentration differences in all SCFAs measured are provided in Figure S4.

Correlation based on Pearson distance between OTU abundances and concentrations of SCFAs (Qiime) is presented as a Cytoscape-visualised Spring Embedded network in Figure 7. Only significant correlations with P-values$<$0.05 were included in the graph. The graph displays a group of OTUs, OTU1, OTU283, OTU615 and OTU3166, all identified as *L. johnsonii* with sequence similarities of 100, 99, 98 and 94% respectively, which are strongly anti-correlated with propionic, butyric, isovaleric and isobutyric acid concentrations. All 4 of these SCFAs were increased in the presence of *Eimeria* and *C. perfringens* together, with either the presence or absence of fishmeal. OTU1713, identified as *L. reuteri* (99% identity), was positively correlated with acetic acid concentrations. An unknown *Clostridium*, closest to *Clostridium methylpentosum* (89% identity), was positively correlated with butyric acid.

The numbers of culturable Coliforms and Enterobacteria were increased in the presence of *Eimeria* while counts of total *Lactobacillus* were not significantly changed (Figure S4 in File S1, Figure 6). pH varied significantly between the groups appearing to be reduced in *Eimeria* containing groups and increased in fishmeal fed groups (Figure S4 in File S1, Figure 6).

Discussion

At present, fishmeal and *Eimeria*, alone or combined, are the most widely used predisposing factors in NE challenge models. The mechanisms of *C. perfringens* interactions with *Eimeria* and fishmeal diet remain poorly understood but one hypothesis is that these factors disrupt the gastrointestinal environment creating disturbances in the resident microbiota and thus allowing the proliferation of *C. perfringens* by either providing nutrients or favourable ecological niches [4]. The data presented here demonstrate, for the first time, that a *C. perfringens* challenge alone is not capable of causing any significant perturbations of intestinal microbiota in birds. However, the predisposing factors *Eimeria* and/or fishmeal are able to have a marked effect on the microbiota composition in the caeca of birds. The strongest influence on alpha and beta diversity of microbiota was recorded when *Eimeria* was used in combination with *C. perfringens*. This is in agreement with previously published studies that investigated mortality of chickens under NE challenge induced with either *Eimeria* or fishmeal [14]. Wu *et al.*, [14] noted the strongest influence on NE induced mortalities when *Eimeria* and fishmeal were combined, while fishmeal alone did not significantly increase

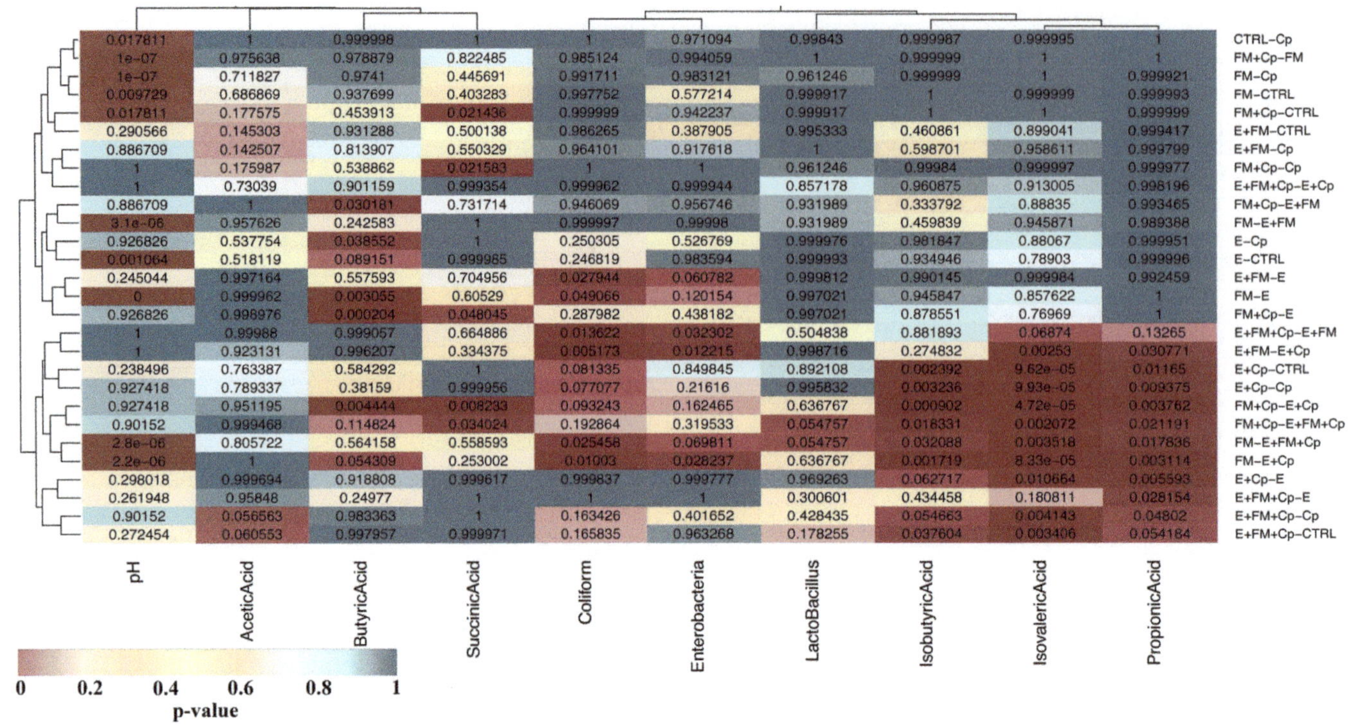

Figure 6. Table of TukeyHSD corrected p-values given in form of a heatmap. ANOVA was calculated for differences between groups for each of the SCFAs, pH and cultured bacterial counts (columns of the heatmap). ANOVA was followed by TukeyHSD honesty test to calculate p-values (shown in each cell of the heatmap) for each to each group-to-group comparison (rows). The heatmap was coloured by p-values according to the key below the graph in order to emphasise significant differences (in dark red). For example the lower right corner cell shows that groups E+FM+Cp and CTRL group (labelled E+FM+Cp – CTRL on the graph) are showing slight differences (TukeyHSD corrected P-value = 0.054184) in concentration of propionic acid. The clustering of heatmap rows and columns was done to identify similarities in SCFA changes between conditions and was based on Euclidean distance and complete agglomeration method in R package ggplot. This identified a hot-spot in the lower right corner of the heatmap of sample comparisons showing significant differences in isobutyric, isovaleric and propionic acid.

mortality of chickens challenged with *C. perfringens*. Although fishmeal had less significant effects on alpha and beta diversity than *Eimeria,* it still caused significant microbiota changes and supported establishment of *C. perfringens* in the cecal community and was thus capable of providing an environment better suited to *C. perfringens* infection.

One of the most surprising findings was that administration of *C. perfringens* on its own did not cause the pathogen to maintain and establish itself. *C. perfringens* was not identified in the 16S sequencing data in any of the birds in the unchallenged control group or the *C. perfringens* challenged group without predisposing factors, while all groups containing predisposing factors, E, FM or E+FM, showed significant presence of *C. perfringens* in all birds post-challenge (Figure 5C and D).

Administration of *C. perfringens* was correlated with an increase in the abundance of OTU146, identified by EzTaxon as 100% identical to *Candidatus* Arthromitus (accession number X80834), recently renamed to *Candidatus* Savagella based on 16S phylogenetic analysis. This group of segmented bacteria are found in gut microbiota of vertebrates like chickens, rodents and fish and are anchored to the gut epithelial cells in the ileum and play an important role in modulating host immune responses [25]. They increase, activate, and coordinate maturation of epithelial lymphocytes [26–28], and induce IgA secreting cells [29]. It was surprising to see this OTU increased only in the *C. perfringens* infected group when predisposing factors were not used but its abundance was not altered in the presence of *C. perfringens* when predisposing factors were also applied. This OTU was detected in only one bird from the three treatment groups containing *Eimeria*; in all other birds in these groups it was absent from the 16S analysis. If *Eimeria* is capable of removing or reducing this immune modulating bacterium to a level lower than the detection limit, its removal could start a chain reaction to unbalance gut mucosal immunity. This could represent a novel way in which *Eimeria* modulates host immunity to increase infectivity. A reduction in *Candidatus* Savagella was not observed in the *Eimeria* group that also had both fishmeal and *C. perfringens*. The group only treated with *C. perfringens* challenge, that strongly induced OTU146, did not develop any clinical symptoms of NE and was capable of suppressing *C. perfringens* establishment in the gut. Whether the increase in *Candidatus* Savagella had any protective role, or was just a coincidental bystander to the challenge needs to be further investigated. Interactions of *Eimeria* and this phylotype are also of potential interest.

The previously reported perturbations in the *Lactobacillus* genus due to *C. perfringens* [5] or predisposing factors [6] were also noted in the present study. *L. acidophilus* (OTU 10, 100% identity, OTU1669, 99.14% identity) and *L. johnsonii* (OTU 823, 98.76% identity) which were previously reported as reduced by NE in a fishmeal challenge model [5,6] were again reduced in the present study when birds were challenged with *C. perfringens* in the presence of fishmeal. However, both of these *Lactobacillus* phylotypes flourished in *C. perfringens* challenged birds in the presence of *Eimeria*. The few other OTUs confidently (>97%) identified as *L. johnsonii* were not reduced by fishmeal but were all consistently induced by *Eimeria* and *C. perfringens*. This, together

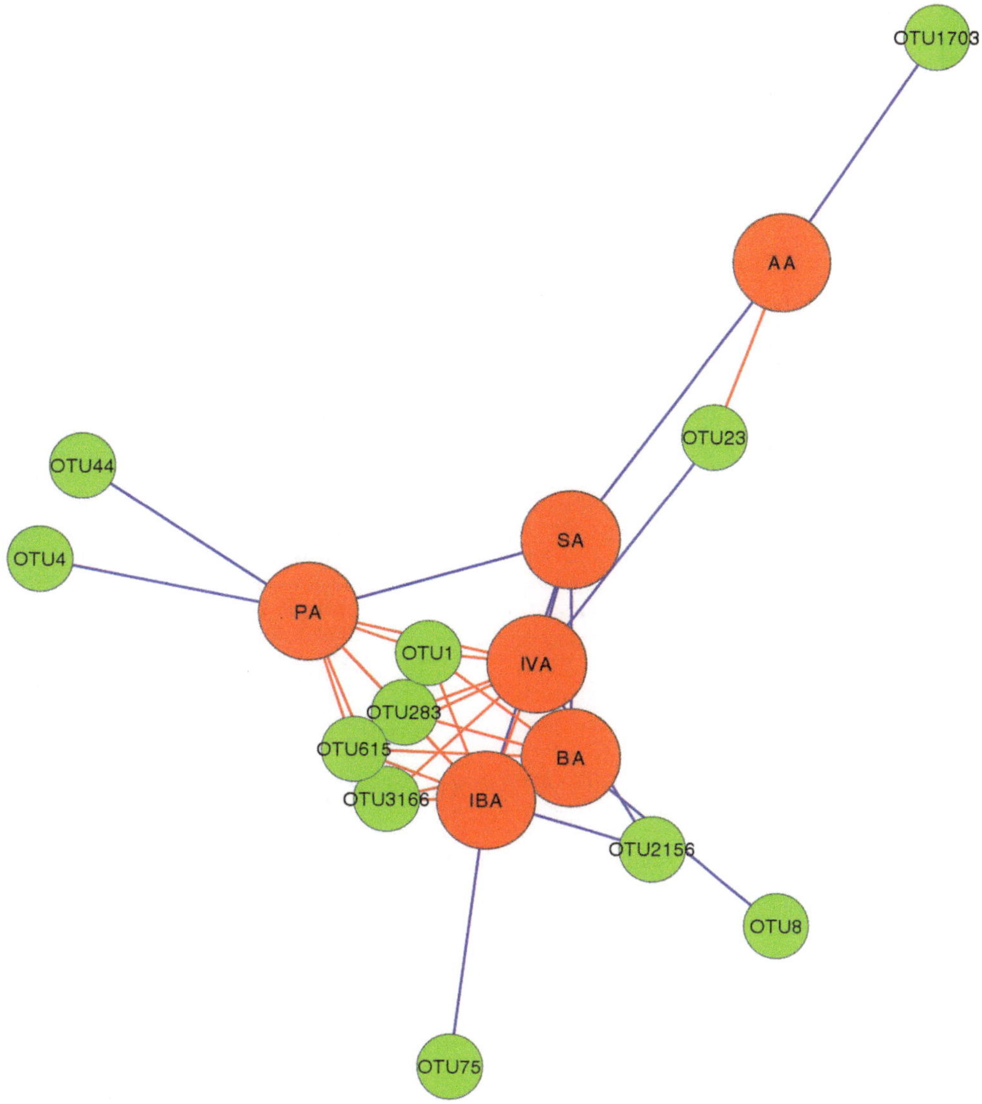

Figure 7. Spring embedded network showing Pearson correlations between SCFA and OTUs (analysed in Qiime). Edge length in the network is proportional to Pearson correlation r value; blue edge is used for negative and red edge for positive correlation. SCFA are represented with big red circles and shortened as AA = acetic Acid, SA = Succinic Acid, IVA = isovaleric Acid, BA = butyric Acid, IVA = IsoValeric Acid and PA = propionic Acid. OTUs are represented with green circles.

with many other phylotype examples (Figure S3), indicate core differences in the influence of *C. perfringens* challenge following the application of *Eimeria* and fishmeal predisposing factors. It is well documented that *Lactobacillus* members have very strict and fastidious requirements for metabolites in their environment, including SCFAs [30]. Groups containing *Eimeria* and/or fishmeal all showed reduced concentrations of acetic acid while isobutyric, butyric, and isovaleric acid concentrations were significantly increased in all groups containing *Eimeria*. Since the presence of *Eimeria* influenced intestinal SCFA concentrations the most, it is likely that SCFA fluctuations influenced some phylotypes including *L. acidophilus* and *L. johnsonii* in the opposite manner to other groups. SCFA vs OTU correlation network analysis indicated that abundances of OTUs corresponding to *L. johnsonii* and *L. reuterii* were strongly correlated with SCFA concentrations, which could also point to another mechanism contributing to *Eimeria*'s influence on NE, as perturbations within genus *Lactobacillus* were previously reported as a response to NE challenge with [6] and without [5] presence of *Eimeria*. This indicates that more than one route can lead to successful *C. perfringens* infection of birds followed by clinical symptoms. Although some of the changes induced in gut microbiota during *C. perfringens* infection have been reproducibly observed across trials it is likely that other aspects of the microbiota perturbations will vary from trial to trial given the very significant differences in the gut microbiota that has been observed in different trials and even within groups of birds [31].

Based on the present study, we can conclude that the pathogenic *C. perfringens* strain used in this study cannot, on its own, establish itself as a member of the chicken cecal microbiota but needs other factors (e.g. fishmeal or *Eimeria* infection) in order to successfully induce the disease. Whether the principal roles of these predisposing factors in the disease models are to change intestinal microbiota and thus intestinal health and metabolite profiles or these microbiota changes are a side effect remains to be further investigated. The data collected to date strongly correlate a compromised microbial community with the ability of *C. perfringens* to cause an infection. It is very likely that other predisposing factors may compromise intestinal health using different molecular strategies. Investigating *C. perfringens* challenge using other predisposing factors, such as targeted immune system compromising, could shed more light on mechanisms of necrotic enteritis onset as well as possible strategies for controlling this important disease.

Supporting Information

File S1 Contains Table S1, Comparison of alpha diversity statistics between treatment groups. The default Qiime settings were used based on a nonparametric two-sample t-test (using 100 times rarefied OTU table and 1000 Monte Carlo permutations to calculate P-values). The upper right section of the matrix, shaded light grey, indicates the p-values for the dominance metric. The lower left section of the matrix, shaded darker grey, indicates the alpha diversity comparison using the observed species metric. P values of less than 0.05 are in bold. Table S2, Detection of statistically significant differences in alpha diversity induced by the different treatments. For each comparison multiple treatment groups were combined. For example, for the *Eimeria* treatment comparison all birds that were treated with *Eimeria*, regardless of fish meal or *C. perfringens* treatment, were compared with all birds that did not receive *Eimeria*. P values of less than 0.05 are in bold. Figure S1, Alpha rarefaction graphs of groups and treatments. Alpha rarefaction measures represented as Observed Species (A and C), Dominance (B and D), Doubles (E), and Equitability (F). The analysis on individual treatment group basis is shown in panels A and B. The analysis of combined data sets (e.g. all with *C. perfringens*, all with *Eimeria* or all with both) are shown in panels C–F and demonstrate the strong influence by the combination of *Eimeria* and *C. perfringens*. Figure S2, Barchart of OTU abundances at a species level. Figure S3, Boxplots of OTUs identified as differential by Ade4 analysis. Continued from main Figure 4. The boxes represent the limits of the second and third quartiles; the whiskers indicate the data within 1.5-fold of the interquartile range; the median is indicated by the horizontal line and the dots are outliers. Note: In order to fit the legend on the x axis the names of two groups are omitted for gray column (E+FM) and for brown column (FM) in boxplots. Figure S4, Boxplots showing SCFA, pH and cultured bacteria across the treatment groups. The blue column in the boxplots represents E+FM+Cp group. The boxes represent the limits of the second and third quartiles; the whiskers indicate the data within 1.5-fold of the interquartile range; the median is indicated by the horizontal line and the dots are outliers.

Acknowledgments

This research was conducted within the Poultry CRC, established and supported under the Australian Government's Cooperative Research Centres Program. We also acknowledge and appreciate help from Dr Mark Geier from (South Australia Research and Development Institute and The University of Adelaide), and Prof Mingan Choct from the Poultry CRC for their input in the design of the animal trial. We thank Honglei Chen for performing the 454 sequencing. The data were analysed using the Isaac Newton High Performance Computing System at Central Queensland University; we wish to acknowledge continuous support in HPC computing provided by Jason Bell.

Author Contributions

Conceived and designed the experiments: SW DS RJM. Performed the experiments: DS SW NR RAS RJM. Analyzed the data: DS SW RJM RAS NR. Contributed reagents/materials/analysis tools: DS SW NR RAS RJM. Contributed to the writing of the manuscript: DS SW RJM.

References

1. Parish WE (1961) Necrotic enteritis in the fowl (*Gallus gallus domesticus*). I. Histopathology of the disease and isolation of a strain of Clostridium welchii. J Comp Pathol 71: 377–393.
2. Van der Sluis W (2000) Clostridial enteritis is an often underestimated problem. World Poultry 16: 42–43.
3. Van Immerseel F, Rood JI, Moore RJ, Titball RW (2009) Rethinking our understanding of the pathogenesis of necrotic enteritis in chickens. Trends Microbiol 17: 32–36.
4. Shojadoost B, Vince AR, Prescott JF (2012) The successful experimental induction of necrotic enteritis in chickens by *Clostridium perfringens*: a critical review. Vet Res 43: 74.
5. Stanley D, Keyburn AL, Denman SE, Moore RJ (2012) Changes in the caecal microflora of chickens following *Clostridium perfringens* challenge to induce necrotic enteritis. Veterinary Microbiology 159: 155–162.
6. Wu SB, Stanley D, Rodgers N, Swick RA, Moore RJ (2014) Two necrotic enteritis predisposing factors, dietary fishmeal and *Eimeria* infection, induce large changes in the caecal microbiota of broiler chickens. Vet Microbiol 169: 188–197.
7. Jerzsele A, Szeker K, Csizinszky R, Gere E, Jakab C, et al. (2012) Efficacy of protected sodium butyrate, a protected blend of essential oils, their combination, and Bacillus amyloliquefaciens spore suspension against artificially induced necrotic enteritis in broilers. Poult Sci 91: 837–843.
8. Timbermont L, Lanckriet A, Dewulf J, Nollet N, Schwarzer K, et al. (2010) Control of *Clostridium perfringens*-induced necrotic enteritis in broilers by target-released butyric acid, fatty acids and essential oils. Avian Pathol 39: 117–121.
9. Wang W, Chen L, Zhou R, Wang X, Song L, et al. (2014) Increased Proportion of *Bifidobacterium* and the *Lactobacillus* group and Loss of Butyrate-producing Bacteria in Inflammatory Bowel Disease. J Clin Microbiol. 52: 398–406.
10. Machiels K, Joossens M, Sabino J, De Preter V, Arijs I, et al. (2013) A decrease of the butyrate-producing species *Roseburia hominis* and *Faecalibacterium prausnitzii* defines dysbiosis in patients with ulcerative colitis. Gut. DOI:10.1136/gutjnl-2013-304833.
11. Furusawa Y, Obata Y, Fukuda S, Endo TA, Nakato G, et al. (2013) Commensal microbe-derived butyrate induces the differentiation of colonic regulatory T cells. Nature 504: 446–450.
12. Mishiro T, Kusunoki R, Otani A, Ansary MM, Tongu M, et al. (2013) Butyric acid attenuates intestinal inflammation in murine DSS-induced colitis model via milk fat globule-EGF factor 8. Lab Invest 93: 834–843.
13. Prescott JF (1979) The prevention of experimentally induced necrotic enteritis in chickens by avoparcin. Avian Dis 23: 1072–1074.
14. Wu SB, Rodgers N, Choct M (2010) Optimized necrotic enteritis model producing clinical and subclinical infection of *Clostridium perfringens* in broiler chickens. Avian Dis 54: 1058–1065.
15. Wu SB, Rodgers N, Choct M (2011) Real-time PCR assay for *Clostridium perfringens* in broiler chickens in a challenge model of necrotic enteritis. Appl Environ Microbiol 77: 1135–1139.
16. Stanley D, Denman SE, Hughes RJ, Geier MS, Crowley TM, et al. (2012) Intestinal microbiota associated with differential feed conversion efficiency in chickens. Appl Microbiol Biotechnol 96: 1361–1369.
17. Lane DJ, editor (1991) 16S and 23S rRNA sequencing.: Wiley, Chichester, UK. p. 115–174.
18. Snell-Castro R, Godon JJ, Delgenes JP, Dabert P (2005) Characterisation of the microbial diversity in a pig manure storage pit using small subunit rDNA sequence analysis. FEMS Microbiol Ecol 52: 229–242.
19. Quinlan AR, Stewart DA, Stromberg MP, Marth GT (2008) Pyrobayes: an improved base caller for SNP discovery in pyrosequences. Nat Methods 5: 179–181.
20. Caporaso JG, Kuczynski J, Stombaugh J, Bittinger K, Bushman FD, et al. (2010) QIIME allows analysis of high-throughput community sequencing data. Nat Methods 7: 335–336.
21. Edgar RC, Haas BJ, Clemente JC, Quince C, Knight R (2011) UCHIME improves sensitivity and speed of chimera detection. Bioinformatics 27: 2194–2200.
22. Chun J, Lee JH, Jung Y, Kim M, Kim S, et al. (2007) EzTaxon: a web-based tool for the identification of prokaryotes based on 16S ribosomal RNA gene sequences. Int J Syst Evol Microbiol 57: 2259–2261.
23. Altschul SF, Madden TL, Schaffer AA, Zhang J, Zhang Z, et al. (1997) Gapped BLAST and PSI-BLAST: a new generation of protein database search programs. Nucleic Acids Res 25: 3389–3402.
24. Chessel D, Dufour AB, Thiolouse J (2004) The ade4 package -I: One table methods. R News 4: 5–10.

25. Thompson CL, Mikaelyan A, Brune A (2013) Immune-modulating gut symbionts are not "*Candidatus* Arthromitus". Mucosal Immunol 6: 200–201.
26. Gaboriau-Routhiau V, Rakotobe S, Lecuyer E, Mulder I, Lan A, et al. (2009) The key role of segmented filamentous bacteria in the coordinated maturation of gut helper T cell responses. Immunity 31: 677–689.
27. Umesaki Y, Okada Y, Matsumoto S, Imaoka A, Setoyama H (1995) Segmented filamentous bacteria are indigenous intestinal bacteria that activate intraepithelial lymphocytes and induce MHC class II molecules and fucosyl asialo GM1 glycolipids on the small intestinal epithelial cells in the ex-germ-free mouse. Microbiol Immunol 39: 555–562.
28. Ivanov, II, Atarashi K, Manel N, Brodie EL, Shima T, et al. (2009) Induction of intestinal Th17 cells by segmented filamentous bacteria. Cell 139: 485–498.
29. Talham GL, Jiang HQ, Bos NA, Cebra JJ (1999) Segmented filamentous bacteria are potent stimuli of a physiologically normal state of the murine gut mucosal immune system. Infect Immun 67: 1992–2000.
30. Sneath PH, Mair NS, Sharpe ME, Holt GH, editors (1986) Bergey's manual of systematic bacteriology: Williams and Wilkins.
31. Stanley D, Geier MS, Hughes RJ, Denman SE, Moore RJ (2013) Highly variable microbiota development in the chicken gastrointestinal tract. PLoS One 8: e84290.
32. Escoufier Y (1987) The duality diagram: a means of better practical applications In Development in numerical ecology; Legendre P, Legendre L, editors. NATO advanced Institute: Springer Verlag. 139–156 p.

8

Local Duplication of Gonadotropin-Releasing Hormone (GnRH) Receptor before Two Rounds of Whole Genome Duplication and Origin of the Mammalian GnRH Receptor

Fatemeh Ameri Sefideh[1], Mi Jin Moon[1], Seongsik Yun[1], Sung In Hong[2], Jong-Ik Hwang[1], Jae Young Seong[1]*

1 Graduate School of Medicine, Korea University, Seoul, Republic of Korea, **2** Department of East-West Integrated Medicine, College of Oriental Medicine, Gachon University, Incheon, Republic of Korea

Abstract

Gonadotropin-releasing hormone (GnRH) and the GnRH receptor (GnRHR) play an important role in vertebrate reproduction. Although many GnRHR genes have been identified in a large variety of vertebrate species, the evolutionary history of GnRHR in vertebrates is unclear. To trace the evolutionary origin of GnRHR we examined the conserved synteny of chromosomes harboring GnRHR genes and matched the genes to linkage groups of reconstructed vertebrate ancestor chromosomes. Consistent with the phylogenetic tree, three pairs of GnRHR subtypes were identified in three paralogous linkage groups, indicating that an ancestral pair emerged through local duplication before two rounds of whole genome duplication (2R). The 2R then led to the generation of six subtypes of GnRHR. Some subtypes were lost during vertebrate evolution after the divergence of teleosts and tetrapods. One subtype includes mammalian GnRHR and a coelacanth GnRHR that showed the greatest response to GnRH1 among the three types of GnRH. This study provides new insight into the evolutionary relationship of vertebrate GnRHRs.

Editor: Hubert Vaudry, University of Rouen, France, France

Funding: This work was supported by grants from the Brain Research Program (2011-0019205) and Basic Science Research Program (2013R1A2A2A01068295) of the National Research Foundation of Korea. The funders had no role in study design, data collection and analysis, decision to publish, or preparation of the manuscript.

Competing Interests: The authors have declared that no competing interests exist.

* E-mail: jyseong@korea.ac.kr

Introduction

Families of neuropeptides and receptors have emerged through evolutionary processes such as gene/chromosome duplications. In particular, two rounds (2R) of whole genome duplication (WGD) during early vertebrate evolution contributed to the expansion of family members [1–8]. Moreover, teleost fish underwent a teleost-specific third round (3R) of genome duplication [6]. In addition to WGD, local tandem duplication of some genes and loss of redundant genes occurred before and after 2R [9–14], therefore the evolutionary scheme of a gene family can be highly complicated. Genome duplication events have produced paralogous chromosomal regions, also called paralogons, that provide a basis for exploring orthologous and paralogous relationships among gene family members as well as predicting gene loss in the paralogons [1,2,3,14,15]. In addition, tracing the family of genes on reconstructed pre-2R vertebrate ancestral chromosomes (*VAC*) is a fast and relatively accurate way to explore relationships among members of a family that contains a large number of paralogous genes [14,16]. In particular, because this method provides a WGD scheme for each ancestral linkage group, gene duplication and/or loss during each step of genome duplication can be traced [16].

The neuropeptide gonadotropin-releasing hormone (GnRH) and its G protein-coupled receptor GnRHR play a pivotal role in the control of reproduction in vertebrates [17,18]. To date, many GnRH and GnRHR genes have been identified in invertebrate and vertebrate species using conventional biochemical and bioinformatics tools [13,19–28]. Most vertebrate species have two or three forms of GnRH in the brain (GnRH1, GnRH2, and GnRH3) [13,19,20,29]. The corresponding genes are likely to have emerged through 2R because the three subtypes of the GnRH gene are on three different paralogons that share common neighbor gene families [13]. Most vertebrate species also possess multiple forms of GnRHR. For example, teleost fish possess four or five isoforms of GnRHR [25,29], whereas amphibian and reptilian species have three forms of GnRHR [23,30]. In our previous study using synteny analysis, we proposed four vertebrate GnRHR clades: non-mammalian GnRHR n1, n2, and n3, and mammalian GnRHR m1. GnRHR n1 and n2 were suggested to have emerged through local duplication before 2R because these genes are on the same linkage group of vertebrate chromosomes [13].

In an extension of our previous study, the present study examined more diverse vertebrate and invertebrate species including lamprey (*Petromyzon marinus*), coelacanth (*Latimeria chalumnae*), spotted gar (*Lepisosteus oculatus*), *Ciona intestinalis*, amphioxus (*Brnachiostoma floridae*), *Caenorhabditis elegans*, and *Drosophila melanogaster*. Synteny analysis and relocation of GnRHR genes and their neighboring genes on vertebrate ancestral linkage groups revealed that three pairs of GnRHRs reside on three paralogous chromosomal regions. When combined with phylogenetic analysis, this observation suggests the presence of six subtypes of vertebrate GnRHRs that arose through local duplication on the same chromosome followed by 2R. The fourth pair of GnRHR was probably lost during 2R. In addition, our study suggests that a coelacanth GnRHR is an ortholog of mammalian GnRHR because the proteins share a high degree of amino acid sequence identity and both receptors show the highest activity in response to GnRH1 among three GnRH types, thus resolving an enduring question regarding the origin of mammalian GnRHR.

Results

Phylogenetic analysis of GnRHR and evolutionary history of the vertebrate *GnRHR* genes

The amino acid sequences of GnRHR from various vertebrate taxa including 13 species (human, mouse, anole lizard, chicken, *Xenopus*, coelacanth, spotted gar, zebrafish, medaka, fugu, stickleback, tetraodon, and lamprey) (Table 1) and invertebrate taxa including 4 species (*C. elegans*, *Drosophila*, *Ciona*, and amphioxus) (Table S1) were retrieved from ENSENBL and NCBI databases. Phylogenetic analysis reveals that vertebrate GnRHRs are grouped monophylogenetically excluding invertebrate GnRHR-like receptors (Figure 1A). To explore the evolutionary relationship among the vertebrate GnRHR lineage, we examined the location of each GnRHR lineage on reconstructed linkage groups of vertebrate ancestors proposed by Nakatani et al. [6]. The Nakatani model suggests the presence of 10–13 pre-2R vertebrate ancestral chromosomes (*VAC*), defined as the *A-J* linkage groups. These *VAC*s then underwent 2R to generate approximately 40 post-2R gnathostome ancestor chromosomes (*GACs A0-J1*). Because chromosomal segments of medaka, chicken, mouse, and human have been matched to these reconstructed linkage groups, the location of a current gene can be traced back to the linkage groups [14,16]. Our data showed that three pairs of GnRHR subtypes (1a–2a, 1b–2b, and 1c–2c) are found in three related *GAC* linkage groups, *GAC A0/C1*, *A4*, and *A5* (Figure 1A). Based on phylogenetic analysis and the gene location on *GACs*, we propose that vertebrate GnRHRs originated from two ancestral *GnRHR* genes designated types 1 and 2 that emerged through a local duplication on the same chromosome before 2R. During 2R each ancestor gene gave rise to subtypes 'a' on *GAC A0/C1*, 'b' on *GAC A4*, and 'c' on *GAC A5*, resulting in six subtypes (1a,b,c and 2a,b,c) of GnRHR in vertebrates. The subtype 1a includes mammalian GnRHR and a coelacanth GnRHR. No ray-finned fish (actinopterygii including spotted gar) GnRHRs belong to the 1a subtype. The subtypes 1b and 1c are included in the same branch. The 1b subtype includes tetrapod and lobe-finned fish (sarcopterygii) receptors whereas the 1c subtype contains only ray-finned fish receptors. This observation may lead to misunderstanding of the origin of these subtypes. For example, 1b and 1c subtype receptors might be considered to be orthologous. However, as 1b and 1c subtype receptors are on different *GACs* (*GAC A4* and *A5*, respectively) they are more likely to be paralogs generated through a second round of WGD. Therefore, it seems likely that the 1b subtype was lost in ray-finned fish and the 1c subtype was lost in lobe-finned fish after 2R. The teleost-specific 3R may have generated an additional form, the 1c′ subtype. The 2a subtype includes only a coelacanth receptor therefore this subtype was lost in other vertebrates. The 2b subtype includes both ray-finned and lobe-finned fish receptors. The evolution of the 2b subtype in teleosts is highly complicated. The teleost-specific 3R might have contributed to generation of the 2b′ subtype, which was followed by local duplication for emergence of the 2b″ subtype. The 2c subtype is composed of human, *Xenopus*, and coelacanth receptors, but no ray-finned fish receptors (Figure 1A).

Based on these results, we propose an evolutionary history of vertebrate GnRHRs. Type 1 and 2 receptors may have emerged through a local duplication on *VAC A* before 2R. During the first round (1R) of WGD, two genes were duplicated on *GAC A0/A1* and *A4/5* linkage groups. According to the Nakatani model, *GAC A2/3* separated from the *GAC A4/5* linkage group by fission after 1R [6] therefore *GAC A2/3* is not discussed here. The *GAC A4/5* linkage group doubled during the second round (2R) of WGD to produce pairs of *GnRHR* on *GACs A4* and *A5*. The second round of WGD may not have generated the fourth GnRHR pair on *GAC A1*. Alternatively, the fourth GnRHR pair on *GAC A1* might have been lost after 2R. After 2R, the 1a subtype gene appears to have moved to the *GAC C1* linkage group, probably through chromosomal rearrangement or a single gene translocation (Figure 1B). Thus, gnathostome ancestors may have six subtypes of GnRHR. Some subtypes of GnRHR have been lost after the divergence of ray-finned and lobe-finned fish. For example, coelacanth lost the 1c subtype and *Xenopus* lacks 1a, 2a, and 1c subtypes. Chicken has only two subtypes, 1b and 2b, and humans possess one functional receptor of the 1a subtype and one nonfunctional pseudogene of the 2c subtype [24]. In early actinopterygians, GnRHRs on *GAC A0/C1* are likely to have disappeared. Thus, spotted gar contains only two GnRHRs (2b and 1c) on *GAC A4* and *A5*. However, GnRHRs on *GACs A4* and *A5* were duplicated through the teleost-specific 3R, followed by loss of some subtypes. Zebrafish contains four subtypes of receptors, 2b, 2b′, 1c, and 1c′. In medaka and tetraodon, the 2c′ subtype was lost but a 2b″ subtype emerged, probably through a local duplication (Figure 1B). Although we propose a scenario for a doublet GnRHR before 2R, a triplet GnRHR before 2R is also possible because the 1a subtype is phylogenetically distinct from 1b and 1c subtypes. Such a scenario involves an additional local duplication, generating three types (1a, 1b/c, and 2a/b/c) before 2R.

Synteny of vertebrate chromosomes containing GnRHRs

To corroborate the gene/genome duplication scheme of the vertebrate GnRHR family, we performed synteny analysis of chromosomal fragments containing GnRHRs. The coelacanth scaffold JH127011 contains the GnRHR 2a subtype and its neighboring genes, which are also found in regions of human chromosomes 5 and 4 that fall into *GAC A0* and *C1*, respectively. It is noteworthy that this region of chromosome 4 contains the GnRHR 1a subtype (Figure 2). Unfortunately, 1a and 2a subtypes are not found in other vertebrate species. The presence of neighbor genes belonging to either *GAC A0* or *C1* in the coelacanth scaffold JH127011 suggests the possibility that the linkage groups including *GAC A0* and *C1* were previously linked. This possibility is partly supported by observations that the paralogous genes *ADAMTS6* and *ADAMTS3* are on either *GAC A0* or *C1* and that some genes in fish, including *ADAMTS3*, *EPHA5*, and *NPFFR2* on *GAC C1*, are on the same chromosomal regions as genes that map on *GAC A0* (Figure 2). An alternative scenario is that GnRHR 1a and some neighbors were translocated to the *GAC C1* linkage group.

The GnRHR 1b and 2b subtypes are on coelacanth scaffolds JH126619 and JH126611, respectively. Neighbor genes on these

Table 1. Classification of vertebrate GnRHR based on phylogenetic and synteny analysis.

Vertebrate species	**Subtype (GAC)**					
	1a (A0/C1)	**1b (A4)**	**1c (A5)**	**2a (A0/C1)**	**2b (A4)**	**2c (A5)**
Human *(H. sapiens)*	**GnRHR (m1)** AAI13547 (Ch4)					**GnRHR (n3/m2)** NR_002328 (Ch1)
Mouse *(M. musculus)*	**GnRHR (m1)** NP_034453 (Ch7)					
Anole lizard *(A. carolinensis)*		**GnRHR (n2)** ENSACAP00000004352 (Scaffold:GL343392)				
Chicken *(G. gallus)*		**GnRHR (n2)** NP_989984 (Ch10)			**GnRHR (n1)** NP_001012627 (Ch10)	
Western clawed frog *(X. tropicalis)*		**GnRHR (n2)** NP_001107548 (Scaffold:GL172999)			**GnRHR (n1)** NP_001107547 (Scaffold: GL172658)	**GnRHR (n3/m2)** NP_001107549 (Scaffold:GL176594)
Coelacanth *(L.chalumnae)*	**GnRHR1a** ENSLACG00000002185 (Scaffold:JH130998)	**GnRHR1b** ENSLACG00000016584 (Scaffold:JH126619)		**GnRHR2a** ENSLACG00000013490 (Scaffold:JH127011)	**GnRHR2b** ENSLACG00000018198 (Scaffold:JH126611)	**GnRHR2c** ENSLACG00000014236 (Scaffold:JH126664)
Spotted gar *(L.oculatus)*			**GnRHR** ENSLOCG00000008760 (Ch LG24)		**GnRHR** ENSLOCG00000014360 (Ch LG3)	
Zebrafish *(D. renio)*			**GnRHR (n3)** NP_001170921 (Ch16)		**GnRHR (n2)** NP_001138451.1 (Ch7)	
			GnRHR′ (n3b) NP_001138452 (Scaffold:Zv-NA22)		**GnRHR′ (n1)** NP_001091663 (Ch18)	
Medaka *(O. latipes)*			**GnRHR (n3)** NP_001098392 (Scaffold:2457)		**GnRHR (n1)** NP_001098393 (Ch6)	
					GnRHR′ (n2) ENSORLP00000015859 (Scaffold:1670)	
					GnRHR″ (n1b) NP_001098352 (Ch3)	
Green pufferfish *(T. nigroviridis)*			**GnRHR (n3)** BAE45702 (Ch_Unrandom)		**GnRHR (n1)** BAE45698 (Ch13)	
			GnRHR′ (n3b) BAE45700 (Ch17)		**GnRHR′ (n2)** ENSORLP00000015859 (Scaffold:1670)	
					GnRHR″ (n1b) BAE45694 (ChUnrandom)	
Stickleback *(G.aculeatus)*			**GnRHR (n3)** ENSGACP00000004101 (Ch20)		**GnRHR (n1)** ENSGACP00000014249 (Ch19)	
			GnRHR′ (n3b) ENSGACP00000000651 (Scaffold:101)		**GnRHR′ (n2)** ENSGACP00000021774 (Ch2)	
					GnRHR″ (n1b) ENSGACP00000019583 (Ch2)	

Table 1. Cont.

Vertebrate species	Subtype (GAC)					
	1a (A0/C1)	1b (A4)	1c (A5)	2a (A0/C1)	2b (A4)	2c (A5)
Fugu (*T. rubripes*)			**GnRHR(n3)** ENSTRUP00000014399 (Scaffold:270)		**GnRHR (n1)** ENSTRUP00000019152 (Scaffold:217)	
			GnRHR′ (n3b) ENSTRUP00000005457 (Scaffold:291)		**GnRHR′ (n2)** ENSTRUP00000014430 (Scaffold:174)	
					GnRHR″ (n1b) ENSTRUP00000018665 (Scaffold:92)	
Lamprey (*P. marinus*)				**GnRHR1** ENSPMAP00000010120 (Scaffold:GL493405)	**GnRHR2** ENSPMAP00000003609 (Scaffold:GL483393)	**GnRHR3** ENSPMAP00000011312 (Scaffold:GL483841)

The subtype annotations were based on phylogeny and location on gnathostome ancestor gene linkage blocks *GAC A0/C1*, *GAC A4*, and *GAC A5*. The accession numbers for NCBI and ENSEMBL and gene location are given below the names of the receptors. The receptor names according to our previous classification [13] are shown in parentheses. The five new coelacanth GnRHRs follow current subtype annotation. ′, product of 3R; ″, product of a local duplication after 3R.

two scaffolds are found on the same chromosomes in human (chromosome 15) and chicken (chromosome 10). The 1b subtype is absent in teleosts. The teleost-specific 3R might have contributed to doubling of the 2b subtype to produce 2b and 2b′ subtypes as these subtypes are found in chromosomal regions that seem to have been duplicated through 3R [6]. In addition, medaka, tetraodon, and stickleback have an additional subtype 2b″ that is likely to have emerged through a local duplication after 3R. In stickleback, the 2b′ and 2b″ subtypes are on the same chromosome (Figure 2). This observation is consistent with the phylogenetic tree (Figure 1A).

Chromosomal regions with GnRHR 1c or 2c subtypes share neighbors in vertebrate chromosomal regions. The 2c subtype is present in coelacanth, human, and *Xenopus*, but not in ray-finned fish. In contrast, the 1c subtype is present in ray-finned fish but absent in lobe-finned fish and tetrapods. There are two 1c subtype genes in teleost fish. As one gene is on a short scaffold with few neighbors, it is unclear whether these genes were generated by the teleost 3R or local duplication (Figure 2).

Many paralogous genes were shared between these linkage groups (Figure 2). For example, *IQGAP*, *ADAMTS*, *MEGF/PEAR*, *RGM/HFE*, and *ARRDC/TXNIP* family genes are commonly present in the three linkage groups. Paralogous genes for *PCSK1*, *ELL2*, *HOMER1*, and *CCNO* on *GAC A0* are present in *GAC A4* and paralogous genes for *SEMA4B*, *RHCG*, *PWX11A*, and *IGF1R* on *GAC A4* are seen in *GAC A5*. This result is consistent with the Nakatani model proposing that the three linkage groups shown in Figure 2 were generated through the 2R.

Subtype-specific motifs in vertebrate GnRHRs

In a search for new GnRHR genes we identified five new genes in coelacanth. Our synteny and phylogenetic analysis revealed that one of these coelacanth GnRHR genes corresponds to mammalian type I GnRHR (the 1a subtype in this study) and three genes correspond to non-mammalian GnRHRs GnRHRn1 (2b), GnRHRn2 (1b), and GnRHRn3 (2c) according to our previous classification [13]. Surprisingly, one coelacanth GnRHR (2a) is unique and cannot readily be compared with other vertebrate GnRHRs. The five coelacanth GnRHRs were aligned with human 1a, *Xenopus* 1b, 2a, 2b, 2c, and zebrafish 1c GnRHRs (Figure 3). Alignment for all amino acid sequences of GnRHR examined in this study is shown in Figure S1. Sequence alignment analysis revealed that all subtypes of GnRHRs share many critical residues involved in ligand binding, binding pocket formation, G protein coupling, and receptor activation (Figure 3). The major difference between types 1 and 2 is found in intracellular loop 3 (IL3). The type 2 receptors have a longer IL3 that contains a highly conserved SKExxLRr/cS motif. The type 1 receptors have subtype-specific residues in IL3: the 1a subtype has a Tr/qVLh/rQDP motif, the 1b subtype contains KQm/lK motif, and the 1c subtype possesses a slightly longer IL3 without pronounced sequence conservation (Figure S1). Because IL3 is involved in G-protein coupling, receptor desensitization, and internalization [31,32], this subtype specificity may result in differences in signaling cascades and down-regulation among receptors. Extracellular loop 3 (EL3) also contains subtype-specific motifs: Sd/eP for 1a, PEY for 1b and 1c, Pe/pS for 2a and 1c, and Sh/qS for 2b. These motifs are known to be involved in ligand specificity [33-36]. Major differences between subtype 1a mammalian GnRHR and other subtype receptors are the absence/presence of the cytoplasmic tail and residue $Asn^{2.50}/Asp^{2.50}$ in transmembrane helix 2 (TMH2) [37-40]. Coelacanth GnRHR1a possesses specific characteristics present in mammalian type I GnRHR (the 1a subtype) – it lacks the cytoplasmic tail and contains $Asn^{2.50}$ in

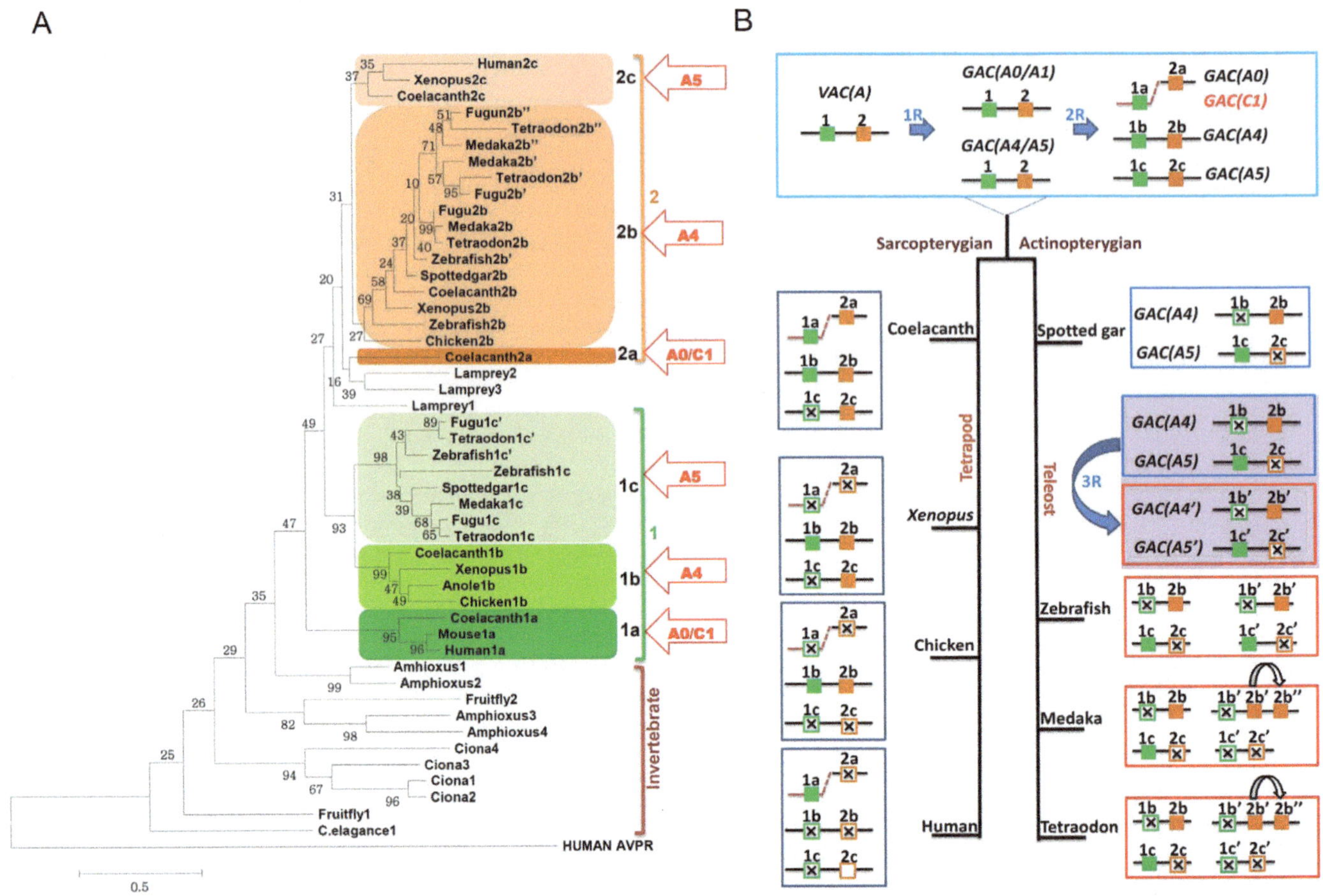

Figure 1. Phylogenetic tree construction for GnRHR-like receptors and evolutionary relationship of vertebrate GnRHRs genes. ***A*,** Amino acid sequences of vertebrate species (human, mouse, chicken, anole lizard, *Xenopus*, coelacanth, spotted gar, zebrafish, medaka, fugu, stickleback, tetraodon, and lamprey) and invertebrate species (*C. elegans*, *Drosophila*, *Ciona*, and amphioxus) were aligned using MUSCLE and the phylogeny tree was generated by MEGA 5.05. The human arginine vasopressin receptor 1a protein sequence was used as an outgroup. The vertebrate GnRHRs are grouped monophylogetically. The vertebrate gene types 1 and 2 are illustrated by green and orange, respectively. The arrows indicate the location of each vertebrate gene type on the ancestral linkage group. ***B*,** Prior to 2R, GnRHR types 1 and 2 emerged as a product of local duplication on the *VAC A*. Following 2R, a, b, and c subtypes of each ancestral type 1 and 2 were produced on *GAC A0*, *GAC A4*, and, *GAC A5* respectively and GnRHR type 1a was translocated to *GAC C1*. During the evolution of vertebrate species some GnRHR subtypes have been lost or/and duplicated. The empty box indicates a pseudogene in a human chromosome. An empty box with a cross indicates loss of the gene.

TMH2. Thus, coelacanth GnRHR 1a may be an ortholog of mammalian type I GnRHR.

Ligand selectivity of coelacanth GnRHR 1a

To further examine functional orthology between coelacanth GnRHR 1a and mammalian type I GnRHR, we examined the ligand selectivity of coelacanth GnRHR 1a. HEK293 cells were transfected with plasmid containing coelacanth GnRHR 1a and the reporter vector SRE-luc or CRE-luc. Cells were then treated with human GnRH1, coelacanth GnRH1, chicken GnRH2, or salmon GnRH3. In response ligand stimulation, cells transfected with coelacanth GnRHR 1a showed an increase in both SRE-luc and CRE-luc activities, indicating that coelacanth GnRHR 1a may be coupled to both $G_{q/11}$- and G_s-mediated signaling pathways (Figure 4). Coelacanth GnRHR 1a responded best to human and coelacanth GnRH1 but poorly to GnRH2 and GnRH3, indicating that coelacanth GnRHR 1a has highest affinity for GnRH1, as does the mammalian type I receptor [33,34].

Discussion

The evolutionary relationship and history of a gene family can be deciphered by conventional phylogenetic analysis and synteny analysis of chromosomal regions containing members of the gene family [5,8,13]. The accumulation of genome sequence information for various invertebrate and vertebrate species has facilitated entire genome comparisons of evolutionarily distant taxa, allowing reconstruction of hypothetical chromosomes of vertebrate or chordate ancestors [6,7]. Recently, relocating gene family members on these reconstructed vertebrate ancestral linkage groups was found to be a complementary tool to examine the evolutionary history of a gene family [14,16]. This method is particularly useful for a gene family with a large number of paralogs that arose before WGD [14]. Because conventional small-scale synteny covers relatively short chromosomal regions, neighbor genes located far from the gene of interest on the chromosome or genes on other chromosomes are often excluded from the analyses. In contrast, the size of the reconstructed ancestral linkage group is much greater than that used for small-scale synteny and the ancestral linkage group also includes genes

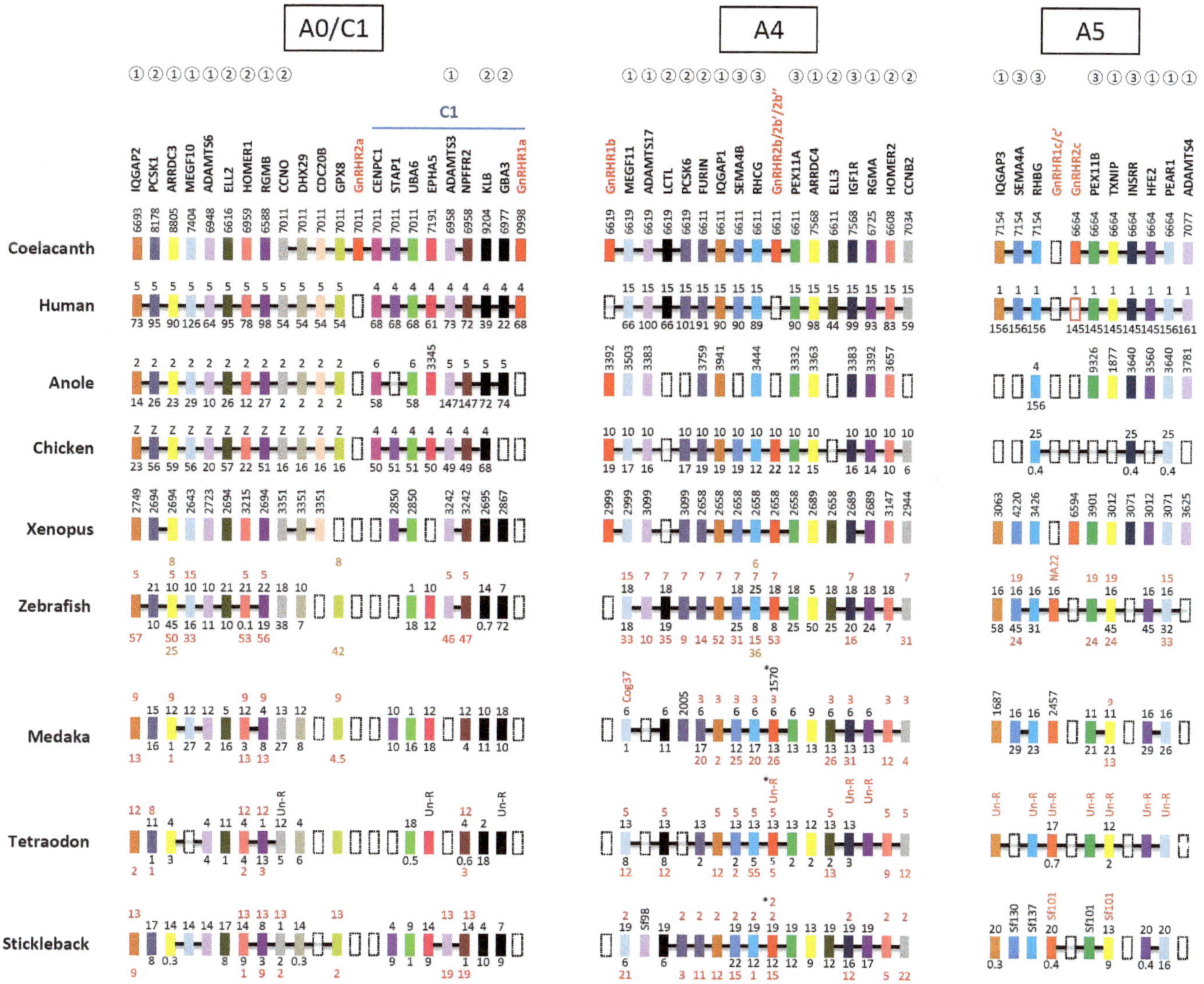

Figure 2. Synteny analysis for chromosome fragments harboring vertebrate GnRHRs. GnRHR and neighboring genes in human, coelacanth, anole, chicken, *Xenopus*, zebrafish, medaka, tetraodon, and stickleback were matched on ancestral linkage groups. The GnRHRs are illustrated in red. Orthologous genes are aligned in the same column and indicated by the same color. The chromosome number and gene location (in megabases) are indicated above and below the indicated genes respectively. For genes located on scaffolds, the gene positions are indicated vertically with only the last four digits of the scaffold number (*e.g.*, JH127011 in coelacanth is indicated as 7011). For teleost species, the duplicated genes are represented by two lines of numbers because of the third round of whole genome duplication. The broken boxes indicate loss or absence of genes. The common paralogs across *GAC A0, GAC A4, GAC A5,* and *GAC C1* are indicated by open circles containing numbers as follows: ① indicates the gene families found on *GACs A0, A4,* and *A5*; ② indicates the gene families observed in *GACs A0* and *A4*; ③ indicates the genes in *GACs A4* and *A5*. In the case of stickleback and medaka, (*) indicates that 2b″ was generated from local gene duplication of 2b′.

clusters that translocated to other chromosomes [14,16]. However, this method suffers from poor resolution in some ancestral linkage groups due to either inaccurate reconstruction because of massive chromosome rearrangements, or a single gene translocation that caused it to move from its authentic chromosomal fragments during or after 2R [14,16]. Thus, combining phylogenic and syntenic analyses is necessary for a better understanding of the evolutionary relationship and history of a gene family [14,16].

By applying the above approaches, we were able to propose an evolutionary history of the GnRHR family in vertebrates. In our previous study, we classified vertebrate GnRHRs into four subtypes, one mammalian 1 subtype (m1) and three non-mammalian subtypes (n1, n2, and n3) [13]. In the present study, through identification of a novel subtype of GnRHR and improved synteny methods, we propose the presence of six subtypes (1a–2c) of GnRHRs in vertebrates. The m1 subtype is equivalent to the 1a subtype that includes a coelacanth GnRHR. The n1 and n2 subtypes are largely shuffled in the present study (Table 1). The tetrapod n2 matches with 1b, whereas teleost n2 belongs to 2b. The tetrapod n1 and teleost n1 are included in the 2b subtype. The n3 group splits into 1c (teleost receptors) and 2c (tetrapod receptors). This confusion is largely due to multiple local duplications of GnRHR before 2R (and after 3R in teleosts) followed by either lobed-finned fish- or ray-finned fish-specific loss of the subtype gene. For example, the n1 and n2 subtypes (1b and 2b in this study) emerged via a local duplication on the same chromosome before 2R, and additional subtypes 2b′ and 2b″ in teleosts arose through 3R and a subsequent local duplication.

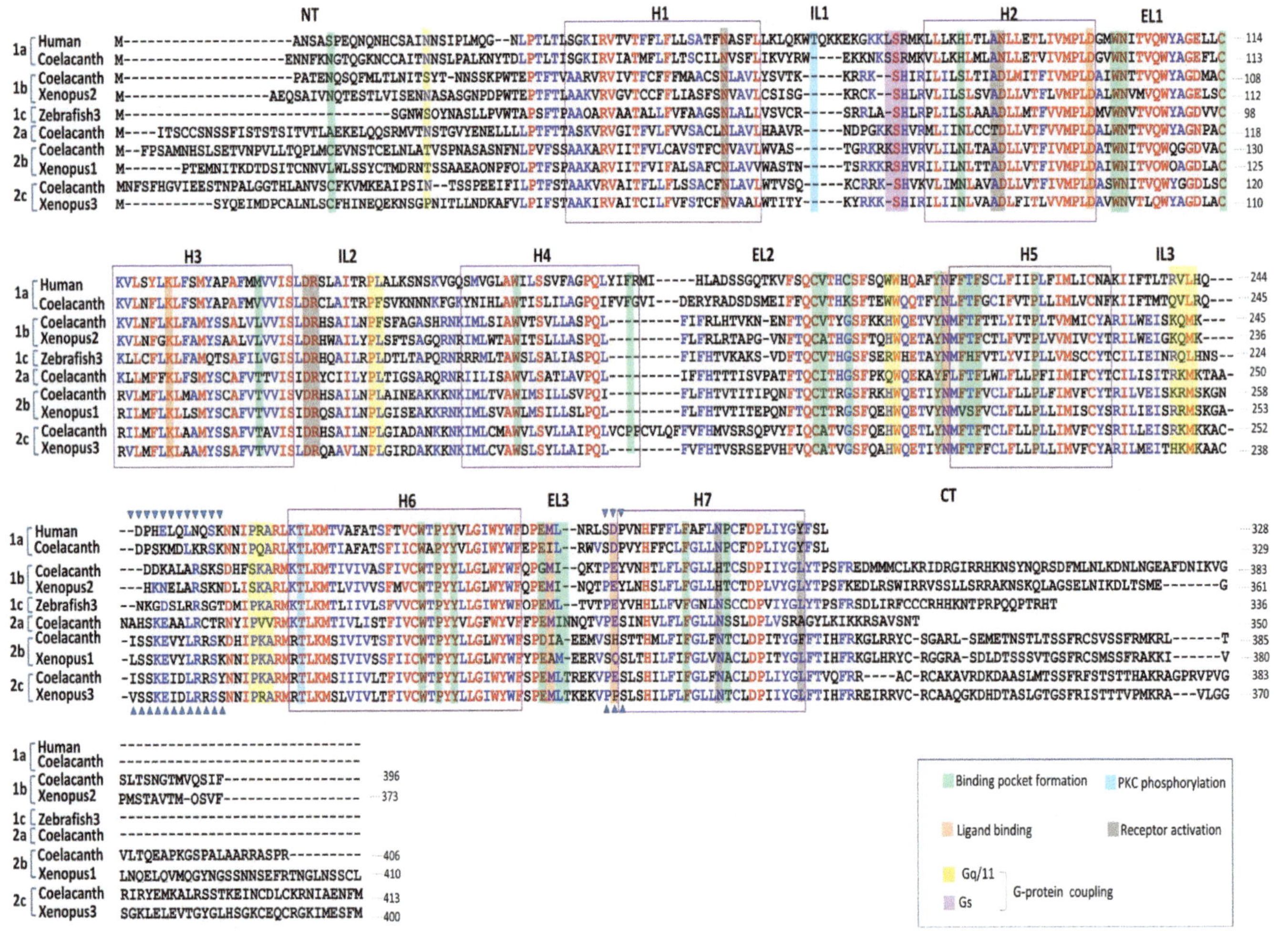

Figure 3. Sequence alignment of coelacanth GnRHRs with vertebrate GnRHRs that represent each subtype. The five coelacanth GnRHRs were aligned with human GnRHR1a, *Xenopus* GnRHR1b, zebrafish GnRHR1c, *Xenopus* GnRHR2b, and *Xenopus* GnRHR2c. Residues with 50% and 90% similarity are indicated in blue and red, respectively. Predicted N terminal (NT), transmembrane helix (H), intracellular loop (IL), extracellular loop (EL) and C-terminal (CT) domains are indicated. The putative residues involved in ligand binding, binding pocket formation, receptor activity, PKC phosphorylation, and G protein coupling are illustrated in different colors. ▼ indicates the subtype-specific motifs.

Thus, our previous synteny failed to explore the fine mechanisms of the emergence of GnRHR subtypes through genome duplications and local duplications [13]. A new GnRHR found in coelacanth is likely to belong to a new subtype 2a.

The phylogenetic trees constructed in our study and by others reveal that the 1a subtype receptors are phylogenetically closer to invertebrate receptors than to other receptors [27] suggesting that, among vertebrate receptors, the 1a subtype receptors are probably closer to an ancestral form of GnRHR. Interestingly, amphioxus has four GnRHRs, two of which are similar to the protostomian GnRHR found in *Drosophila* and *C. elegans* whereas the other two are similar to vertebrate GnRHR [27,41]. Indeed, a recent study showed that the vertebrate-like amphioxus GnRHRs exhibited a high affinity to vertebrate GnRHs but not to protostomian GnRHs, whereas protostomian-like amphioxus GnRHRs had poor affinity to vertebrate GnRHs [27]. Thus, amphioxus contains two GnRHR lineages, vertebrate-like GnRHR and protostomian-like GnRHR. The protostomian GnRHRs were not found in the basal vertebrate lamprey. Instead, lamprey contains three receptors which are likely to belong to type 2 receptors. As the scaffolds containing lamprey GnRHRs are short and do not have any neighbors, syntenic analysis to explore the evolutionary position of these genes is impossible.

Our chromosome analysis showed that three pairs of the subtypes (1a–2a, 1b–2b, and 1c–2c) are present on three paralogous chromosomal regions. Although pairs of the subtype are on the same chromosomes, members in each pair are phylogenetically distant; instead, the phylogeny tree shows a close relationship among type 1 subtypes (1a, 1b, and 1c) and type 2 subtypes (2a, 2b, and 2c). This indicates that a local duplication of GnRHR occurred before 2R and that consecutive chromosome duplications have contributed to the generation of three pairs. The fourth pair was probably lost after 2R. There is accumulating evidence for local duplication gene families before 2R. In the case of somatostatin and its paralogous genes cortistatin, urotensin II, and urotensin II-like peptide, two pairs of the genes are on two paralogous chromosomes [11]. The neuropeptide Y receptor (NPYR) triplet is proposed to have existed before 2R [9]. In addition, prolactin-releasing hormone receptors, which are phylogenetically very close paralogous receptors for NPYR, are also in the near vicinity of NPYR on the same chromosomes [10]. The secretin-like receptors and their peptides genes are also clustered on paralogous chromosomes [14], showing that paralogous genes

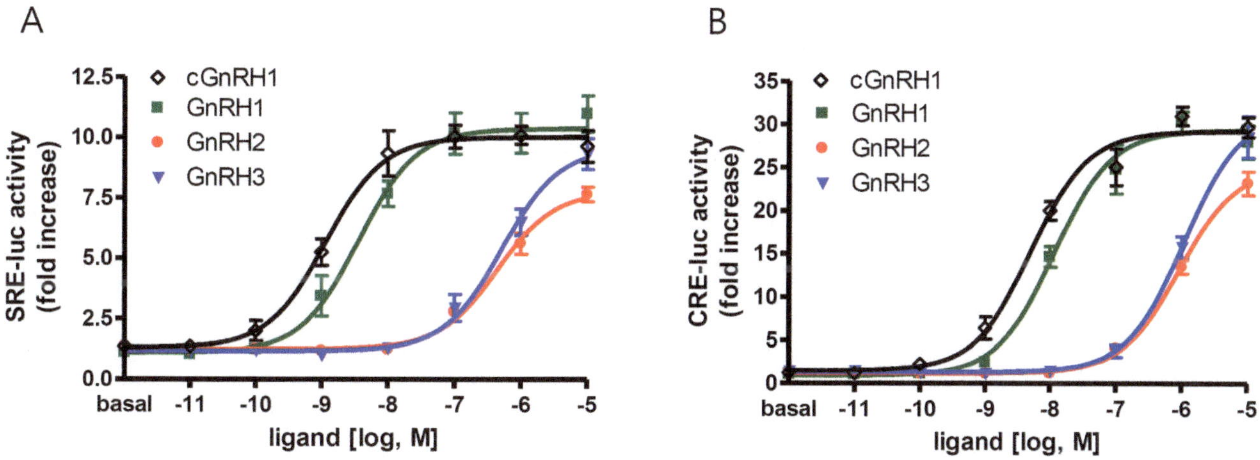

Figure 4. Activity of GnRH peptides with coelacanth GnRHR 1a. Plasmid containing coelacanth GnRHR 1a sequence was co-transfected into HEK293T cells with SRE-luc (*A*) or CRE-luc (*B*) vector in 48-well plates. Forty-eight hours after transfection, cells were treated with the indicated concentrations of peptides (◇ coelacanth (c) GnRH1; ■ GnRH1; ● GnRH2; ▼ GnRH3) for 6 h, and luciferase activity was examined.

that arose through local duplications reside in the near vicinity on the same chromosomes or on reconstructed ancestral chromosomes.

The origin of type 1 mammalian GnRHR has been questioned because orthologs of the mammalian receptor have not been found in other vertebrates and the structure of the mammalian receptor is quite different from that of other receptor subtypes [13,27,42]. In our study, we found that a coelacanth receptor is similar to the mammalian receptor based on amino acid sequence. Like mammalian GnRHR, this coelacanth receptor lacks the C-terminal cytoplasmic tail, has conserved $Asn^{2.50}/Asp^{7.49}$ residues in TMH2 and THM7, and harbors an Sd/eP motif in ECL3. The presence or absence of the C-terminal cytoplasmic tail is important for receptor down-regulation and internalization [37]. For example, addition of the C-terminal cytoplasmic tail to mammalian GnRHR greatly enhances the internalization and desensitization rates [37]. Furthermore, the C-terminal cytoplasmic tail is likely to be involved in signaling pathway. Deletion of the C-terminal tail from bullfrog GnRHR-1 remarkably decreased its ability to induce G_s-mediated adenylyl cyclase (AC)/protein-kinase A (PKA) signaling. In contrast, addition of this motif to mammalian GnRHR improved its ability to induce the AC/PKA-linked signaling pathway [38]. Interaction of the $Asn^{2.50}$ residue in TMH2 with the $Asp^{7.49}$ residue in TMH7 of mammalian GnRHR is essential for receptor conformation and activation whereas non-mammalian receptors have $Asp^{2.50}/Asp^{7.49}$ in both TMH2 and TMH7 [39,40]. The GnRH binding residues (i.e. Asp^{98}, Asn^{102}, Lys^{121}, Asn^{212}, Trp^{280}, Trp^{289}, and Tyr^{290}) of mammalian GnRHR-1 are highly conserved among vertebrate GnRHRs [43–47]. Thus, a mammalian GnRHR-specific motif, the Sd/eP motif in ECL3, was considered to be important for high affinity toward GnRH1 [33–35]. Indeed, our study shows that the coelacanth receptor with the SDP motif responded best to human and coelacanth GnRH1 but poorly to GnRH2 and GnRH3. In particular, differences in the specific domains (SD/EP, PEY, and PPS) at the ECL3 have been used for classification of GnRHR [36,42]. Taken together, these findings indicate that the coelacanth receptor is a functional ortholog of the mammalian type 1 GnRHR, thus the 1a subtype receptor is no longer unique to mammals.

In summary, the evolutionary history of the GnRHR represents repetitions of continuous duplications and losses within a gene family during metazoan evolution. In particular, during emergence of early vertebrates, at least two GnRHRs appear to have been generated through local duplication. This doublet was amplified as three pairs through WGD, followed by loss of redundant members before the divergence of ray-finned and lobed-finned fish. Evolution of GnRHR in teleosts is more complicated than that of tetrapods due to teleost-specific 3R, local duplication after 3R, and loss of genes before or after 3R. Because of the complexity of GnRHR evolutionary history, a combination of phylogenetic analysis, small-scale synteny, and relocating gene family on the reconstructed ancestor chromosome is required for better understanding of the evolutionary history of the gene family. This issue will be further clarified when improved genome data of other vertebrate and invertebrate species are available.

Materials and Methods

Phylogeny of the GnRHR family

ENSEMBE (http://www.ensembel.org) and GenBank (http://www.ncbi.nlm.nih.gov/Entrez/) databases were used to retrieve all annotated amino acid sequences for GnRHR of vertebrates including lamprey, spotted gar, zebrafish, medaka, fugu, stickleback, tetraodon, coelacanth, anole lizard, *Xenopus*, chicken, mouse, and human, and of invertebrates including *C. elegans*, *Drosophila*, *Ciona*, and amphioxus [26,27,30,41,48–51]. Orthologous or paralogous genes from vertebrate and invertebrate species were identified through research tools provided by the ENSEMBEL database. To obtain additional sequences other than the well-annotated query sequences, a TBLASTN algorithm was performed against a genome database of selected species [14]. The phylogenetic analysis of GnRHR sequences was accomplished as previously described [14]. The MUSCLE algorithm with default settings was used to align the sequences as implemented in MEGA 5.05. A maximum likelihood phylogenetic tree was created following the Jones-Taylor-Thornton model with a confidence level of 100 replicate bootstrap samples.

Synteny analysis and location of GnRHR genes on reconstructed ancestral linkage group

For synteny analysis, contig views of genome regions surrounding the GnRHR loci were compared. The exact map location of orthologs/paralogs of neighboring genes was obtained from the ENSEMBLE database [14]. Next, the chromosomal segments of three taxa (medaka, chicken, and human) with a reliable synteny were matched with vertebrate ancestral linkage groups according to the Nakatani model [6] as described previously [14,16]. The Nakatani model provides vertebrate ancestral linkage blocks displayed on individual human chromosomes compared with the corresponding chromosome locations of medaka, chicken, and mouse [6]. Comparison of results from each taxon resolved the locations of the gene blocks at consecutives stages of vertebrate genome evolution.

Chemicals and hormones

All chemicals were obtained from Sigma-Aldrich (St. Louis, MO, USA) unless otherwise stated. Restriction enzymes were obtained from New England Biolabs (Ipswich, MA, USA). Human (hu) GnRH1, coelacanth GnRH1 (pyroEYWSYDLRPG-NH2), chicken GnRH2, and salmon GnRH3 were synthesized by AnyGen (Gwangju, Korea). The purities of the synthesized peptides were greater than 98% based on high-performance liquid chromatography. All peptides were dissolved in distilled water and then diluted in media to the desired working concentrations.

Plasmid constructs

The pcDNA3.1 expression vector was purchased from Invitrogen Corp. (San Diego, CA, USA). The CRE-luc vector containing four copies of the cyclic AMP-responsive element (CRE; TGACGTCA), and the SRE-luc vector containing a single copy of the serum response element (SRE, CCATATTAGG) were purchased from Stratagene (La Jolla, CA, USA). The cDNA for coelacanth GnRHR 1a was synthesized by GenScript (Piscataway, NJ, USA). The cDNA was incorporated into the *EcoR*I and *Xho*I sites of pcDNA3.1 and the resulting construct was verified by sequencing.

Cell transfection and luciferase assay

HEK293T cells (American Type Culture Collection, Manassas, VA, USA) were maintained in Dulbecco's modified Eagle's medium (DMEM) supplemented with 10% fetal bovine serum, 100 U/ml penicillin G, and 100 µg/ml streptomycin (Invitrogen). Cells were seeded in 48-well plates at a density of 1.4×10^4 cells per well 1 day before transfection. A mixture containing 75 ng of CRE-luc (or SRE-luc), 75 ng of the coelacanth GnRHR 1a plasmid, and 2 µl of Effectene reagent (Qiagen, Chatsworth, CA, USA) was prepared and added to each well according to the manufacturer's instructions. Approximately 48 h after transfection, cells were treated with the respective ligands for 6 h. For SRE-luc analysis, cells were maintained in serum-free DMEM for at least 16 h before ligand treatment. Cells were lysed by addition of 100 µl lysis buffer and the luciferase activity in 40 µl of cell extract was determined on a luciferase assay system according to the standard protocol for the Synergy 2 Multi-Mode Microplate Reader (BioTek, Winooski, VT, USA).

Data analysis

Data analysis was performed by nonlinear regression with a sigmoidal dose-response. The agonist concentrations that induced half-maximal stimulation (EC_{50}) were calculated with GraphPad PRISM4 software (GraphPad Software Inc., San Diego, CA, USA). All data were presented as mean ± S.E. of at least three independent experiments.

Supporting Information

Figure S1 Sequence alignment of vertebrate GnRHRs. GnRHRs from human, coelacanth, anole, chicken, *Xenopus*, zebrafish, medaka, tetraodon, fugu, and stickleback are shown. Residues with 50% and 90% similarity are indicated in blue and red respectively. Predicted N terminal (NT), transmembrane helix (H), intracellular loop (IL), extracellular loop (EL), and C terminal (CT) domains are indicated.

Table S1 The accession numbers for NCBI and ENSEMBL of *C. elegans*, *Drosophila*, *Ciona*, and amphioxus GnRHRs are given beneath receptor's name as well as gene location in brackets.

Author Contributions

Conceived and designed the experiments: FAS MJM SY SIH JIH JYS. Performed the experiments: FAS MJM SY. Analyzed the data: FAS MJM SY SIH JYS. Contributed reagents/materials/analysis tools: JIH JYS. Wrote the paper: FAS JIH JYS.

References

1. Lundin LG (1993) Evolution of the vertebrate genome as reflected in paralogous chromosomal regions in man and the house mouse. Genomics 16: 1–19.
2. Fredriksson R, Lagerström MC, Lundin L-G, Schiöth HB (2003) The G-protein-coupled receptors in the human genome form five main families. Phylogenetic analysis, paralogon groups, and fingerprints. Molecular pharmacology 63: 1256–1272.
3. Larhammar D, Lundin L-G, Hallböök F (2002) The human Hox-bearing chromosome regions did arise by block or chromosome (or even genome) duplications. Genome research 12: 1910–1920.
4. Lee LT, Siu FK, Tam JK, Lau IT, Wong AO, et al. (2007) Discovery of growth hormone-releasing hormones and receptors in nonmammalian vertebrates. Proceedings of the National Academy of Sciences 104: 2133–2138.
5. Lee YR, Tsunekawa K, Moon MJ, Um HN, Hwang J-I, et al. (2009) Molecular evolution of multiple forms of kisspeptins and GPR54 receptors in vertebrates. Endocrinology 150: 2837–2846.
6. Nakatani Y, Takeda H, Kohara Y, Morishita S (2007) Reconstruction of the vertebrate ancestral genome reveals dynamic genome reorganization in early vertebrates. Genome research 17: 1254–1265.
7. Putnam NH, Butts T, Ferrier DE, Furlong RF, Hellsten U, et al. (2008) The amphioxus genome and the evolution of the chordate karyotype. Nature 453: 1064–1071.
8. Larsson T, Olsson F, Sundstrom G, Lundin L-G, Brenner S, et al. (2008) Early vertebrate chromosome duplications and the evolution of the neuropeptide Y receptor gene regions. BMC evolutionary biology 8: 184.
9. Tostivint H, Joly L, Lihrmann I, Parmentier C, Lebon A, et al. (2006) Comparative genomics provides evidence for close evolutionary relationships between the urotensin II and somatostatin gene families. Proceedings of the National Academy of Sciences of the United States of America 103: 2237–2242.
10. Wraith A, Törnsten A, Chardon P, Harbitz I, Chowdhary BP, et al. (2000) Evolution of the neuropeptide Y receptor family: gene and chromosome duplications deduced from the cloning and mapping of the five receptor subtype genes in pig. Genome research 10: 302–310.
11. Lagerström MC, Fredriksson R, Bjarnadóttir TK, Fridmanis D, Holmquist T, et al. (2005) Origin of the prolactin-releasing hormone (PRLH) receptors: evidence of coevolution between PRLH and a redundant neuropeptide Y receptor during vertebrate evolution. Genomics 85: 688–703.
12. Daza DO, Sundström G, Bergqvist CA, Larhammar D (2012) The evolution of vertebrate somatostatin receptors and their gene regions involves extensive chromosomal rearrangements. BMC evolutionary biology 12: 231.
13. Kim D-K, Cho EB, Moon MJ, Park S, Hwang J-I, et al. (2011) Revisiting the evolution of gonadotropin-releasing hormones and their receptors in vertebrates: secrets hidden in genomes. General and comparative endocrinology 170: 68–78.
14. Hwang J-I, Moon MJ, Park S, Kim D-K, Cho EB, et al. (2013) Expansion of Secretin-Like G Protein-Coupled Receptors and Their Peptide Ligands via Local Duplications Before and After Two Rounds of Whole-Genome Duplication. Molecular biology and evolution 30: 1119–1130.
15. Um HN, Han JM, Hwang JI, Hong SI, Vaudry H, et al. (2010) Molecular coevolution of kisspeptins and their receptors from fish to mammals. Annals of the New York Academy of Sciences 1200: 67–74.

16. Yegorov S, Good S (2012) Using paleogenomics to study the evolution of gene families: origin and duplication history of the relaxin family hormones and their receptors. PloS one 7: e32923.
17. Matsuo H, Baba Y, Nair R, Arimura A, Schally A (1971) Structure of the porcine LH-and FSH-releasing hormone. I. The proposed amino acid sequence. Biochemical and biophysical research communications 43: 1334–1339.
18. Reinhart J, Mertz L, Catt K (1992) Molecular cloning and expression of cDNA encoding the murine gonadotropin-releasing hormone receptor. The Journal of biological chemistry 267: 21281–21284.
19. Powell J, Zohar Y, Elizur A, Park M, Fischer W, et al. (1994) Three forms of gonadotropin-releasing hormone characterized from brains of one species. Proceedings of the National Academy of Sciences 91: 12081–12085.
20. White RB, Eisen JA, Kasten TL, Fernald RD (1998) Second gene for gonadotropin-releasing hormone in humans. Proceedings of the National Academy of Sciences 95: 305–309.
21. Fernald RD, White RB (1999) Gonadotropin-releasing hormone genes: phylogeny, structure, and functions. Frontiers in neuroendocrinology 20: 224–240.
22. Millar R, Lowe S, Conklin D, Pawson A, Maudsley S, et al. (2001) A novel mammalian receptor for the evolutionarily conserved type II GnRH. Proceedings of the National Academy of Sciences 98: 9636–9641.
23. Wang L, Bogerd J, Choi HS, Seong JY, Soh JM, et al. (2001) Three distinct types of GnRH receptor characterized in the bullfrog. Proceedings of the National Academy of Sciences 98: 361–366.
24. Morgan K, Conklin D, Pawson AJ, Sellar R, Ott TR, et al. (2003) A transcriptionally active human type II gonadotropin-releasing hormone receptor gene homolog overlaps two genes in the antisense orientation on chromosome 1q. 12. Endocrinology 144: 423–436.
25. Moncaut N, Somoza G, Power DM, Canário AV (2005) Five gonadotrophin-releasing hormone receptors in a teleost fish: isolation, tissue distribution and phylogenetic relationships. Journal of molecular endocrinology 34: 767–779.
26. Tello JA, Rivier JE, Sherwood NM (2005) Tunicate gonadotropin-releasing hormone (GnRH) peptides selectively activate Ciona intestinalis GnRH receptors and the green monkey type II GnRH receptor. Endocrinology 146: 4061–4073.
27. Tello JA, Sherwood NM (2009) Amphioxus: beginning of vertebrate and end of invertebrate type GnRH receptor lineage. Endocrinology 150: 2847–2856.
28. Silver MR, Kawauchi H, Nozaki M, Sower SA (2004) Cloning and analysis of the lamprey GnRH-III cDNA from eight species of lamprey representing the three families of Petromyzoniformes. General and comparative endocrinology 139: 85–94.
29. Kah O, Lethimonier C, Somoza G, Guilgur L, Vaillant C, et al. (2007) GnRH and GnRH receptors in metazoa: a historical, comparative, and evolutive perspective. General and comparative endocrinology 153: 346–364.
30. Ikemoto T, Park M (2005) Identification and molecular characterization of three GnRH ligands and five GnRH receptors in the spotted green pufferfish. Molecular and cellular endocrinology 242: 67–79.
31. Karges B, Karges W, de Roux N (2003) Clinical and molecular genetics of the human GnRH receptor. Human reproduction update 9: 523–530.
32. Naor Z, Huhtaniemi I (2012) Interactions of the GnRH receptor with heterotrimeric G proteins. Frontiers in neuroendocrinology.
33. Wang C, Yun O, Maiti K, Kim KK, Chae CH, et al. (2004) Position of Pro and Ser near Glu7. 32 in the extracellular loop 3 of mammalian and nonmammalian gonadotropin-releasing hormone (GnRH) receptors is a critical determinant for differential ligand selectivity for mammalian GnRH and chicken GnRH-II. Molecular Endocrinology 18: 105–116.
34. Li JH, Choe H, Wang AF, Maiti K, Wang C, et al. (2005) Extracellular loop 3 (EL3) and EL3-proximal transmembrane helix 7 of the mammalian type I and type II gonadotropin-releasing hormone (GnRH) receptors determine differential ligand selectivity to GnRH-I and GnRH-II. Molecular pharmacology 67: 1099–1110.
35. Flanagan CA, Becker II, Davidson JS, Wakefield IK, Zhou W, et al. (1994) Glutamate 301 of the mouse gonadotropin-releasing hormone receptor confers specificity for arginine 8 of mammalian gonadotropin-releasing hormone. Journal of Biological Chemistry 269: 22636–22641.
36. Flanagan CA, Chen C-C, Coetsee M, Mamputha S, Whitlock KE, et al. (2007) Expression, structure, function, and evolution of gonadotropin-releasing hormone (GnRH) receptors GnRH-R1SHS and GnRH-R2PEY in the teleost, Astatotilapia burtoni. Endocrinology 148: 5060–5071.
37. Heding A, Vrecl M, Bogerd J, McGregor A, Sellar R, et al. (1998) Gonadotropin-releasing hormone receptors with intracellular carboxyl-terminal tails undergo acute desensitization of total inositol phosphate production and exhibit accelerated internalization kinetics. Journal of Biological Chemistry 273: 11472–11477.
38. Oh DY, Song JA, Moon JS, Moon MJ, Kim JI, et al. (2005) Membrane-proximal region of the carboxyl terminus of the gonadotropin-releasing hormone receptor (GnRHR) confers differential signal transduction between mammalian and nonmammalian GnRHRs. Molecular Endocrinology 19: 722–731.
39. Zhou W, Flanagan C, Ballesteros JA, Konvicka K, Davidson JS, et al. (1994) A reciprocal mutation supports helix 2 and helix 7 proximity in the gonadotropin-releasing hormone receptor. Molecular pharmacology 45: 165–170.
40. Flanagan CA, Zhou W, Chi L, Yuen T, Rodic V, et al. (1999) The functional microdomain in transmembrane helices 2 and 7 regulates expression, activation, and coupling pathways of the gonadotropin-releasing hormone receptor. Journal of Biological Chemistry 274: 28880–28886.
41. Lindemans M, Liu F, Janssen T, Husson SJ, Mertens I, et al. (2009) Adipokinetic hormone signaling through the gonadotropin-releasing hormone receptor modulates egg-laying in Caenorhabditis elegans. Proceedings of the National Academy of Sciences 106: 1642–1647.
42. Morgan K, Millar RP (2004) Evolution of GnRH ligand precursors and GnRH receptors in protochordate and vertebrate species. General and comparative endocrinology 139: 191–197.
43. Davidson JS, McArdle CA, Davies P, Elario R, Flanagan CA, et al. (1996) Asn102 of the gonadotropin-releasing hormone receptor is a critical determinant of potency for agonists containing C-terminal glycinamide. Journal of Biological Chemistry 271: 15510–15514.
44. Flanagan CA, Rodic V, Konvicka K, Yuen T, Chi L, et al. (2000) Multiple interactions of the Asp2. 61 (98) side chain of the gonadotropin-releasing hormone receptor contribute differentially to ligand interaction. Biochemistry 39: 8133–8141.
45. Hövelmann S, Hoffmann SH, Kühne R, ter Laak T, Reiländer H, et al. (2002) Impact of aromatic residues within transmembrane helix 6 of the human gonadotropin-releasing hormone receptor upon agonist and antagonist binding. Biochemistry 41: 1129–1136.
46. Millar RP, Lu Z-L, Pawson AJ, Flanagan CA, Morgan K, et al. (2004) Gonadotropin-releasing hormone receptors. Endocrine Reviews 25: 235–275.
47. Seong JY, Wang L, Yun O, Maiti K, Li JH, et al. (2003) Ala/Thr201 in extracellular loop 2 and Leu/Phe290 in transmembrane domain 6 of type 1 frog gonadotropin-releasing hormone receptor confer differential ligand sensitivity and signal transduction. Endocrinology 144: 454–466.
48. Hauser F, Søndergaard L, Grimmelikhuijzen CJ (1998) Molecular cloning, genomic organization and developmental regulation of a novel receptor from drosophila melanogaster structurally related to gonadotropin-releasing hormone receptors from vertebrates. Biochem Bioph Res Co 249: 822–828.
49. Kusakabe T, Mishima S, Shimada I, Kitajima Y, Tsuda M (2003) Structure, expression, and cluster organization of genes encoding gonadotropin-releasing hormone receptors found in the neural complex of the ascidian Ciona intestinalis. Gene 322: 77–84.
50. Kakar SS, Musgrove LC, Devor DC, Sellers JC, Neill JD (1992) Cloning, sequencing, and expression of human gonadotropin releasing hormone (GnRH) receptor. Biochem Bioph Res Co 189: 289–295.
51. Joseph NT, Aquilina-Beck A, MacDonald C, Decatur WA, Hall JA, et al. (2012) Molecular cloning and pharmacological characterization of two novel GnRH receptors in the lamprey (Petromyzon marinus). Endocrinology 153: 3345–3356.

SDF-1 Chemokine Signalling Modulates the Apoptotic Responses to Iron Deprivation of Clathrin-Depleted DT40 Cells

Alena Pance[3]*, Frank R. Morrissey-Wettey[1], Helen Craig[1], Alison Downing[2], Richard Talbot[2], Antony P. Jackson[1]*

1 Department of Biochemistry, Hopkins Building, University of Cambridge, Cambridge, United Kingdom, **2** Roslin Institute, Roslin, Midlothian, Scotland, United Kingdom, **3** The Wellcome Trust Sanger Institute, Hinxton, Cambridge, United Kingdom

Abstract

We have previously deleted both endogenous copies of the clathrin heavy-chain gene in the chicken pre B-cell-line DT40 and replaced them with clathrin under the control of a tetracycline-regulatable promoter (Tet-Off). The originally derived cell-line DKO-S underwent apoptosis when clathrin expression was repressed. We have also described a cell-line DKO-R derived from DKO-S cells that was less sensitive to clathrin-depletion. Here we show that the restriction of transferrin uptake, resulting in iron deprivation, is responsible for the lethal consequence of clathrin-depletion. We further show that the DKO-R cells have up-regulated an anti-apoptotic survival pathway based on the chemokine SDF-1 and its receptor CXCR4. Our work clarifies several puzzling features of clathrin-depleted DT40 cells and reveals an example of how SDF-1/CXCR4 signalling can abrogate pro-apoptotic pathways and increase cell survival. We propose that the phenomenon described here has implications for the therapeutic approach to a variety of cancers.

Editor: Qiang Wang, Cedars-Sinai Medical Center, United States of America

Funding: The work was supported by the following: Department of Biochemistry, University of Cambridge, BBSRC, and Marie Curie Fellowship (FRMW). The funders had no role in study design, data collection and analysis, decision to publish, or preparation of the manuscript.

Competing Interests: The authors have declared that no competing interests exist.

* Email: apj10@cam.ac.uk (APJ); alena.pance@sanger.ac.uk (AP)

Introduction

Clathrin plays a fundamental role in membrane trafficking pathways in eukaryotic cells. It is responsible for receptor-mediated endocytosis of selected molecules from the plasma membrane and the transport of some lysosomal enzymes from the *trans*-Golgi network to the lysosome [1]. The chicken pre-B cell-line DT40 was originally isolated as an avain-leukosis virus-derived chicken B-lymphocyte cell-line [2]. It exhibits an extraordinarily high rate of homologous recombination, and this property greatly facilitates gene targeting [3]. The DT40 cell-line has thus become established as an important tool for the study of a wide range of cell-biological phenomena [4]. To understand the function of clathrin in more detail, we inactivated both endogenous copies of the clathrin gene in DT40 and replaced them with clathrin under the control of the Tet-Off inducible promoter. In the presence of doxycycline, clathrin expression was strongly inhibited and this allowed the functional consequences of clathrin-depletion to be investigated in a vertebrate cell context. The originally generated cell-line conditionally deficient in clathrin expression was designated DKO-S (*d*ouble *k*nock*o*ut cells, *s*ensitive to clathrin-depletion). In this cell-line, we found that clathrin-depletion induced apoptosis. We also described a variant derived from DKO-S that did not die in the absence of clathrin. We designated this cell-line DKO-R (*d*ouble *k*nock*o*ut cells *r*esistant to clathrin-depletion) [5]. We have used both of these DKO cell-lines to study clathrin function [5,6,7,8,9].

The apoptotic response of clathrin-depleted DT40 cells is particularly curious. Clathrin expression has been dramatically reduced in other vertebrate cell-lines such as HeLa cells without the activation of apoptosis, or indeed without inducing any form of cell death [10]. Why then does clathrin-depletion in DT40 cells differ? The distinct phenotype of the DKO-R variant raises further questions. What adaptations has this variant acquired to overcome the apoptotic response to clathrin-depletion shown by its DKO-S parent? Here we show that iron deficiency is a major apoptotic signal stemming from clathrin depletion. We furthershow that the resistant cell-line DKO-R has increased survival under these conditions due to endogenous expression of the chemokine SDF-1 and the autocrine stimulation of a survival pathway based on its receptor CXCR-4. We show that this surprisingly small change can explain all the known phenotypic differences between DKO-S and DKO-R cells.

Materials and Methods

Cell culture and materials

Except where stated, all reagents were purchased from Sigma, Poole, UK. All cell-lines were maintained in RPMI 1640 media, 0.2% (wt/vol) Na_2HCO_3, 1% (wt/vol) L-glutamine with 10% (vol/vol) heat-treated foetal calf serum (FCS) and between 0 and 2% (vol/vol) heat-treated chicken serum as indicated in the text. Serum and media were purchased from Gibco, Paisley, UK. Cells were maintained at 37°C and with 5% CO_2. Some batches of bovine serum contain the protease dipeptidylpeptidase IV (CD26) that destroys SDF-1 activity [11]. To avoid this complication for experiments using SDF-1, the media was supplemented with the selective CD26 inhibitor diprotin A (0.1 mM) [12]. Cell numbers were counted with a haemocytometer after Trypan Blue staining. Fully iron-saturated chicken transferrin (conalbumin from Sigma) was produced by incubating 10 mgs of protein in 1 ml of 0.1 mg/ml ferric ammonium citrate in phosphate buffered saline (PBS) pH 7.2 for 3 hours at room temperature, then dialysing the protein overnight at 4°C against PBS [13]. Iron-saturated chicken transferrin was stored in 0.1 ml aliquots at −20°C until use. Apotransferrin was produced by dialysing chicken transferrin against two overnight changes of 0.1 M sodium citrate, 0.1 M sodium acetate buffer pH 4.5 at 4°C, followed by an overnight dialysis at 4°C against PBS [14]. Aliquots (0.1 ml) were stored at −20°C until used.

Electrophoresis and western blotting

Cells were lysed in PBS with 0.1% Triton X-100 (vol/vol) and 1× protease inhibitor cocktail (Boehringer Ingelheim, Bracknell, UK). Total protein was determined using the BCA protein assay kit (Pierce, Cramlington, UK) with bovine serum albumin as standard. Protein (about 50–80 μg cell extract; about 1–2 μg partially purified chicken transferrin) was separated by sodium dodecyl sulphate (SDS) polyacrylamide gel electrophoresis in gels of 8% acrylamide [15]. For western blots, proteins in the gel were transferred to Hybond C membrane (Amersham Biosciences, Chalfont St.Giles, UK). Blots were blocked by incubation for 1 hour in PBS, 0.1% Triton X-100 and 5% powdered milk, then incubated overnight at 4°C with primary antibody (typically 0.1–1 μg/ml) diluted into PBS, 0.1% (vol/vol) Triton X100 and 5% (vol/vol) FCS. Specific signal was detected using horseradish peroxidase-labelled second antibodies and enhanced chemiluminescence (Pierce). To confirm protein loading, nitrocellulose was stained with 0.1% amido black in 10% acetic acid, 45% methanol and destained with 10% acetic acid, 45% methanol. Clathrin was detected using mouse monoclonal antibody TD1 [16]. Chicken transferrin was detected using mouse monoclonal antibodies [17]. Transferrin receptor was detected using mouse monoclonal antibody H68.4 (Invitrogen).

Apoptosis assays

Cells with apoptotic bodies were counted on a fluorescent microscope following staining with 1 μg/ml Hoechst 33342 [5]. Caspase 3 activity was determined as described [18]. Cells were centrifuged at 12,000 rpm for 8 minutes, washed twice in PBS and lysed in 20 mM HEPES pH 7.4, 10 mM KCl, 250 mM sucrose, 1.5 mm $MgCl_2$, 0.5 mM EDTA, 0.5 mM EGTA and protease inhibitor cocktail (Roche, Welwyn Garden City, UK). Samples were incubated with 14 μM acetyl-DEVD-AMC substrate for 40 minutes and fluorescence at 450 nm determined. The rate of reaction was linear over this time period. For inhibitor studies, a 1 mM stock of inhibitor (AMD3100, CCX771 or CCX704) in DMSO was diluted into at final concentration for the assays of 0.5 μM. The same volume of DMSO used in the experimental samples was added to control cells.

Partial purification protocols

Saturated ammonium sulphate solution was added slowly to 30 ml heat-treated chicken serum at 4°C. Precipitates were redisolved in 3 ml PBS (to give a nominally 10× stock), dialysed overnight against PBS and sterilised by filtration through a 0.45 micron filter [19]. Separate fractions corresponding to proteins precipitated by 0–40%, 40–80% and 80–100% saturated ammonium sulphate were prepared and frozen in aliquots at −20°C until used. DKO-S cells were seeded into the wells of a 24 well plate at 1×10^4/ml in 2 ml in medium lacking chicken serum and supplemented with 0.1 μg/ml doxycycline to repress clathrin expression. Wells were supplemented with 0.01 ml sterile ammonium sulphate fractions and cell numbers counted after 3 days in those wells showing evidence of cell growth. The ammonium sulphate fraction promoting the strongest growth was loaded onto a Sephadex G-200 column maintained at 4°C and pre-calibrated with high and low molecular weight standards kit (Pharmacia, Sandwich, UK). Elution flow was maintained at 1 ml/min with PBS, collecting 3 ml fractions. Each fraction from the column was filter sterilized and 0.1 ml added to the DKO-S cell bioassay as described above. Positive fractions were pooled, concentrated by ultrafiltration to a final volume of 5 ml and dialysed against 50 mM Tris buffer pH 7.5. The sample was applied to a Mono Q HR 5/5 anion exchange column at room temperature and eluted by Fast-Protein Liquid Chromatography (FPLC) with a linear gradient of 0 − 1 M NaCl in 50 mM Tris buffer pH 7.5. Aliquots (0.1 ml) from each fraction were examined by SDS polyacrylamide gel electrophoresis and stained with Coomassie Briliant Blue R-250 (Bio Rad, Hemel Hempstead, UK). The remaining samples of each column fraction were dialysed against PBS, filter sterilised and 0.1 ml aliquots added to the DKO-S bioassay.

Mass spectrometry of gel excised fractions

Coomassie-stained proteins within the gel pieces were reduced, carboxyamidomethylated, and digested to peptides using trypsin on a MassPrepStation (Waters, Manchester, UK). The resulting peptides were applied to a LC-MS/MS column. For LC-MS/MS, the reverse phase liquid chromatographic separation of peptides was achieved with a PepMap C18 reverse phase, 75 mm i.d., 15-cm column (LC Packings, Amsterdam) on a capillary LC system (Waters) attached to QTof2 (Waters) mass spectrometer or the same column attached to a Dionex Dual Gradient LC system attached to a QSTAR XL (Applied Biosystems, Framingham, MA, USA). The MS/MS fragmentation data achieved was used to search the National Center for Biotechnology Information database using the MASCOT search engine (http://www.matrixscience.com).

Microarray analysis

We used the 13,209 EST chicken microarray designed by the collaboration between Fred Hutcheson Cancer Research, University of Delaware and ARK Genomics (Roslin Institute) [20]. Full details are available from ArrayExpress ('ARK-Genomics G. gallus 13 K v 4.0', accession number: A-MEXP-831). The contents for the array were selected from a clustering of all chicken EST information available in 2003. A single representative of each cluster was selected and supplemented with a range of singleton expressed sequence tags (ESTs) that targeted known genes and some that were known to show differential expression in immune tissues. This array gives a broad coverage of genes from the chicken transcriptome being sourced from over 39 different EST libraries, representing 20 different adult tissues and stages of developmental growth.

Detailed protocols for the microarray analysis are available from the website www.ark-genomics.org (RNA extraction, RNA QC, Amino-allyl labelling, dye coupling, fluorescent labelling QC and hybridisation). Total RNA was prepared from DKO-S and DKO-R cell-lines using two stages, initial extraction was with Trizol (Invitrogen, Paisley, UK) followed by RNAeasy (Qiagen, Crawley, UK). The purified RNAs were quality tested using an Agilent Bioanalyser 2100 (Agilent UK) with all samples having a RIN number in excess of 7.0 which we have found to be acceptable for microarray analysis [20]. The total RNA (20 μg per sample) was tagged with amino-allyl UTP using the Fairplay II kit (Stratagene, UK) according to the manufacturers protocol with the exception that the tagged cDNA was precipitated overnight at −20°C. The precipitate was resuspended in coupling buffer (0.1 M carbonate buffer pH 9.0) and the appropriate Cy3 or Cy5 mono-reactive dye added (GE Healthcare, UK) as required by the experiment. Two fluorescent labels were prepared from each total RNA sample and labelled with different dyes. Samples from DKO-S and DKO-R cells were randomly paired for hybridisation analysis with reciprocal dye combinations for each pair. Hybridisations and washes were carried out overnight on GenTac Hybridisation stations (Genomics Solutions, Huntingdon, UK) as outlined in the protocol. The dried slides were scanned in a Scanarray 5000 XL scanner (GSI Lumonics) at constant laser power of 80% and 78% for Cy3 and Cy5 respectively.

Data was extracted from the slide using BlueFuse software (BlueGnome, Cambridge, UK). Features with poor confidence information (confidence <0.30, flagged D and E) were eliminated from the analysis. M v A plots [where $M = \log_2 (Cy5/Cy3)$ and $A = 1/2*[\log_2(Cy5) + \log_2(Cy3)]$ of the data for each slide (data not shown) were suitably linear to require only a simple global normalisation of the data. Analysis was performed using GeneSpring software (Agilent UK) on the fused data (mean of replicate values for features on individual slides) from the BlueFuse program. The data was filtered with a probability of 5% with a false discovery rate (FDR) [21] of 15%. The resulting list of differentially expressed genes was then re-annotated using the EST sequence from the feature to update the information available on each cDNA target on the array.

The microarray data described in this manuscript has been deposited with the Gene Expression Omnibus (GEO) data repository under the accession number GSE57328

RT-PCR

Total RNA was isolated with the 'Absolutely RNA' kit from Stratagene, following the manufacturer's instructions. RNA (1 μg) was used for cDNA synthesis using an Moloney Murine Leukemia Virus (MMLV) reverse transcriptase and random primers (Promega). One μL of RT reaction was used for the PCR following the protocol: 1 min 94°C and 20 cycles of amplification by 1 min 94°C, 1 min 55°C, 1 min 72°C, and finishing with 5 min at 72°C. Amplified products were visualised in 1% agarose with ethidium bromide. The following primers were used:

Actin 5′-attcctatgtgggcgacgag-3′ F, 5′-tggatagcaacgtacatggc-3′ R (259 bps)

SDF-1 5′-gcctgacttaccgatgcc-3′ F, 5′-ggccaactccaaacccatc-3′ R (333 bps)

CXCR4 5′-ccttgccattctggtctgtgg-3′ F, 5′-ccgggcaagacaagtcc-tacc-3′ R (367 bps)

For real time PCR, the following primers were used:

Cyclophilin A 5′-gcgagaagggatttggctacaaggg-3′F, 5′-ggatttgc-caccagtgccgttgtg-3′R (102 bp)

SDF-1 5′-cttcgagagcaacgtggcgag-3′F, 5′-gcacacttgcttgctgttgctc-3′R (112 bp)

CXCR4 5′-ggcagcatggacggtttgg-3′F, 5-gcacggctctccatagtctcc-3′R (108 bp)

CXCR7 5′-cctcgtccagcataaccaatgg-3′F, 5′-ccacgctcatgcatgc-cag-3′R (113 bp)

Tf 5′-cgagaagggtgatgtggc-3′F, 5′-ggcagagcaactcaaagtc-3′R (118 bp)

TfR 5′-cagttggagtgctggagact-3′F, 5′-gggctggcagaaaccttg-3′R (147 bp)

For amplification with SYBR Green PCR master mix, following the settings recommended by the manufacturer.

Statistical tests

Apoptotic responses for cells grown either with or without clathrin expression were determined using two-tailed unpaired Student's t-test.

Results

Iron-deprivation induces apoptosis in DT40 cells

Addition of 0.1 μM doxycycline to the media of both DKO-S and DKO-R cells completely repressed clathrin expression (Figure 1). DT40 cells are typically grown in media supplemented with 10% foetal-calf serum (FCS) and 1% chicken serum [3]. We previously showed that when DKO-S cells were seeded into this standard medium in the presence of doxycycline, the clathrin-depleted cells died by apoptosis after 3–4 days, reflecting the decline in the level of clathrin over this period. The cells died more quickly when clathrin-depleted DKO-S cells were grown in the presence of 10% FCS, but only 0.25% chicken serum [5]. This suggests that chicken serum contains a factor required by DKO-S cells that becomes growth limiting in the absence of clathrin. To investigate the nature of this factor, we first extended the growth experiments to include a wider range of chicken serum concentrations (0 to 5%) (Figure S1A and S1B). The inhibitory effect of clathrin-depletion on cell growth was particularly dramatic at low levels of chicken serum (0.25%). When seeded into medium lacking chicken serum altogether, DKO-S cells grew noticeably less well even when expressing clathrin, and they needed a seeding density of at least 2×10^4 cells/ml to grow. In the absence of clathrin, DKO-S cells in this medium died rapidly. By contrast we found that at chicken serum concentrations higher than normally used (up to 5%), DKO-S cells increasingly survived clathrin-depletion (Figure S1A). Presumably, at this high concentration the increased availability of the potential factor helped the cells to survive longer when clathrin expression was repressed. When the same experiment was conducted for the DKO-R cell-line we found a similar pattern, but with the striking difference that DKO-R cells required less chicken serum to survive clathrin-depletion compared to DKO-S cells (Figure S1B). For both clathrin-depleted DKO-S and R cells, reduction in the level of chicken serum increased apoptosis as measured both by caspase activity and nuclear condensation, but the DKO-S cell-line was markedly more sensitive to this effect compared to DKO-R cells as the chicken serum levels were reduced (Figure 2A and B). This suggests that the response of these two cell-lines to clathrin-depletion reflects a similar underlying mechanism, but with a quantitative difference in sensitivity to restriction of the chicken serum factor. Hence, at the level of chicken serum that we routinely used (1%), the DKO-S cells typically died but the DKO-R cells survived in the absence of clathrin.

In order to identify this putative factor, chicken serum was fractionated with ammonium sulphate and the capacity of the different fractions to support growth was examined. For this experiment, DKO-S cells were seeded in a multiwell plate at 1×10^4 cells/ml in medium without chicken serum (see materials and methods), together with doxycycline to repress clathrin expression. Under these conditions, clathrin-depleted DKO-S cells did not grow (Figure S1A). The ammonium sulphate fractions from chicken serum were added to these cells to give an equivalent chicken serum concentration of about 5%. Only the 40–80% ammonium sulphate fraction supported growth under these conditions (Figure S2A). Gel filtration of this fraction on G-200

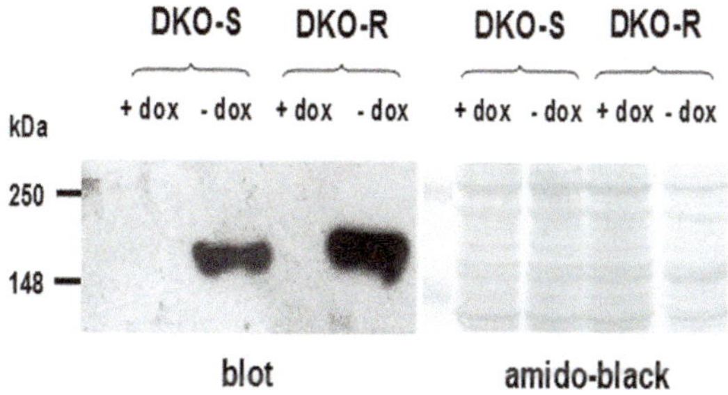

Figure 1. Western blot showing the complete repression of clathrin expression in DKO-S and DKO-R cells when grown in the presence of 0.1 μM doxycycline (dox). Cells were grown for 72 hours in media with or without doxycycline as indicated. Following development of the blot, the nitrocellulose was stained with amido black to detect total protein.

Sepharose eluted the growth activity as a broad peak between the 69 and 150 kDa size marker (Figure S2B). Subsequent FPLC ion-exchange chromatography of this gel-filtration fraction produced a single sharp leading peak of growth-supporting biological activity separated from most of the other proteins (Figure 3A). When analysed by SDS PAGE, this peak yielded two major protein bands of apparent molecular weight of about 80 kDa and 60 kDa (Figure 3B). Each of these proteins was separately excised from the gel and analysed by mass spectrometry (MS) sequencing. The lower molecular weight band was identified as vitamin D binding protein [22]. Purified samples of this protein did not support the growth of clathrin-depleted DKO-S cells in the absence of chicken serum (data not shown) even at the highest concentration used. The higher molecular weight band, which did support growth, was identified as chicken transferrin, and this identification was further confirmed by western blotting (Figure 3C).

Purified iron-saturated chicken transferrin mimicked the effect of full chicken serum both on cell growth, apoptotic response and sensitivity to clathrin-depletion od DKO-S cells (Figures 4A, B, C). These cells survived clathrin-depletion if they were grown in standard medium without chicken serum, supplemented with concentrations of fully iron-saturated chicken transferrin of 10 μg/ml or higher (Figure 4A). At lower concentrations, (eg 2 μg/ml shown in Figure 4B), clathrin-depleted DKO-S cells died, but DKO-R cells survived (Figure 4B). Using quantitative western blotting, the level of transferrin in our chicken serum was estimated at about 0.5 mg/ml (data not shown) so that 10 μg/ml corresponds to the level of chicken transferrin present in media supplemented with 2% chicken serum. The degree of iron saturation in commercial chicken serum is unknown, but if it is similar to human serum transferrin (about 30% iron-loaded) [23], then this value is consistent with the observed quantitative effects of chicken serum on the two clathrin-depleted cell-lines. Although the DKO-S and -R cells were always grown in media with 10% FCS, it should be noted that, as with other mammalian transferrins [24], bovine transferrin binds relatively weakly to the chicken transferrin receptor (FRW/APJ data not shown). So in these experiments it is likely to be the chicken serum that supplies the majority of the iron. When supplemented with chicken apotransferrin, from which iron had been removed by prior chelation and dialysis [14], growth of clathrin-depleted DKO-S cells was significantly reduced (Figure 4A). It has been reported that FCS contains high levels of iron stores [25], which could supply some intake into the cells *via* coupling to apotransferrin and could explain the residual growth under this condition. By contrast, growth was completely abolished for clathrin-depleted DKO-S cells with apotransferrin (Figure 4A). The role of transferrin and iron in cell survival was confirmed with deferoxamine, a powerful and highly specific iron chelator that is known to prevent iron uptake into cells, and which induced apoptosis of DKO-S cells [26] (Figure 4C).

Does the differential survival of clathrin-depleted DKO-S and R cells reflect differences in transferrin receptor (TfR) expression? A quantitative RT-PCR analysis showed similar levels of TfR mRNA in DKO-R and DKO-S (Figure 5A). Likewise, western blotting confirmed similar levels of TfR protein in the two cell-lines (Figure 5B). These results are consistent with our previous

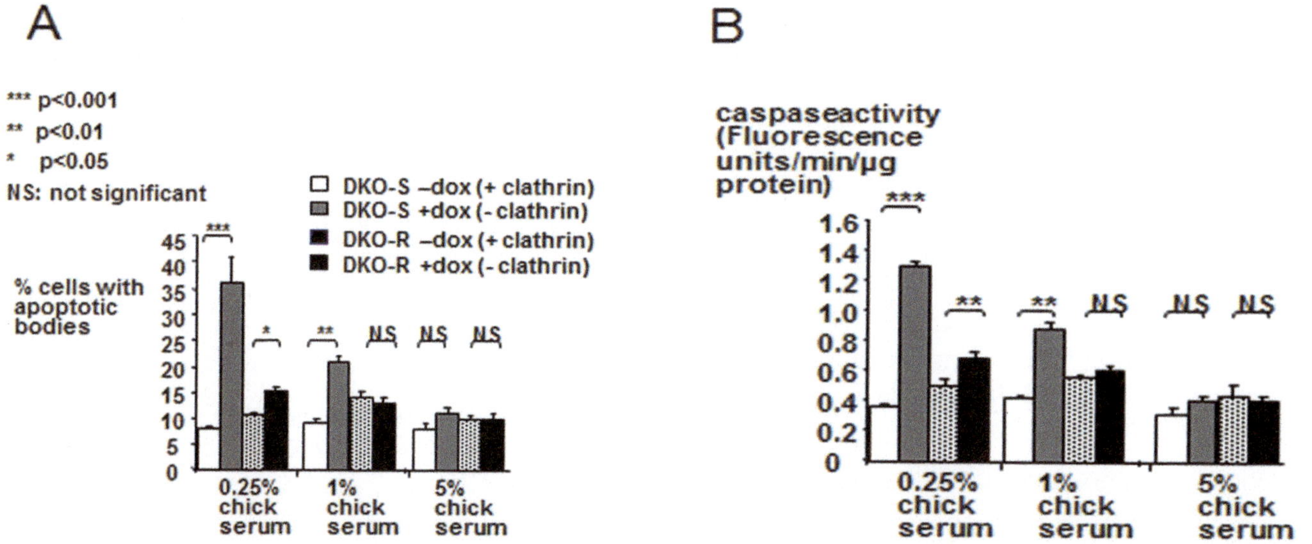

Figure 2. DKO-S cells show a higher apoptotic response to clathrin-depletion than DKO-R cells. (A) The proportion of apoptotic cells and (B) caspase activity were measured as described in materials and methods for DKO-S and DKO-R cells grown with or without 0.1 μM doxycycline (dox) and in media supplemented with increasing concentrations of chicken serum are as indicated. Values are means of three measurements +/− standard deviation. Statistically significant differences, with p values, are indicated.

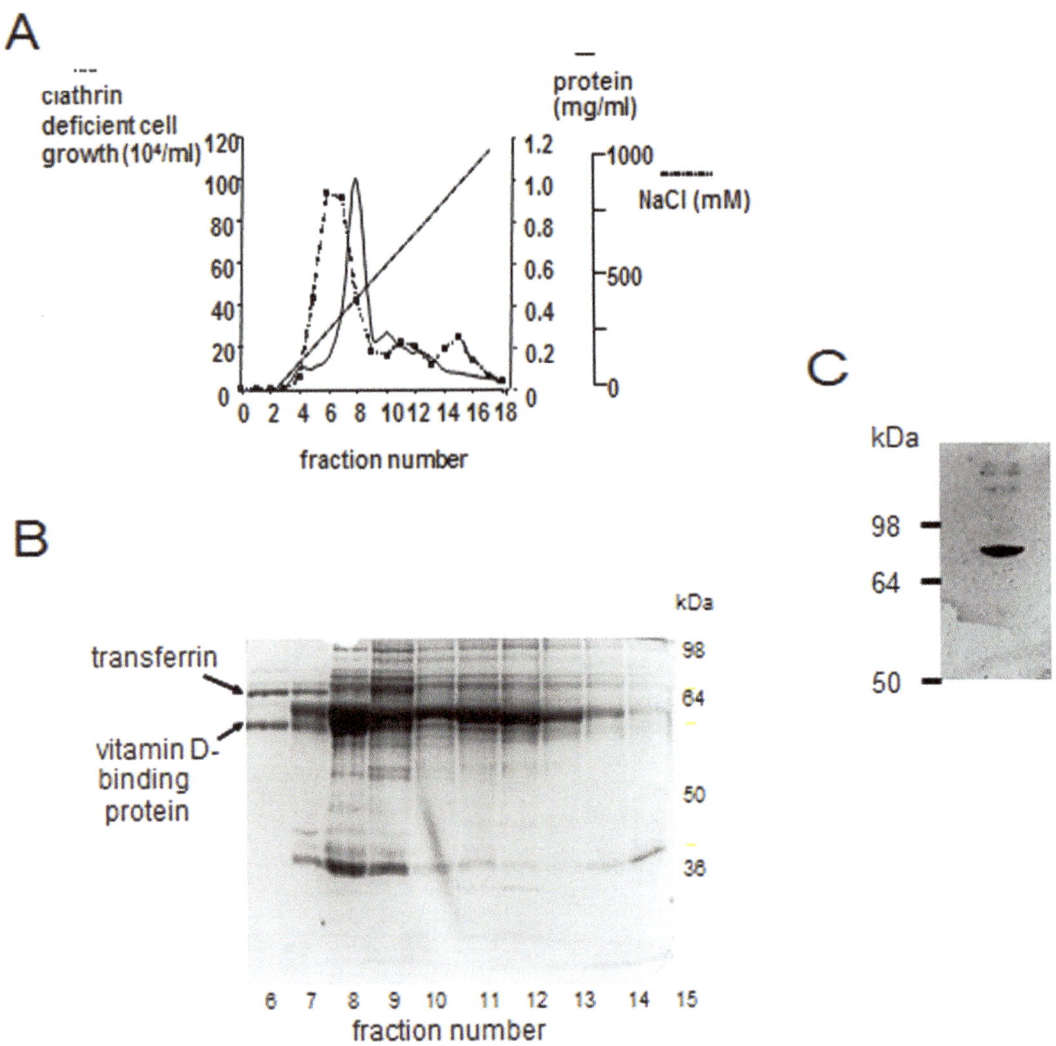

Figure 3. Identification of the putative chicken survival factor as transferrin. (A) FPLC separation of the positive fraction from the gel filtration step showing separation of the main bioactivity peak from major protein fractions. In each case, cell growth after 72 hours was determined as described in materials and methods. (B) SDS polyacrylamide gel electophoresis of the fractions from the FPLC column. Fraction 6, which contains the major bioactivity peak contains only two major proteins identified as vitamin D binding protein and transferrin. (C) Western blot of FPLC fraction 6 using anti-(chicken transferrin) monoclonal antibody.

report showing that the rates of transferrin internalisation into DKO-S and DKO-R cells are similar and reduced to similar levels when clathrin is depleted [8]. An alternative possibility is that DKO-R cells synthesise their own transferrin, which could then support survival. However, neither cell line expresses detectable levels of transferrin mRNA (Figure 5C) so the difference between DKO-S and DKO-R does not rely on changes in expression of the transferrin iron uptake pathway. Hence, the lower apoptotic sensitivity shown by the DKO-R cells must result from an additional mechanism.

Endogenous expression of SDF-1 is responsible for DKO-R resistance to clathrin-depletion-induced apoptosis

Since the distinctive phenotypes of the DKO-S and R cells are stable [5], they could reflect changed gene expression profiles. To search for the pathway responsible for cell survival, we compared the global patterns of mRNA expression between the two cell-lines using an EST chicken microarray [20] (see Materials and Methods). There was a limited number of statistically significant differences between DKO-S and DKO-R cells (Table S1). This is to be expected, since the DKO-R cell-line derives from the DKO-S parent [5]. One ribosomal protein was up-regulated in DKO-S cells, but the physiological significance of this is unclear. On the other hand, several genes were up-regulated in DKO-R cells by a factor of two-fold or more compared to DKO-S cells (Figure 6 and Table S1). Figure 6A shows these genes in decreasing order of significance and from these, groups of functionally related genes have been highlighted in Figure 6B. Strikingly, 65% of the up-regulated genes in DKO-R cells whose function is known, are components of the pathways implicated in signalling, trafficking and cell interaction. Of these genes, the chemokine receptor CXCR4 was of particular interest. CXCR4 is a serpentine G-protein coupled receptor that is commonly expressed on lymphocyte cell-lines, including B and pre-B-cells [27]. When activated by its ligand, stromal cell-derived factor 1 (SDF-1, CXCL12), the CXCR4 receptor stimulates calcium entry, MAP kinase and Akt-dependent pathways [28] (Figure 6C). Indeed, in previous work we found constitutively active Akt and ERK1/2 in DKO-R cells

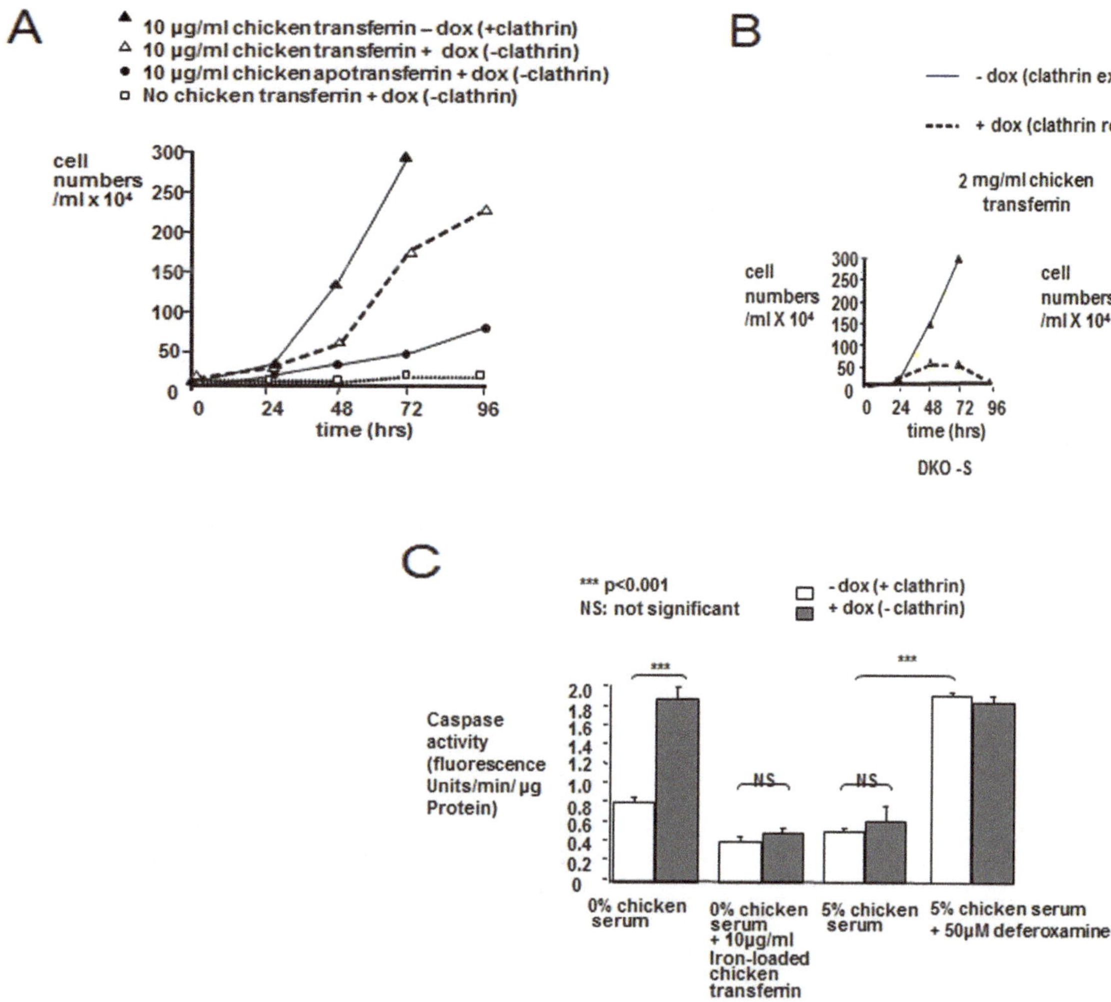

Figure 4. Purified chicken transferrin reproduces the effect of full chicken serum on the cell growth and apoptotic response of DKO-S cells to clathrin-depletion. (A) Fully iron-loaded transferrin, but not apoptransferrin rescues clathrin-depleted DKO-S cells. DKO-S cells were seeded at 2×10^4 cells/ml in media lacking chicken serum and treated as indicated. Cell growth was monitored as described in Figure 1. (B) Clathrin-depleted DKO-R cells require less chicken transferrin for survival. Cell growth was monitored as described in the legend to Figure 1. (C) Caspase activity in clathrin-expressing or clathrin-depleted DKO-S cells treated with 10 µM iron-loaded transferrin or 50 µM deferoxamine as indicated. Cells were seeded into flasks at (2×10^4 cells/ml) in treated media and caspase activity measured 72 hours later. Values are means of three measurements +/− standard deviation.

[5], which is consistent with the activation of CXCR4 signalling. These pathways in turn modulate actin cytoskeletal rearrangements, enhanced integrin expression, and stimulate chemotaxis towards SDF-1 secreting cells [29,30,31], Several genes potentially connected to these pathways were up-regulated in DKO-R cells including MAP kinase kinase 3, integrin β5, actin capping protein and Tara, a regulator of actin rearrangement (Figure 6 and Table S1). Crucially in the present context, SDF-1/CXCR4 signalling has been implicated in cell survival with a predominantly anti-apoptotic effect in lymphocyte cell-lines [32,33,34]. SDF-1 was not present in the microarray data set, so to confirm and extend the microarray results, we examined CXCR4 and SDF-1 mRNA expression in DKO-S and DKO-R cells by qualitative and quantitative RT-PCR. Both cell-lines expressed CXCR4, although there was a higher expression in DKO-R compared to DKO-S cells and SDF-1 was detectable in DKO-R cells, but not DKO-S (Figure 7A). Consistent with the microarray data and the qualitative RT-PCR, there was a significant increase in CXCR4 mRNA in DKO-R cells compared to DKO-S cells. Strikingly, SDF-1 expression showed an 7.5 fold increase in DKO-R cells compared to DKO-S (Figure 7B). Wild-type DT40 cells expressed SDF-1 mRNA at a level comparable to the DKO-S cell-line and the differential expression of CXCR4 and SDF-1 in these cell lines was independent of the presence of clathrin in the cells (Figure S3).

It has previously been shown that recombinant human SDF-1 can activate CXCR4 signalling on DT40 cells [35]. Treatment of clathrin-depleted DKO-S cells with recombinant human SDF-1α significantly reduced apoptosis at a chicken serum concentration (1%) that was normally lethal for these cells (Figure 7C). The selective activation of CXCR4 signalling in DKO-S cells led to a more DKO-R-like phenotype in their response to clathrin-depletion. The reciprocal experiment was performed with the drug AMD3100 which is a highly selective inhibitor of CXCR4 signalling [36,37]. At a concentration of 5 µg/ml, AMD3100 did not affect apoptotic behaviour of clathrin-expressing DKO-R cells in medium containing 1% chicken serum. However, when clathrin expression was repressed in DKO-R cells, under conditions where

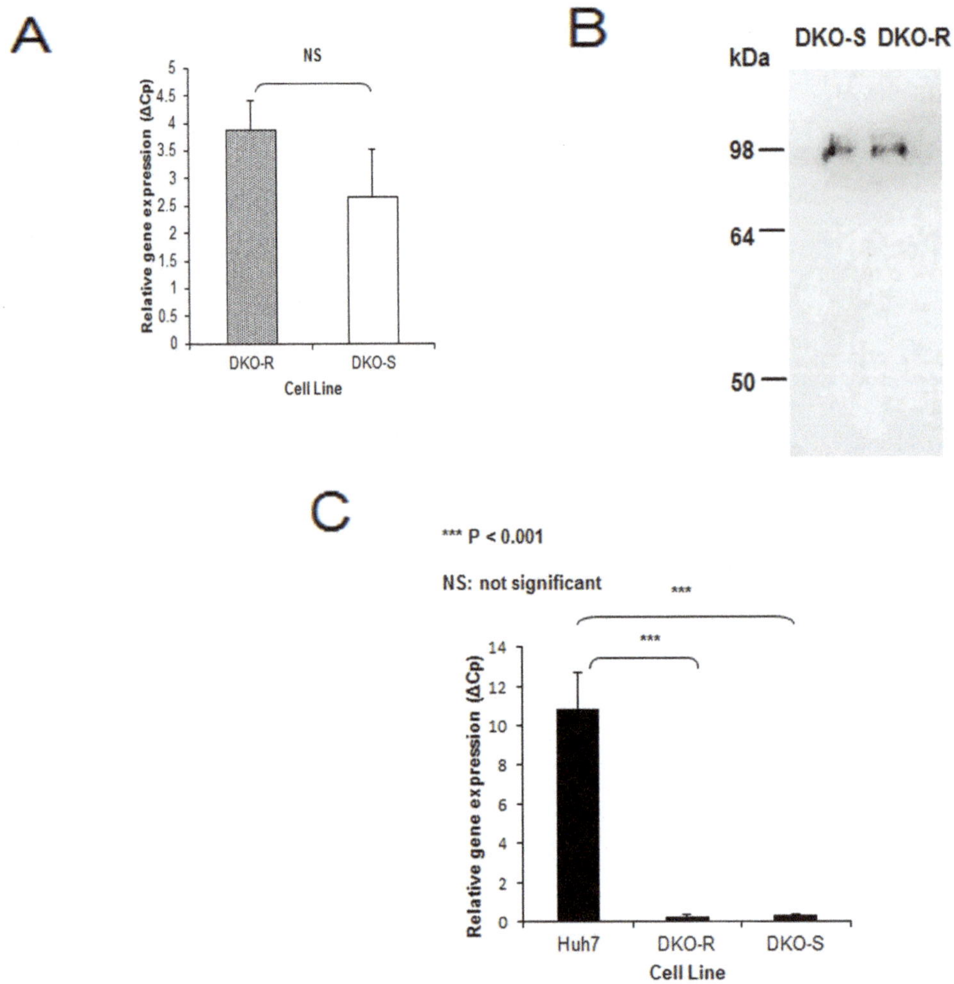

Figure 5. Analysis of the expression of transferrin and its receptor. (A) Quantitative RT-PCT of the transferrin receptor in both cell lines. (B) Western blot for the transferrin receptor in DKO-R and DKO-S cells. (C) Quantitative RT-PCR of transferrin in a control hepatic human cell line (Huh7) and DKO-R and DKO-S cells. Statistically significant differences, with p values, are indicated.

they normally survived (ie 1% chicken serum), the AMD3100-treated, clathrin-depleted DKO-R cells now underwent apoptosis (Figure 7D).

Although SDF-1 is the only ligand for CXCR4, it can also bind another receptor in this family, CXCR7 [38]. In order to assess the participation of CXCR7-mediated signalling, we examined CXCR7 expression in both cell lines. The levels of CXCR7 were similar between DKO-R and DKO-S and approximately 100 fold lower than the levels of CXCR4 (note the different ordinance scales in Figure 8A compared to Figure 7B). In order to assess the potential role of CXCR7 we investigated the effect of a highly specific inhibitor: CCX771 [39] and an inactive close analogue compound CCX704 on the apoptotic response of DKO-R cells to clathrin-depletion. In contrast to the CXCR4 inhibitor AMD3100, neither CCX771 nor CCX704 had any effect on caspase activity (Figure 8B). Although a small increase in apoptosis was observed, this was the same with both the active and inactive CXCR7 antagonists and was not accompanied by an increase in caspase activity. Taken together, our data indicates that DKO-R cells, unlike the DKO-S cells, can operate an anti-apoptotic autocrine pathway, due to the simultaneous expression of SDF-1 ligand and its receptor CXCR4.

Discussion

Our initial observation that clathrin-depletion in DKO-S cells induced apoptosis is surprising because in mammalian cells, RNAi-mediated clathrin knockdown does not produce the same effect [10,40]. However, proliferation and survival of some tumour cell lines are correlated with transferrin uptake [41]. In particular, iron restriction is known to induce apoptosis in activated T-lymphocytes and the promyelocytic cell-line HL60 [42]. Furthermore, a monoclonal antibody that blocks transferrin binding to its receptor induced apoptosis in adult T-cell leukaemia cells [43]. As with DT40, these are all fast growing lymphocyte-derived cells, suggesting that a relatively high apoptotic sensitivity to iron deficiency may be a common feature of this type of cell-line. A comparison of several human and mouse cell-lines with regards to sensitivity to iron deprivation showed that cell-lines of haematopoietic origin are indeed particularly sensitive to iron restriction. Interestingly HeLa cells, commonly used in assays of clathrin-function have a relatively high resistance to apoptotic stimuli [44].

Iron is a cofactor for key enzymes required for purine and pyrimidine synthesis, the tricarboxylic acid cycle and the mitochondrial electron transport chain [45]. Thus in fast growing cells, iron deficiency may limit both DNA synthesis and the

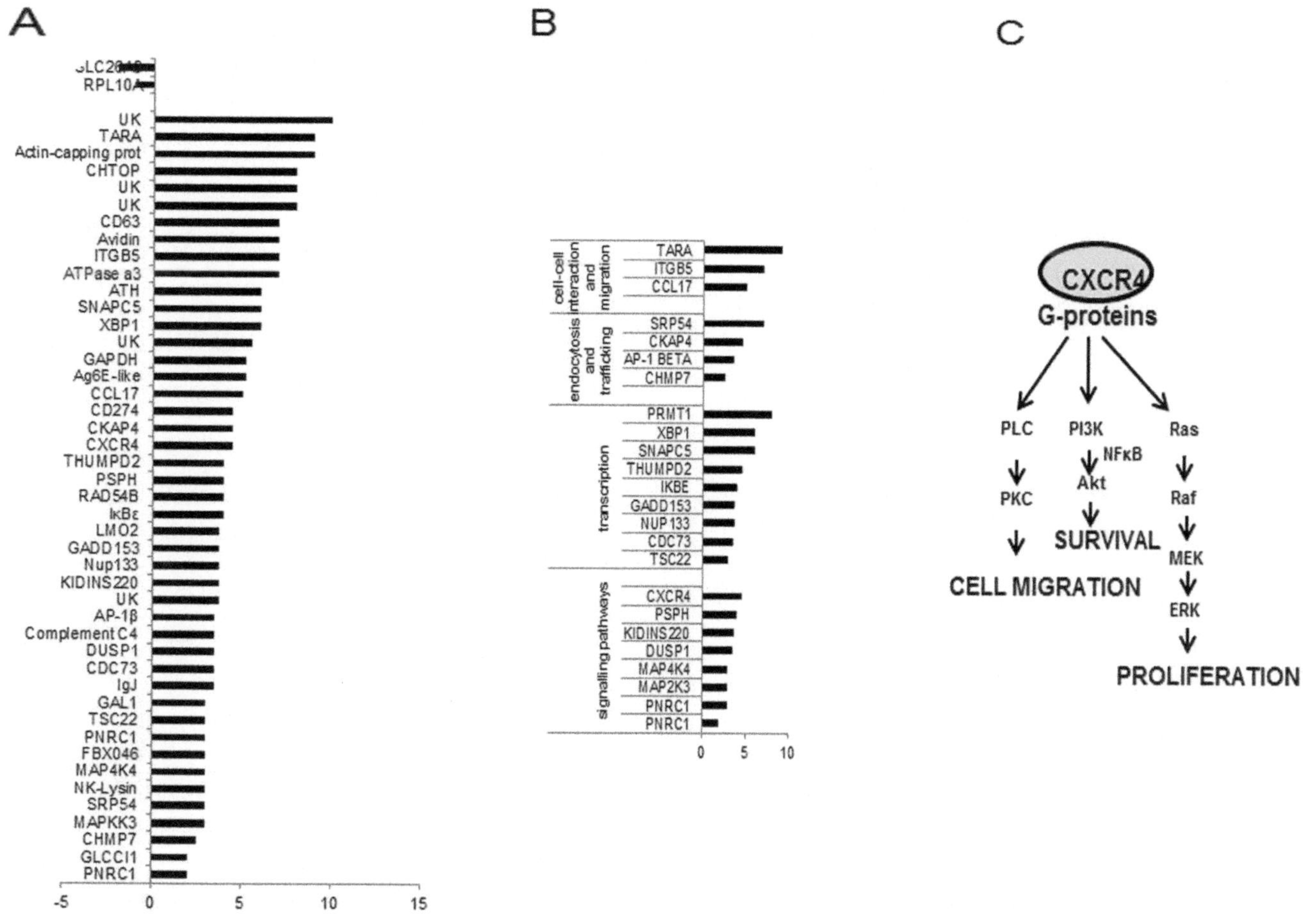

Figure 6. Microarray analysis of the gene expression profiles of DKO-s and DKO-R cells. (A) differentially expressed genes ordered in descending significance according to the P value UK: unknown. (B) functional clusters of genes of processes implicated in cell fate. (C) depiction of the CXCR4 signalling pathway.

capacity to generate ATP from aerobic respiration. Iron restriction reduces transcription of the cell cycle control protein p21(WAF1/CIP1) [46], downregulates anti-apoptotic Bcl-2, up-regulates the pro-apoptotic Bax [47] and activates a mitochondrial caspase pathway [48]. Clathrin-depletion in the DT40 cells reduced, but did not abolish transferrin uptake [5,8]. This clathrin-independent residual transferrin uptake probably accounts for the survival of clathrin-depleted DKO-S cells when grown in media with high levels of chicken serum. We have found that some batches of chicken serum are better than others at supporting the growth of clathrin-depleted DKO-S cells [8], and this correlates with the level of transferrin (APJ, data not shown). Additionally, in cells with increased requirements for iron due to their rapid proliferation rate, such as neoplastic cells, alternative routes of iron uptake to transferrin have been observed. Thus non-receptor-mediated pinocytosis has been suggested as a significant mechanism of iron uptake in human hepatoma and melanoma cell-lines [49].

The different apoptotic thresholds shown by clathrin-depleted DKO-S and DKO-R cells is a notable example of how cells can modulate their apoptotic response to iron deficiency depending on the activity of other signals. We propose that the DKO-R cell-line has induced an autocrine loop mediated by the anti-apoptotic chemokine SDF-1 and its receptor CXCR4. Thus the DKO-R cells have enhanced an important survival pathway that helps to damp down the apoptotic signal generated by partial iron restriction. Our work suggests that SDF-1/CXCR4 autocrine signalling can play an important role in regulating tumour survival [32] and is consistent with the observation that activation of this pathway reduces apoptosis in serum-starved murine embryonic stem cells [12]. High expression of CXCR4 was associated with carcinoma, migration, proliferation and metastasis [50]. The DT40 cell-line was derived from a pre B-cell [2] and indeed, SDF-1 was initially named 'Pre B-cell growth-stimulating factor' in recognition of its role in promoting the survival of pre B-cells *in vitro* [51]. In T cells, activated CXCR4 stimulates both MAP kinase and Akt-dependent pathways [34,52]. We showed that phospho-Akt is much more abundant in DKO-R than DKO-S and though a decrease is observed in both lines after clathrin depletion, this decrease is less prominent in DKO-R and Akt activity remains much higher than in DKO-S. We also examined ERK1/2 showing that it is constitutively active in DKO-R cells [5]. As Akt and ERK are pivotal to the CXCR4 signalling pathway, and since CXCR4 only binds SDF-1 [53], the constitutive stimulation of these enzymes in DKO-R cells is consistent with an autocrine effect of endogenously synthesised SDF-1. In agreement with our observations, a dramatic increase in Akt and ERK1/2 phosphorylation in response to SDF-1 stimulation has been noted in MEF cells and this activation was inhibited by the CXCR4 inhibitor AMD3100 but not by a CXCR7 inhibitor [54].

SDF-1 activated CXCR4 receptors modulate integrin signalling, promote chemotaxis towards SDF-1 secreting cells and

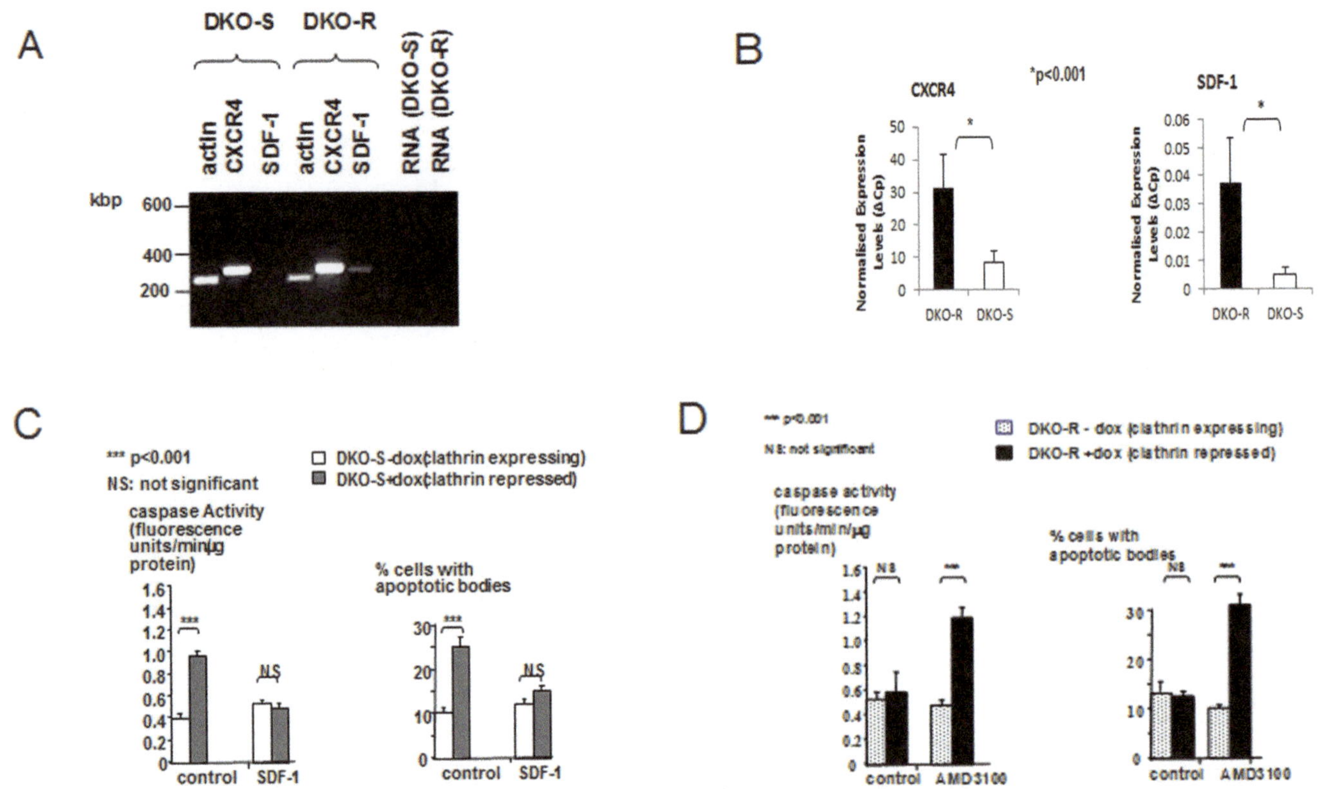

Figure 7. RT-PCR for CXCR4, SDF-1 and CXCR7 in DKO-S and DKO-R cells. (A) standard RT-PCR as described in materials and methods followed by agarose gel migration. Controls (RNA) for genomic DNA contamination in which the RT-PCR reaction was conducted without prior treatment with reverse transcriptase are shown. (B) real time PCR from cDNA obtained from both cell-lines, results are expressed as ΔCp normalising the levels of expression to Cyclophilin A. (C) Caspase activity and percentage of apoptosis of clathrin-expressing and clathrin-repressed DKO-S cells in the presence or absence of 20 nM recombinant human SDF-1α. Values are means of four determinations +/− standard deviation. (D) Caspase activity and percentage of apoptosis of clathrin-expressing and clathrin-repressed DKO-R cells in the presence or absence of 5 μM AMD3100. In both (C) and (D), cells were grown in standard DT40 medium with 1% chicken serum. Values are means of four determinations +/− standard deviation. Statistically significant differences, with p values, are indicated.

induce major actin cytoskeletal rearrangements [28]. It is possible that some of these changes could affect additional aspects of the DKO-R phenotype. For example, it has been observed that receptor-mediated endocytosis of the B-cell receptor (but not other receptors) is significantly less clathrin-dependent in DKO-R cells compared to DKO-S cells [8]. It will now be interesting and

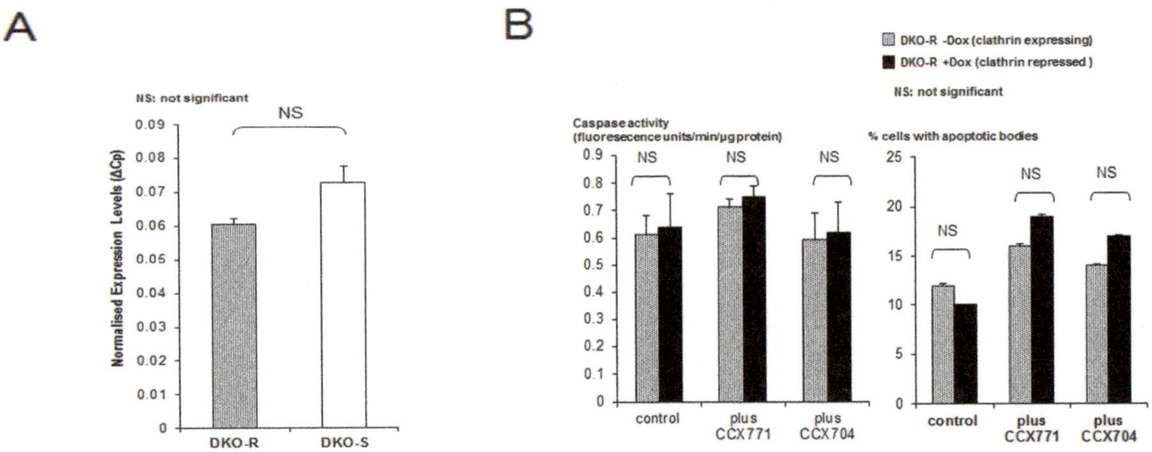

Figure 8. CXCR7 signaling is not responsible for the apoptotic-resistace shown by clathrin-depleted DKO-R cells. (A) Quantitative RT-PCR for CXCR7 in both cell lines. (B) Caspase activity and percentage of apoptosis of clathrin-expressing and clathrin-repressed DKO-R cells in the presence or absence of 0.5 μM CCX771 and inactive analog CCX704. Cells were grown in standard DT40 medium with 1% chicken serum. Values are means of four determinations +/− standard deviation.

important to investigate whether SDF-1 signalling can explain this unusual result. Evidently, the altered expression of only a small number of genes is enough to produce the DKO-R phenotype and several of these are directly related to the SDF-1 signal pathway. In prostate tumour cell-lines, SDF-1 signalling up-regulates the expression of CXCR4 and other downstream targets of its signalling pathway [55]. If this is also true for DT40, then the primary change that produced the DKO-R phenotype could have been an up-regulation of SDF-1 expression. This is supported by our observation that wild-type DT40 cells do not express SDF-1 (Figure S3). The DKO-R cells were originally isolated from an overgrown population of DKO-S cells, and it seems likely that this condition selected for an enhanced anti-apoptotic phenotype. We have subsequently identified other cells derived from DKO-S that are similarly resistant to clathrin-depletion, although in these cases, the molecular mechanism has not been investigated. It appears that such variants are not uncommon in DT40 populations and this may in turn have important implications for the use of DT40 to study apoptotic pathways.

Our results provide a worked example of how the phenotypic consequences of gene inactivation are contingent upon the wider physiological background and how this needs to be taken into account when interpreting gene knockout experiments. Furthermore, many tissue-culture cells possess great plasticity to adapt to their environment *via* genetic changes, and these adaptations can have an impact on the phenotype generated by research manipulations. Our results further emphasise that cell survival depends on a balance of positive and negative signals that can be independently modulated. A number of therapeutic strategies for the treatment of leukaemia and other lymphocyte-derived tumours have been proposed and are currently undergoing clinical trials. Several of these aim to stimulate apoptosis by blocking transferrin endocytosis [43,56], or prevent iron uptake using chelating agents [57]. Moreover, the up-regulation of SDF-1/CXCR4 expression is a known mechanism used by some tumour cells that contributes to chemotherapy resistance [30]. In this context, the relative ease with which the DKO-R cells emerged from the DKO-S background should raise a cautionary note, as it implies a simple mechanism by which cells can escape from such therapies. Adaptive changes based on CXCR4-SDF-1 regulation and signalling may be important factors in the resistance to chemotherapy.

Supporting Information

Figure S1 Figure S1A: growth of DKO-S cells in increasing levels of chicken serum, as indicated. Figure S1B: growth of DKO-R cells in increasing levels of chicken serum as indicated.

Figure S2 Cell growth of clathrin-deficient DKO-S cells. (A) in ammonium sulfate fractionated chicken serum. (B) in G-200 Sepharose filtered fractions of the 40–80% ammonium sulphate fraction.

Figure S3 Effect of doxycycline on expression of CXCR4 and SDF-1. Wild-type DT40 cells as well as the DKO-R and DKO-S clones were grown with or without 0.1 μM doxycycline (DOX) for 72 hours prior RNA extraction. The levels of CXCR4 and SDF-1 expression were assessed by qRT-PCR normalising to cyclophilin A.

Table S1 Microarray data showing genes differentially expressed in DKO-S and DKO-R cells. For genes upregulated in DKO-R cells, CXCR4 and other components of pathways known to be modified by activated CXCR4 signalling are shaded.

Acknowledgments

We thank Dr Caroline Le Bousse-Kerdilès and Dr Jean-Jacques Lataillade (Institut André Lwoff, Villejuif, France) for the gift of recombinant human SDF-1 and Mark Penfold at Chemocentrix for the generous provision of CCX771 and CCX704. We thank Dr Kathryn Lilley and the proteomics facility in the Biochemistry department for their sequence analysis of partially purified samples. We thank Dr Anne Mason (Department of Biochemistry, University of Vermont College of Medicine) for the monoclonal antibodies against chicken transferrin. We thank Dr Beatrice Scharlb for help with the protein purification procedures.

Author Contributions

Conceived and designed the experiments: APJ AP FRMW RT. Performed the experiments: AP FRMW HC AD APJ. Analyzed the data: AP RT APJ. Contributed reagents/materials/analysis tools: AP RT APJ. Wrote the paper: APJ AP. Revision of manuscript: FRMW HC AD RT.

References

1. Edeling MA, Smith C, Owen D (2006) Life of a clathrin coat: insights from clathrin and AP structures. Nat Rev Mol Cell Biol 7: 32–44.
2. Baba TW, Giroir BP, Humphries EH (1985) Cell lines derived from avian lymphomas exhibit two distinct phenotypes. Virology 144: 139–151.
3. Buerstedde JM, Takeda S (1991) Increased ratio of targeted to random integration after transfection of chicken B cell lines. Cell 67: 179–188.
4. Winding P, Berchtold MW (2001) The chicken B cell line DT40: a novel tool for gene disruption experiments. J Immunol Methods 249: 1–16.
5. Wettey FR, Hawkins SF, Stewart A, Luzio JP, Howard JC, et al. (2002) Controlled elimination of clathrin heavy-chain expression in DT40 lymphocytes. Science 297: 1521–1525.
6. Jackson AP, Flett A, Smythe C, Hufton L, Wettey FR, et al. (2003) Clathrin promotes incorporation of cargo into coated pits by activation of the AP2 adaptor micro2 kinase. J Cell Biol 163: 231–236.
7. Diaz-Griffero F, Jackson AP, Brojatsch J (2005) Cellular uptake of avian leukosis virus subgroup B is mediated by clathrin. Virology 337: 45–54.
8. Stoddart A, Jackson AP, Brodsky FM (2005) Plasticity of B cell receptor internalization upon conditional depletion of clathrin. Mol Biol Cell 16: 2339–2348.
9. Neumann-Staubitz P, Hall SL, Kuo J, Jackson AP (2010) Characterization of a temperature-sensitive vertebrate clathrin heavy chain mutant as a tool to study clathrin-dependent events in vivo. PLoS One 5: e12017.
10. Motley A, Bright NA, Seaman MN, Robinson MS (2003) Clathrin-mediated endocytosis in AP-2-depleted cells. J Cell Biol 162: 909–918.
11. Buckley SJ, Collins PJ, O'Connor BF (2004) The purification and characterisation of novel dipeptidyl peptidase IV-like activity from bovine serum. Int J Biochem Cell Biol 36: 1281–1296.
12. Guo Y, Hangoc G, Bian H, Pelus LM, Broxmeyer HE (2005) SDF-1/CXCL12 enhances survival and chemotaxis of murine embryonic stem cells and production of primitive and definitive hematopoietic progenitor cells. Stem Cells 23: 1324–1332.
13. Karin M, Mintz B (1981) Receptor-mediated endocytosis of transferrin in developmentally totipotent mouse teratocarcinoma stem cells. J Biol Chem 256: 3245–3252.
14. Aisen P, Leibman A, Zweier J (1978) Stoichiometric and site characteristics of the binding of iron to human transferrin. J Biol Chem 253: 1930–1937.
15. Laemmli UK (1970) Cleavage of structural proteins during the assembly of the head of bacteriophage T4. Nature 227: 680–685.
16. Nathke IS, Heuser J, Lupas A, Stock J, Turck CW, et al. (1992) Folding and trimerization of clathrin subunits at the triskelion hub. Cell 68: 899–910.
17. Mason AB, Brown SA, Church WR (1987) Monoclonal antibodies to either domain of ovotransferrin block binding to transferrin receptors on chick reticulocytes. J Biol Chem 262: 9011–9015.
18. Xue L, Fletcher GC, Tolkovsky AM (1999) Autophagy is activated by apoptotic signalling in sympathetic neurons: an alternative mechanism of death execution. Mol Cell Neurosci 14: 180–198.
19. Ausubel FM, Brent R, Kingston RE, Moore DA, Seidman JG, et al. (2002) Current protocols in molecular biology. John Wiley and Sons.

20. Burnside J, Neiman P, Tang J, Basom R, Talbot R, et al. (2005) Development of a cDNA array for chicken gene expression analysis. BMC Genomics 6: 13.
21. Hochberg Y, Benjamini Y (1990) More powerful procedures for multiple significance testing. Stat Med 9: 811–818.
22. Bouillon R, Van Baelen H, Tan BK, De Moor P (1980) The isolation and characterization of the 25-hydroxyvitamin D-binding protein from chick serum. J Biol Chem 255: 10925–10930.
23. Beilby J, Olynyk J, Ching S, Prins A, Swanson N, et al. (1992) Transferrin index: an alternative method for calculating the iron saturation of transferrin. Clin Chem 38: 2078–2081.
24. Buchegger F, Trowbridge IS, Liu LF, White S, Collawn JF (1996) Functional analysis of human/chicken transferrin receptor chimeras indicates that the carboxy-terminal region is important for ligand binding. Eur J Biochem 235: 9–17.
25. Kakuta K, Orino K, Yamamoto S, Watanabe K (1997) High levels of ferritin and its iron in fetal bovine serum. Comp Biochem Physiol A Physiol 118: 165–169.
26. Hann HW, Stahlhut MW, Hann CL (1990) Effect of iron and desferoxamine on cell growth and in vitro ferritin synthesis in human hepatoma cell lines. Hepatology 11: 566–569.
27. Horuk R (2001) Chemokine receptors. Cytokine Growth Factor Rev 12: 313–335.
28. Kucia M, Jankowski K, Reca R, Wysoczynski M, Bandura L, et al. (2004) CXCR4-SDF-1 signalling, locomotion, chemotaxis and adhesion. J Mol Histol 35: 233–245.
29. Lataillade JJ, Domenech J, Le Bousse-Kerdiles MC (2004) Stromal cell-derived factor-1 (SDF-1)\CXCR4 couple plays multiple roles on haematopoietic progenitors at the border between the old cytokine and new chemokine worlds: survival, cell cycling and trafficking. Eur Cytokine Netw 15: 177–188.
30. Burger JA, Kipps TJ (2002) Chemokine receptors and stromal cells in the homing and homeostasis of chronic lymphocytic leukemia B cells. Leuk Lymphoma 43: 461–466.
31. Ganju RK, Brubaker SA, Meyer J, Dutt P, Yang Y, et al. (1998) The alpha-chemokine, stromal cell-derived factor-1alpha, binds to the transmembrane G-protein-coupled CXCR-4 receptor and activates multiple signal transduction pathways. J Biol Chem 273: 23169–23175.
32. Lataillade JJ, Clay D, Bourin P, Herodin F, Dupuy C, et al. (2002) Stromal cell-derived factor 1 regulates primitive hematopoiesis by suppressing apoptosis and by promoting G(0)/G(1) transition in CD34(+) cells: evidence for an autocrine/paracrine mechanism. Blood 99: 1117–1129.
33. Burger JA, Tsukada N, Burger M, Zvaifler NJ, Dell'Aquila M, et al. (2000) Blood-derived nurse-like cells protect chronic lymphocytic leukemia B cells from spontaneous apoptosis through stromal cell-derived factor-1. Blood 96: 2655–2663.
34. Suzuki Y, Rahman M, Mitsuya H (2001) Diverse transcriptional response of CD4(+) T cells to stromal cell-derived factor (SDF)-1: cell survival promotion and priming effects of SDF-1 on CD4(+) T cells. J Immunol 167: 3064–3073.
35. Guinamard R, Signoret N, Ishiai M, Marsh M, Kurosaki T, et al. (1999) B cell antigen receptor engagement inhibits stromal cell-derived factor (SDF)-1alpha chemotaxis and promotes protein kinase C (PKC)-induced internalization of CXCR4. J Exp Med 189: 1461–1466.
36. De Clercq E (2003) The bicyclam AMD3100 story. Nat Rev Drug Discov 2: 581–587.
37. Hatse S, Princen K, Bridger G, De Clercq E, Schols D (2002) Chemokine receptor inhibition by AMD3100 is strictly confined to CXCR4. FEBS Lett 527: 255–262.
38. Burns JM, Summers BC, Wang Y, Melikian A, Berahovich R, et al. (2006) A novel chemokine receptor for SDF-1 and I-TAC involved in cell survival, cell adhesion, and tumor development. J Exp Med 203: 2201–2213.
39. Zabel BA, Wang Y, Lewen S, Berahovich RD, Penfold ME, et al. (2009) Elucidation of CXCR7-mediated signaling events and inhibition of CXCR4-mediated tumor cell transendothelial migration by CXCR7 ligands. J Immunol 183: 3204–3211.
40. Caldieri G, Capestrano M, Bicanova K, Beznoussenko G, Baldassarre M, et al. (2012) Polarised apical-like intracellular sorting and trafficking regulates invadopodia formation and degradation of the extracellular matrix in cancer cells. Eur J Cell Biol 91: 961–968.
41. Seligman PA, Kovar J, Gelfand EW (1992) Lymphocyte proliferation is controlled by both iron availability and regulation of iron uptake pathways. Pathobiology 60: 19–26.
42. Hileti D, Panayiotidis P, Hoffbrand AV (1995) Iron chelators induce apoptosis in proliferating cells. Br J Haematol 89: 181–187.
43. Moura IC, Lepelletier Y, Arnulf B, England P, Baude C, et al. (2004) A neutralizing monoclonal antibody (mAb A24) directed against the transferrin receptor induces apoptosis of tumor T lymphocytes from ATL patients. Blood 103: 1838–1845.
44. Kovar J, Valenta T, Stybrova H (2001) Differing sensitivity of tumor cells to apoptosis induced by iron deprivation in vitro. In Vitro Cell Dev Biol Anim 37: 450–458.
45. Richardson DR (2005) Molecular mechanisms of iron uptake by cells and the use of iron chelators for the treatment of cancer. Curr Med Chem 12: 2711–2729.
46. Gazitt Y, Reddy SV, Alcantara O, Yang J, Boldt DH (2001) A new molecular role for iron in regulation of cell cycling and differentiation of HL-60 human leukemia cells: iron is required for transcription of p21(WAF1/CIP1) in cells induced by phorbol myristate acetate. J Cell Physiol 187: 124–135.
47. Yuan J, Lovejoy DB, Richardson DR (2004) Novel di-2-pyridyl-derived iron chelators with marked and selective antitumor activity: in vitro and in vivo assessment. Blood 104: 1450–1458.
48. Greene BT, Thorburn J, Willingham MC, Thorburn A, Planalp RP, et al. (2002) Activation of caspase pathways during iron chelator-mediated apoptosis. J Biol Chem 277: 25568–25575.
49. Heath JL, Weiss JM, Lavau CP, Wechsler DS (2013) Iron deprivation in cancer – potential therapeutic implications. Nutrients 5: 2836–2859.
50. Yang YC, Lee ZY, Wu CC, Chen TC, Chang CL, et al. (2007) CXCR4 expression is associated with pelvic lymph node metastasis in cervical adenocarcinoma. Int J Gynecol Cancer 17: 676–686.
51. Nagasawa T, Kikutani H, Kishimoto T (1994) Molecular cloning and structure of a pre-B-cell growth-stimulating factor. Proc Natl Acad Sci U S A 91: 2305–2309.
52. Vlahakis SR, Villasis-Keever A, Gomez T, Vanegas M, Vlahakis N, et al. (2002) G protein-coupled chemokine receptors induce both survival and apoptotic signaling pathways. J Immunol 169: 5546–5554.
53. Qin S, Rottman JB, Myers P, Kassam N, Weinblatt M, et al. (1998) The chemokine receptors CXCR3 and CCR5 mark subsets of T cells associated with certain inflammatory reactions. J Clin Invest 101: 746–754.
54. McGinn OJ, Marinov G, Sawan S, Stern PL (2012) CXCL12 receptor preference, signal transduction, biological response and the expression of 5T4 oncofoetal glycoprotein. J Cell Sci 125: 5467–5478.
55. Kukreja P, Abdel-Mageed AB, Mondal D, Liu K, Agrawal KC (2005) Up-regulation of CXCR4 expression in PC-3 cells by stromal-derived factor-1alpha (CXCL12) increases endothelial adhesion and transendothelial migration: role of MEK/ERK signaling pathway-dependent NF-kappaB activation. Cancer Res 65: 9891–9898.
56. Trowbridge IS, Lopez F (1982) Monoclonal antibody to transferrin receptor blocks transferrin binding and inhibits human tumor cell growth in vitro. Proc Natl Acad Sci U S A 79: 1175–1179.
57. Dayani PN, Bishop MC, Black K, Zeltzer PM (2004) Desferoxamine (DFO) – mediated iron chelation: rationale for a novel approach to therapy for brain cancer. J Neurooncol 67: 367–377.

10

Analysis of Micro-Rearrangements in 25 Eukaryotic Species Pairs by SyntenyMapper

Stefanie Kaufmann[1], Dmitrij Frishman[1,2,3]*

1 Department of Genome Oriented Bioinformatics, Technische Universität München, Freising, Bavaria, Germany, **2** Institute of Bioinformatics and Systems Biology, German Research Center for Environmental Health, Neuherberg, Bavaria, Germany, **3** Department of Bioinformatics, St Petersburg State Polytechnical University, St Petersburg, Russia

Abstract

High-quality mapping of genomic regions and genes between two organisms is an indispensable prerequisite for evolutionary analyses and comparative genomics. Existing approaches to this problem focus on either delineating orthologs or finding extended sequence regions of common evolutionary origin (syntenic blocks). We propose SyntenyMapper, a novel tool for refining predefined syntenic regions. SyntenyMapper creates a set of blocks with conserved gene order between two genomes and finds all minor rearrangements that occurred since the evolutionary split of the two species considered. We also present TrackMapper, a SyntenyMapper-based tool that allows users to directly compare genome features, such as histone modifications, between two organisms, and identify genes with highly conserved features. We demonstrate SyntenyMapper's advantages by conducting a large-scale analysis of micro-rearrangements within syntenic regions of 25 eukaryotic species. Unsurprisingly, the number and length of syntenic regions is correlated with evolutionary distance, while the number of micro-rearrangements depends only on the size of the harboring region. On the other hand, the size of rearranged regions remains relatively constant regardless of the evolutionary distance between the organisms, implying a length constraint in the rearrangement process. SyntenyMapper is a useful software tool for both large-scale and gene-centric genome comparisons.

Editor: Shoba Ranganathan, Macquarie University, Australia

Funding: This work was supported by the German Research Foundation (DFG, www.dfg.de) International Research Training Group 'Regulation and Evolution of Cellular Systems' (GRK 1563). Publication was supported by the Technische Universität München within the funding programme Open Access Publishing. The funders had no role in study design, data collection and analysis, decision to publish, or preparation of the manuscript.

Competing Interests: The authors have declared that no competing interests exist.

* Email: d.frishman@wzw.tum.de

Introduction

The most basic step in comparative genomics is to find functional genetic elements (genes, pseudogenes, repeats, regulatory sequences) as well as entire genome regions that are conserved between two species. The finding of matching genomic regions is central to tracing the evolutionary history that led from a common ancestor to the contemporary genome sequences via a succession of evolutionary events, such as gene duplications and translocations. Establishing equivalent locations between genomes is also an important prerequisite for comparing position-specific functional, structural, and evolutionary features measured by modern high-throughput techniques, such as transcriptionally active regions, chromatin accessibility, replication domains and single nucleotide polymorphisms (SNPs).

Finding corresponding locations in two different genomes usually involves the identification of syntenic regions, which represent the longest sequence stretches of common evolutionary origin and consist of a number of conserved genome regions, often with interspersed short segments of lower or no similarity [1]. The order of these equivalent syntenic regions is different in both genomes due to an unknown number of large rearrangement events that occurred after the species diverged from the last common ancestor. Based on their extent, rearrangements are usually (somewhat arbitrarily) subdivided into two classes: i) macro-rearrangements, which involve multi-megabase sized intra- and interchromosomal relocation of large syntenic blocks, and ii) micro-rearrangements [1], i.e. re-ordering of smaller segments (below 1Mb) within a syntenic region.

The distinction between finding large regions of common origin and rearrangements of gene order at a much finer scale is intrinsically ill defined. In addition, each of these tasks has its own complications. While looking for long genomic blocks in two genomes that have evolved from the same sequence, one must allow for gaps and ignore micro-rearrangements. The search for orthologs is hampered by the presence of paralogous families and by local similarity hits covering individual domains of multi-domain proteins. Below we give a general overview of the most common types of methods for the identification of equivalent genomic locations using synteny, as illustrated in Figure 1.

Sequence-based methods

The most widely used approach to syntenic block detection is based on whole-genome sequence alignments. For example, ENSEMBL Compara [2,3] starts with short local alignment seeds with a perfect match in both organisms and elongates them until

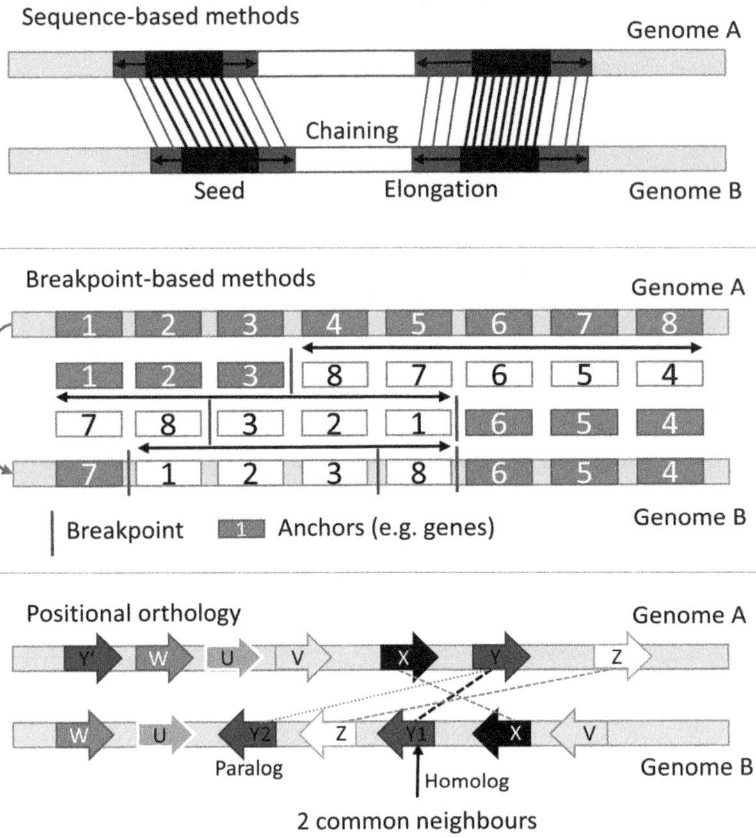

Figure 1. Overview of different approaches for identifying orthologous regions in two genomes. Sequence-based methods (e.g. ENSEMBL Compara) start with short local alignments that are extended to longest possible alignments over gaps. Breakpoint-based methods use orthologous elements (called 'anchors') to find the minimum number of rearrangements that transforms one genome into the other. Positional orthology tries to distinguish orthologs from paralogs by analyzing gene neighborhoods.

the similarity score falls below a predefined threshold. This procedure produces a set of medium length alignments with a low number of gaps and mismatches. Pairs of such alignments that are located sufficiently close to each other are then chained to create extended aligned stretches of common evolutionary origin. A similar approach was published by Liao et al. [4] who introduced pairs of unique 16-mers as a substitute for local alignments. This allows for a much faster searching for orthologous regions than whole-genome alignments. The method is designed to find the longest regions with a common ancestor in two genomes and is thus appropriate for analyzing large-scale genomic rearrangement events, but not for comparisons at the gene level.

Breakpoint-based methods

These methods [1] divide both genomes to be compared into homologous elements, e.g. genes that can be matched between them. The goal is to find the smallest combination of translocations, inversions and duplications explaining today's genomes. One example of a breakpoint-based method for the detection of syntenic blocks is the GRIMM genome rearrangements Web server [5], which is based on the popular algorithm by Hannenhalli and Pevzner [6,7]. GRIMM is able to distinguish between macro- and micro-rearrangements and relies on an initial alignment of orthologous elements. However, since GRIMM's main goal is the reconstruction of evolutionary events, it focuses on finding macro-rearrangements and the most important micro-rearrangements within them while discarding small rearrangements. While it is a well-suited method for the detection of macro-rearrangements, it fails to reconstruct a complete evolutionary history on the level of genes. Additionally, GRIMM is not able to deal with gene duplication in a genome (the so called 'word problem'). Another method, also based on the Hannenhalli-Pevzner algorithm, is Cinteny [8], which focuses on the detection of syntenic regions at different sensitivities.

Positional orthology

Positional orthology is an umbrella term for all ortholog prediction methods that rely on gene neighborhood, such as localSynteny [9] or MSOAR [10,11]. They aim to produce a one-to-one mapping of genes by taking the direct neighbors of all orthologs into account and attempt to delineate orthologs based on the evolutionary time point of their creation. This leads to a mapping with higher probabilities for the resulting orthologs to fulfill similar functions in their species. The main drawback of these methods is their definition of gene neighborhood, which is composed of the adjacent genes on both sides. Only a subset of direct neighbors is thus used to define the orthology of the genes in question, although consideration of a larger segment of genes, which lies in a conserved order in both genomes could greatly improve the prediction.

All types of approaches focus on one partial aspect of the evolutionary relationship between two species, even though they are highly interdependent, and no single approach, applied separately, is adequate for comparing quantitative or qualitative properties along eukaryotic chromosomes. Comparative genomics studies focusing on genes and their immediate environment (i.e. intergenic regions, regulatory elements, adjacent genes) usually only compare orthologs. If the immediate linear environment of the gene is important for the comparison of species, considering pairs of orthologs independently from each other is not sufficient. For example, the expression of Homeobox (Hox) genes is determined by their order on the chromosome [12,13]. Another example are lamina- associated domains (LAD) which, when located in the intergenic region between two genes, determine the subnuclear localization of the entire genomic region. Features such as LADs are known to correlate with hetero- and euchromatin [14] and hence also influence gene expression, which, again, demonstrates the importance of the linear environment in comparative genomics.

Syntenic regions, originally defined as segments of conserved gene order, would seem to be the perfect basis for comparing both genes and their neighborhoods between two species, but there are very few regions of continuous similarity between mammalian genomes. Instead, a more general term syntenic blocks is often used [1] to describe conserved regions that are interrupted by local micro-rearrangements and therefore do not lend themselves to straightforward comparison of genes and their environments. Refinement of such regions formed by macro-rearrangements and delineation of maximal length blocks of conserved gene order are required to allow for comparison of genes and regulatory elements in conserved neighborhoods.

In this work we propose a new method, SyntenyMapper, which aims to reconcile all three types of approaches discussed above by combining the search for completely conserved blocks of orthologous genes with the identification of microrearrangements within syntenic blocks. Using pre-calculated syntenic regions and orthologous genes as input, SyntenyMapper finds rearranged regions of conserved gene order within syntenic blocks. It is thus well suited for a gene-based comparison of genomes, since it not only allows for consideration of the genomic properties of orthologous genes, but also of their conserved gene neighborhood.

SyntenyMapper can be best compared with a class of orthology-based tools suitable for the identification of small blocks of conserved gene order, or collinear blocks, which usually work on a genome-wide scale. Similar to our tool, CYNTENATOR [15], MCScanX [16] and i-ADHoRe [17] identify regions of conserved gene order by applying alignment techniques to a set of ortholog anchors such as genes. These methods are in principle suitable for identifying all micro-rearrangements of gene order in a genome and are comparable to SyntenyMapper when applied to syntenic regions (see the Results section for a detailed comparison). However, in contrast to these methods, SyntenyMapper is designed to take into account the hierarchical structure of the genome and aims to find *all* exact micro-rearrangements within predefined syntenic blocks, independent of the number of elements they contain. CYNTENATOR, i-ADHoRe and MCScanX are less precise, allowing for gaps and mismatches of ortholog pairs. Our tool, however, delineates small blocks of perfectly conserved order that are ideal for comparison of closely related genomes and analyzing evolutionary rearrangement events in a region of interest. Through the use of predefined syntenic regions, the complexity of the task is greatly reduced and SyntenyMapper is thus able to find all small rearrangements within seconds.

Additionally, SyntenyMapper implements a preprocessing step to create a set of syntenic one-to-one orthologs. It thus also has a lot in common with positional orthology methods. However, SyntenyMapper relies on known orthology relationships and filters many-to-many groups according to gene order on the chromosome. The conservation of gene order in one large and conserved segment is thus the main guide for creating a one-to-one orthology mapping. SyntenyMapper expands and combines existing approaches for a more detailed assessment of evolutionary history.

SyntenyMapper is available as a stand-alone software repository via the Galaxy [18,19,20] platform's tool shed (https://toolshed.g2.bx.psu.edu, repository name "synteny_mapper") and as source code on our website (http://webclu.bio.wzw.tum.de/syntenymapper). Pre-computed results for the syntenic regions and orthologs from the ENSEMBL Compara database [2,3] can be accessed and downloaded at our website as well.

Material and Methods

SyntenyMapper

SyntenyMapper takes as input a set of syntenic regions and a set of one-to-one orthologs between two genomes of interest. Duplications of genes leads to presence of one-to-many and many-to-many co-orthologs, which are converted to one-to-one orthologs using the following pre-processing procedure (see Figure 2):

- Genes are grouped into one-to-many and many-to-many ortholog groups
- Each one-to-many group is reduced to a single one-to-one ortholog pair with the highest sequence identity
- Asymmetric many-to-many groups (those containing n genes in the genome A and m genes in the genome B, with $n \neq m$) are converted to symmetric many-to-many groups. For example, if $n = m + \delta$, exactly δ genes will be removed from the genome A based on an ascending ranking according to the average percent sequence identity of each gene to all other genes in the group.
- Many-to-many groups, all of which are now symmetric, are split into individual one-to-one orthologous pairs. For any many-to-many group consisting of n genes $\{a_1, a_2, ..., a_n\}$ in genome A and m genes $\{b_1, b_2, ..., b_m\}$ in genome B this is achieved by considering only orthology relationships between the genes with the same sequential number (i.e. a_1 with b_1, a_2 with b_2, etc.).

This pre-processing procedure aims to identify syntenic orthologs among groups of orthologous genes, i.e. those genes among a set of duplicated genes that are located at equivalent genomic positions with respect to their neighbors. For this reason, gene order is considered as the main factor for resolving many-to-many groups. In one-to-many groups sequence identity is used as a rough measure to identify the most recent ancestor gene.

As an example, Figure 2A shows two syntenic regions, the genes they harbor, and the pairwise orthologous relationships obtained from an external source, such as ENSEMBL [2,3]. Genes without orthologs (e.g. gene a_2) are excluded from consideration. Gene a_{10} from genome A has two orthologs in the genome B (one-to-many group). Genes a_4, a_8 and a_9 in the genome A as well as genes b_3 and b_5 in the genome B form asymmetric many-to-many orthologous groups. All remaining genes have only one ortholog. After conducting the pre-processing steps described above, the same syntenic regions look as depicted in Figure 2B. Gene a_2 has been removed and gene a_{10} now only has one ortholog with the highest sequence identity (gene b_9). The asymmetric many-to-many group has first been converted to a symmetric one by removing the gene a_9, and then split into ortholog pairs according to the gene order, resulting in one-to-one orthologous gene pairs b_3-$a_4$and b_5-a_8.

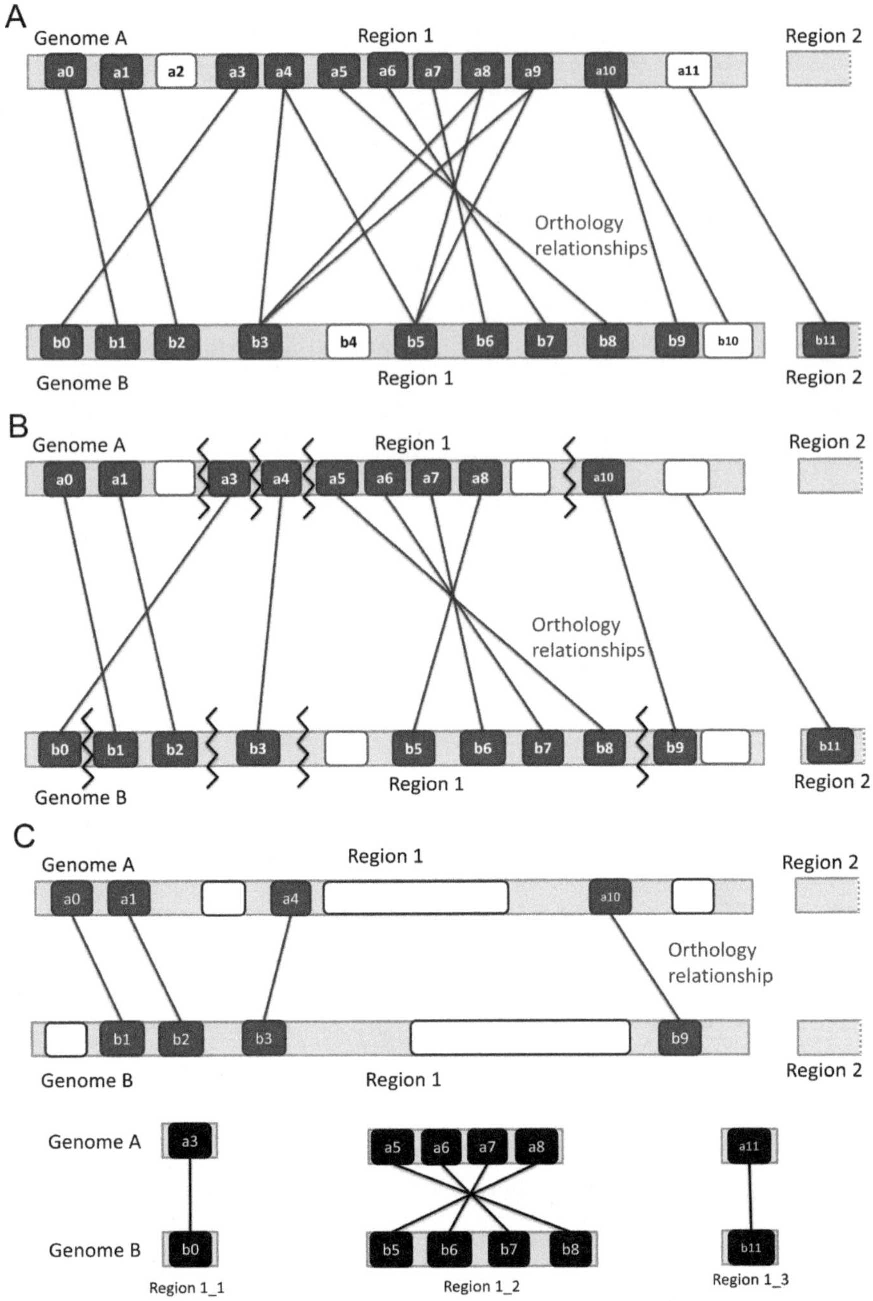

Figure 2. Detection of collinear blocks by SyntenyMapper. A: Illustration of a syntenic region between two species, with numbered boxes representing genes and connecting lines representing orthology relationships. Gene a_{11} and gene b_{11} have no orthologs in their syntenic regions, but are orthologous to each other. Genes a_2 and b_4 have no orthologs. B: During pre-processing one-to-many (genes a_{10} and b_9, b_{10}) and asymmetric many-to-many (genes a_5,a_6,a_7,a_8,a_9 and b_5,b_6,b_7,b_8), groups are first converted into symmetric groups by excluding genes with the lowest sequence identity to the rest of the group (genes a_9 and b_{10}), and subsequently paired as one-to-one orthologs based on gene order. Breakpoints (zig-zag lines) are identified as described in the Methods section. C: Using breakpoints, SyntenyMapper defines rearranged segments, shown in black, as new syntenic regions 1_1 to 1_3 within the long original region.

Given the resulting dataset of one-to-one orthologs, SyntenyMapper identifies two types of evolutionary events - translocation (genes a_3 and b_0 in Figure 2) and inversion of gene order (genes a_5, a_6, a_7, a_8 and b_5, b_6, b_7, b_8). A **translocated** segment is a chromosomal region that breaks off from its original position and reinserts into the genome at another position in one species; during an **inversion** the region inverts its direction before reinsertion. SyntenyMapper finds these events by searching for breakpoints, or locations of unconserved neighborhoods of two genes, in the reference genome A by using orthology relationships to genome B as a guide.

A **breakpoint** $\left(a_i/b_j,a_{i+1}/b_l\right)$ is defined by two orthologous gene pairs a_i, b_j and a_{i+1}, b_l if $j \pm 1 \neq l$, where genes a_i, a_{i+1} are from the reference genome A and genes b_j, b_l are from the genome B. In Figure 2B, breakpoints are marked in both genomes. When a rearranging genomic region reinserts into genome B at a new position, **two breakpoints** emerge in A, one at each end, as illustrated in Figure 3. Consequently, the genes between two subsequent breakpoints in A and their orthologs in B either form a so-called **block**, i.e. a set of genes within a translocated or inversed segment, or belong to a non-rearranged part of the original syntenic region that is enclosed between two blocks. To distinguish blocks from syntenic regions with conserved gene order that were not subject to rearrangement, SyntenyMapper looks up the two breakpoints preceding and following $(a_i/b_j,a_{i+1}/b_l)$ in the genome B. If there is no breakpoint preceding and/or following $(a_i/b_j,a_{i+1}/b_l)$, the start and/or end positions of the syntenic region are taken as reference points. The set of these three breakpoints or reference points defines two adjacent segments of genes. The length of both segments is compared and the shorter segment is defined as a new block and a new syntenic region, which lies within the longer original syntenic region.

The choice of a reference genome is arbitrary as each translocated segment in B with respect to A is also a translocated segment in A with respect to B. As seen in Figure S1, breakpoint definition with B as a reference genome leads to the definition of the same block as was found using A as a reference genome (Figure 3).

Within translocated blocks, the direction of genes is identical in both species, while inversed blocks show opposite orientation of genes. The pseudocode of the SyntenyMapper algorithm to find breakpoints and blocks is shown in Figure S2.

In the only step that involves all synteny regions, distant translocations, the so called 'external orthologs', are identified by searching for orthologs of those genes without orthologs in their own syntenic blocks. In Figures 2B, C gene a_{11} in the syntenic region 1 of the genome A and gene b_{11} in the syntenic region 2 of the genome B do not have orthologs in their own syntenic regions, but are orthologous of each other. These two genes are paired and excluded from their respective syntenic regions to define a new one.

Figure 2C shows syntenic regions refined by SyntenyMapper. Each gene now has a single syntenic orthologous partner while inversed and translocated blocks are redefined as new syntenic regions. Genes or groups of genes that were removed from their syntenic region during one of the prior steps will be termed 'excluded regions' in the following sections.

SyntenyMapper is implemented in Java and integrated in the Galaxy platform [18,19,20] for easy use and accessibility. Since each syntenic region is treated separately, SyntenyMapper computes micro-rearrangements fast and is able to analyze the human and mouse genomes in under one minute on a standard Linux workstation. Pre-computed results for ENSEMBL Compara syntenic regions data can be downloaded from our website (http://webclu.bio.wzw.tum.de/syntenymapper). The user can also analyze own data using the SyntenyMapper tool within the Galaxy environment if they match the required format described in detail in the help section. Syntenic regions from sources other than ENSEMBL should be defined in a similar manner, i.e. they should represent the longest possible regions evolved from a common sequence in the ancestor. Refined syntenic regions can be visualized using the linear or circular representations implemented in Circos [21] using the tool provided within the SyntenyMapper's Galaxy repository. Additionally, SyntenyMapper generates two output files containing a) coordinates of all syntenic regions, both original and newly defined during the mapping, marked as caused by either an internal or an external micro-rearrangement, and b) syntenic orthologs for each syntenic region.

TrackMapper

TrackMapper, also implemented in Java, allows users to directly compare so called feature tracks from two species, given a mapping from SyntenyMapper. The tool accepts as input any positional genomic features, such as binding sites or signal intensities, in the generally accepted BED format. In a BED file each line corresponds to one genomic element and contains genomic position (chromosome number, start and end coordinates) as well as an optional signal weight in columns 1–4, respectively. For each gene left after SyntenyMapper preprocessing, TrackMapper calculates the average coverage, *i.e.* the percentage of the gene's base pairs overlapping with the feature (e.g. a LINE repeat) if no signal weight is given, or the average value of the feature if a signal weight is given. These values often represent the strength of a signal, such as the height of a histone modification peak or the expression value. The vector of average coverage values for each gene is then converted into Z-scores by subtracting the mean and dividing by standard deviation. Let z_A and z_B be the vectors of feature Z-scores for syntenic one-to-one orthologs found by SyntenyMapper in genomes A and B, respectively. The measure of similarity between any two feature tracks, calculated as $z=|z_A-z_B|$, can be downloaded or further analyzed with other Galaxy Tools, which provide a wide range of plotting tools, such as distribution histograms, and statistical

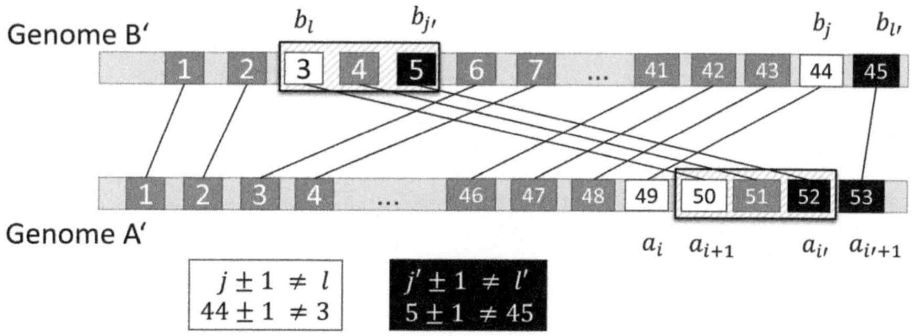

Figure 3. Breakpoint definition in SyntenyMapper. Illustration of two breakpoints emerging at both ends of a translocated segment a_3,a_4,a_5 in genome *A* and b_{50},b_{51},b_{52} in genome *B* (hatched box). By definition a breakpoint is constituted by two orthologous gene pairs a_i/b_j and a_{i+1},b_l if $j\pm1\neq l$, as shown in the boxes underneath the schema. The second breakpoint is described by $a_{i'}/b_{j'}$ and $a_{i'+1}/b_{l'}$. White and black boxes mark the four genes forming the first $(a_2/b_2,a_3/b_{50})$ and the second $(a_5/b_{52},a_6/b_3)$breakpoint, respectively. *A* is used as reference genome to define the block formed by a micro-rearrangement as the genes that lie between the adjacent breakpoints in *A*, in this case a_2, a_3 and a_5,a_6. The genes between these two breakpoints and their orthologs in *B* form a block.

analyses, such as correlation tests. Additionally, TrackMapper provides the vector mean as a compact similarity measure between the two tracks over all genes.

Currently, a widely used tool for mapping of tracks between species is LiftOver [22], which was not designed for the purpose of comparing two genomes and is also asymmetrical, in that it converts a feature track from one reference species to the other. By contrast, TrackMapper is able to directly compare feature tracks from two species on the gene level without defining one genome as a source and the other as a target.

Test data: syntenic regions and orthologs from human and mouse

Data on syntenic regions and orthologs in *Homo sapiens* and *Mus musculus* (assemblies hg19 and mm10, respectively) were obtained from ENSEMBL Compara (version 73) [3]. We downloaded 356 syntenic regions with a mean length of 7.63 mB and 6.89 mB in human and mouse, respectively, and the complete set of ENSEMBL protein-coding genes containing 23,618 and 22,769 unique genes in human and mouse with mean lengths of 59.8 kB and 44.3 kB, respectively. In *Homo sapiens*, an average of 55.10 genes fall into each synteny region, while in *Mus musculus* each syntenic region contains 58.40 genes on average. 27,453 pairwise orthology relationships between protein-coding genes were also downloaded from ENSEMBL.

To test the performance of TrackMapper in analyzing the conservation of genomic feature tracks we obtained ENCODE data for three histone modifications (H3k4me1, H3k4me3, H3k9ac) for human (Broad Institute, embryonic stem cells) and mouse (Ren Lab, ES-E14) [23]. Coordinates were converted to the most recent human (hg19) and mouse (mm10) genome assemblies using LiftOver [22]. For randomization we created n elements of the same length as the original peaks at random positions on each chromosome, with n being the number of histone modification peaks on this chromosome.

Calculation of sequence similarity between syntenic regions

We determined sequence similarity between ENSEMBL syntenic regions using our own implementation of the linear runtime trie-based sequence comparison algorithm proposed by Rieck and Laskov [24]. A trie is a tree structure similar to a suffix tree, with the distinction that for a finite set of strings, every string is represented in the path from the root to one of the leaves. Long sequences such as syntenic regions are converted into finite sets of strings by splitting them into overlapping k-mers (in our case k was set to 6). They are inserted into a trie by iterating over each 6-mers' characters and, starting from the root of the trie, following the edge with the corresponding character to the next node until no such edge exists and one or more new edges need to be inserted.

The algorithm then makes use of the trie's maximum depth of k by performing a parallel depth-first search on the tries of the two sequences. A distance score is calculated for each node using the inner function m, which compares the number of occurrences of the string represented by that node in both sequences. The score is accumulated over the whole trie using the outer function $\oplus$. In our implementation, we used the sum $\sum$ as outer function $\oplus$ and the Manhattan distance as inner function m (Equation 1).

$$m = |\phi(x) - \phi(y)| \quad (1)$$

where x,y are trie nodes and $\phi(x)$ returns the number of occurrences of the string readable from the root of the trie to x in the sequence.

Comparison with CYNTENATOR, i-ADHoRe and MCScanX

We compared SyntenyMapper with the latest versions of CYNTENATOR [15] (November 2012), i-ADHoRe 3.0 [17] and MCScanX [16] (May 2012). For each ENSEMBL syntenic region we used as input the actual gene order order and sequence identity values between the corresponding ENSEMBL orthologs. CYNTENATOR was run on each syntenic region with default parameters and homology type BLAST to consider identities, and a simple guide tree containing only human and mouse. We ran i-ADHoRe with the suggested gap size and cluster gap size of 15, probability cutoff 0.001, q-value 0.9, and anchor points 3. For MCScanX, the program MCScanX_h was used with default parameters.

Results

SyntenyMapper: a novel tool for refining syntenic orthologs

In this work we propose a new comparative genomics tool for the identification of micro-rearrangements within syntenic regions that were shaped by macro-rearrangements between species. SyntenyMapper complements the set of one-to-one orthologs from ENSEMBL by finding syntenic one-to-one orthologs among one-to-many/many-to-many orthologous groups and uses them to identify deletions, inversions, local and distant translocations within syntenic regions, further refining the definition of these regions. As a result, SyntenyMapper provides the user with a set of evolutionary building blocks with completely conserved gene order between two species.

The tool is easily accessible through the Galaxy Platform and can be used to analyze both user-supplied syntenic regions as well as those obtained from ENSEMBL Compara. The resulting refined syntenic regions and their associated annotation tracks can be interactively visualized using the circular Circos representation [21] or a linear plot created with an R script (for an example see Figure S3), and analyzed with our own track-comparison tool called TrackMapper.

Detection of micro-rearrangements between human and mouse genomes

To illustrate the performance of the SyntenyMapper approach, we applied it to syntenic regions and orthologs between the human and mouse genome obtained from ENSEMBL Compara. Syntenic region length is highly correlated between these species (Figure S4).

As seen in Table 1, the majority of protein-coding ENSEMBL genes (70.07%) have exactly one ortholog within their syntenic region. The second largest subset (12.30%) is constituted by those genes that do not have any orthologs and are hence not treated by SyntenyMapper. Genes in many-to-many groups within one syntenic region comprise only 2.30% of the total gene number; most of these groups are asymmetric. Finally, genes only having orthologs in another syntenic region (external orthologs) make up a mere 1.27% of the data. All other types of orthologous relationships, such as genes with orthologs in regions not covered by syntenic regions, represent less than 2% of all cases and are ignored by the current version of SyntenyMapper.

During the rearrangement detection process, SyntenyMapper implements a pre-processing step to find syntenic ortholog pairs among the set of orthologous genes. While converting one-to-many and many-to-many ortholog groups into one-to-one

Table 1. Frequency of different cases of orthologous relationships for a given gene in a syntenic region between human and mouse.

Type of orthologous relationship	#Genes
No ortholog	5,705 (12.30%)
One internal ortholog	32,505 (70.07%)
Many internal orthologs	1,062 (2.29%)
One external ortholog	487 (1.05%)
Many external orthologs	105 (0.23%)
Many in- and external orthologs	204 (0.44%)
One ortholog in a syntenic-block-free region	99 (0.21%)
Many orthologs in a syntenic-block-free region	15 (0.03%)
Many orthologs: internal, external, and in syntenic-block-free regions	166 (0.36%)

Italic font indicates classes of genes that are covered by SyntenyMapper. Internal orthologs: Orthologous genes that lie in the same syntenic region. External orthologs: Orthologous genes that lie in different syntenic regions. Syntenic-block-free region: Genomic region that is not covered by ENSEMBL syntenic regions.

orthologs, a total of 941 genes (2.1% of all human and mouse genes) are removed as non-syntenic. As all relationships of these genes are non-syntenic as well, a total of 10,840 relationships from the original set of 27,453 ENSEMBL Compara orthologs are eliminated with the non-syntenic genes that formed them.

SyntenyMapper finds 16,613 syntenic ortholog pairs between human and mouse and detects 2,898 blocks that were subject to micro-rearrangements within or between the original 356 syntenic regions. There are three different types of syntenic regions obtained after this analysis: i) original regions, which are identical to the input regions except for excluded non-syntenic genes (356, 10.94%), ii) internally translocated regions that represent blocks created by micro-rearrangements within the syntenic region (2,817, 86.57%), and iii) externally translocated regions that represent one or more neighboring genes that were translocated between syntenic regions (81, 2.49%).

Most frequent are internal micro-rearrangements, but blocks caused by these contain only 1.52 genes on average, while the majority of genes (73.68%) still lie within original syntenic regions. We can thus conclude that often blocks consisting of just one or two genes disturb the conservation of gene order within a syntenic region. Regions translocated over large distances are rare and, in the specific case of human/mouse comparison presented here, almost always contain only a single gene. Genes within one syntenic region lie within a linear distance of around 7 to 8mB from each other. Hence, the proximity of genes within a syntenic region leads to more frequent rearrangements compared to large linear distances. Linear proximity correlates with spatial proximity, which has been shown to be one of the triggers for rearrangements [25].

One major advantage of our approach is its ability to refine regions formed by macro-rearrangements, which are large-scale intra- or inter-chromosomal translocations, through the consideration of all micro-rearrangements, whereby short segments change their positions within syntenic regions [26]. SyntenyMapper uses pre-calculated syntenic regions, for example from ENSEMBL, which are created in such a way that their length is maximal, disregarding small rearrangements within them (see introduction). Identification of micro-rearrangements can greatly improve our understanding of evolutionary events shaping extant genomes and is instrumental for comparing the properties of regions of conserved gene order between two species.

Figure 4 shows a syntenic region with the same orientation in human and mouse, with most of the genes having syntenic one-to-one orthology relationships. However, the order of genes is disrupted by a translocation of a large block containing seven genes located in the beginning of the human region and in the end of the mouse region. The order and direction of genes within this block is preserved. Interestingly, there is a sizeable gap between syntenic orthologs and translocated genes on the human chromosome, which may imply that the translocation happened in *Homo sapiens* after human-mouse divergence.

SyntenyMapper is also able to identify a small-scale rearrangement with the majority of genes within the syntenic region in mouse lying on the reverse strand, even though the region is annotated as situated on the forward strand (Figure S5). In human, all genes lie on the forward strand, implying that an inversion occurred in mouse. Our approach recognizes this inversion of multiple genes and redefines it as a new syntenic region.

These examples illustrate the difficulties in comparing genome regions that evolved from the same sequence due to recent genome rearrangements that make any linear comparison impossible. Our method enables the user to refine syntenic regions and to discover micro-rearrangements at the level of individual genes. The analysis is not restricted to translocations within one region and also considers those genes that lie within other syntenic regions.

As an example, Figure S6 shows the relationship between two pairs of syntenic regions that share one orthologous gene pair. These rare external translocations (592, 1.27% of all genes) of genes out of their syntenic region almost always involve single genes in the human/mouse comparison. We hypothesize that translocations of single genes over large linear distances are favored by short spatial distances between the chromosomal regions involved, as has been shown for cancer cells [25]. All rearrangements illustrated in this section were not found by ENSEMBL Compara and cannot be directly inferred from orthology relationships, stressing the value of SyntenyMapper for comparative genomics.

To demonstrate the usefulness of TrackMapper for comparing feature tracks between genomes analyzed histone modifications, which are known to be largely conserved between mouse and human [27]. Using histone modification data from ENCODE we applied TrackMapper to calculate the measure that quantifies the difference in the extent to which genes overlap with histone

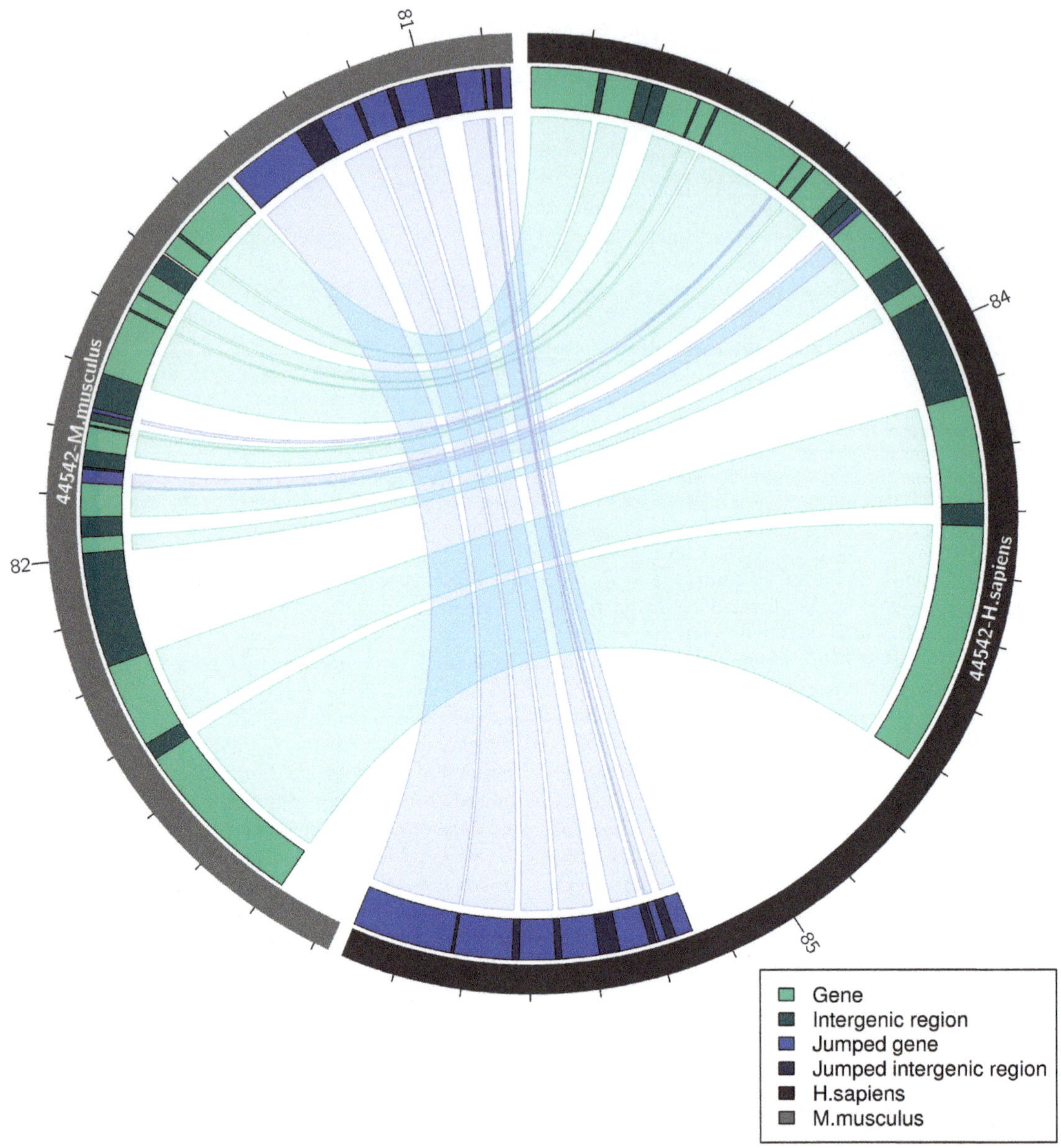

Figure 4. Visualization of SyntenyMapper results for a syntenic region in human and mouse. The region (ENSEMBL identifier 44542) is illustrated in human as a dark grey ideogram (right) and in mouse as a light grey ideogram (left). Ticks are placed at 100 kB distance and the numbers represent positions in mB on the human and mouse chromosomes 15 and 7, respectively. The Circos circular plot illustrates the positions of genes/ intergenic regions for one syntenic region in both species and the correspondence between them. Micro-rearrangements are illustrated by color-coding, with syntenic orthologs and out-of-order genes shown in grey and black, respectively, while the intergenic regions between syntenic orthologs and between out-of-order genes are shown in white. A large block of seven genes (black) was translocated in either human or mouse. In the Galaxy version of the plots, gene annotations are given as labels and as direct links to ENSEMBL through clicks onto the gene track.

modification peaks in human and mouse. For all three histone modifications considered here (see *Methods*) the difference measures are low, with a respective mean of 0.77, 0.63 and 0.70 for H3k4me1, H3k4me3 and H3k9ac. We ran TrackMapper on mouse data and randomized human histone modification peaks, to receive significantly higher difference value distributions (Wilcoxon rank sum test p-value $<2.2e\text{-}16$ in all three cases) with means of 0.98, 1.00 and 1.02, respectively. Of special interest are genes with very low difference scores, which can be easily identified using TrackMapper's tabular output (File S1). There are 171 ortholog pairs with a very low H3k4me3 difference score (below 0.01). TrackMapper is thus a convenient tool for in-depth analysis of feature conservation at the gene-level.

Pre-computed ENSEMBL Compara species comparison

ENSEMBL Compara provides syntenic regions and orthologs for 25 pairs of eukaryotic species, with 16 of them involving human. We conducted a large-scale analysis of micro-rearrangements within these syntenic regions using SyntenyMapper and calculated the number of micro-rearrangements within and between syntenic regions as well as the average number of genes involved in these events (Table S1).

Among the most closely related species pairs are human *vs* chimp (*P. troglodytes*) and mouse *vs* rat (*R. norvegicus*). Both of them share a high number of orthologs, however, the number of ENSEMBL syntenic regions differs vastly: while human and chimp share only 139 syntenic regions, there are 554 ones between mouse and rat. Because the average syntenic region length between human and chimp is about four times the size of syntenic regions in mouse and rat (22mB and 4.8mB, respectively), the percentage of the genomes covered is similar (human *vs* chimp: 87.76%, mouse *vs* rat: 94.64%).

Using branch lengths of the UCSC species tree [28] (available for all species pairs considered in this study except for those involving gorilla, pig, orangutan, common marmoset and turkey) we analyzed the correlation between the evolutionary distance and micro- and macro-rearrangement related genome features. In general, one would expect more closely related species to share a low number of very long syntenic regions, and an increase in the number and a decrease in the average length of syntenic regions with the growing evolutionary distance. Indeed, for species pairs separated by short or medium evolutionary distance, this expectation is true and the average syntenic region length and their number exhibit a negative exponential correlation (Figure 5A). However, more distantly related species, such as human and platypus, contain fewer ENSEMBL syntenic regions than would be expected based on this exponential correlation pattern. Strong deviation from this correlation pattern observed for the species pairs involving platypus as well as in the lizard vs chicken comparison is caused by the very low sequence similarity between these species, which leads to a low coverage of the genomes by syntenic regions (e.g. human *vs* platypus: only 21% of the genome is covered, see Table S2). Two other distant species pairs - human *vs* chicken and mouse *vs* chicken – are more in line with the general trend, but due to significant differences in genome size (human genome 3.1 gB, mouse genome 2.7 gB, chicken genome 1.1 gB), they also show a low genome synteny coverage of the respective longer genomes.

Because of SyntenyMappers's gene-based approach, the number of detected internal and external micro-rearrangements is dependent of the number of orthologs, which is higher for closely related species. As seen in Figure 5B, the average number of internal micro-rearrangements (per syntenic region), ranging between 0 and 30, increases with the increasing average syntenic region length and decreasing evolutionary distance. This implies that the number of micro-rearrangements depends on the size of the syntenic regions that harbor them, which is in turn correlated with evolutionary distance, as illustrated in Figure 5A.

While the total number of micro-rearrangements indirectly depends on the degree of relationship between the genomes, there is no correlation between the number of micro-rearrangements (internal or external) per mB and evolutionary distance (Figure S7). We also found only a slight positive correlation between sequence distance and the number of internal micro-rearrangements (Pearson correlation coefficient 0.22). In particular, low sequence similarity does not necessarily lead to a high number of micro-rearrangements (Figure S8).

The higher numbers of micro-rearranged regions per syntenic region in more closely related species are thus mainly due to the greater length of syntenic regions. By contrast, the size of micro-rearranged regions (i.e. the number of genes they contain) does not show any dependence on the syntenic region length and the evolutionary distance (Figure 5C), because the mechanisms of transposition, which is the main cause of small-scale translocations, are the same in all species.

External translocations between syntenic regions are less common, with the average number per syntenic region ranging between 0 and 4 for all species pairs. Overall there is a slight tendency for longer syntenic regions in more related species to contain a higher number of such external micro-rearrangements (Figure 5D). In almost all cases, only a single gene is subject to an external micro-rearrangement, regardless of the size of the synteny regions or the evolutionary distance (Figure 5E). However, with the exception of mouse and platypus, which harbor on average only 1.0 external micro-rearranged genes per syntenic region, all distantly related species pairs (mouse vs chicken, human vs platypus, human vs chicken, chicken vs lizard) have somewhat longer external translocations (average>1.05). Larger external micro-rearrangements (1.3 genes in external micro-rearrangements per syntenic region) are especially common between chicken (*G. gallus*) and wild turkey (*M. gallopavo*). In particular, SyntenyMapper was able to detect a group of six consecutive genes that was translocated between two syntenic regions in these organisms (see Figure S9). As the only closely related species pair with sharing relatively large external translocations, chicken and turkey genomes behave very differently in this aspect. Cases like this can be easily identified with SyntenyMapper, allowing for detailed genome comparison and further analysis based on the produced mapping.

Comparison with existing methods

SyntenyMapper is the first tool that was developed to detect micro-rearrangements in the form of blocks of conserved gene order within macro-rearranged regions. However, available software for detection of collinear blocks (i.e. sets of genes with conserved order in two or more species) can be applied to ENSEMBL syntenic regions as well, although no rearrangements between syntenic regions can be detected using this approach.

We detected collinear blocks between human and mouse with SyntenyMapper (discarding single-gene regions), CYNTENATOR, i-ADHoRe and MCScanX.

CYNTENATOR applies the Smith-Waterman algorithm to genomes represented by strings of genes, with homologies provided in the form of BLASTP output, and identifies local alignments, which represent blocks of conserved gene order in both species. The main advantage of this method is its handling of multiple genomes, when provided with a guide phylogenetic tree that can be obtained from other sources.

Since there is no gold standard annotation of syntenic regions, we have to rely on a qualitative comparison of the results. We have identified several reasons for discrepancies between CYNTENATOR and SyntenyMapper:

CYNTENATOR is not designed to detect external micro-rearrangements when applied to syntenic regions. However, this makes up for only a small percentage of the discrepancies: in only 8 of 356 syntenic regions (2.25%) CYNTENATOR misses just the external rearrangements. A larger problem is that CYNTENATOR, in contrast to our method, is unable to detect inversed collinear blocks of any size. Such inversions are common and occur in 170 out of 356 (47.75%) of all syntenic regions, including cases where the complete region is inversed in the second species (see Figure S10 for an example). In contrast, we have identified only one syntenic region where SyntenyMapper misses a collinear block detected by CYNTENATOR because two genes in this block overlap.

Other minor differences affect only the length of collinear blocks and are mainly caused by different definitions. Due to the usage of the Smith-Waterman alignment algorithm for aligning gene strings, CYNTENATOR sometimes mismatches non-orthologous

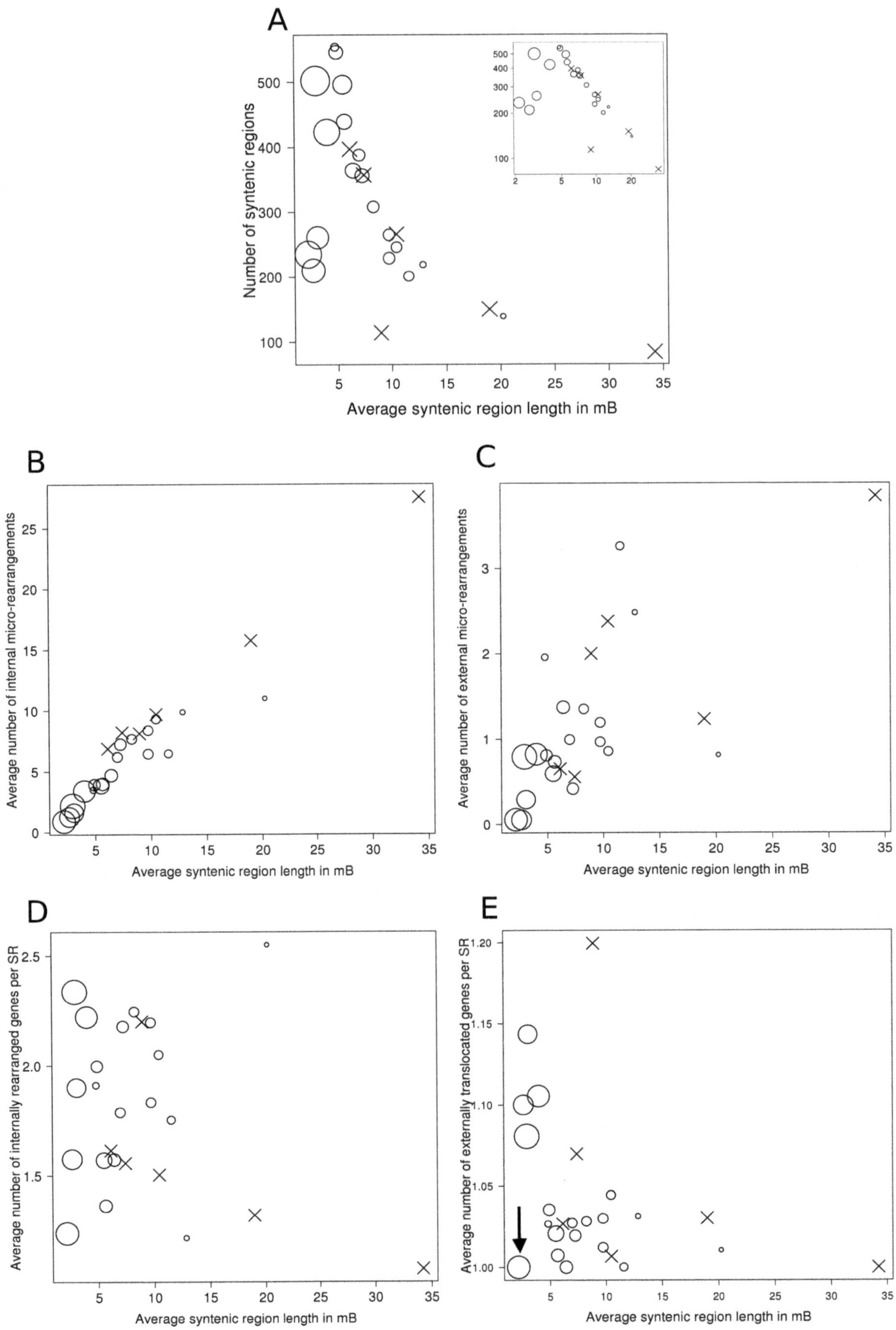
A
Number of syntenic regions
Average syntenic region length in mB
B
Average number of internal micro-rearrangements
Average syntenic region length in mB
C
Average number of external micro-rearrangements
Average syntenic region length in mB
D
Average number of internally rearranged genes per SR
Average syntenic region length in mB
E
Average number of externally translocated genes per SR
Average syntenic region length in mB

Figure 5. Relationship of syntenic region length, evolutionary distance and other features. Dependence of synteny features on the average syntenic region length (x axis) and evolutionary distance (circle size, inferred from branch lengths in Miller et al (2007), calculated as the average number of substitutions per site). Crosses correspond to the species pairs with no distance information available. A) Negative exponential correlation between the number of syntenic regions and their average length (inset: logarithmic axis scales). Closely related species (small circles) tend to have fewer, longer syntenic regions. Distant species (large circles) tend to have high numbers of very short syntenic regions. B) The average number of internal micro-rearrangements per syntenic region strongly correlates with syntenic region length and evolutionary distance. Evolutionary distant pairs of species share short syntenic regions with few internal micro-rearrangements. C) No clear correlation between syntenic region length and rearrangement number can be observed for external micro-rearrangements. D) The size of internal micro-rearrangements (average number of genes involved) does not correlate with the syntenic region length and evolutionary distance. E) Similarly, the number of genes involved in external translocations is generally independent of the syntenic region length. However, with the exception of mouse and platypus (average number of genes in externally translocated regions: 1.0, marked by arrow), distant species pairs tend to have somewhat longer externally translocated regions (average>1.05).

genes, and includes gaps when genes without orthologs occur. SyntenyMapper, while also allowing for the presence of genes without orthologs, will fragment a collinear block that is disrupted by a pair of non-orthologs into two blocks. Additionally, overlapping genes are excluded by our method. When we compare results from CYNTENATOR and SyntenyMapper, we thus often find apparently shorter but equivalent collinear blocks in the results from our method.

Another minor difference is caused by different definitions of collinear blocks. Our definition of a refined syntenic region provides for rearrangements that are embedded within a backbone of conserved gene order that ideally spans the whole syntenic region. In such a case, SyntenyMapper defines two collinear blocks, a small one embedded within a larger one, while CYNTENATOR will define three consecutive blocks.

Furthermore, CYNTENATOR fragments a large collinear block into two blocks if it is disturbed by external single-gene rearrangements, sometimes for no apparent reason (see Figure S11 for an example). SyntenyMapper is thus better suited for identifying all collinear blocks in a syntenic region, including inversions.

Another widely used tool for genome comparison is i-ADHoRe, which detects collinearity on the basis of a gene homology matrix. Blocks of conserved gene order are identified as dense diagonals and the corresponding genes are then aligned using the Needleman-Wunsch algorithm, a greedy graph strategy or a new algorithm named GG2. In this process, gaps are introduced if necessary to produce blocks with as many homologous pairs as possible. The software is well suitable for multi-genome comparisons.

Like CYNTENATOR, i-ADHoRe can be applied to syntenic regions and produces results that are comparable with SyntenyMapper. The main difference between the methods is the insertion of gaps and mismatches in i-ADHoRe alignments to create longer blocks, while our method creates a separate block if it is disrupted by a non-orthologous gene pair. The design goal of i-ADHoRe to detect collinear blocks that contain as many orthologs as possible comes at the expense of frequently missing small rearrangements that are partially embedded in larger ones.

For example, in a syntenic region comprising 11 genes, three of which are translocated within the region, SyntenyMapper correctly identifies the translocation (see Figure S12) while i-ADHoRe ignores it and defines it as a gap. Overall, both methods detect the same amount of collinear blocks in most syntenic regions (222, 62.36%), although mismatches in i-ADHoRe can result in longer detected regions. In the majority of the remaining cases (68, 19.10%) i-ADHoRe misses one or more regions due to mismatches (as described above) or inability to detect external micro-rearrangements.

We have investigated cases where SyntenyMapper detects fewer collinear blocks than i-ADHoRe (43, 12.08%). Besides the implementation differences, where our tool defines a backbone of genes with embedded micro-rearrangements while other tools define multiple adjacent blocks, we have also found that i-ADHoRe tends to disrupt collinear blocks if they are interrupted by a longer stretch of genes without orthologs. By contrast, SyntenyMapper ignores genes without orthologs when defining blocks of conserved gene order. From these results we conclude that, while both methods provide a similar functionality and largely consistent results, SyntenyMapper is better suited for a very detailed analysis of genome rearrangements that requires exact definitions of conserved gene order blocks, without mismatches and gaps. i-ADHoRe and CYNTENATOR, on the other hand, are applicable to more than two genomes and can provide a good overview of less stringent collinear blocks.

MCScanX is another software package that includes not only methods for the identification of collinear blocks. Like CYNTENATOR it requires BLASTP output or a list of orthologous genes as input, and uses a dynamic programming approach to find chains of collinear gene pairs in the two genomes. Its main advantage is the large set of downstream analysis tools, which includes four different visualization modes for the results, classification of duplicated genes into specific classes, and detection of whole genome duplication events.

When investigating reasons for discrepancies between SyntenyMapper and MCScanX, it became apparent that the latter method fails to handle duplicates correctly. For a one-to-many ortholog group it appears as if MCScanX detects multiple overlaying collinear blocks, where a single gene is contained in more than one such block and paired with different orthologs. SyntenyMapper uses a pre-processing procedure based on gene order and sequence similarity to identify one-to-one orthologs among sets of duplicated genes. As a consequence, each gene is associated with a single gene in the other genome, allowing for overlap-free definition of collinear blocks. MCScanX appears to keep one-to-many or many-to-many groups and defines blocks with genes in conserved order regardless of whether or not these genes are already present in other blocks. This behavior leads to significant overlapping between collinear blocks.

Per definition, a single gene cannot be part of two or even more collinear blocks. From these results we conclude that MCSCanX cannot provide the same functionality as SyntenyMapper, CYNTENATOR or i-ADHoRe.

Discussion

SyntenyMapper is a new rapid tool for comparative genomics that enables analysis of micro-rearrangements, detection of positional orthology, and direct comparison of genomic features between two species. Previously developed methods focus on finding regions caused by either macro- or micro-rearrangements on a global scale and use either whole-genome alignments or homologous elements alone to define these. By contrast, we identify micro-rearrangements within large synteny regions by focusing on the conservation of gene order. This combination of alignments and homologous elements allows us to find large blocks with conserved gene order that can be seen as the smallest evolutionary building blocks within largely conserved regions. The analysis of these numerous internal rearrangements can provide additional insights into evolutionary history and serves as a better basis for comparative genomics analyses than the original syntenic regions alone.

We have applied SyntenyMapper to 25 species pairs using syntenic regions and ortholog sets from ENSEMBL Compara. As expected, closely related species contain few but long syntenic regions, compared to a high number of short regions in distant pairs. The number of internal micro-rearrangements is proportional to the size of the synteny region they reside in, which in turn depends on the degree of relationship between the genomes. However, the density of micro-rearrangements, i.e. the number of micro-rearrangements per mB, does not correlate with the evolutionary distance. We found that similar sequences tend to have fewer micro-rearrangements, but the correlation is weak.

More distant species pairs tend to have short to medium syntenic regions harboring between 0 and 10 internal micro-rearrangements while more closely related organisms with long syntenic regions (over 10 mB length) contain between 10 and 25 micro-rearrangements. External syntenic regions are rare, with only 0 to 4 such translocations per syntenic region in all genome pairs, and show only a slight trend for a higher number in longer regions. We speculate that external translocations occur only under very specific circumstances, when distant genome regions are spatially close.

There is no correlation between the number of internally translocated genes in a micro-rearranged block and syntenic region length or evolutionary distance, implying that the transposition mechanism acts regardless of evolutionary history. While macro-rearrangements arise by complex processes involving chromosome double strand breaks [25], small-scale rearrangements are most likely caused by cut-and-paste DNA transposition [29]. Our results show that there are constraints that limit the total length of the translocated genome region. DNA transposons are often used as vector elements in biotechnology, and it has been reported that the efficiency of transposition decreases with increasing cargo size [30,31,32]. We show that the average cargo of transposons in higher eukaryotic genomes comprises between 1 and 2.5 genes for translocations over short linear distances, and between 1 and 1.2 genes for more distant translocations. This implies that the length constraints of transposable elements are also dependent on the linear distance between the source and the target position in the genome. This insight could be valuable for biotechnology, where ways to overcome the length limitations in transposons are searched for [32,33]. External translocations are also not correlated with the evolutionary distance or syntenic region length, but longer externally translocated regions appear to occur only in distant species pairs.

In general, we conclude that syntenic regions between the genomes of closely related species are longer and contain more micro-rearrangements of genes due to their length. More distant species pairs contain a higher number of short and less similar syntenic regions with fewer micro-rearrangements. The density and size of these is largely independent of the evolutionary distance and only slightly influenced by sequence similarity.

SyntenyMapper creates a one-to-one mapping of genes between species similar to positional orthology methods. Based on this mapping, TrackMapper is able to directly compare quantitative and qualitative features of genes, such as values representing the relative time point of replication or the overlap with long terminal repeats, and calculate a similarity measure for each pair of orthologs and the complete set of genes.

Beyond comparative genomics, identification of micro-rearrangements may be instrumental in understanding disease mechanisms. A number of diseases caused by micro-rearrangements are known, including the DiGeorge syndrome or Miller-Dieker lissencephaly [34].

Supporting Information

Figure S1 Effect of reversing the reference genome used in the example shown in Figure 5. The reference genome used here for the definition of breakpoints is A′ (=B in Figure 5). The detected breakpoints are $(a_{49}/b_{44}, a_{50}/b_3)$ (white boxes) and $a_{52}/b_5, a_{53}/b_{45}$ (black boxes). Based on the adjacent breakpoints in the new reference genome A′, the same translocated segment (hatched box) is detected as in Figure 2.

Figure S2 Pseudocode of the SyntenyMapper algorithm to find rearranged segments. SyntenyMapper uses externally defined syntenic regions and one-to-one orthologs as input to find maximum length blocks of conserved gene order (termed blocks). It iterates over all genes in genome A and identifies breakpoints according to the definition given in the *Methods* section, using the helper function $j(i)$, which returns the index of gene i's ortholog in genome B. SyntenyMapper identifies the two breakpoints preceding and following the detected breakpoint $(a_{i-1}/b_{j(i-1)}, a_i/b_{j(i)})$, because each pair of adjacent breakpoints encloses either a rearranged genomic segment or the region between two rearranged segments, as described in *Methods*. To distinguish these two cases, lengths of both segments defined by the three adjacent breakpoints are compared and the shorter of the two is defined as a block resulting from a micro-rearrangement with respect to the longer original syntenic region. The type of the rearrangement (translocation or inversion) is detected based on gene order within this block.

Figure S3 Linear representation of a syntenic region (ENSEMBL identifier 44542) produced by SyntenyMapper. Upper half shows genes in mouse, lower half genes in human. Green genes are those with conserved order, translocated or overlapping genes are colored blue. To better see these overlapping genes, conserved order and translocated genes are depicted in independent lines and a combined line, marked in the legend on the right and left edge of the plot.

Figure S4 Comparison of syntenic region length in human and mouse. The regression line is shown as dotted line (Pearson correlation coefficient 0.9932).

Figure S5 A syntenic region (ENSEMBL identifier 44514) in human (dark grey) and mouse (light grey) containing a large inversed segment, illustrated in blue and only one ortholog with the same orientation as the syntenic region (green). Ticks are placed at 100 kB distance and the numbers show the position on chromosomes 13 (human) and 14 (mouse) in mB.

Figure S6 Translocation of a single gene from the human region 44801 to the mouse region 44598, shown with red line. Ticks are placed at 100 kB distance and the numbers show the positions in mB on chromosomes X in human and mouse (region 44801) as well as on chromosomes 19 in human and 7 in mouse (region 44598).

Figure S7 Average number of micro-rearrangements (internal and external) per megabase covered by syntenic regions versus evolutionary distance. No correlation can be observed.

Figure S8 Syntenic regions (SR) with low sequence similarity (high distance score) show a trend to contain more internal micro-rearrangements per megabase (Pearson correlation coefficient 0.22). Outliers with extremely high sequence distance are not shown.

Figure S9 A translocation involving six consecutive genes between two syntenic regions in chicken (*G. gallus*, dark grey) and wild turkey (*M. gallopavo*, light grey), marked by red lines. Ticks are placed at 100 kB distance and the numbers show the positions in mB on chromosomes 6 in chicken and 8 in turkey (region 47198) as well as on chromosomes 17 in chicken and 19 in turkey (region 47135).

Figure S10 An example of an inversed syntenic region between human and mouse where CYNTENATOR detects no collinear block despite eleven genes lying in the same order in both genomes.

Figure S11 An example of a syntenic region between human and mouse where CYNTENATOR fragments the existing collinear block into two blocks (location of split marked red in both species) despite lack of genes disrupting the gene order.

Figure S12 Example of a syntenic region (ENSEMBL identifier 44459) including a micro-rearrangement of three genes that is correctly identified by SyntenyMapper but ignored as a gap by i-ADHoRe.

Table S1 Statistics of pre-computed synteny mapping for ENSEMBL Compara (version 73).

Table S2 Evolutionary distance and genome coverage by syntenic regions for all species pairs. SR: Syntenic region.

File S1 List of human and mouse orthologs with significantly high similarity in H3k4me3 peak density (TrackMapper difference score below 0.01).

Acknowledgments

We thank Boris Joffe for useful discussions.

Author Contributions

Conceived and designed the experiments: SK DF. Performed the experiments: SK. Analyzed the data: SK. Wrote the paper: SK DF.

References

1. Pevzner P, Tesler G (2003) Genome rearrangements in mammalian evolution: lessons from human and mouse genomes. Genome Res 13: 37–45.
2. Vilella AJ, Severin J, Ureta-Vidal A, Heng L, Durbin R, et al. (2009) EnsemblCompara GeneTrees: Complete, duplication-aware phylogenetic trees in vertebrates. Genome Res 19: 327–335.
3. Flicek P, Ahmed IM, Amode MR, Barrell D, Beal K, et al. (2013) Ensembl 2013. Nucleic Acids Res 41: D48–55.
4. Liao BY, Chang YJ, Ho JM, Hwang MJ (2004) The UniMarker (UM) method for synteny mapping of large genomes. Bioinformatics 20: 3156–3165.
5. Tesler G (2002) GRIMM: genome rearrangements web server. Bioinformatics 18: 492–493.
6. Hannenhalli S, Pevzner PA (1995) Transforming men into mice (polynomical algorithm for genomic distance problem). In: 36th Annual Symposium on Foundations of Computer Science (Milwaukee, WI, 1995). Los Alamitos: IEEE Computer Society Press. pp.581–92.
7. Hannenhalli S, Pevzner PA (1999) Transforming cabbage into turnip: polynomial algorithm for sorting signed permutations by reversals. J ACM 46: 1–27.
8. Sinha AU, Meller J (2007) Cinteny: flexible analysis and visualization of synteny and genome rearrangements in multiple organisms. BMC Bioinformatics 8: 82.
9. Jun J, Mandoiu II, Nelson CE (2009) Identification of mammalian orthologs using local synteny. BMC Genomics 10: 630.
10. Fu Z, Chen X, Vacic V, Nan P, Zhong Y, et al. (2007) MSOAR: a high-throughput ortholog assignment system based on genome rearrangement. J Comput Biol 14: 1160–1175.
11. Shi G, Zhang L, Jiang T (2010) MSOAR 2.0: Incorporating tandem duplications into ortholog assignment based on genome rearrangement. BMC Bioinformatics 11: doi:10.1186/1471-2105-11-10.
12. Pearson JC, Lemons D, McGinnis W (2005) Modulating Hox gene functions during animal body patterning. Nat Rev Genet 6: 893–904.
13. Wellik DM (2007) Hox patterning of the vertebrate axial skeleton. Dev Dyn 236: 2454–2463.
14. Guelen L, Pagie L, Brasset E, Meuleman W, Faza MB, et al. (2008) Domain organization of human chromosomes revealed by mapping of nuclear lamina interactions. Nature 453: 948–951.
15. Rödelsperger C, Dieterich C (2010) CYNTENATOR: Progressive Gene Order Alignment of 17 Vertebrate Genomes. PLoS ONE 5: doi:10.1371/journal.-pone.0008861.
16. Wang Y, Tang H, DeBarry JD, Tan X, Li J, et al. (2012) MCScanX: a toolkit for detection and evolutionary analysis of gene synteny and collinearity. Nucleic Acids Res 40: doi:10.1093/nar/gkr1293.
17. Proost S, Fostier J, De Witte D, Dhoedt B, Demeester P, et al. (2011) i-ADHoRe 3.0 – fast and sensitive detection of genomic homology in extremely large data sets. Nucleic Acids Research 40: doi:10.1093/nar/gkr955.
18. Giardine B, Riemer C, Hardison RC, Burhans R, Elnitski L, et al. (2005) Galaxy: a platform for interactive large-scale genome analysis. Genome Res 15: 1451–1455.
19. Blankenberg D, Von Kuster G, Coraor N, Ananda G, Lazarus R, et al. (2010) Galaxy: a web-based genome analysis tool for experimentalists. Curr Protoc Mol Biol 19: 1–21.
20. Goecks J, Nekrutenko A, Taylor J (2010) Galaxy: a comprehensive approach for supporting accessible, reproducible, and transparent computational research in the life sciences. Genome biology 11: doi: 10.1186/gb-2010-11-8-r86.
21. Krzywinski MI, Schein JE, Birol I, Connors J, Gascoyne R, et al. (2009) Circos: An information aesthetic for comparative genomics. Genome Research 19: doi: 10.1101/gr.092759.109.
22. Hinrichs AS, Karolchik D, Baertsch R, Barber GP, Bejerano G, et al. (2006) The UCSC Genome Browser Database: update 2006. Nucleic Acids Res 34(Database issue): 590–598.
23. Consortium TEP (2004) The ENCODE (ENCyclopedia Of DNA Elements) Project. Science 306: 636–640.
24. Rieck K, Laskov P (2008) Linear-Time Computation of Similarity Measures for Sequential Data. J Mach Learn Res 9: doi = 10.1.1.130.8262.
25. Mani RS, Chinnaiyan AM (2010) Triggers for genomic rearrangements: insights into genomic, cellular and environmental influences. Nat Rev Genet 11: 819–829.
26. Peng Q, Pevzner PA, Tesler G (2006) The fragile breakage versus random breakage models of chromosome evolution. PLoS Comput Biol 2: doi:10.1371/journal.pcbi.0020014.
27. Woo Y, Li W (2012) DNA replication timing and selection shape the landscape of nucleotide variation in cancer genomes. Nature communications 3: doi: 10.1038/ncomms1982.
28. Miller W, Rosenbloom K, Hardison RC, Hou M, Taylor J, et al. (2007) 28-Way vertebrate alignment and conservation track in the UCSC Genome Browser. Genome Res 17: 1797–1808.

29. Muñoz-López M, García-Pérez JL (2010) DNA Transposons: Nature and Applications in Genomics. Curr Genomics 11: 115–128.
30. Izsvak Z, Ivics Z, Plasterk RH (2000) Sleeping Beauty, a wide host-range transposon vector for genetic transformation in vertebrates. J Mol Biol 302: 93–102.
31. Ding S, Wu X, Li G, Han M, Zhuang Y, et al. (2005) Efficient transposition of the piggyBac(PB) transposon in mammalian cells and mice. Cell 122: 473–83.
32. Balciunas D, Wangensteen KJ, Wilber A, Bell J, Geurts A, et al. (2006) Harnessing a high cargo-capacity transposon for genetic applications in vertebrates. PLoS Genet 2: doi: 10.1371/journal.pgen.0020169.
33. Zayed H, Izsvak Z, Walisko O, Ivics Z (2004) Development of hyperactive sleeping beauty transposon vectors by mutational analysis. Mol Ther 9: 292–304.
34. Rosenberg C, Knijnenburg J, Bakker E, Vianna-Morgante AM, Sloos W, et al. (2006) Array-CGH detection of micro rearrangements in mentally retarded individuals: clinical significance of imbalances present both in affected children and normal parents. J Med Genet 43: 180–186.

11

PB1-F2 Attenuates Virulence of Highly Pathogenic Avian H5N1 Influenza Virus in Chickens

Olivier Leymarie[1], Carissa Embury-Hyatt[2], Christophe Chevalier[1], Luc Jouneau[1], Marco Moroldo[3], Bruno Da Costa[1], Yohannes Berhane[2], Bernard Delmas[1], Hana M. Weingartl[2,4*], Ronan Le Goffic[1*]

1 Unité de Virologie et Immunologie Moléculaires, Unité de Recherche UR892, Institut National de la Recherche Agronomique, Jouy-en-Josas, France, **2** National Centre for Foreign Animal Disease, Canadian Food Inspection Agency, Winnipeg, Manitoba, Canada, **3** Centre de Ressources Biologiques pour la Génomique des Animaux Domestiques et d'Intérêt Economique, Institut National de la Recherche Agronomique, Jouy-en-Josas, France, **4** Department of Medical Microbiology, University of Manitoba, Winnipeg, Manitoba, Canada

Abstract

Highly pathogenic avian influenza virus (HPAIV) is a permanent threat due to its capacity to cross species barriers and generate severe infections and high mortality in humans. Recent findings have highlighted the potential role of PB1-F2, a small accessory influenza protein, in the pathogenesis process mediated by HPAIV in mammals. In this study, using a recombinant H5N1 HPAIV (wt) and its PB1-F2-deleted mutant (ΔF2), we studied the effects of PB1-F2 in a chicken model. Unexpectedly, when using low inoculation dose we observed that the wt-infected chickens had a higher survival rate than the ΔF2-infected chickens, a feature that contrasts with what is usually observed in mammals. High inoculation dose had similar mortality rate for both viruses, and comparison of the bio-distribution of the two viruses indicated that the expression of PB1-F2 allows a better spreading of the virus within chicken embryos. Transcriptomic profiles of lungs and blood cells were characterized at two days post-infection in chickens inoculated with the wild type (wt) or the ΔF2 mutant viruses. In lungs, the expression of PB1-F2 during the infection induced pathways related to calcium signaling and repressed a large panel of immunological functions. In blood cells, PB1-F2 was associated with a gene signature specific for mitochondrial dysfunction and down-modulated leucocytes activation. Finally we compared the effect of PB1-F2 in lungs of chickens and mice. We identified that gene signature associated to tissue damages is a PB1-F2 feature shared by the two species; by contrast, the early inhibition of immune response mediated by PB1-F2 observed in chickens is not seen in mice. In summary, our data suggest that PB1-F2 expression deeply affect the immune response in chickens in a way that may attenuate pathogenicity at low infection dose, a feature differing from what was previously observed in mammal species.

Editor: Michael C. W. Chan, Centre of Influenza Research, The University of Hong Kong, Hong Kong

Funding: This work was partially funded by the Conseil regional d'Île-de-France through DIM Malinf ("Domaine d'Intérêt Majeur Maladies Infectieuses, parasitaires et nosocomiales émergentes", Grant#: dim100157) and by the OECD Co-operative Research Programme (Contract No.: TAD/PROG 67049). OL was supported by "DIM Malinf" doctoral fellowships awarded by the "Conseil regional d'Île-de-France". The funders had no role in study design, data collection and analysis, decision to publish, or preparation of the manuscript.

Competing Interests: The authors have declared that no competing interests exist.

* Email: ronan.legoffic@jouy.inra.fr (RLG); Hana.Weingartl@inspection.gc.ca (HMW)

These authors contributed equally to this work.

Introduction

Since 1997, H5N1 highly pathogenic avian influenza virus (HPAIV) is an omnipresent public health threat [1]. This concern is based on capacity of such virus to cross the species barrier from their avian hosts to humans. Waterfowl and shorebirds constitute the natural hosts of H5N1 HPAIV; infected wild aquatic birds usually develop relatively mild symptoms and limited disease. In ducks, infection is usually asymptomatic [2,3]. Nevertheless, when the virus is transmitted to poultry, mortality rate can reach 100%. The ability of H5N1 HPAIV to cross species barriers and spread to humans has been reported in 15 countries and confirmed by World Health Organization (WHO). The total number of cases confirmed by WHO is 650, with case fatality rate of 60% [4]. However, seroprevalence study among poultry workers suggested that H5N1 HPAIV could also cause infections with only mild symptoms in humans [5]. Human-to-human H5N1 HPAIV transmission has not been described yet, but recent works designed to address the questions of transmissibility and adaptation of H5N1 HPAIV to the human host identified important determinants in the HA-encoding segment [6,7].

Influenza A virus belongs to the *Orthomyxoviridae* family, and its genome consists of eight negative strand RNA segments encoding up to 14 proteins [8,9]. Viral determinants conferring host adaptation can be acquired through segment exchange between strains. This gene reassortment ability provides genome plasticity facilitating the crossing of species barriers [10,11]. The PB1-encoding segment from the H1N1 influenza viruses responsible for the 1957 and 1968 pandemics was shown to have an avian origin [10]. This segment was also demonstrated to exert an important role in the pathogenesis mediated by the 1918 pandemic influenza virus [12]. In addition to the PB1 component of the polymerase complex, this segment 2 also encodes the N40 protein, a N-truncated version of PB1 lacking transcriptase function, and PB1-F2, a pro-apoptotic protein [13,14]. PB1-F2 drew attention in recent years since a number of reports associated its expression with an increase of virus pathogenicity [15–21]. When looking at the prevalence of a functional PB1-F2 in strains of various origins, its expression appears unequally distributed: for example 96% of avian strains encodes a full-length PB1-F2 while only 7% of human H1N1 isolates express a functional PB1-F2 [22,23]. Thus, several reports suggest that the loss of a functional PB1-F2 could be beneficial for the virus when it crosses the species barrier to spread through humans [22,24–26]. Consequently, the loss of PB1-F2 could be an adaptation process of the virus to mammalian hosts in order to confer optimized replicative efficiencies and viral fitness [27]. On the contrary, PB1-F2 from a highly virulent avian strain could be acquired by a circulating human strain through segment exchange, and then contribute to increased virulence associated with seasonal influenza viruses.

PB1-F2 was first described in 2001 [13]. This 90 amino-acid long protein is encoded by an alternative open reading frame (ORF) overlapping the PB1 ORF. In mammals, PB1-F2 can induce apoptosis of immune cells [13] and promote inflammation in a strain-dependent manner [17,19,27,28]. PB1-F2 triggers apoptosis by disturbing the mitochondrial membrane potential, an event that can lead to cytochrome c release and subsequent activation of caspases [29]. Inflammation induction is triggered by an exacerbation of the NF-κB transcription factor activity [19,30]. The molecular basis of this exacerbation is currently unknown but the propensity of PB1-F2 to form β-sheet structures and amyloid fibers are suspected to play an important role in this process [31]. PB1-F2 has also been described to up-regulate the viral polymerase activity [32], but this property is strain-specific and has no impact on the pathogenesis [33].

In mammals, PB1-F2 behaves as a virulence factor [15]. A recombinant WSN/1933 (H1N1) mutant lacking PB1-F2 has been shown to be less virulent than its wild-type (wt) counterpart [19]. Such effects on the mortality are not always visible, especially when highly pathogenic H5N1 strains are studied due to the extreme 50% lethal doses (LD50) of these viruses [34]. However, in mice models, the high LD50 can be by-passed using Mx+/+ transgenic mice [20]. Varga and co-workers described the inhibition of type I interferon (IFN) by PB1-F2; they showed that PB1-F2 antagonizes the function of MAVS through disruption of the mitochondrial membrane potential [18,35,36]. On the other hand we observed an exacerbation of the IFN expression when PB1-F2 was expressed during WSN/1933 infection [30]. This feature correlates well with the pro-inflammatory properties of PB1-F2. The sequence polymorphism of PB1-F2 that dictates the pro-inflammatory properties of PB1-F2 may explain the observed differences [28].

In this study, we compared the pathological process mediated by a H5N1 HPAIV unable to express PB1-F2 with its PB1-F2-expressing counterpart in chickens to elucidate the role of PB1-F2 in an avian host. Survival curves, bio-distribution and host responses to both viruses were analyzed in order to determine and analyze the impact of PB1-F2 expression in this host. Unexpectedly, and in contrast to what is observed in mammals, PB1-F2 attenuates virulence in chicken. Using functional genomics tools, we delineated the impact of PB1-F2 in the lungs of infected chickens. Finally we compared these effects with what we previously observed in mouse infected with the same H5N1 HPAIV couple [34].

Results

Viral distribution of wild-type and PB1-F2 deleted viruses in chicken embryos

The recombinant influenza A/duck/Niger/2090/2006(H5N1) (herein named Nig06) and its PB1-F2 knocked out counterpart (named ΔF2) were previously produced [34]. To study the effects of PB1-F2 expression in the chicken host, we first performed histological investigations to characterize the bio-distribution of Nig06 and ΔF2 viruses within chicken embryos. Examination of embryos at 24 hours post inoculation by immunohistochemistry showed that the viral antigen was more widespread in the wt group as compared to the ΔF2-virus group. In examined tissues of most of the embryos including the brain, heart, spleen, liver, lung, kidney, spinal cord, bone and skeletal muscle, there was weak to moderate immunostaining in the ΔF2 group whereas extensive to widespread immunostaining was observed in the wt group (Fig. 1). In both groups antigen was primarily observed in endothelial cells in all tissues. Some spread to surrounding parenchyma including hepatocytes, neurons, skeletal muscle, cardiomyocytes and pneumocytes was observed in both groups but was more pronounced in the wt group. In both groups there was consistently strong immunostaining in the chorioallantoic membrane. At the 18 and 48 hour timepoints post-inoculation, there were no differences observed between the two groups. In summary, these data suggest that PB1-F2 expression may accelerate the systemic spreading of the virus, as previously described [20].

Mortality associated with PB1-F2 from Nig06

To determine the role of PB1-F2 in highly pathogenic AIV pathogenesis, we first aimed to characterize the impact of PB1-F2 on the mortality in adult 8 weeks old white leghorn chickens. Chickens were challenged using 1000 plaque forming units (PFU) of wt Nig06 ($n = 10$) or ΔF2 Nig06 ($n = 10$). As shown in Fig. 2A, this amount of virus killed 90% of the chickens. Death of the animals occurred between days 3 and 8 post-infection (pi) and the mean time of death is 4 days pi. No differences could be observed between the 2 types of viruses. Remarkably, we found that wt Nig06-infected chickens ($n = 20$) had a higher survival rate than ΔF2 Nig06-infected chickens ($n = 20$): 50% *vs.* 15% respectively in survival experiments using a lower viral dose of 100 PFU (Fig. 2B). The chicken LD_{50} was estimated to be of $10^{2.05}$ PFU for the wt Nig06, and of $10^{1.62}$ PFU for the ΔF2 Nig06. These results suggest that the expression of PB1-F2 in birds infected with low dose of HPAIV could be beneficial for the avian host survival.

Replication and shedding of wt and ΔF2 Nig06

To further characterize the role of PB1-F2 in the pathogenic process exerted by the viral infection, we investigated whether PB1-F2 could influence the spreading of the virus by quantifying the tissue distribution of the virus using qRT-PCR after 2 days pi (Fig. 3A). The amounts of viral copy number of wt and ΔF2 viruses were roughly the same in trachea, lung, spleen and thymus tissues. However, in the blood of ΔF2-infected chicken, although the difference is not statistically significant ($p = 0.17$), we observed a higher amount of virus as compared to wt-infected chicken virus. Such differences are also observed in heart, liver, kidney and brain but to a lesser extent. In contrast, in the pancreas (not statistically significant) and in the intestine, we detected a higher amount of viral copies in the wt-infected chicken. Importantly, the difference observed in the intestine is statistically significant ($p<0.05$), and suggests that PB1-F2 could influence the enteric tropism of the virus, though, as the difference between the two conditions is less than one log viral copy number, this result could be statistically significant but biologically non relevant. We next compared the shedding capacities of the wt and the ΔF2 viruses. Oropharyngeal and cloacal swabs were taken at day 2 pi for virus copy number quantification. The analysis of swabs from wt-infected chickens revealed a higher number of positive samples (7/10 vs. 4/10 for the ΔF2 group), yet, when looking at the amount of viral RNA

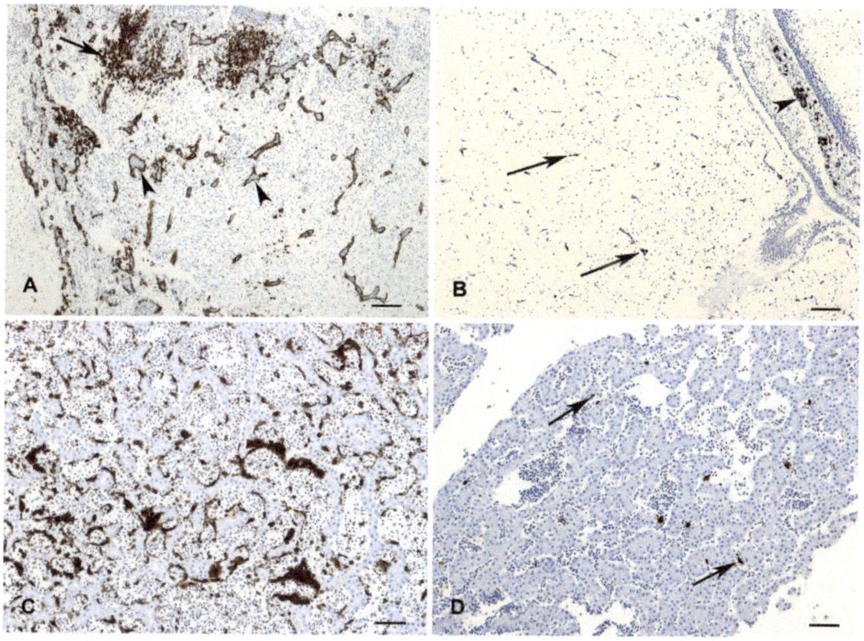

Figure 1. Immunohistochemical detection of influenza A antigen in chicken embryos at 24 hours post-inoculation. (A) Brain; Wt group. Extensive immunostaining was observed in endothelial cells (arrowheads) and well as multifocal areas of brain parenchyma involving neurons (arrow). (B) Brain; ΔF2 group. There were occasional small foci of endothelial (arrows) and parenchymal (arrowhead) staining. (C) Liver; Wt group. There is extensive immunostaining of sinusoidal lining cells as well as scattered hepatocytes. (D) Liver, ΔF2 group. There was mild immunostaining of individual sinusoidal lining cells (arrows).

detected within the positive individual swabs, no differences could be evidenced between the two types of infection (Fig. 3B and 3C). In order to confirm the qRT-PCR virus RNA quantification data, we attempted virus isolation on oral swabs by plaque assay method to quantify the virus shedding (Figure S1).

Impact of PB1-F2 on the expression profiles of representative genes of the host response

Prior to characterization of the global transcriptome of the infected-chickens, we first explored the impact of PB1-F2 on the host response by using qRT-PCR assays. We focused on several gene representatives of the inflammatory and immune responses: STAT1, β2M, TLR4, IFNAR1, CTLA-4, CCL5, TLR7, HSPA2, IL2RG, TLR6 and BSL2L1. The two inoculum doses were then compared (Fig. 4). Surprisingly, despite the outcome of the survival curves, the differences between wt- and ΔF2-infected chickens were larger and statistically more significant in the 1000 PFU group (p value: 0.0006 *vs.* 0.0331). Consequently, the 1000 PFU inoculum dose was chosen for further global transcriptomic analysis.

Overview of differences in gene expression following infection with wt or ΔF2 Nig06

To determine how PB1-F2 modulates virus pathogenicity, we investigated the overall host response to wt- and ΔF2-Nig06

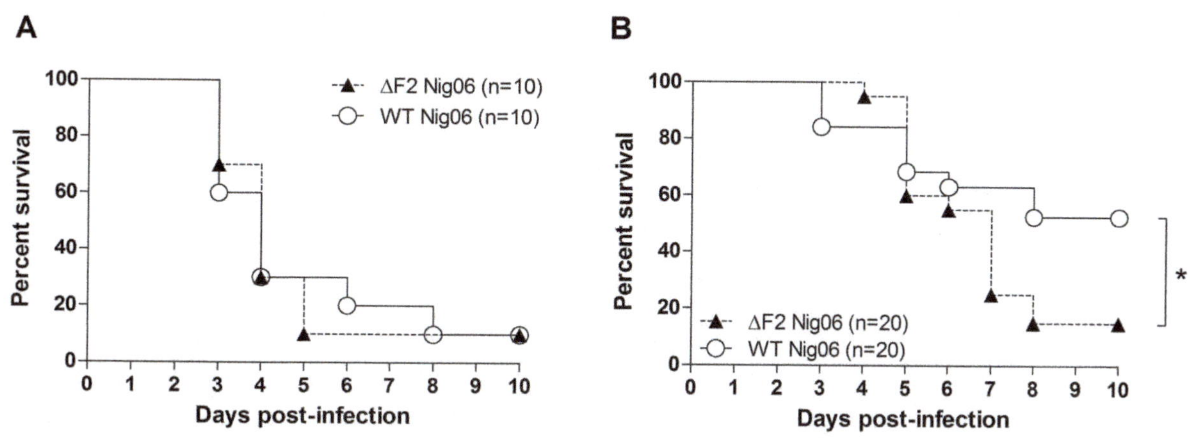

Figure 2. Characterization of the mortality induced by the wt and ΔF2 Nig06 HPAIV. Survival curves of chickens infected with wt or ΔF2 Nig06 virus. The chickens were inoculated via nares with 0.5 PBS containing 1000 (A) or 100 (B) PFU. The chickens were observed for 10 days after challenge.

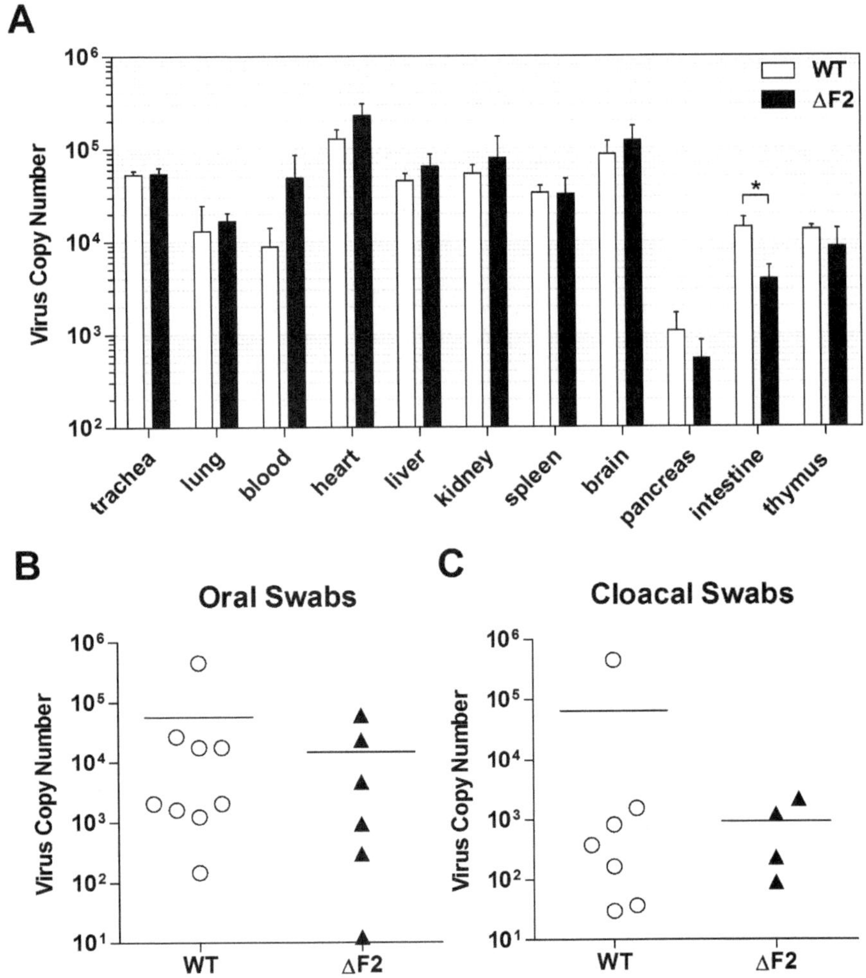

Figure 3. Tissue distribution and shedding of the wt and ΔF2 Nig06 HPAIV. (A) Viral titers of the indicated organs were measured by qRT-PCR at day 2 pi with 1000 PFU of wt or ΔF2 Nig06 virus. (B) Oral and (C) cloacal swabs were collected at day 2 pi to detect and quantify viral shedding using qRT-PCR.

infection. Microarray analyses of RNA samples extracted from lungs and blood samples of wt- or ΔF2-infected chicken were carried out. Two groups of 5 White Leghorns chickens were intranasally infected using 1000 PFU of each virus. After 2 days pi, blood samples were collected; chickens were euthanized at the same day and lungs were collected. Total RNA were extracted, processed and analyzed using the Agilent Chicken (V2) Gene Expression Microarray (4×44 K). Each probe signals were normalized and statistically treated as described in the materials and methods section. To identify outliers arrays, hierarchical correlation clustering (uncentered with average linkage) of the entire set of samples was carried out. As a consequence, one chicken was excluded in each group of the functional analysis. The 8 remaining chicken specimens showed a strong "compartment" effect: lungs and blood samples displayed a clear distinct clustering (Fig. 5A). Remarkably, within each "compartment" cluster, the 2 viral infections also constitute 2 separate clusters, indicating a clear effect of PB1-F2 during the Nig06 infection of chickens. In order to illustrate the global variance by which different sample sets correlate, arrays data from each samples were subjected to principal component analysis (Fig. 5B). As for the hierarchical correlation clustering, the 4 sets of samples clustered in distinct localized areas, indicating different gene expression profiles in lung and blood in response to wt or ΔF2 viruses. Collectively, these data indicate a potent effect of PB1-F2 during the chicken response to Nig06 infection, and also a tissue specific-effect of PB1-F2.

Analysis of the impact of PB1-F2 expression in Nig06-infected chickens lungs

The functional consequences of PB1-F2 expression during Nig06 infection of lungs was addressed by analyzing the functions associated with the differentially expressed genes. Regulated genes in the group of wt-infected chickens were directly compared to regulated genes from the group of ΔF2-infected chicken to generate 2 sets of genes: genes up-regulated and genes down-regulated in presence of PB1-B2. We selected genes that were at least 2 fold different in their expression between wt- and ΔF2-infected chicken (adjusted p-value<0.05). Figure 6A represents the distribution of the genes, among the 3848 regulated genes, half of them appear up-regulated in the presence of PB1-F2 and half of them appear down-regulated. We then explored the functional consequences of PB1-F2 expression by using ontological annotations of the differentially expressed genes. The set of genes up-regulated during wt Nig06 infection revealed a strong association of PB1-F2 to "Calcium Signaling" pathways: Glutamate Receptor Signaling, GABA Receptor Signaling, G-Protein Coupled Receptor

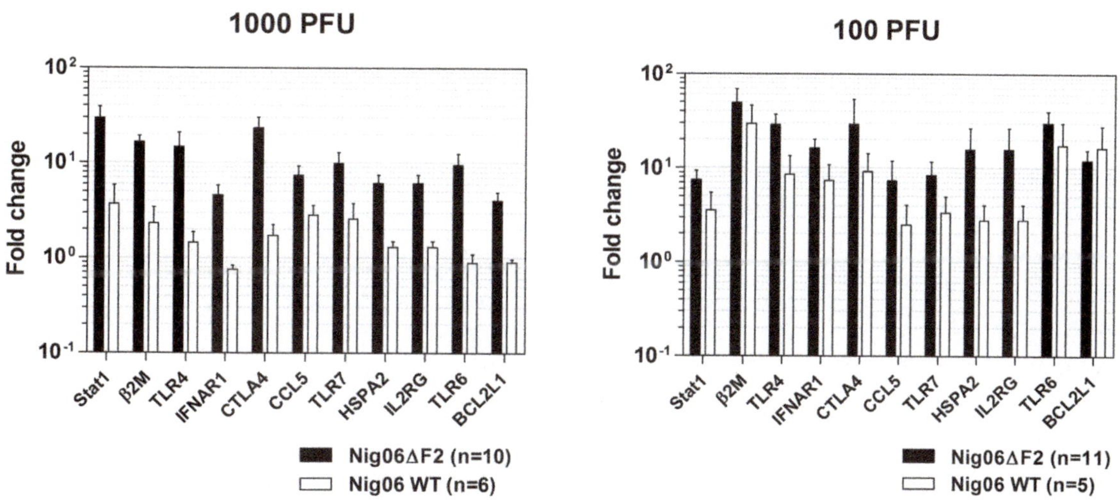

Figure 4. Impact of PB1-F2 on expression profiles of several genes representative of the host response. Total RNA isolated from lungs of chickens infected with 1000PFU (A) and (B) (day 2 pi) were reverse-transcribed and used to quantify expression of several host response markers by qPCR: signal transducer and activator of transcription 1 (STAT1, Gene ID: 424044), beta-2-microglobulin (β2M, Gene ID: 414830), toll-like receptor 4 (TLR4, Gene ID: 417241), interferon (alpha, beta and omega) receptor 1 (IFNAR1, Gene ID: 395665), cytotoxic T-lymphocyte-associated protein 4 (CTLA-4, Gene ID: 424106), chemokine (C-C motif) ligand 5 (CCL5, Gene ID: 417465), toll-like receptor 7 (TLR7, Gene ID: 418638), heat shock 70 kDa protein 2 (HSPA2, Gene ID: 423504), interleukin 2 receptor gamma (IL2RG, Gene ID: 395199), toll-like receptor 6 (TLR6, Gene ID: 771173), and B-cell CLL/lymphoma 2-like 1 (BCL2L1, Gene ID: 373954). Gene expressions were normalized with the β-actin gene (Gene ID: 396526) expression level and presented as fold increase relative to mock-treated chickens. Data are means ± SEM obtained from the indicated number of chickens.

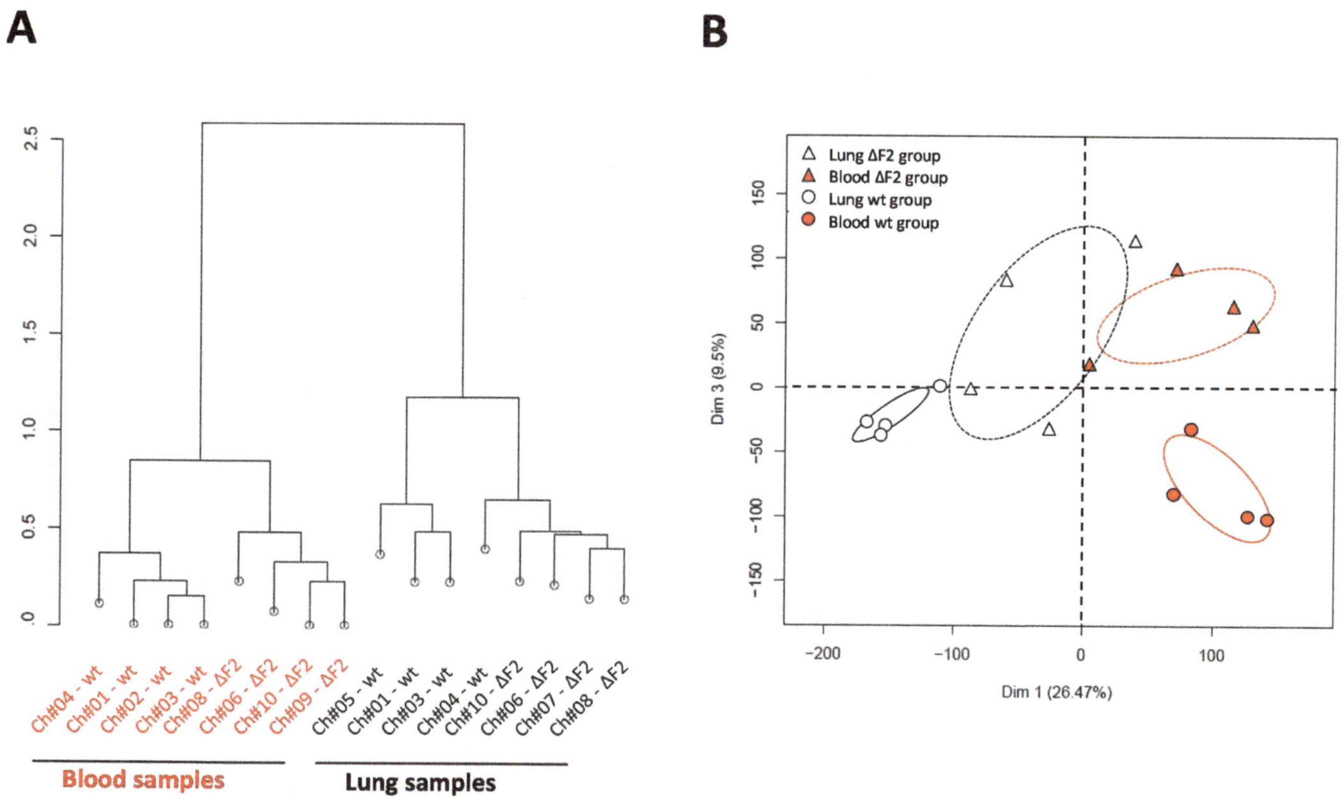

Figure 5. Correlation clustering and principal component analysis of microarray data. The expression value for each gene from lung and blood tissues of wt and ΔF2-infected chickens were used for the analysis. (A) The expression distance was measured between all pairs of arrays and represented as a tree. (B) The principal component analysis of the expression values was made to represent the variability between arrays. X-axis represents the first dimension (Dim 1, 26.47% of the variance) which separates the tissue samples (lung *vs.* blood), y-axis represent the third dimension (Dim 3, 9.5% of the variance) which separates the viral infections (wt *vs.* ΔF2). Clusters of samples on the PCA plot present a strong correlation of expression signals.

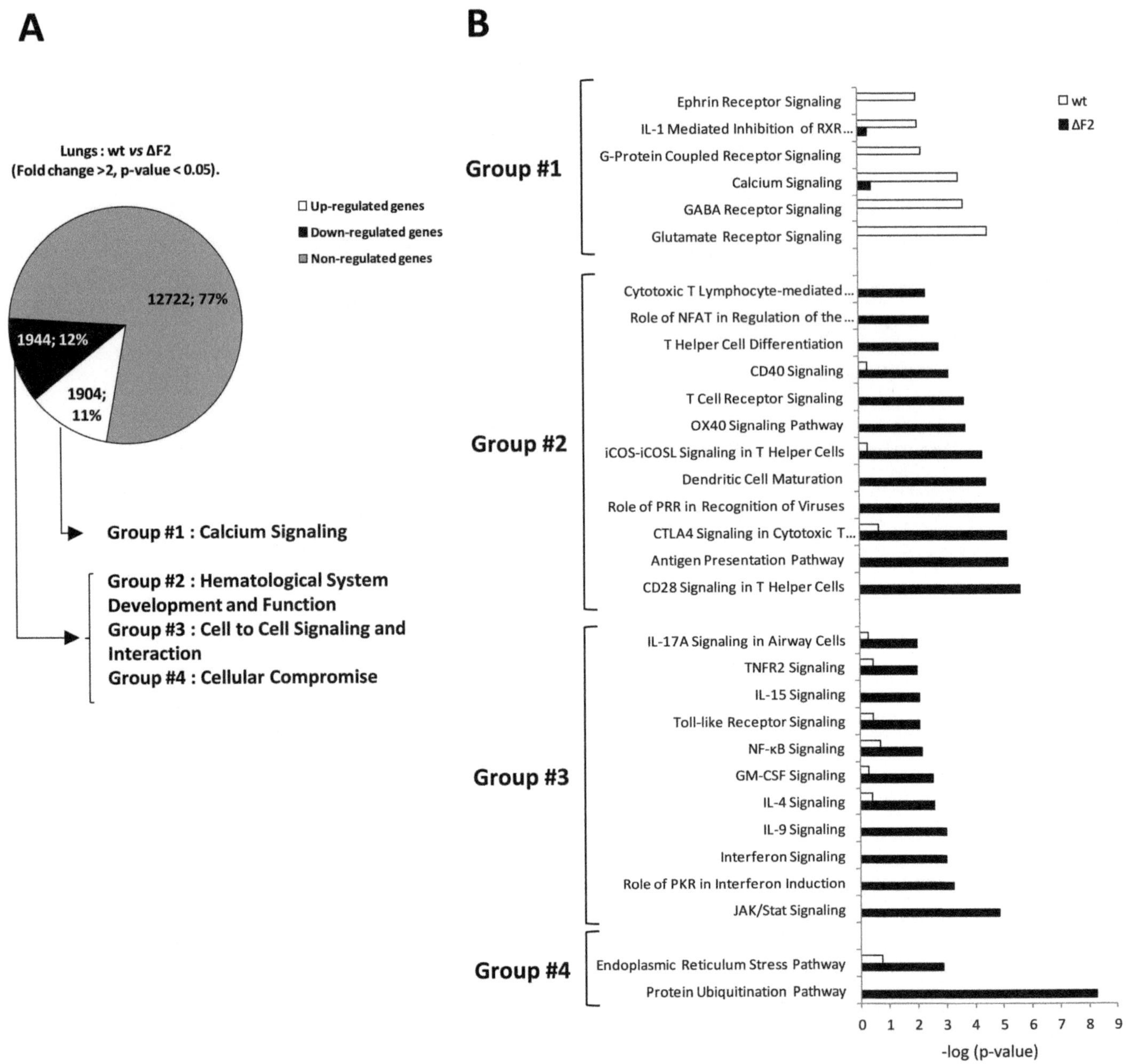

Figure 6. Global analysis of PB1-F2-dependant gene expression changes in the lungs of influenza infected chickens at day 2 pi. (A) Distribution of genes differentially regulated between wt- and ΔF2-infected chicken lungs. Major functions according to GO annotated function are indicated for each category of regulated genes. (B) Canonical pathways associated to differentially expressed genes were compared using Ingenuity Pathways Analysis. Canonical pathways are ranked using the p-value obtained using the right-tailed Fisher's exact test, it represents the probability of each biological function to be involved in the group of analyzed genes.

Signaling (Fig. 6B). This suggests that PB1-F2 could disturb intracellular calcium stores and interfere with pathways in which calcium is involved. Logically, when looking at the heat map representative of this pathway (Fig. 7A), we observed that most of the genes were down-regulated in the absence of PB1-F2 except few genes playing important role in calcium homeostasis: ITPR2, ATP2B1, ASPH and CREB3. ITPR2 and ATP2B1 are two Ca^{2+} pumps localized within the endoplasmic reticulum (ER) [37,38]. ASPH is an aspartate-hydroxylase regulating the Ca^{2+} release from the ER [39]. CREB3 is a ER-bound transcription factor activated by Ca^{2+} signaling and involved in inflammatory gene expression [40]. Overall, the analysis of this group of genes revealed that PB1-F2 expression modulates Ca^{2+} signaling pathways within the lungs of infected chicken.

The set of genes down-regulated by PB1-F2 (*i.e.* up-regulated in the ΔF2-infected chicken lungs) can be divided into 3 different main functions: "Hematological System Development and Function", "Cell to Cell Signaling and Interaction" and "Cellular Compromise" (Fig. 6A). The cluster of genes associated with "Hematological System Development and Function" (group #2, Fig. 6A and 6B) illustrates the strong impact of PB1-F2 on immune cells. PB1-F2 expression suppressed the activation of multiple pathways essential for the mobilization and activation of dendritic cells and lymphocytes: CD40, OX40, iCOS, CTL4 and CD28 signaling pathways. This strong effect is linked to the regulation of the group #3 of genes which is involved in "Cell to Cell Signaling and Interaction". It is composed of genes regulating the signal transduction of several cytokines including NF-kB and interferon signaling pathways. Heat maps of representative genes of these 2 main functions are shown in figures 7B and 7C.

The expression of PB1-F2 also down-regulate a cluster of genes functionally associated to "cellular compromise". Two canonical pathways are linked to these genes: "ER Stress Pathway" and "Protein Ubiquitination Pathway". These two functional categories illustrate the virulence factor properties of PB1-F2 during influenza virus infection. As shown in figure 7D, we found that the expression of PB1-F2 during the infection represses the entire gene cluster representative of the two pathways with the exception of ERN1. Interestingly, ERN1 (also known as IRE1) is a transmembrane protein resident of the ER which is implicated in the sensing of unfolded proteins in the lumen of the ER. Activation of ERN1 leads to a potent transcriptional response triggering growth arrest and apoptosis [41]. Collectively, these transcriptomic data on the lung response associated to PB1-F2 revealed a potent effect of PB1-F2 on the host response within chicken airways, and particularly on genes involved in Ca^{2+} homeostasis and ER stress pathways.

Analysis of the impact of PB1-F2 expression in blood of Nig06-infected chickens

As illustrated in Fig. 2A, HPAIV are able to spread systemically in chicken. To gain insight into the functions of PB1-F2 beyond the respiratory tract, we studied the host response of chicken blood cells. RNA samples were collected before infection and at day 2 pi. Each RNA sample from blood of infected chicken was directly compared to RNA sample from the same chicken before infection using a dual-color hybridization design. Four chickens in each group (wt- and ΔF2-infected) were used to identify the genes activated during the host response. The PB1-F2-dependant gene profile in blood cells was very different from the profile obtained in lungs: the set of up-regulated genes was restricted to 81 genes, representing only 0.5% of the analyzed genes (Fig. 8A). The number of down-regulated genes was comparable to that observed in the lungs (7.9%). The 81 PB1-F2-up-regulated genes are strongly associated to "Mitochondrial Dysfunction" and "Glucocorticoid Receptor Signaling" pathways (Fig. 8B). The mitochondrial dysfunction pathway appears very interesting since PB1-F2 is mainly localized to the mitochondria [13,42,43] and is able to permeabilize mitoplasts (Christophe Chevalier, unpublished data). Among those 81 genes, a number of genes encoded by the mitochondrial genome are present (Fig. 8C, left panel). The relative levels of expression of 3 mitochondrial genes: *COX1*, *COX2* and *COX3* were confirmed in blood samples using quantitative PCR (Fig. 8D). The ontological analyses of down-regulated genes showed that PB1-F2 down-regulates activation of leukocytes (Leukocyte Extravasation Signaling, p38 MAPK Signaling, Wnt/β-catenin Signaling; Fig. 8B). A heat map of representative genes implicated in these biological processes is represented in fig. 8C (right panel).

Taken together, these blood cells transcriptomic data suggest a strong induction of mitochondrial genes transcription mediated by PB1-F2 and a down-regulation of leukocyte activation which could be due to an alteration of the mitochondria integrity. The loss of the mitochondrial membrane potential could also explain the inhibition of leukocytes activation as previously described [36].

Comparison of Nig06 PB1-F2 functions in chicken and mouse infected lungs

Since the Nig06 is able to infect mammals and birds, we compared the host response associated with PB1-F2 in the lungs of mice and chickens after 2 days pi. We used the chicken data obtained in the present study and the mouse data published in a previous work [34]. We generated two sets of genes by directly comparing wt- and ΔF2-infected animals. The median up- and median down-regulated genes were selected using an adjusted p-value$<$0.05 (Fig. 9A and 9B), then we compared these two groups of genes in an ontological analysis. The functional classification of the genes regulated by PB1-F2 in chicken and mouse revealed major differences in the host response. In chickens, genes associated with "inflammatory response" and "immunological disease" correspond with 25% and 15% of the regulated-genes respectively, whereas in mice these functions are underrepresented with only 2% and 5% (Fig. 9C and 9D). When comparing the canonical pathways associated with the genes deregulated by PB1-F2 in both species, we identified host-specific PB1-F2 functions. As shown in Fig. 9E, in chicken, PB1-F2 regulated numerous inflammatory and immune pathways. Importantly, most of these pathways were down-regulated by the expression of PB1-F2 during the infection. For example, in chicken, the majority of the genes implicated in "CTLA4 Signaling in Cytotoxic T Lymphocytes" were down-regulated, suggesting that this specific function is down-modulated by PB1-F2 or that the cell type involved in this pathway is depleted by infection with PB1-F2 expressing virus (Fig 10A). On the contrary, in mouse, only few canonical pathways were regulated by PB1-F2 at this time-point. In particular, we found that PB1-F2 upregulated the expression of genes associated with "PPARα/RXRα Activation", a pathway exerting anti-inflammatory functions (Fig. 10B). Presumably as a consequence of this, a delay in the triggering of the immune response is observed in mouse infected by the PB1-F2-expressing Nig06 virus [34]. Our data also indicate that PB1-F2 expression triggers host responses shared by avian and mammal hosts. Among these responses, we found "Aldosterone Signaling", "PDGF Signaling" and "eNOS signaling" pathways which illustrate the damages caused by PB1-F2 within the epithelium, connective tissue and endothelium respectively (Fig. 10C-E).

In summary, PB1-F2 from Nig06 exerts different functions in mouse and chicken. In lungs of the avian host, PB1-F2 strongly decreases the inflammation response whereas its impact is mild in mice. However, the epithelial cells damage provoked by PB1-F2 expression appears to be a feature shared by both species.

Discussion

Highly pathogenic H5N1 AIV infections among domestic poultry have become endemic in several countries in Asia and in Egypt [44]. An AIV is defined as "highly pathogenic" when it causes at least 75% mortality in 8-week-old naïve chickens intravenously infected [2], or if its hemagglutinin contains polybasic cleavage site [45]. Most highly pathogenic AIV provoke multi-organ failure, including hemorrhage in the intestinal and respiratory systems and lymphoid necrosis. In this work, we analyzed the contribution of PB1-F2 in the pathology of chickens infected by a highly pathogenic AIV isolated in Niger in 2006 [34]. Unexpectedly, at low inoculum dose, the PB1-F2-expressing virus infection resulted in a reduced mortality in comparison to the ΔF2 virus. This feature contrasts with what is observed in mammals since PB1-F2 usually increases pathology in mice models [15,17–19,27,34]. To characterize the functional causes of this observation, we explored the host responses of the infected chickens in two

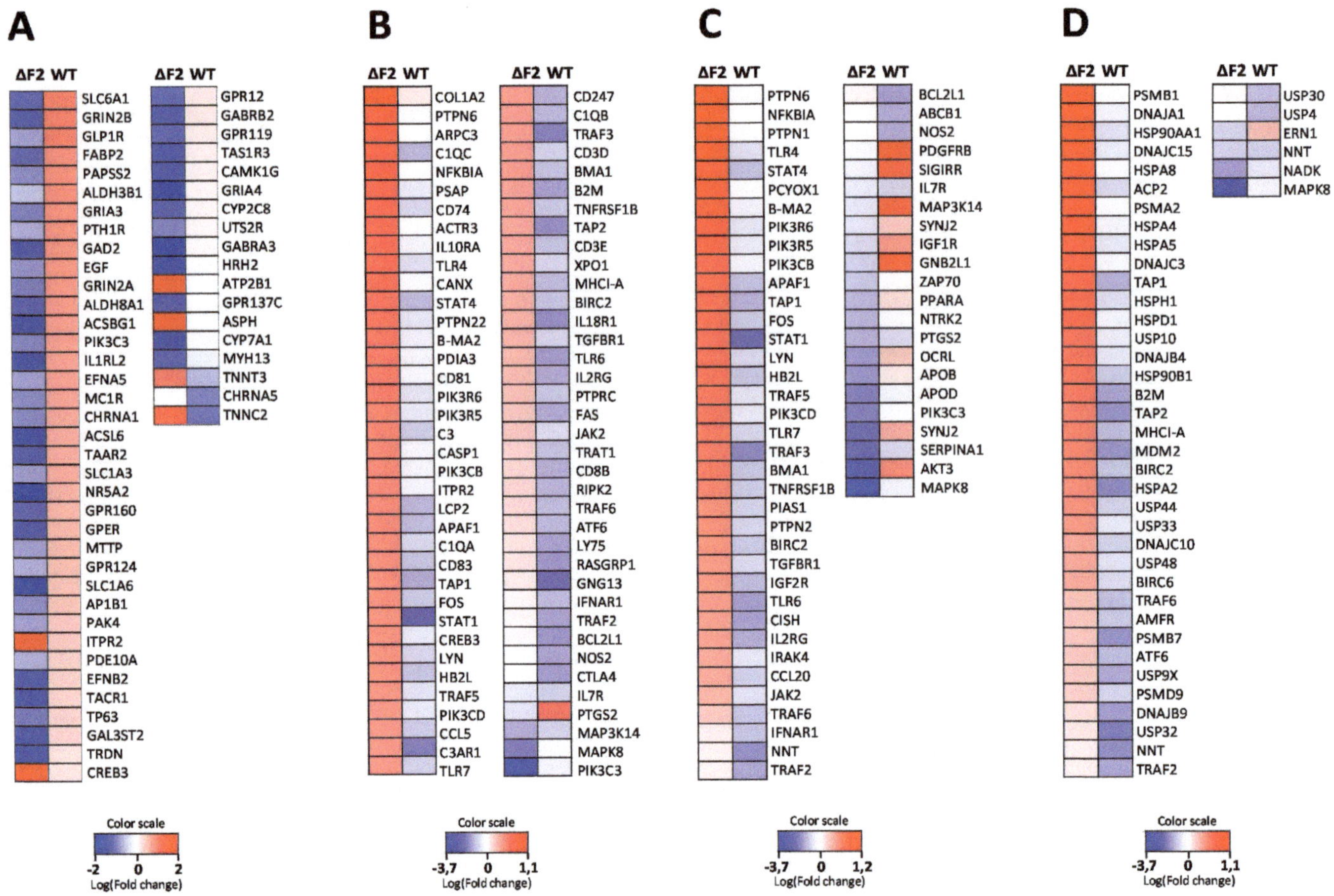

Figure 7. Heat maps of selected genes in the lungs of ΔF2- and wt-infected chickens at day 2 pi. Genes shown in red are upregulated and genes in blue are downregulated. Data are expressed in Log base 2 ratio. (A) Heat map of genes related to "Calcium Signaling pathway". (B) Heat map of genes related to "Hematological System Development and Function". (C) Heat map of genes related to "Cell to Cell Signaling and Interaction". (D) Heat map of genes related to "Cellular Compromise".

tissues: lung and blood. By comparing the genes differentially expressed in presence or absence of PB1-F2 during infection, we were able to identify genes signatures associated with this protein.

In lungs, PB1-F2 expression increases the transcription of genes involved in calcium signaling and alters the ER integrity to induce a ER-stress pathway. The ER stress response, also known as the unfolded protein response, is regulated by several enzymes including ERN1 (also known as IRE1). ERN1 activity has been shown to be important during the viral cycle of influenza virus [46]. The up-regulation of ERN1 in presence of PB1-F2 is related to the ability of PB1-F2 to misfold and aggregate in membrane environments [31]. The cellular Ca^{2+} concentration dynamics plays a critical role in epithelium homeostasis, and prolonged decrease of Ca^{2+} concentration within the ER triggers multiple cellular cascades that can ultimately lead to cell death [47]. A multitude of factors regulate the Ca^{2+} fluxes, including cytokines and reactive oxygen metabolites, but the strong membrane affinity of PB1-F2 and its capacity to alter membrane integrity [31,48] supports the hypothesis that PB1-F2 itself could modify Ca^{2+} fluxes and then generate a gene signature in relation with "calcium signaling". Importantly, Ueda and colleagues previously characterized the apoptosis induction of duck epithelial cells infected by a highly pathogenic H5N1 AIV through an extracellular Ca^{2+} influx mechanism [49]. This Ca^{2+} imbalance results in an excess of Ca^{2+} transport into the mitochondria, inducing a loss of mitochondrial membrane potential and apoptosis. Alternatively, the mitochondrial Ca^{2+} overload can occur through ER-mitochondria direct transfer, a mechanism facilitated by ER sensitization [50].

Interestingly, we identified a mitochondrial dysfunction gene signature associated to PB1-F2 expression in blood of infected-chickens. Mitochondrial dysfunction occurs when the ROS-mediated oxidative stress overpowers the antioxidant defense system. In parallel, inhibition of pathways relative to leukocyte activation was also evidenced in the presence of PB1-F2 (Fig. 8C). These two concomitant events are reminiscent of the fact that PB1-F2 was shown to inhibits immune response by decreasing the mitochondrial membrane potential [36]. Hence, PB1-F2 could trigger mitochondrial dysfunction in immune cells and may consequently deplete leukocytes through apoptosis induction in the infected host. This mechanism can be amplified through cytokine secretion such as CTLA-4 (Fig 4 and Fig 7). CTLA-4 is expressed by T-cells and has been described to play a crucial role in the immunomodulatory properties of these cells [51].

It is worth noting that the helicase RIG-I is absent in the chicken genome [52]. This is of first importance since PB1-F2 has been described to inhibit the type I interferon induction in mammals by binding to MAVS, the RIG-I adaptor protein allowing signal transduction [35,36]. Thus, it seems unlikely that PB1-F2 acts in this way in the chicken host. In contrast to chickens, ducks express a functional form of RIG-I [52]. This

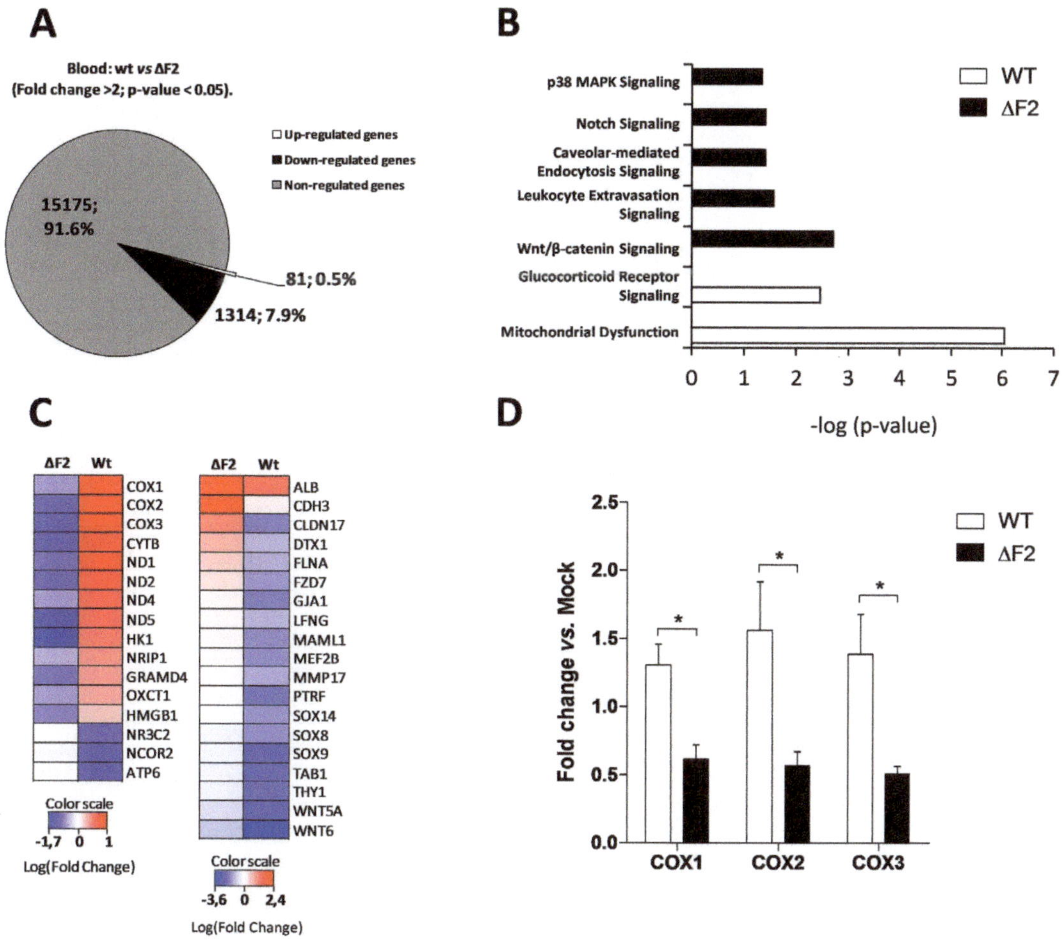

Figure 8. Global analysis of PB1-F2-dependant gene expression changes in the blood of influenza infected chickens. (A) Distribution of genes differentially regulated between wt- and ΔF2-infected chicken blood samples. (B) Canonical pathways associated to differentially expressed genes were compared using Ingenuity Pathways Analysis. Canonical pathways are ranked using the p-value obtained with the right-tailed Fisher's exact test, it represents the probability of each biological function to be involved in the group of analyzed genes. (C) Heat maps of genes related to "Mitochondrial Dysfunction" (left panel) and to "Leukocyte activation pathways" (right panel). Genes shown in red are upregulated and genes in blue are downregulated. Data are expressed in Log base 2 ratio. (D) RT-PCR quantifications of COX1, COX2 and COX3 mitochondrial gene expressions in blood of wt- and ΔF2-infected chickens at day 2 pi. Gene expressions were normalized with the β-actin gene expression level and presented as fold increase relative to mock-infected chickens. Data are means ± SD of 4 chickens. *: $p<0.05$.

differential expression of RIG-I between chickens and ducks is probably a key component that could explain the opposite PB1-F2 phenotype observed in these two species. Indeed, Schmolke and collaborators demonstrated that the deletion of PB1-F2 caused a delayed onset of pathologic signs and systemic spreading of virus [20]. These data in conjunction with previous findings in other studies support the hypothesis that the detrimental effect of PB1-F2 on the host could be mediated by the activated form of MAVS (*i.e.* filamentous form, [53]). The absence of RIG-I in the chicken genome imply that MAVS is probably less activated during infection and consequently reduce the negative effects of PB1-F2.

Essentially, no difference was observed in the outcome of the infection between the wt and the ΔF2 H5N1 virus using the dose of 1000 PFU. This would be consistent with the highly pathogenic genotype and phenotype of the virus due to multibasic cleavage site of the hemagglutinin. Interestingly, notable difference in the outcome of the infection was observed at an inoculation dose of 100 PFU, with the wt inoculated chickens being the survivors. Despite the molecular signatures associated with PB1-F2, it is still difficult to explain why the wt Nig06 is less virulent than the ΔF2 virus at a low dose. Analysis of gene regulation indicated that numbers of genes are strongly down regulated in the wt inoculated birds. While some of the genes are linked to pathogenesis, the overall combined effect of this lack of upregulation may have led to reduced mortality in this inoculation group of birds. It cannot be excluded that the role of PB1-F2 in birds is to attenuate the influenza virus to allow survival of the reservoir host, since almost all known avian isolates express this protein [22,23], which appears to be excluded upon adaptation of the virus to a mammalian host, where gene upregulation caused by PB1-F2 contributes to pathogenesis [17,19,27,28]. The down regulation of immune and inflammatory pathways in presence of PB1-F2 is associated to a better survival rate of infected chickens; this suggests that the host response could be implicated in the pathogenesis as previously described in mice models [54]. However, the molecular profiles of ΔF2-infected chickens and the cytokine analysis did not show aberrant cytokines production (data not shown) as described in the "cytokine storm" observed in human acute respiratory distress syndrome [55]. Nevertheless, a recent work by Kuchipudi and collaborators studied the kinetic of

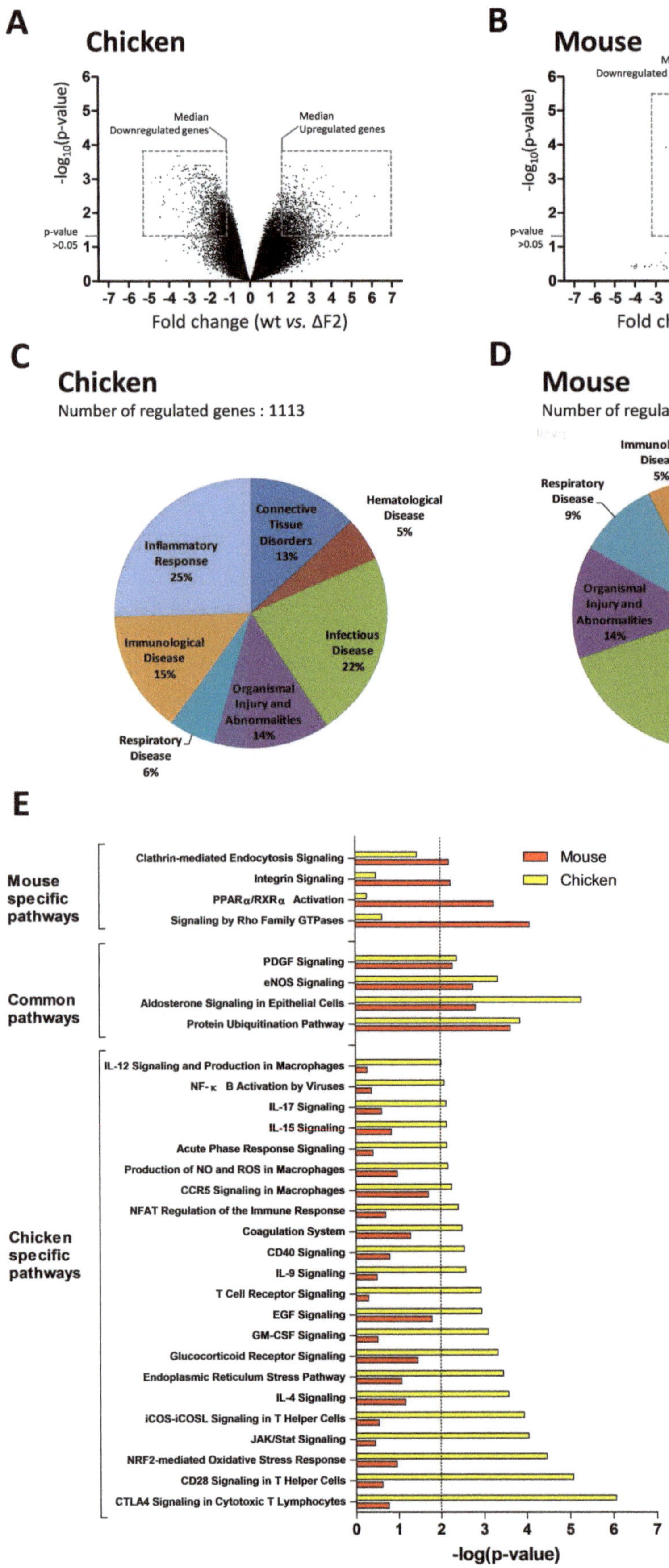
A
Chicken
-log10(p-value)
Median
Downregulated genes
Median
Upregulated genes
p-value
>0.05
Fold change (wt vs. ΔF2)
B
Mouse
Median
Downregulated genes
Median
Upregulated genes
-log10(p-value)
p-value
>0.05
Fold change (wt vs. ΔF2)
C
Chicken
Number of regulated genes : 1113
Connective Tissue Disorders 13%
Hematological Disease 5%
Infectious Disease 22%
Organismal Injury and Abnormalities 14%
Respiratory Disease 6%
Immunological Disease 15%
Inflammatory Response 25%
D
Mouse
Number of regulated genes : 1163
Inflammatory Response 2%
Immunological Disease 5%
Respiratory Disease 9%
Connective Tissue Disorders 13%
Hematological Disease 20%
Infectious Disease 37%
Organismal Injury and Abnormalities 14%
E
Mouse
Chicken
Mouse specific pathways
Clathrin-mediated Endocytosis Signaling
Integrin Signaling
PPARα/RXRα Activation
Signaling by Rho Family GTPases
Common pathways
PDGF Signaling
eNOS Signaling
Aldosterone Signaling in Epithelial Cells
Protein Ubiquitination Pathway
Chicken specific pathways
IL-12 Signaling and Production in Macrophages
NF-κ B Activation by Viruses
IL-17 Signaling
IL-15 Signaling
Acute Phase Response Signaling
Production of NO and ROS in Macrophages
CCR5 Signaling in Macrophages
NFAT Regulation of the Immune Response
Coagulation System
CD40 Signaling
IL-9 Signaling
T Cell Receptor Signaling
EGF Signaling
GM-CSF Signaling
Glucocorticoid Receptor Signaling
Endoplasmic Reticulum Stress Pathway
IL-4 Signaling
iCOS-iCOSL Signaling in T Helper Cells
JAK/Stat Signaling
NRF2-mediated Oxidative Stress Response
CD28 Signaling in T Helper Cells
CTLA4 Signaling in Cytotoxic T Lymphocytes
-log(p-value)

Figure 9. Comparison of Nig06 PB1-F2 impact on the lung host-response in chicken and mouse. (A) Scatter plot comparing wt-infected chickens vs. ΔF2-infected chicken lung transcriptomes at day 2 pi. Genes selected for ontological analysis are highlighted. (B) Scatterplot comparing wt-infected mice vs. ΔF2-infected mice lung transcriptomes at day 2 pi. (C) Distribution of major GO functions associated to genes regulated by PB1-F2 in infected chicken lungs. (D) Distribution of major GO functions associated to genes regulated by PB1-F2 in infected mouse lungs. (E) Canonical pathways associated to differentially expressed genes in chicken and mouse were compared using Ingenuity Pathways Analysis and ranked with the p-value obtained using the right-tailed Fisher's exact test.

cell death induction in avian species infected with AIV and provided a link between the rapid induction of apoptosis and resistance to virus [56]. As a consequence, AIV could have evolved a mechanism implying PB1-F2 to delay the death of the host in order to have time to efficiently spread.

By comparing the host responses regulated by PB1-F2 in chicken and mouse using the same H5N1 wt- and mutant viruses, we were able to identify common and differentially regulated pathways in both hosts. The identified functions suggest that PB1-F2 expression provokes damages to the infected lungs in both species. PB1-F2 has affinity for hydrophobic environments and is able to disturb membrane integrity [31,48,57], this property is likely to induce damages to the epithelium structure and to alter ion channels control of fluid and electrolyte transport across epithelium. Consequently, the pathway "Aldosterone Signaling in Epithelial Cells" is regulated by PB1-F2 since it integrates genes implicated in ions flux and water retention in epithelia. Such genes like ASIC1, SCNN1A and SCNN1B (ENaCα and β) encode ion channels; their expressions are upregulated by PB1-F2 in chicken lungs (Fig. 9C) and suggest a perturbation of the electrodiffusion of the apical membrane of epithelial cells.

As a consequence of epithelial tissue integrity alteration, the wt Nig06 is able to spread more efficiently in infected embryos and also in intestine of infected chickens even if the biological relevance of the intestine viral replication data are questionable. Given that fecal-to-oral transmission is the most common mode of spread between birds, the aptitudes attributed to PB1-F2 to increase the biodispersion of the virus through the host organs could provide an advantage to avian viruses that express PB1-F2. This can explain why 96% of the avian virus genomes encode a functional PB1-F2. On the contrary, as PB1-F2 promotes inflammation in mammals [19,27,34] and facilitates secondary bacterial pneumonia [17,21], the loss of PB1-F2 functions could be beneficial for an adaptation of the virus to the mammal hosts. This loss of function is particularly visible in the H1N1 influenza viruses isolated in humans: only 7% of the recently isolated viruses express a full length PB1-F2 [23].

In summary, the present study shed in light the complexity of PB1-F2 functions. PB1-F2 has strain specificity, cell type specificity and host specificity. Further research to identify relationship between specific PB1-F2 structural motif and pathogenesis is needed, a better understanding of the chicken antiviral responses is also necessary.

Materials and Methods

Ethics statement

All animal work was carried out in compliance with Canadian Council on Animal Care guidelines and was approved by the

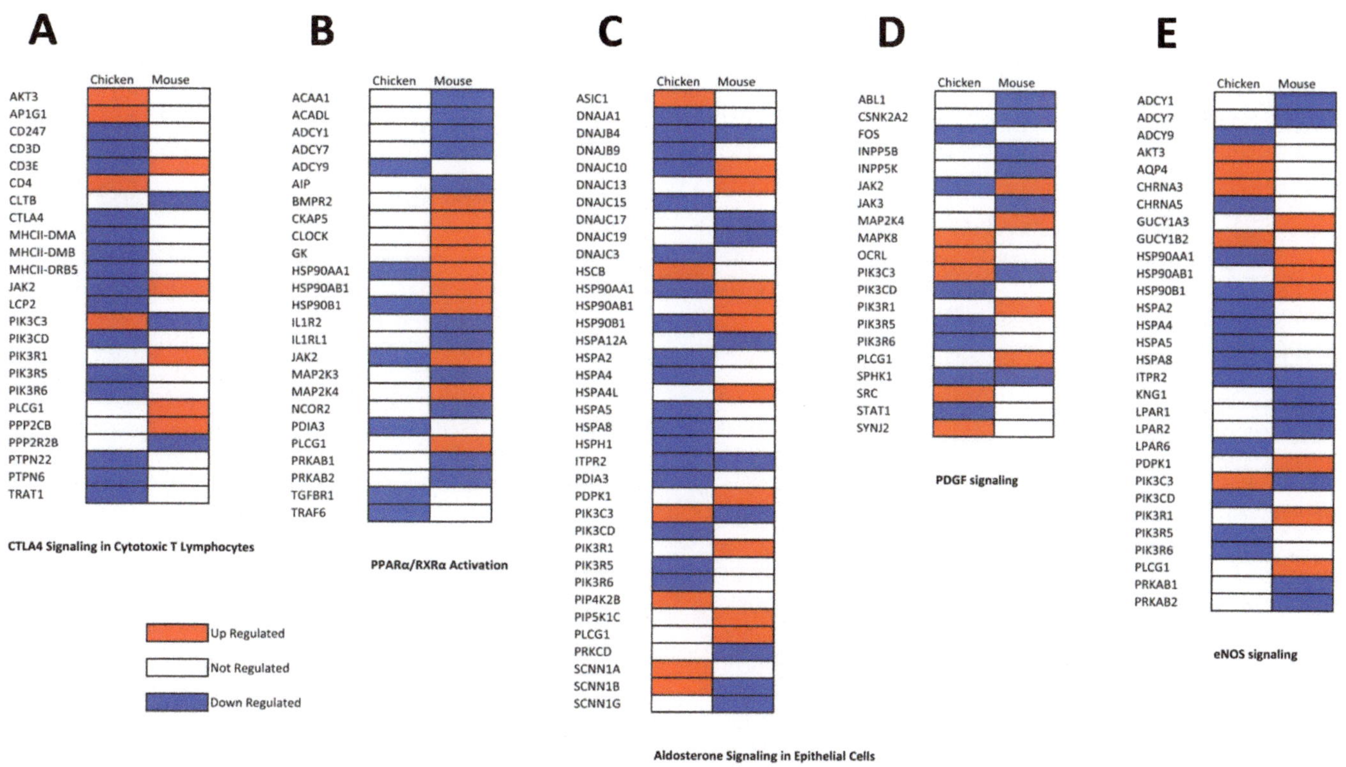

Figure 10. Heat maps of selected genes showing differential regulation in response to PB1-F2 in lungs of chicken and mouse at day 2 pi. Genes are representative of "CTLA4 Signaling in Cytotoxic T Lymphocytes" (A), "PPARα/RXRα Activation" (B), "Aldosterone Signaling" (C), "PDGF Signaling" (D) and "eNOS signaling" (E). Genes shown in red are up-regulated and those shown in blue are down-regulated in presence of PB1-F2.

Table 1. Primers used in real time PCR assays.

Gene name	Gene ID	Primer sequences		Tm	Product length
STAT1	424044	sense	GCAGGGAACAGAACAAATGAGG	62.23	129
		antisense	TGACAATGATGGGAAGTGATGTGG	63.47	
β2M	414830	sense	GAAGGCAGTTGCGCTGGTGG	64.56	158
		antisense	TGGTGATCCTGGGTGGGTGG	63.71	
TLR4	417241	sense	AATCCCAAACACCACCCTGG	60.18	198
		antisense	AGGTGCTGGAGTGAATTGGC	60.61	
IFNAR1	395665	sense	AGCAGAGAGGAATGCATCGG	59.89	91
		antisense	TCAAGACAACAGTCAGCGCA	60.18	
CTLA-4	424106	sense	TGCCGAAGTAATGGAAGTGACTC	63.01	149
		antisense	ATTTCAGTGAACTTGTCGCCTGTC	64.12	
CCL5	417465	sense	TCTCCATCCTCCTGGTTGCC	61.27	73
		antisense	CACACGGTTGTATCAGCCCC	61.02	
TLR7	418638	sense	ATCTTTCAGAGGTGGCTGCAC	60.61	120
		antisense	TTTTGGGAAACCAACGTCCT	57.85	
HSPA2	423504	sense	ATCATGTCTGGCAAAGGGCCG	63.34	172
		antisense	TGGCAGCATCCCCGATGAGG	64.50	
IL2RG	395199	sense	TCGTCAAGTACAAGAGCAACAAGG	63.58	179
		antisense	CCCAGAAGACAGGCACACTC	62.95	
TLR6	771173	sense	TCTGACGACATTTATCAAGGCA	57.80	107
		antisense	ATGGTCATCATCTCCCCAGA	57.50	
BSL2L1	373954	sense	GTTCGAGCATCCGACGTGAG	63.67	143
		antisense	ATTCACTACCTGCTCAAAGCTCTG	63.20	
β-actin	396526	sense	TTGCTGACAGGATGCAGAAG	60.14	141
		antisense	ACATCTGCTGGAAGGTGGAC	60.12	

Animal Care Committee at the Canadian Science Centre for Animal and Human Health.

Viruses

Influenza A/duck/Niger/2090/2006 (H5N1) was used in this study. Wild type (wt) and PB1-F2 knockout (ΔF2) viruses were produced by reverse genetics system using a bidirectional transcription plasmid derived from pHW2000 [58]. The viruses were prepared as previously described [34] and titrated on Madin Darby canine kidney (MDCK) cells.

Embryos histological analysis

Ten days old embryos were fixed in 10% neutral phosphate buffered formalin, routinely processed and sectioned at the level of the brain, thorax, abdomen and legs as well as the chorioallantoic membrane. For immunohistochemistry, paraffin tissue sections were quenched for 10 minutes in aqueous 3% H_2O_2 then pretreated with proteinase K for 15 minutes. The primary antibody was a mouse monoclonal antibody specific for influenza A nucleoprotein (NP) (F26NP9, produced in-house) and was used at a 1:10,000 dilution for one hour. They were then visualized using a horseradish peroxidase labelled polymer, Envision + system (anti-mouse) (Dako, USA), reacted with the chromogen diaminobenzidine (DAB). The sections were then counter stained with Gill's hematoxylin. Slides were examined and the extent of immunostaining was scored as weak (less than 20 cells staining), mild 1+ (< 25% of the section staining), moderate 2+ (25–50% of the section staining), extensive 3+ (51 to 75% of the section staining) or widespread 4+ (>75% of the section staining).

Infection of chickens with wt or ΔF2 Nig06 and sample collection

Specific pathogen free (SPF) white Leghorn chickens at 40 days old were obtained from Fallowfield, Ottawa CFIA laboratory. They were floor housed in heated BSL3 animal cubicles and allowed 1 week of acclimatization before the start of experiments. Ten to 20 chickens per group were inoculated intranasally with 10^2 or 10^3 PFU per chicken of either wt or ΔF2 Nig06 H5N1 in 0.5 ml sterile PBS distributed into both nares for the survival experiments. Cloacal and oropharyngeal swabs were collected from each chicken on day 0 (prior to challenge) and at predetermined time points post challenge. Chickens were monitored daily for clinical signs including: depression, apathy, ruffled feathers, respiratory distress, hemorrhages and necrosis on the face, eyes, nares, combs, wattles, feet and legs. Clinical signs were scored as normal, mildly depressed, depressed and severely depressed. For animal welfare reasons, severely depressed chickens were humanely euthanized with intravenous injection of sodium pentobarbital (240 mg/ml). In second set of experiments targeting the host response, five chickens per group were inoculated intranasally with 10^3 PFU per chicken of either wt or ΔF2 Nig06 H5N1 in 0.5 ml sterile PBS distributed into both nares. Blood was collected from the wing vein of anaesthetized chickens on days 0 and 2 post infection (pi). At 2 days pi, chickens were euthanized with intravenous injection of sodium pentobarbital

(240 mg/ml), and tissue samples were collected. Swabs, trachea, lung, blood, heart, liver, kidney, spleen, brain, pancreas, intestine and thymus were stored at -70 °C.

RNA extraction and qRT-PCR

RNA was isolated from swabs, bloods and lungs homogenates using the TRIzol-chloroform method according to the manufacturer's instructions (Invitrogen). RNA quality was checked on a Bioanalyzer 2100 (Agilent Technologies) and samples with a RNA Integrity Number (RIN) score between 7 and 9 were used in microarray or qRT-PCR experiments. Viral loads in swabs and tissues homogenates were determined by qRT-PCR assay specific for the influenza A M1 gene [59] with primers and probes that were modified to detect the Nig06 IAV: forward primer, 5′- CTT CTA ACC GAG GTC GAA ACG TA -3′; reverse primer, 5′-GGT GAC AGG ATC GGT CTT GTC TTT-3′; probe, 5′-TET-TCA GGC CCC CTC AAA GCC GAG-BHQ-3′ as previously described [34]. The mRNA levels of host genes were assayed using the Mastercycler realplex sequence detector (Eppendorf) and the double strand specific dye SYBR Green system (Applied Biosystems). Details of the primers are provided in Table 1. The PCR conditions and cycles were as follows: initial DNA denaturation 10 min at 95°C, followed by 40 cycles at 95°C for 15 sec, followed by an annealing step at 60°C for 15 sec, and then extension at 72°C during 30 sec. Each point was performed in triplicate. To ensure that the primers produced a single and specific PCR amplification product, a dissociation curve was performed at the end of the PCR cycle. Relative quantitative evaluation was performed by the comparative ΔΔCt method. The mean ΔCt obtained in mock-infected chickens for each gene was used as calibrator, after normalization to endogenous control β-actin. The results are presented as an n-fold difference relative to calibrator ($RQ = 2^{-\Delta\Delta C_t}$).

Microarray experiments

Transcriptional profiling was performed using the Agilent-026441 Gallus gallus Oligo Microarray (v2), 4×44Kslides (GEO accession: GPL15357). A dual color design was used to provide direct comparisons between infected lungs [infected-by-wt-virus/infected-by-ΔF2-virus], and between infected bloods and mock-infected bloods [infected-by-wt-virus/mock-infected] and [infected-by-ΔF2-virus/mock-infected]. To reduce potential experimental biases, RNA samples were collected from 5 different chickens for each experimental condition (Mock, wt-infected, ΔF2-infected). A total of 24 samples were analyzed, corresponding to 6 microarray slides. Fluorescently labeled cRNAs were obtained using the two colors Low Input Quick Amp Labeling Kit (Agilent Technologies) and starting from 100 ng of total RNA for each sample. supplemented with known synthetic RNA (two-color RNA spike-in kit, Agilent Technologies). cRNAs were subsequently purified using RNeasy Mini Spin columns (Qiagen) and the purified cRNAs were then run onto a Bioanalyzer 2100 using RNA 6000 Nano Chip (Agilent technologies). cRNA yields and specific activities were measured using a NanoDrop 2000 (Thermo Scientific). An equal amount of 800 ng of cyanine 3 and cyanine 5 labeled cRNA were hybridized for each sample. The hybridization and the washing steps were performed following the manufacturer's recommendations. The arrays were scanned using an Agilent G2505C scanner, and the scan protocol used a resolution of 5 µm and a 20 bit dynamic range. The resulting .tiff images were analyzed using the Feature Extraction software version 10.7.3.1 (Agilent) using the GE2_107_Sep09 protocol. For each channel, the median of the signal intensity was used without background subtraction. Data were analyzed to define genes that are differentially expressed between wt-infected and ΔF2-infected samples. Differentially expressed genes were identified with a False Discovery Rate (FDR) equal to 5%. Microarray data are available in the Gene Expression Omnibus (GEO) database (http://www.ncbi.nlm.nih.gov/geo/) under GEO accession number GSE56506.

Transcriptomic analysis

For functional analysis the data files resulting from differential analysis were imported into GeneSpring GX 12.1 software (Agilent Technologies). Hierarchical clustering analysis was performed to analyze cellular genes that were differentially expressed during infection (Euclidian distance, average linkage). For further analysis, data files were uploaded into the Ingenuity Pathways Analysis (IPA) software (Ingenuity Systems).

Statistical analysis

Survival of chickens was compared using Kaplan-Meier analysis and log-rank test. qRT-PCR quantification are expressed as the mean ± standard error of the mean (SEM) of at least four chickens, and statistical analyzes were performed using the paired Student T test. Correlation clustering and principal component analysis were performed on normalized data using the FactoMineR package. Ontological analysis made with IPA used the right-tailed Fisher's exact test to calculate a p-value determining the probability that each biological function and disease assigned to that data set is due to chance alone.

Supporting Information

Figure S1 Virus isolation by plaque assay on MDCK cells from oral swabs of chickens infected with 1000 PFU collected at 2 dpi (wt n = 15; ΔF2 n = 15) and at 4 dpi (wt n = 7; ΔF2 n = 5). No live virus could be detected in swabs from 6 chickens in the wt-infected condition at day 2 pi, and from 9 chickens in the ΔF2-infected condition at day 2 pi.

Acknowledgments

We thank Jérôme Lecardonnel for technical assistance in microarrays hybridization.

Peter Marszal, Greg Smith and Tyler Hill are gratefully acknowledged for technical assistance in molecular biology experiments. We also thank all the CFIA/NCFAD staff for technical assistance in animal experiments, in particular Kim Azaransky, Jaime Bernstein, Christine De Graff, Maggie Forbes, Michelle French, Cory Nakamura, Marlee Phair and Kevin Tierney.

Author Contributions

Conceived and designed the experiments: OL HMW RLG. Performed the experiments: OL CEH CC YB HMW RLG. Analyzed the data: OL CEH CC LJ BD HMW RLG. Contributed reagents/materials/analysis tools: BDC MM. Wrote the paper: HMW RLG.

References

1. Yen HL, Webster RG (2009) Pandemic influenza as a current threat. Curr Top Microbiol Immunol 333: 3–24.
2. Cardona CJ, Xing Z, Sandrock CE, Davis CE (2009) Avian influenza in birds and mammals. Comp Immunol Microbiol Infect Dis 32: 255–273.

3. Kim JK, Negovetich NJ, Forrest HL, Webster RG (2009) Ducks: the "Trojan horses" of H5N1 influenza. Influenza Other Respir Viruses 3: 121–128.
4. WHO (2013) http://www.who.int/influenza/human_animal_interface/H5N1_cumulative_table_archives/en/index.html.Accessed 2014 Jan 24.
5. Wang TT, Parides MK, Palese P (2012) Seroevidence for H5N1 influenza infections in humans: meta-analysis. Science 335: 1463.
6. Herfst S, Schrauwen EJ, Linster M, Chutinimitkul S, de Wit E, et al. (2012) Airborne transmission of influenza A/H5N1 virus between ferrets. Science 336: 1534–1541.
7. Imai M, Watanabe T, Hatta M, Das SC, Ozawa M, et al. (2012) Experimental adaptation of an influenza H5 HA confers respiratory droplet transmission to a reassortant H5 HA/H1N1 virus in ferrets. Nature 486: 420–428.
8. Jagger BW, Wise HM, Kash JC, Walters KA, Wills NM, et al. (2012) An overlapping protein-coding region in influenza A virus segment 3 modulates the host response. Science 337: 199–204.
9. Wise HM, Hutchinson EC, Jagger BW, Stuart AD, Kang ZH, et al. (2012) Identification of a novel splice variant form of the influenza A virus M2 ion channel with an antigenically distinct ectodomain. PLoS Pathog 8: e1002998.
10. Kawaoka Y, Krauss S, Webster RG (1989) Avian-to-human transmission of the PB1 gene of influenza A viruses in the 1957 and 1968 pandemics. J Virol 63: 4603–4608.
11. Scholtissek C, Rohde W, Von Hoyningen V, Rott R (1978) On the origin of the human influenza virus subtypes H2N2 and H3N2. Virology 87: 13–20.
12. Pappas C, Aguilar PV, Basler CF, Solorzano A, Zeng H, et al. (2008) Single gene reassortants identify a critical role for PB1, HA, and NA in the high virulence of the 1918 pandemic influenza virus. Proc Natl Acad Sci U S A 105: 3064–3069.
13. Chen W, Calvo PA, Malide D, Gibbs J, Schubert U, et al. (2001) A novel influenza A virus mitochondrial protein that induces cell death. Nat Med 7: 1306–1312.
14. Wise HM, Foeglein A, Sun J, Dalton RM, Patel S, et al. (2009) A complicated message: Identification of a novel PB1-related protein translated from influenza A virus segment 2 mRNA. J Virol 83: 8021–8031.
15. Zamarin D, Ortigoza MB, Palese P (2006) Influenza A virus PB1-F2 protein contributes to viral pathogenesis in mice. J Virol 80: 7976–7983.
16. Conenello GM, Zamarin D, Perrone LA, Tumpey T, Palese P (2007) A single mutation in the PB1-F2 of H5N1 (HK/97) and 1918 influenza A viruses contributes to increased virulence. PLoS Pathog 3: 1414–1421.
17. McAuley JL, Hornung F, Boyd KL, Smith AM, McKeon R, et al. (2007) Expression of the 1918 influenza A virus PB1-F2 enhances the pathogenesis of viral and secondary bacterial pneumonia. Cell Host Microbe 2: 240–249.
18. Conenello GM, Tisoncik JR, Rosenzweig E, Varga ZT, Palese P, et al. (2011) A single N66S mutation in the PB1-F2 protein of influenza A virus increases virulence by inhibiting the early interferon response in vivo. J Virol 85: 652–662.
19. Le Goffic R, Leymarie O, Chevalier C, Rebours E, Da Costa B, et al. (2011) Transcriptomic Analysis of Host Immune and Cell Death Responses Associated with the Influenza A Virus PB1-F2 Protein. PLoS Pathog 7: e1002202.
20. Schmolke M, Manicassamy B, Pena L, Sutton T, Hai R, et al. (2011) Differential Contribution of PB1-F2 to the Virulence of Highly Pathogenic H5N1 Influenza A Virus in Mammalian and Avian Species. PLoS Pathog 7: e1002186.
21. Iverson AR, Boyd KL, McAuley JL, Plano LR, Hart ME, et al. (2011) Influenza virus primes mice for pneumonia from Staphylococcus aureus. J Infect Dis 203: 880–888.
22. Zell R, Krumbholz A, Eitner A, Krieg R, Halbhuber KJ, et al. (2007) Prevalence of PB1-F2 of influenza A viruses. J Gen Virol 88: 536–546.
23. Chakrabarti AK, Pasricha G (2013) An insight into the PB1F2 protein and its multifunctional role in enhancing the pathogenicity of the influenza A viruses. Virology.
24. DeLuca DS, Keskin DB, Zhang GL, Reinherz EL, Brusic V (2012) PB1-F2 Finder: scanning influenza sequences for PB1-F2 encoding RNA segments. BMC Bioinformatics 12 Suppl 13: S6.
25. Dundon WG (2012) Variability among the neuraminidase, non-structural 1 and PB1-F2 proteins in the influenza A virus genome. Virus Genes 44: 363–373.
26. Pasricha G, Mishra AC, Chakrabarti AK (2012) Comprehensive global amino acid sequence analysis of PB1F2 protein of influenza A H5N1 viruses and the influenza A virus subtypes responsible for the 20th-century pandemics. Influenza Other Respi Viruses.
27. McAuley JL, Chipuk JE, Boyd KL, Van De Velde N, Green DR, et al. (2010) PB1-F2 proteins from H5N1 and 20 century pandemic influenza viruses cause immunopathology. PLoS Pathog 6: e1001014.
28. Alymova IV, Green AM, van de Velde N, McAuley JL, Boyd KL, et al. (2011) Immunopathogenic and antibacterial effects of H3N2 influenza A virus PB1-F2 map to amino acid residues 62, 75, 79, and 82. J Virol 85: 12324–12333.
29. Zamarin D, Garcia-Sastre A, Xiao X, Wang R, Palese P (2005) Influenza virus PB1-F2 protein induces cell death through mitochondrial ANT3 and VDAC1. PLoS Pathog 1: e4.
30. Le Goffic R, Bouguyon E, Chevalier C, Vidic J, Da Costa B, et al. (2010) Influenza A Virus Protein PB1-F2 Exacerbates IFN-{beta} Expression of Human Respiratory Epithelial Cells. J Immunol 185: 4812–4823.
31. Chevalier C, Al Bazzal A, Vidic J, Fevrier V, Bourdieu C, et al. (2010) PB1-F2 influenza A virus protein adopts a beta-sheet conformation and forms amyloid fibers in membrane environments. J Biol Chem 285: 13233–13243.
32. Mazur I, Anhlan D, Mitzner D, Wixler L, Schubert U, et al. (2008) The proapoptotic influenza A virus protein PB1-F2 regulates viral polymerase activity by interaction with the PB1 protein. Cell Microbiol.
33. McAuley JL, Zhang K, McCullers JA (2010) The effects of influenza A virus PB1-F2 protein on polymerase activity are strain specific and do not impact pathogenesis. J Virol 84: 558–564.
34. Leymarie O, Jouvion G, Hervé P, Chevalier C, Lorin V, et al. (2013) Kinetic characterization of PB1-F2-mediated immunopathology during highly pathogenic avian H5N1 influenza virus infection. PLoS One 8: e57894.
35. Varga ZT, Ramos I, Hai R, Schmolke M, Garcia-Sastre A, et al. (2011) The influenza virus protein PB1-F2 inhibits the induction of type i interferon at the level of the MAVS adaptor protein. PLoS Pathog 7: e1002067.
36. Varga ZT, Grant A, Manicassamy B, Palese P (2012) Influenza Virus Protein PB1-F2 Inhibits the Induction of Type I Interferon by Binding to MAVS and Decreasing Mitochondrial Membrane Potential. J Virol 86: 8359–8366.
37. Di Leva F, Domi T, Fedrizzi L, Lim D, Carafoli E (2008) The plasma membrane Ca2+ ATPase of animal cells: structure, function and regulation. Arch Biochem Biophys 476: 65–74.
38. Foskett JK, White C, Cheung KH, Mak DO (2007) Inositol trisphosphate receptor Ca2+ release channels. Physiol Rev 87: 593–658.
39. Srikanth S, Jew M, Kim KD, Yee MK, Abramson J, et al. (2012) Junctate is a Ca2+-sensing structural component of Orai1 and stromal interaction molecule 1 (STIM1). Proc Natl Acad Sci U S A 109: 8682–8687.
40. Audas TE, Li Y, Liang G, Lu R (2008) A novel protein, Luman/CREB3 recruitment factor, inhibits Luman activation of the unfolded protein response. Mol Cell Biol 28: 3952–3966.
41. Xu C, Bailly-Maitre B, Reed JC (2005) Endoplasmic reticulum stress: cell life and death decisions. J Clin Invest 115: 2656–2664.
42. Yamada H, Chounan R, Higashi Y, Kurihara N, Kido H (2004) Mitochondrial targeting sequence of the influenza A virus PB1-F2 protein and its function in mitochondria. FEBS Lett 578: 331–336.
43. Gibbs JS, Malide D, Hornung F, Bennink JR, Yewdell JW (2003) The influenza A virus PB1-F2 protein targets the inner mitochondrial membrane via a predicted basic amphipathic helix that disrupts mitochondrial function. J Virol 77: 7214–7224.
44. Brown IH (2010) Summary of avian influenza activity in Europe, Asia, and Africa, 2006–2009. Avian Dis 54: 187–193.
45. OIE-WAHID (2012) Infection with viruses of notifiable avian influenza. Terrestrial Animal Health Code, Chapter 10-4.
46. Hassan IH, Zhang MS, Powers LS, Shao JQ, Baltrusaitis J, et al. (2011) Influenza A viral replication is blocked by inhibition of the inositol-requiring enzyme 1 (IRE1) stress pathway. J Biol Chem 287: 4679–4689.
47. Hajnoczky G, Davies E, Madesh M (2003) Calcium signaling and apoptosis. Biochem Biophys Res Commun 304: 445–454.
48. Henkel M, Mitzner D, Henklein P, Meyer-Almes FJ, Moroni A, et al. (2010) The proapoptotic influenza A virus protein PB1-F2 forms a nonselective ion channel. PLoS One 5: e11112.
49. Ueda M, Daidoji T, Du A, Yang CS, Ibrahim MS, et al. (2010) Highly pathogenic H5N1 avian influenza virus induces extracellular Ca2+ influx, leading to apoptosis in avian cells. J Virol 84: 3068–3078.
50. Hajnoczky G, Csordas G, Das S, Garcia-Perez C, Saotome M, et al. (2006) Mitochondrial calcium signalling and cell death: approaches for assessing the role of mitochondrial Ca2+ uptake in apoptosis. Cell Calcium 40: 553–560.
51. Vignali DA, Collison LW, Workman CJ (2008) How regulatory T cells work. Nat Rev Immunol 8: 523–532.
52. Barber MR, Aldridge JR, Jr., Webster RG, Magor KE (2010) Association of RIG-I with innate immunity of ducks to influenza. Proc Natl Acad Sci U S A 107: 5913–5918.
53. Xu H, He X, Zheng H, Huang LJ, Hou F, et al. (2014) Structural basis for the prion-like MAVS filaments in antiviral innate immunity. Elife 3: e01489.
54. Le Goffic R, Balloy V, Lagranderie M, Alexopoulou L, Escriou N, et al. (2006) Detrimental contribution of the Toll-like receptor (TLR)3 to influenza A virus-induced acute pneumonia. PLoS Pathog 2: e53.
55. Tisoncik JR, Korth MJ, Simmons CP, Farrar J, Martin TR, et al. (2012) Into the eye of the cytokine storm. Microbiol Mol Biol Rev 76: 16–32.
56. Kuchipudi SV, Dunham SP, Nelli R, White GA, Coward VJ, et al. (2012) Rapid death of duck cells infected with influenza: a potential mechanism for host resistance to H5N1. Immunol Cell Biol 90: 116–123.
57. Chanturiya AN, Basanez G, Schubert U, Henklein P, Yewdell JW, et al. (2004) PB1-F2, an influenza A virus-encoded proapoptotic mitochondrial protein, creates variably sized pores in planar lipid membranes. J Virol 78: 6304–6312.
58. Hoffmann E, Krauss S, Perez D, Webby R, Webster RG (2002) Eight-plasmid system for rapid generation of influenza virus vaccines. Vaccine 20: 3165–3170.
59. Spackman E, Senne DA, Myers TJ, Bulaga LL, Garber LP, et al. (2002) Development of a real-time reverse transcriptase PCR assay for type A influenza virus and the avian H5 and H7 hemagglutinin subtypes. J Clin Microbiol 40: 3256–3260.

12

Early Expression of Hypocretin/Orexin in the Chick Embryo Brain

Kyle E. Godden, Jeremy P. Landry, Natalya Slepneva, Paola V. Migues¤, Maria Pompeiano*

Department of Psychology, McGill University, Montreal, Quebec, Canada

Abstract

Hypocretin/Orexin (H/O) neuropeptides are released by a discrete group of neurons in the vertebrate hypothalamus which play a pivotal role in the maintenance of waking behavior and brain state control. Previous studies have indicated that the H/O neuronal development differs between mammals and fish; H/O peptide-expressing cells are detectable during the earliest stages of brain morphogenesis in fish, but only towards the end of brain morphogenesis (by ~85% of embryonic development) in rats. The developmental emergence of H/O neurons has never been previously described in birds. With the goal of determining whether the chick developmental pattern was more similar to that of mammals or of fish, we investigated the emergence of H/O-expressing cells in the brain of chick embryos of different ages using immunohistochemistry. Post-natal chick brains were included in order to compare the spatial distribution of H/O cells with that of other vertebrates. We found that H/O-expressing cells appear to originate from two separate places in the region of the diencephalic proliferative zone. These developing cells express the H/O neuropeptide at a comparatively early age relative to rodents (already visible at 14% of the way through fetal development), thus bearing a closer resemblance to fish. The H/O-expressing cell population proliferates to a large number of cells by a relatively early embryonic age. As previously suggested, the distribution of H/O neurons is intermediate between that of mammalian and non-mammalian vertebrates. This work suggests that, in addition to its roles in developed brains, the H/O peptide may play an important role in the early embryonic development of non-mammalian vertebrates.

Editor: Hubert Vaudry, University of Rouen, France, France

Funding: This work was supported by the G. W. Stairs Fund, the McGill Startup funds and the RGP0004/2013 Human Frontiers Science Program grant to MP. The funders have no role in study design, data collection and analysis, decision to publish, or preparation of the manuscript.

Competing Interests: The authors have declared that no competing interests exist.

* Email: maria.pompeiano@mcgill.ca

¤ Current address: Biomedical Sciences, University of Edinburgh, Edinburgh, Scotland, United Kingdom

Introduction

Hypocretins/Orexins (H/Os) are neuropeptides produced by a relatively small number of neurons in the vertebrate hypothalamus (hypocretin 1 and 2 and orexin A and B are independently-coined names that refer to the same peptides) [1], [2]. H/O peptides and their precursors are strongly conserved among higher vertebrates [3], with chicken sequences clustering closely with those of mammals and other tetrapods, while fish sequences are less conserved [4]. The location of H/O neurons in the hypothalamus is also conserved in all vertebrates examined thus far [3]. Mammalian H/O neurons are contained within the dorsal and lateral hypothalamus [5–7]. In amphibians, reptiles and fishes, H/O neurons show a more restricted medial periventricular distribution [4], [8–10]. In birds, H/O neurons show a distribution pattern that is intermediate between that of mammals and other tetrapods. They are located medially within the paraventricular hypothalamic nucleus, extending into the lateral hypothalamic area [11–13] (the terminology used throughout the present paper follows the nomenclature of [14]).

H/O neurons play a critical functional role in the regulation of behavioral arousal and brain state changes in mammals. H/O neurons are generally active during waking and virtually silent during sleep [15–17], and promote sleep-to-waking transitions [18]. They also regulate several other physiological functions, stimulating locomotion, feeding, food reward, metabolism, thermogenesis, the neuroendocrine axis, respiration, and the cardiovascular sympathetic and gastrointestinal vagal systems [19]. It has therefore been suggested that H/O neurons act as global activators of a broad range of brain systems [20–22]. The conservation of the distribution pattern of H/O fibers also suggests a conservation of H/O function among vertebrates [8–10]. H/Os induce arousal in neonatal chickens [23] and larval zebrafish [24], and stimulate feeding and locomotion in fish [4].

Mammalian embryos do not show any signs of a waking-like state being present before birth [25]. Accordingly, they appear to produce H/O peptides late in the gestation period, presumably in preparation for post-natal life. H/O neurons are first detected at about 80-85% of the gestation period in rats [26], [27]. If H/O peptides function primarily after birth, one might expect precocial mammalian species like sheep to start their H/O expression at roughly the same proportion of the way through embryonic development as altricial mammalian species like rats. Sheep fetuses show a good number of H/O neurons and high cerebrospinal fluid levels of H/O by about 85% of gestation [28], suggesting that H/O expression may actually start at earlier embryonic ages in sheep. However, no work to date has directly addressed this question. Fish embryo brains start expressing H/O mRNA between the cleavage and segmentation stages [29–31], approximately midway between zygote formation and their larval stage, and it is therefore likely that these peptides are being released at earlier developmental stages than in mammals [32], [33]. Since signs of sleep behavior do not appear until well into the larval stage at about 5 days post-fertilization [24], (an)other role(s) for H/O in fish embryo development is(are) likely. It has previously been suggested that H/Os may be involved "in the complex energy balance during the hatching process" [30]. A direct role in brain embryonic developmental processes also cannot be excluded.

Bird embryos, unlike those of mammals but like those of many fish, are biologically independent from physiological changes that may occur in their mother's body during their entire incubation period. While previous researchers have examined the embryonic development of chicken hypothalamic peptidergic systems [34–37], no information has previously been made available about the development of H/O. We therefore investigated H/O expression in the brains of chick embryos using immunohistochemistry. We were particularly interested in whether H/O neurons in bird embryos emerge at relatively earlier developmental stages (as in fish embryos) or later stages (as in mammalian embryos).

Embryos were examined at ages ranging from embryonic day (E) 3 (~14% of gestation) until the day before hatching (E20, ~95% of the way through gestation). We extended our neuroanatomical studies to post-natal day (P) 1 and P21 chicks to examine possible differences between pre- and post-natal brains. By E3, the diencephalon is clearly distinguishable in the anterior part of the neural tube [38]. Neurogenesis starts around E4 (~19% of gestation), when cells abandon the proliferative ventricular zone and form a less dense, post-proliferative mantle zone [39]. Cells then disperse in the mantle zone following migration [40]. Our work thus covers a time span that includes the major neuronal production and migration phases of the chick hypothalamus.

Methods

Ethics statement

The experimental protocol for the use of chick embryos was submitted to the McGill University Animal Compliance Office, which, after consultation with the McGill University Animal Care Committee, issued a written waiver stating that according to Canadian and McGill University animal care guidelines, no formal approval was necessary to perform these experiments. McGill Standard Operating Procedures were followed to minimize any possible suffering by embryos. The experimental use and care of P1 and P21 chicks was approved by the McGill University Animal Care Committee.

Tissue collection

Fertilized chicken eggs (Bovans brown; Couvoir Simetin, Mirabel, QC) were incubated in a commercial egg incubator (Brinsea Octagon, Brinsea Products Inc., Titusville, FL) using constant conditions (37.5°C; 60% relative humidity). Some eggs were incubated until hatching and the chicks were sacrificed within 24 hours after hatching. Brown P21 chicks were commercially obtained (Couvoir Simetin). Embryos were deeply anesthetized by exposing the egg to isoflurane vapors. P1 and P21 chicks were also deeply anesthetized with isoflurane. E3, E4, E5 and E6 embryos were extracted from the egg and immersion fixed in 10% formalin/PBS for 24 hrs at 4°C. Older embryos (E8, E10, E12, E14, E16, E18 and E20) and P1 and P21 chicks were transcardially perfused with Howard Ringer's solution (123 mM NaCl, 1.5 mM, 5 mM KCl; 2 min) and then with 10% formalin/1× chick embryology PBS (150 mM NaCl, 2.8 mM KH_2PO_4, 7.2 mM K_2HPO_4; 10 min) using a peristaltic pump set at a flow rate appropriate for each age (1–15 mL/min). The heads were kept in 10% formalin/1× chick embryology PBS at 4°C overnight. Brains from E10–E20 embryos and P1 and P21 chicks were extracted from the skull. The basal part of the skull containing the pituitary gland was retained for E12, E16 and E20 embryos.

Whole embryos (ages E3–E6), heads (age E8) and the isolated brains and skull bases (ages E10–E20, P1, P21) were cryoprotected in 10% sucrose/1× chick embryology PBS for 1 day and in 30% sucrose/1× chick embryology PBS for 2–3 days until they sank. They were then frozen at -65°C and cut into 40 µm thick coronal sections at a cryostat (Leica CM3050; Leica Microsystem Canada, Richmond Hill, ON). All sections were collected and deposited on glass slides and kept at −65°C.

We examined the brains from E3–E8 with n = 3 embryos for each age, from E10–E20 with n = 4 embryos for each age and from P1 and P21 with n = 4 and n = 2 chicks, respectively. The pituitary gland was examined at E6 (when it first became distinguishable) with n = 3 embryos, E8 (n = 3), E12 (n = 2), E16 (n = 3) and E20 (n = 4).

Immunohistochemistry, quantification procedures and statistical analyses

Immunohistochemical staining of every other section was performed following standard protocols. Slides were incubated with blocking solution containing 10% normal horse serum, 2% bovine serum albumine, 0.5% Triton X-100 in 1×PBS (137 mM NaCl, 1.5 mM KCl, 8 mM Na_2HPO_4, 2.7 KH_2PO_4, pH 7.4; 1 hour at room temperature, RT), a goat polyclonal anti-H1/OA primary antibody (Santa Cruz Biotechnologies, sc-8070; 1:500 in blocking solution; overnight at RT), a biotinylated secondary antibody (Vector Labs; 1:500 in blocking solution; 1 hour at RT), the avidin-peroxidase complex (Vector Labs; 1:200 in 1×PBS containing also 0.5% Triton X-100; 1 hour at RT) and 3,3′-diaminobenzidine (Sigma) as a revelation system. Omission of the primary antibody or preincubation of the primary antibody with the blocking peptide (Santa Cruz Biotechnologies, sc-8070P; following company protocol) did not yield any labeling. The primary antibody also recognizes H2/OB but does not recognize the precursor protein (Technical Service, Santa Cruz Biotechnology, Inc.; personal communication and antibody datasheet).

All quantification procedures were conducted blindly with reference to the source of the sections. The total number of labeled cells was estimated using a Leica DM6000 B microscope with the 20X objective lens and the computer-assisted optical fractionator method of stereology using Stereo Investigator (Version 10.04.2, MicroBrightField, Inc., Williston, VT). Within each brain section, contours were traced around clusters of labeled cells in the hypothalamus. Each contour was quantified in its entirety using side by side counting frames. Following set inclusion and exclusion boundaries on each counting frame reduced the possibility of counting the same cell twice. Sections that were damaged or lost were considered missing. The total number of cells was then extrapolated taking into account the sections that were not labeled. Kruskal-Wallis ANOVAs with posthoc tests corrected for multiple comparisons [41] were used to evaluate the significance of differences among mean cell number values at the various developmental stages.

The cranio-caudal extension of the H/O hypothalamic area was estimated by multiplying the total number of sections containing H/O neurons by 2 (we labeled every other slide) and by the 40 µm section thickness. Kruskal-Wallis ANOVAs with posthoc tests corrected for multiple comparisons [41] were used to evaluate the statistical significance of differences among mean extension values at the various developmental stages.

Antibody specificity

The supplier has not validated the primary antibody used in this study (sc-8070) by Western blot in any animal species. It has been used for immunohistochemical studies in both mammalian and non-mammalian species. In some of these species, the antibody specificity was established by comparison with another antibody of known specificity [42]. In other cases, the immunostaining was accompanied by a Western blot using an antibody against prepro-H/O [43]. In one case, the antibody was reported to have "passed the Western blotting test" but details were not provided about the test [44]. The low molecular weight and low expression levels of the H/O peptides makes their visualization with Western blot challenging. We are not aware of any other published Western blot analysis using the same antibody we used here (sc-8070) in any animal species. Using a different antibody from ours, H1/OA was detectable in the hypothalamus of transgenic mice overexpressing prepro-H/O, while no band was seen in wild-type mice [45].

The specificity of the antibody used here in chicken embryo brains is suggested by the sequence analysis described below. We were also able to demonstrate it directly by Western blot analysis [46].

Sequence analysis. The anti-H1/OA primary antibody was raised against a 19 residue peptide mapping at the C-terminus of the human H1/OA (aminoacids 48–66 of the human precursor protein). The immunogen shares 84% sequence identity with both H1/OA and H2/OB of *Gallus gallus* origin (protein accession # NP_989516.1). The immunogen sequence was entered into DELTA-BLAST [47] and the only sequence in the *Gallus gallus* proteome producing significant alignments is that of prepro-H/O (protein accession # NP_989516.1), at the level of amino acids 43–61 (E value 2e-9; corresponding to the C-terminus of the H1/OA sequence) and 74–91 (E value 1e-8; corresponding to the C-terminus of the H2/OB sequence). This analysis suggests that the sequence recognized by the antibody is very specific to the two H/O peptides.

Western blot analysis. Fertilized chicken eggs (Bovans brown; Couvoir Simetin, Mirabel, QC) were incubated as above. E20 embryos in the egg ($n = 8$) were anesthetized with isoflurane, extracted from the egg and decapitated. The brains were quickly extracted and frozen at −75°C. The hypothalamus was dissected from the frozen brain on a cryostat in two different ways: a) the whole posterior hypothalamus ($n = 4$); b) a more precise dissection of the posterior hypothalamus excluding areas in its dorsolateral part and in its more posterior parts which do not contain H/O cells ($n = 4$). Brain sections were cut just before and after dissection, fixed and then stained with Cresyl Violet to confirm the proper dissection of the hypothalamus.

Each dissected hypothalamus was homogenized in ice-cold HEPES-buffered sucrose buffer (20 mM HEPES, 320 mM Sucrose, 1.0 mM EDTA, 2.0 mM EGTA, pH 7.4) supplemented with protease inhibitor cocktail (Pierce). Synaptosomes were prepared by a sucrose-density gradient centrifugation method [48]. Protein concentration from total homogenate and synaptosomal fraction was determined by a bicinchonic acid assay (Pierce). Samples (40 µg of total protein/lane) were mixed with 2X loading Sample buffer (200 mM Tris-HCl pH 6.8, 40% glycerol, 2% SDS, 0.04% Coomasie blue, 2% β-mercaptoethanol), incubated at 37°C for 15 min and loaded on a Tricine 10–20% gel (BioRad) for SDS-PAGE with Tris-Tricine SDS running buffer [49]. Blocking peptide solutions (sc-8070P; 0.1 µg/lane) were treated with the same protocol and loaded on separate lanes. Proteins were transferred onto PVDF membranes (0.2 uM pore size, Millipore) at 4°C and at 20 V for 18 h. Membranes were blocked with 3% BSA in Tris-buffered saline containing 0.1% Tween 20 (TBS-T) and incubated with the anti-H1/OA antibody (sc-8070; 1:500) in TBS-T for 1 hour at RT. After 3 washes in TBS-T, the membranes were incubated with HRP-conjugated anti-goat secondary antibody (Millipore; 1:5000) in TBS-T for 1 h at RT, followed by 3 washes in TBS-T. Membranes were treated with enhanced chemiluminiscence (ECL) Plus Western blotting substrate (Pierce) or SuperSignal West Femto Chemiluminescent Substrate (Pierce) and subsequently exposed to autoradiography film or scanned with a Storm Laser Scanner (Molecular Dynamics).

We inconsistently detected a faint band at ~3 kDa corresponding to the processed H/O peptides in the fresh synaptosomal fraction, but never in the total homogenate obtained from dissected whole hypothalamus. H/O peptide concentration in the adult rat hypothalamus is about 10^{-6} g/g of total proteins [50]. We loaded 40 µg of total hypothalamic protein/lane and we were not able to detect a consistent H/O band using a sensitive revelation system that has a detection limit of 40 pg of protein/lane. This suggests that H/O levels in the chick E20 posterior hypothalamus are lower than in the adult rat and below the detection limit for Western blot analysis.

With the more precise dissection of the hypothalamus, we were able to reliably obtain a band at ~3 kDa (Figure 1, left panel). The antibody did not recognize any other protein from the tissue extracts including the chicken pro-H/O, in agreement with the antibody data sheet and information provided (Santa Cruz Biotechnology, Inc. Technical Service). It recognized the 19 amino-acid blocking peptide as a ~1.5–2 kDa band (Figure 1, left panel). Preincubation of the primary antibody with the blocking peptide (sc-8070P; following company protocol) did not yield any band (Figure 1, right panel).

Results

Neuronal and glial precursors and differentiating cells can be distinguished during development based on ultrastructural features observed with electron microscopy [51], or by the expression of selective markers [52]. Until E4-E5, cells in the proliferative ventricular zone are still capable of division and considered undifferentiated [51]. Once they stop dividing, cells leave the ventricular zone and move to the developing mantle zone where they undergo migration and differentiation [39]. Since we did not perform either one of the above-mentioned analyses to assess the developmental status of H/O-labeled cells, we refer to them as "cells" at earlier ages. Starting from E10 inclusive, we call them

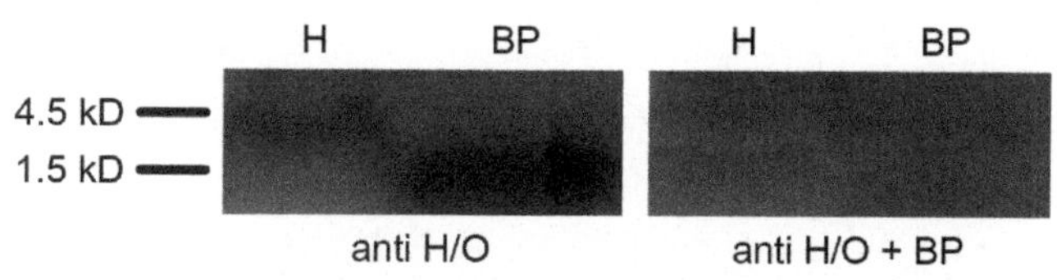

Figure 1. Western blot analysis of the anti-H1/OA antibody in the chick embryo hypothalamus. Synaptosomal preparations from the dissected hypothalamus from an E20 chick embryo (H; 40 µg of proteins) and the blocking peptide (BP; 10 µg) were loaded. The anti-H1/OA antibody binds to a hypothalamic peptide (~3 kDa) and to the blocking peptide (~1.5–2 kDa) (anti H/O; left panel). Preincubation of the anti H1/OA antibody with the blocking peptide does not yield any band (anti H/O + BP; right panel).

"neurons" because of the presence of H/O-positive varicose terminals (axons) in the hypothalamus.

The overall developmental pattern of H/O cells

Cells start producing H/O peptide at extremely early ages in chicken embryos. H/O cells were already detectable by E3, the youngest age we examined. We counted ~1000 labelled cells at this age (14% of P1 values; Table 1). We were not able to reliably count H/O cells at the ages of E4-E6, because labeled cells became very densely packed and often indistinguishable as independent entities using light microscopy in our immersion fixed preparations. We systematically quantified labeled cell numbers starting from E8 (Table 1, Figure 2, A), the youngest age at which embryos were perfused. The estimated number of H/O cells was already high at E8 and E10 (~4000–4500; 62–67% of P1 values), with a significant increase to ~5500 (77% of P1 values; E12), ~6000 (87% of P1 values; E14), ~6500 (95% of P1 values; E16) by about 3/4 of the way through the incubation period. Values were still high at ~6200 at E18 (91% of P1 values). A decrease (significant with respect to E16) was then seen at E20 (~5800 H/O cells; 85% of P1 values) while the value at P1 reached ~6900 H/O cells. The cranio-caudal spatial extent of the hypothalamic area containing H/O cells was also estimated for all ages (Table 1; Figure 2, B). At E3 it was about 0.5 mm, significantly increasing over the period including E6 and E8, when a value of about 1.5 mm was obtained. A significant increase was later seen at E14, when a plateau was reached at a value of about 2 mm. (Our examination of the P21 chicks was limited to the description of H/O neuronal distribution; no H/O neuron counts were performed at this later age).

From E3-E6, cells begin expressing H/O peptides before they migrate from the ventral proliferative zone, and change the orientation of their neurites as they migrate laterally

At **E3**, H/O cells were seen at medial locations in the ventral part of the ventricular zone of the diencephalon and distributed in clusters (Figure 3, A). The cranio-caudal level corresponds to that of the optic stalk. Labeled cells were seen in the outer third/half of the thickness of the ventricular zone. They were round in shape with a big nucleus surrounded by a thin and unevenly labeled cytosol. Some of these cells also showed short labeled neurites that ran towards the outer surface of the neural tube. From here, these labeled neurites were occasionally seen turning in a laterodorsal direction. At **E4** and **E5**, labeled cells were seen concentrated in two discrete groups in the diencephalic wall, one along the ventral midline and the other more dorsally at about 1/3 of the total ventrodorsal extension of the diencephalic wall (Figure 3, B). H/O cells had a roundish shape, were more strongly labeled than at E3, and had short, strongly-labeled neurites. Cranially, H/O cells first appeared at the level of the optic stalk (levels d, c and b of plate 84 in [38]). They were located in the outer third/half of the diencephalic wall at more anterior and ventral levels with mostly radially-oriented neurites. More posteriorly and more dorsally, a few labeled cells were seen in the diencephalic wall with radially-oriented neurites (Figure 3, B). Most H/O cells were seen just outside the ventricular zone of the diencephalon intermingled with fibers and unlabeled cells in the developing mantle zone. The orientation of their labeled neurites changed from strictly radial (closest to the diencephalic wall) to a variety of directions (more laterally) (Figure 3, B).

By **E6**, H/O cells were still roundish in shape and their neurites were longer than at younger ages (except at the most cranial and medial levels). Starting cranially at the level of the optic nerves, strongly labeled cells were seen along the midline in the ventral part of the diencephalic wall, between the ventricular zone and a thick fiber layer corresponding to the developing optic chiasm

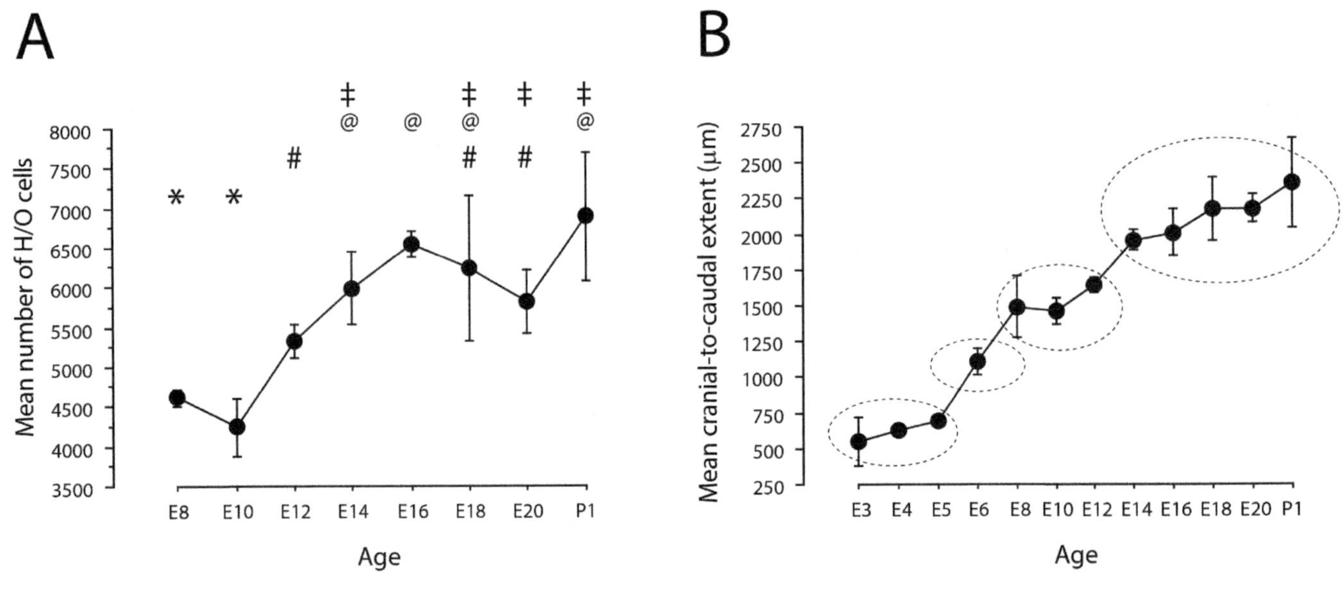

Figure 2. Mean number of H/O neurons (A) and their cranio-caudal spatial extent (in μm) (B) in the brains of embryos at different ages. Bars represent ± 1 SEM and n = 4 for all ages, except for incubation periods of 8 days or less, where n = 3. For each graph, points that do not share symbols above them are significantly different from each other at the $p<0.05$ level, two-tailed, corrected for multiple comparisons (Kruskal-Wallis ANOVA; H = 15.96, df = 6, $p = 0.014$ in A; H = 33.05, df = 10, $p = 0.0003$ in B).

Table 1. Total number (mean per animal) of H/O positive cells found in the entire hypothalamus, and cranio-caudal spatial extent (in μm) of the hypothalamic area containing H/O cells at different ages.

Age	n	Total number of H/O cells (mean ± SEM)	Cranio-caudal extent (μm; mean ± SEM)
E3	3	964 ± 417	547 ± 170
E4	3	nc	627 ± 35
E5	3	nc	693 ± 35
E6	3	nc	1107 ± 93
E8	3	4614 ± 114	1493 ± 218
E10	4	4242 ± 359	1460 ± 89
E12	4	5333 ± 217	1640 ± 52
E14	4	5994 ± 450	1960 ± 69
E16	4	6544 ± 164	2010 ± 162
E18	4	6236 ± 913	2180 ± 222
E20	4	5825 ± 392	2180 ± 100
P1	4	6889 ± 812	2360 ± 314

n: number of animals; nc: not collected; SEM: Standard Error of the Mean.

(Figure 3, C). Their neurites had a radial orientation. More caudally, H/O cells were not strongly labeled and were present more dorsally and bilaterally in the thicker mantle zone of the ventral part of the diencephalon. Their neurites had a radial orientation. At the caudalmost levels, a patch of strongly labeled H/O cells was seen bilaterally in the diencephalic wall, above the third ventricle enlargement (Figure 3, D). The medial-most cells (closer to the proliferative zone) were generally less strongly labeled than the more lateral cells, and their labeled neurites had a radial orientation. The more laterally-located cells had neurites extending in diverse directions.

From E8-E20, H/O cells populate the developing hypothalamus

At **E8**, the optic chiasm becomes prominent and marks the most cranial location at which H/O cells were seen. At this level, labeled cells were seen around the ventral tip of the 3rd ventricle, just outside the densely packed circumventricular proliferative zone. A few cells were seen more dorsally and bilaterally, along the ventral half of the 3rd ventricle. These cells had neurites that were oriented in a ventro-dorsal direction. About 200–300 μm more caudally, a bigger concentration of H/O cells was seen bilaterally half-way up the 3rd ventricle with neurites oriented in different directions. A few cells were present also in ventrolateral locations with neurites oriented in a dorsomedial-to-ventrolateral direction. H/O cells were rather roundish and not very strongly labeled at these cranial-most levels. More caudally, H/O cells were still seen in great numbers bilaterally next to the 3rd ventricle about half way up, with neurites oriented in different directions. A great number of labeled cells were also seen extending in ventrolateral directions with neurites oriented in dorsomedial-to-ventrolateral directions. More strongly-labeled cells with elongated shapes and strongly-labeled neurites were seen at these more caudal and ventrolateral locations.

By **E10** and **E12**, a small number of labeled neurons remained close to the circumventricular proliferative zones (Figure 4, top panel). A few labeled neurons were found scattered bilaterally along the 3rd ventricle; these were more concentrated at more dorsal levels (Figure 4, top two panels), with neurites oriented in different directions. At E12, these neurons were much more abundant than at E10. More caudally, labeled neurons also extended in a ventrolateral direction, with neurites oriented in dorsomedial-to-ventrolateral directions. The area containing labeled neurons had an inverted V shape, with the vertex located in the middle third of the 3rd ventricle (Figures 4, bottom panel and 5, A). H/O neurons showed an elongated shape with strongly-labeled cell bodies and neurites (Figure 5, C). H/O-positive varicose terminals were first seen in the hypothalamus at E10.

At **E14**, the hippocampal (pallial) commissure became visible above the 3rd ventricle. Starting from this age, H/O neurons were found starting just posterior to it. H/O neurons showed multiple labeled neurites, and were bigger and rounder than at earlier ages, especially in ventrolateral and posterior locations. Cranial H/O neurons were seen in small numbers mostly in a medial position lining the ventral half of the 3rd ventricle at **E16** (Figure 4, first panel from the top) and **E18**. Neurons here had their main neurites oriented in a dorsoventral direction. At more caudal levels, a high concentration of labeled neurons was seen lateral to the 3rd ventricle at **E16** (Figure 4, second and third panels from the top) and **E18**. These neurons had their main neurites oriented in various directions. From here, H/O neurons also extended in a ventrolateral direction, filling an area with an inverted V shape (Figure 4, second-fourth panels from the top), with neurites oriented in the same direction.

At **E20**, a few labelled cells were still seen around the ventral end of the 3rd ventricle (Figure 6, top panel). There appeared to be more H/O neurons than at earlier ages located at the most anterior levels, lining the ventral half of the 3rd ventricle, corresponding to the developing rostral part of the hypothalamic paraventricular nucleus (Figure 6, top two panels). At more posterior levels, H/O neurons were seen in regions corresponding to the magnocellular and parvocellular parts of the developing paraventricular nucleus, and in the periventricular stratum. From here, labeled neurons extended ventrolaterally into an area that included the developing posterior hypothalamic nucleus and lateral hypothalamic area, filling an area with an inverted V shape (Figures 5, B and 6, bottom two panels). There also appeared to be more H/O neurons in ventrolateral locations at E20 than at earlier ages. H/O neurons showed a more roundish shape and a stronger labeling than at E10 (Figure 5, D).

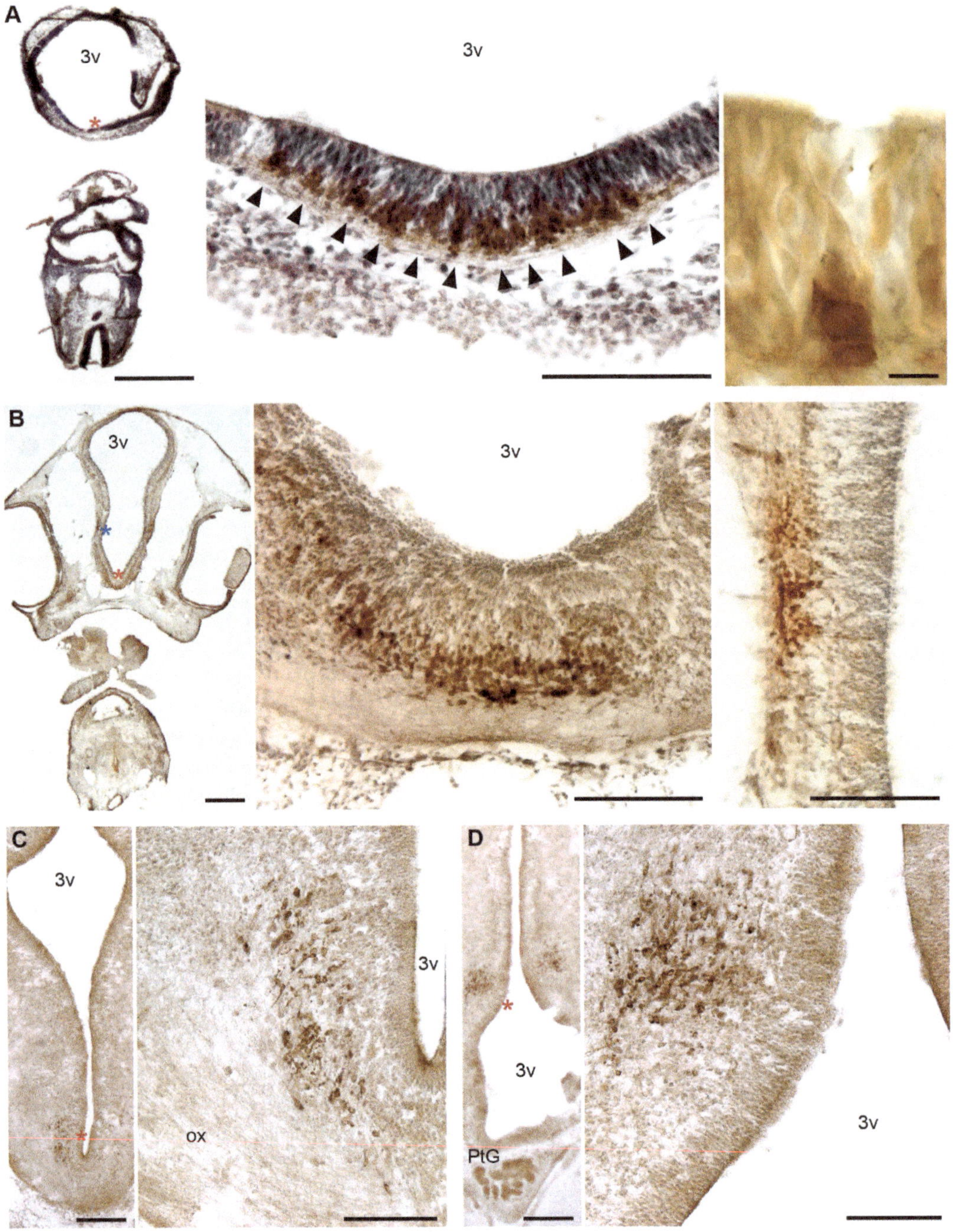

Figure 3. H/O cells in chick embryos at earlier ages (E3–E6). H/O cells appear brown. In A, the left panel shows a low-magnification view of an E3 embryo coronal section stained for H/O and counterstained with Cresyl Violet. The star indicates the ventral part of the diencephalic vesicle that is shown at higher magnification in the middle panel. H/O cells appear grouped in clusters (arrows). The right panel show one of these clusters of labelled cells at higher magnification in a consecutive section that was not counterstained with Cresyl Violet. In B, the left panel shows a low-magnification view of an E4 embryo coronal section stained for H/O. The stars indicate two locations in the ventral part of the diencephalic vesicle that are shown at higher magnification in the central (red star) and right (blue star) panels. In C and D, the left panels show a low-magnification view of an E6 embryo coronal section stained for H/O at two different levels. At more anterior levels (C), the star indicates a labeled ventral region that is shown at higher magnification in the right panel. At more posterior levels (D), the star indicates a labeled region in a more dorsal location, shown at higher magnification in the right panel. 3v: 3rd ventricle; ox: optic chiasm; PtG: pituitary gland. Scale bars are 500 μm (A–D, left panels), 10 μm (A, right panel), and 100 μm (A–D, other panels).

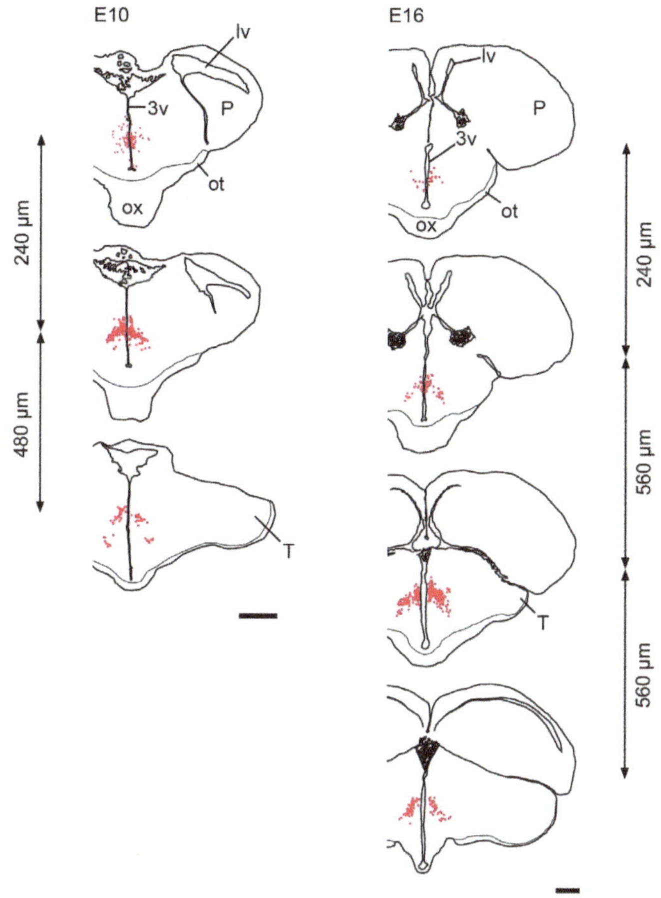

Figure 4. Distribution of H/O neurons (red dots) in the hypothalamus of E10 (left column) and E16 chick embryos (right column). The most cranial level is shown on top and the most caudal one on the bottom. The distance between consecutive levels is indicated on the side. 3v: 3rd ventricle; lv: lateral ventricle; ot: optic tract; ox: optic chiasm; P: pallium; T: tectum. Scale bars are 1 mm.

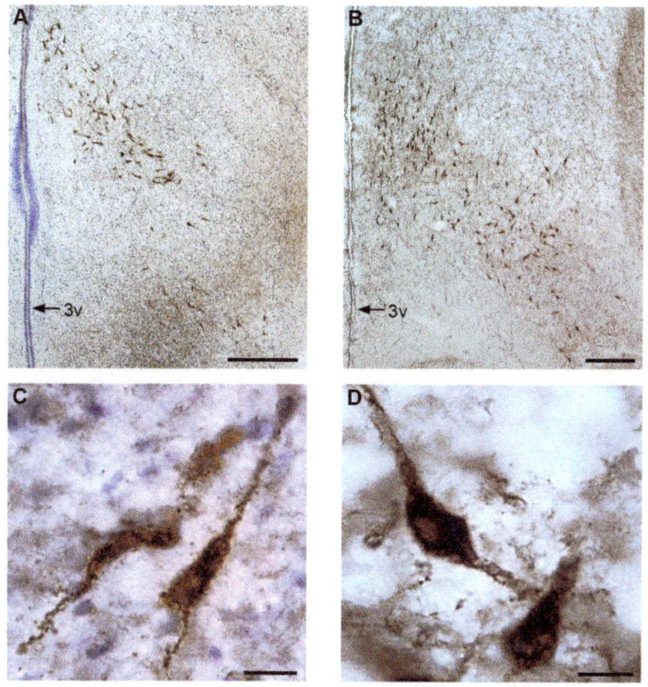

Figure 5. H/O neurons in E10 and E20 chicken embryos. H/O neurons appear brown. Coronal sections of the caudal portions of the hypothalamus show the distribution of labeled neurons in a representative E10 embryo at low (A) and at high magnification (C) and in a representative E20 embryo at low (B) and at high magnification (D). The sections from the E10 embryo were counterstained with Cresyl Violet to better identify the brain structures. The inverted V-shape distribution of H/O neurons is evident at both ages. Labeled neurons appear bigger and more strongly labeled at E20 than E10. 3v: 3rd ventricle. Scale bars are 200 µm (A, B) and 10 µm (C, D).

At P1 and P21, the spatial distribution of H/O neurons is unchanged with respect to E20

At **P1**, the spatial distribution of H/O neurons was similar to what was described at E20, including a few labelled cells around the ventral end of the 3rd ventricle.

At **P21**, brain size was substantially increased with respect to E20 and P1, but the spatial distribution of H/O neurons in the posterior hypothalamus was the same. At more anterior levels, labelled neurons were found in a medial location close to the 3rd ventricle in the paraventricular hypothalamic nucleus and in the periventricular stratum (Figure 6, top two panels). At more posterior levels, labelled neurons were distributed in ventrolateral locations corresponding with the posterior hypothalamic nucleus and lateral hypothalamic area, filling an area with an inverted V shape (Figure 6, bottom two panels). No H/O neurons were detected around the ventral end of the 3rd ventricle.

H/O labeling did not enter the developing pituitary gland

A few H/O labeled cells were seen in the infundibulum at E6. This is not surprising, since this structure is continuous with the one lining the ventral part of the 3rd ventricle, where H/O neurons appear to come from. At E6, a few labeled cells were also seen in the epithelium of the distal part of Rathke's pouch, in close proximity to the developing pituitary gland. Despite a careful search, we could not detect any labeled fibers in the pituitary gland at any of the ages we examined. Well-stained H/O varicose fibers were seen in the infundibulum at E12, E16 and E20.

Discussion

Using an anti-H1/OA antibody whose molecular specificity was confirmed with Western blot analysis, we have quantified the development of H/O-positive cells in the brain of chick embryos. In agreement with the present results, H/O neurons have previously been described in post-natal chickens at similar locations using in-situ hybridization [11],[53] (compare Figure 6, bottom two panels with Figure 3 from [11] and Figure 1 from [53]).

By E3, five regions can be distinguished in the anterior part of the neural tube (telencephalon, diencephalon, mesencephalon, metencephalon and myelencephalon), the telencephalic vesicles are developing, and the cranial and cervical flexures have appeared in the chick embryo [38]. Neurogenesis then starts around E4 (~19% of gestation), when cells abandon the proliferative ventricular zone and form a less dense, post-proliferative mantle zone [39]. Cells then disperse in the mantle zone following radial and tangential migration [40]. Hypothalamic neurons are generated mostly from the ventricular zone lining the third ventricle in the embryonic diencephalon [54]. The hypothalamus is generated with an outside-inside pattern, with three successive but overlapping waves of neurons giving origin to the

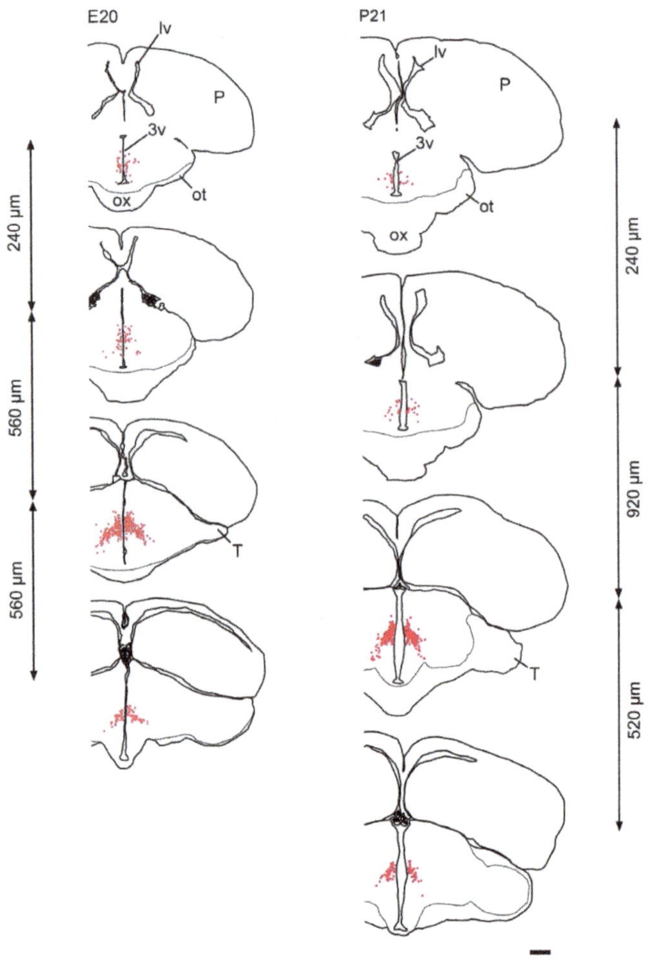

Figure 6. Distribution of H/O neurons (red dots) in the hypothalamus of E20 chick embryos (left column) and P21 chicks (right column). The most cranial level is shown on top and the most caudal one on the bottom. The distance between consecutive levels is indicated on the side. 3v: 3rd ventricle; lv: lateral ventricle; ot: optic tract; ox: optic chiasm; P: pallium; T: tectum. Scale bar is the same for both columns and is 1 mm.

lateral/reticular, the core and the midline hypothalamus, respectively [54]. Previous work on the neuroendocrine system in the posterior hypothalamus of chick embryos has described how different types of parvocellular and magnocellular neurons are first detected starting around E5 [55]. The present work thus covers a time span that includes the major neuronal production for and migration into the chick hypothalamus.

The main result from the present work is that H/O cells appear to be the first neurochemically distinct population to become detectable in the developing chick embryo hypothalamus (by E3 or earlier). These cells start producing H/O when they are still in the ventricular zone.

Chicken H/O neurons appear to originate from 2 different locations in the diencephalic proliferative zone

Chicken H/O cells are already detectable by E3 in the external part of the ventricular zone of the 3rd ventricle. Previous work has shown that the initial migration of neurons from this proliferative zone is strictly radial, with non-radial migration seen only outside of the ventricular zone starting from E5 in the developing chick diencephalon [56]. The location of the labeled cells at E3–E4 should therefore indicate their site of origin in the proliferating diencephalic wall. It appears that there are 2 separate locations in the proliferative epithelium lining the 3rd ventricle where H/O cells originate: an anterior/ventral/medial location and a more posterior/dorsal/bilateral location. Based upon the position and morphology of labeled cells around these proliferative zones, the ventromedial zone seems to still generate H/O cells until at least P1. The present results cannot exclude the possibility that they may also generate cells (perhaps for a more prolonged period of time) that do not start expressing H/O peptide until later on, as seen in rats [26], [27], [57]. This early start of H/O production in the chick diencephalon should facilitate the identification of possible H/O-neuronal fate determinants.

Migrating H/O cells appear to follow two different migratory paths

Since this study used only coronal brain sections, it is only possible to make inferences about the migration of H/O cells in the dorsoventral direction (observable within sections) but not in the cranio-caudal direction (going between sections). Previous observations suggest that neurites of developing hypothalamic neurons appear "at the time and place of non-radial migration" [56], and that cells migrate along the direction assumed by their cellular processes [56]. The orientation of the neurites should therefore indicate the direction of cell migration. Chicken embryo H/O cells originating from the ventromedial proliferative zone thus appear to migrate dorsally along the 3rd ventricle; these may represent the main source of the most medial (and anterior) group of H/O neurons. These H/O neurons may also reach more dorsal positions and contribute to the intermediate dorsal concentration of H/O neurons, together with the neurons originating from the more dorsal proliferative zone. H/O cells in this intermediate dorsal group show neurites with different orientations, some in the dorsoventral direction and others in a mediolateral direction (within a single section). H/O cells originating from the more dorsal proliferative zone might instead represent the main source of the more caudal neurons concentrated in the ventrolateral locations in the hypothalamus. Since the ventromedial proliferative zone seems to produce H/O cells until later developmental times, the consequence is that H/O neurons in the intermediate dorsal position (corresponding in part to the paraventricular hypothalamic nucleus) would be generated later than those in the ventrolateral position (corresponding to the lateral hypothalamic area). This would be in accordance with what has been observed in rats [54].

Interestingly, the two patterns of migrations proposed here for H/O cells (in a ventral-to-dorsal direction along the 3rd ventricle and in a dorsomedial-to-ventrolateral direction) have been described for cells giving rise to other hypothalamic areas in mice [58]. An alternative hypothesis is that H/O cells could migrate just laterally from their site of origin in the ventromedial proliferative zone and reach the ventrolateral locations. This hypothesis is contradicted by the complete lack of H/O cells showing neurites oriented in mediolateral directions within this area or present in intermediate positions between the ventromedial proliferative zone and ventrolateral positions. However, in order for the migratory pathway of H/O cells to be established with certainty, further experiments using specific neuronal markers for tracking cell movements in vivo will be necessary. Early expression of H/O provides a tool for the identification of this cell population in chick embryos.

Chickens appear to produce more H/O neurons at earlier times in embryonic development than rats do

The present experiments showed that chicken H/O neurons express peptide from the earliest ages examined (E3, 14% of the embryonic period) and that the number of H/O neurons increases during chick embryonic development up to a maximal value of about 6500 around age E16 (about 75% of the fetal period). A similar number of H/O cells were seen at P1. At E20, we observed a small decrease in H/O cells which was significant with respect to E16 (but not to E18 or P1). Further experiments are needed in order to ascertain whether cell death could contribute to this phenomenon.

Among mammals, the development of H/O neurons has been mostly studied in rats; the data vary among studies. Wistar rats appear to reach a maximum of ~2500 H/O neurons during the 9th–10th postnatal week in one study [59] and to have ~6700 neurons in another study (rats of 200–250 g) [60]. Values of 3500–4000 have been reported for "adult" Sprague-Dawley rats [61], an unidentified strain [62] and Flinders Sensitive and Flinders Resistant Line rats [63]. Most of these values are notably lower than those we obtained in chick embryos, suggesting that H/O neurons may play a more prominent role in the development of bird embryos with respect to mammalian embryos (see below).

In rats, H/O neurons are generated in one sharp peak around E12 [64] (~55% of gestation) but they only become detectable by immunohistochemistry starting at E18 (~82% of gestation) using an anti-prepro-peptide antibody [27], or E19 (~86% of gestation) using an anti-H2/OB antibody [26], or after P10 using an anti-H1/OA antibody [57]. At these stages the H/O neurons are already well-developed, as demonstrated by the contemporaneous detection of labelled fibers in the hypothalamus and locus coeruleus [26], [27]. While an exact determination of when the H/O neurons that function in the developed brain are generated in chick embryos requires birthdating experiments, H/O peptides are clearly being produced at earlier ages than in rats.

Comparison with the development of H/O neurons in non-rodent mammalian and non-mammalian species

As mentioned in the Introduction, sheep fetuses show a sizeable number of H/O neurons by about 85% of gestation [28]. The presence of high cerebrospinal fluid levels of H/O at the same age suggests that H/O expression actually starts at earlier embryonic ages in sheep; however, no work to date has addressed this question. Similarly, in another relatively precocial species, the pig, prepro-H/O mRNA is detectable in fetuses at 93% of gestation but no younger ages were examined. More research is needed into the development of H/O neurons in precocial mammals, like sheep and guinea pigs, to understand whether H/O expression in embryos varies as a function of developmental pattern.

Although H/O expression was first found here at the segmentation stage in chick embryos, in fish it has been reported to start earlier, in stages ranging from the cleavage stage in the Atlantic cod [31], to the neurula stage in the orange-spotted grouper [30] and the segmentation stage in zebrafish [29]. Future work is needed to demonstrate how early H/O expression actually starts in chickens and other birds.

H/O neurons in chickens are distributed differently within the hypothalamus than in other animal species

In adult vertebrates, H/O neurons are mostly found in the hypothalamus, but differences occur among different species. In chickens, the majority of H/O neurons are distributed in a dorsomedial position in the paraventricular and posterior hypothalamic nuclei. A lower density of H/O neurons is found extending in a ventrolateral position (into the lateral hypothalamic area). A smaller but significant number of neurons is present in ventromedial positions lining the 3rd ventricle, especially at more anterior levels of the posterior hypothalamus. This distribution is consistent with the one previously described in chickens [11] and other birds [12], [13].

In reptiles, amphibians and fish, hypothalamic H/O neurons are primarily arranged in medial locations, lining the 3rd ventricle, in both the anterior and posterior portions [4], [9], [10]. Fish deviate from other vertebrates in having major extra-hypothalamic populations of H/O neurons [65]. In most mammals, H/O neurons are concentrated in the lateral hypothalamus and are lacking in medial periventricular locations [1], [66]. Our observations lend support to the previously-stated idea that the avian anatomical H/O pattern may be intermediate between that of amphibians and mammals [11]. Like reptiles, amphibians and fish, chickens present a medial periventricular H/O neuronal population. Like mammals, chickens present H/O neurons in dorsomedial and ventrolateral locations, although they are missing a dorsolateral extension. How differences in anatomical location may be reflected in the functional organization of chicken H/O neurons requires further investigation.

What functions might the H/O peptides serve in embryos?

Previous studies have strongly suggested that the adult function of H/O peptides is similar in birds and mammals. In fact, intracerebroventricular administration of H1/OA increases arousal [23], possibly by activating the monoaminergic systems in chickens [67]. This makes the differing embryonic patterns in the expression of this peptide all the more interesting.

Since the antibody used in this work appears to recognize only the active H/O peptides, the present results suggest that H/O may be released during very early developmental stages in chick embryos. There are some preliminary indications that H/O may play a role in brain development in higher vertebrates. H/O peptides seem to promote synaptogenesis and neuronal maturation [68], [69] as well as neuronal survival [70]. Early expression and release of H/O may thus facilitate the precocial development of circuits underlying all different functions regulated by H/O [19], including circuits involved in eventually maintaining a waking state.

If this is the case, one might expect that H/O would be produced earlier in precocial than in altricial species, since they require such circuits to mature more rapidly. A confirmation or refutation of this hypothesis in precocial (like the sheep) and altricial (like the rat) mammals also awaits further experiments.

Possible role(s) of H/O in the regulation of metabolism and body temperature

While chicks are precocial at birth [71], the precocity of H/O expression observed here in embryos appears rather extreme, more akin to the pattern seen in fish [32], where, in adults, H/O has been linked to arousal state regulation, locomotion, foraging/reward-seeking behavior, feeding, and sexual behavior [4], [65]. The most likely intersection of these traits with bird embryos may be in the domains of controlling food absorption from the yolk (feeding) and modulation of spontaneous embryonic movements (locomotion and body temperature control).

One possible role in development is based on the involvement of H/O in energy homeostasis [72]. In adult rats, H/O neurons act as sensors for relevant metabolites and hormones, thus integrating information about nutritional status [19]. They then trigger appropriate physiological responses (arousal, locomotion and food intake) [19], [73]. H/O increases nutrient uptake and utilization in muscle and adipose tissue, and some of these effects may be mediated directly [74]. H/O also increases energy expenditure and body temperature. In adult birds, H/O may regulate energy balance under extreme conditions [75].

H/O could be controlling physiological functions essential for chick (and other non-mammalian) embryos related to obtaining nutrients from stored yolk and to their utilization. These effects may be indirectly mediated through the autonomic nervous system and neuroendocrine axes. H/O could reach the pituitary and control the production of pituitary hormones [76]. Once in the hypothalamo-hypophyseal portal system, H/O could also affect peripheral tissues directly. H/O receptors are expressed in the pituitary and peripheral organs in adult chickens [77]. It would be especially interesting to know whether they are also expressed in the embryonic yolk sac membrane.

In birds, heat production starts prenatally, and is essential for the transition from ectothermy to endothermy [78]. Heat is generated through non-shivering thermogenesis in muscle and liver (birds do not have brown adipose tissue) and is controlled by thyroid hormones [78]. Interestingly, TRH and thyroid hormones are produced early in chick embryos [55], [79]. While H/O plays an important role in inducing brown adipose tissue differentiation and thermogenesis in rodents [80], a role for H/O in non-shivering thermogenesis in birds has not been investigated.

We recently demonstrated that cFos expression in H/O neurons is affected by hypoxia in chick embryos and could be orchestrating the embryo response to hypoxia [81]. Similarly, H/O could be modulating chick embryo responses to hypothermia or other insults.

In summary, this study has demonstrated a very early production of H/O neuropeptides in chick embryo brains, and a relatively rapid early proliferation of H/O neurons in the hypothalamus. We suggest that the relatively early developmental production of H/O in chick embryos is related to the fact that they are self-sufficient and cannot depend on maternal production of H/O or other regulatory factors, or on nutrients of maternal origin.

Acknowledgments

We thank Evan Balaban for help with the statistical analysis and for critically reading the manuscript.

Author Contributions

Conceived and designed the experiments: KEG JPL NS PVM MP. Performed the experiments: KEG JPL NS PVM MP. Analyzed the data: MP. Contributed reagents/materials/analysis tools: MP. Wrote the paper: KEG JPL NS PVM MP.

References

1. de Lecea L, Kilduff TS, Peyron C, Gao X-B, Foye PE, et al. (1998) The hypocretins: hypothalamus-specific peptides with neuroexcitatory activity. Proc Natl Acad Sci U S A 95: 322–327.
2. Sakurai T, Amemiya A, Ishii M, Matsuzaki I, Chemelli RM, et al. (1998) Orexins and orexin receptors: a family of hypothalamic neuropeptides and G-protein-coupled receptors that regulate feeding behavior. Cell 92: 573–585.
3. Wong KKY, Ng SYL, Lee LTO, Ng HKH, Chow BKC (2011) Orexins and their receptors from fish to mammals: a comparative approach. Gen Comp Endocrinol 171: 124–130.
4. Matsuda K, Azuma M, Kang KS (2012) Orexin system in teleost fish. Vitam Horm 89: 341–361.
5. Nambu T, Sakurai T, Mizukami K, Hosoya Y, Yanagisawa M, et al. (1999) Distribution of orexin neurons in the adult rat brain. Brain Res 827: 243–260.
6. Hahn JD (2010) Comparison of melanin-concentrating hormone and hypocretin/orexin peptide expression patterns in a current parceling scheme of the lateral hypothalamic zone. Neurosci Lett 468: 12–17.
7. Kruger JL, Dell L-A, Pettigrew JD, Manger PR (2010) Cellular location and major terminal networks of the orexinergic system in the brain of five microchiroptean species. J Chem Neuroanat 40: 256–262.
8. Galas L, Vaudry H, Braun B, van den Pol AN, de Lecea L, et al. (2001) Immunohistochemical localization and biochemical characterization of hypocretin/orexin-related peptides in the central nervous system of the frog *Rana ridibunda*. J Comp Neurol 429: 242–252.
9. López JM, Domínguez L, Moreno N, González A (2009) Comparative immunohistochemical analysis of the distribution of orexins (hypocretins) in the brain of amphibians. Peptides 30: 873–887.
10. Domínguez L, Morona R, Joven A, González A, López JM (2010) Immunohistochemical localization of orexins (hypocretins) in the brain of reptiles and its relation to monoaminergic systems. J Chem Neuroanat 39: 20–34.
11. Ohkubo T, Boswell T, Lumineau S (2002) Molecular cloning of chicken prepro-orexin cDNA and preferential expression in the chicken hypothalamus. Biochim Biophys Acta 1577: 476–480.
12. Singletary KG, Deviche P, Strand C, Delville Y (2006) Distribution of orexin/hypocretin immunoreactivity in the brain of male songbird, the house finch, *Carpodacus mexicanus*. J Chem Neuroanat 32: 81–89.
13. Phillips-Singh D, Li Q, Takeuki S, Ohkubo T, Sharp PJ, et al. (2003) Fasting differentially regulates expression of agouti-related peptide, pro-opiomelanocortin, prepro-orexin, and vasoactive intestinal polypeptide mRNAs in the hypothalamus of the Japanese quail. Cell Tissue Res 313: 217–225.
14. Puelles L, Martinez de-la-Torre M, Paxinos G, Watson C, Martinez S (2007) The chick brain in stereotaxic coordinates. New York: Academic Press. 267 p.
15. Lee MG, Hassani OK, Jones BE (2005) Discharge of identified orexin/hypocretin neurons across the sleep-waking cycle. J Neurosci 25: 6716–6720.
16. Mileykowskiy BY, Kiyashchenko LI, Siegel JM (2005) Behavioral correlates of activity in identified hypocretin/orexin neurons. Neuron 46: 787–798.
17. Takahashi K, Lin JS, Sakai K (2008) Neuronal activity of orexin and non-orexin waking-active neurons during wake-sleep states in the mouse. Neuroscience 153: 860–870.
18. Carter ME, Brill J, Bonnavion P, Huguenard JR, Huerta R, et al. (2012) Mechanism for hypocretins-mediated sleep-to-wake transitions. Proc Natl Acad Sci U S A 109: E2635–E2644.
19. Li J, Hu Z, de Lecea L (2014) The hypocretins/orexins: integrators of multiple physiological functions. Br J Pharmacol 171: 332–350.
20. Hagan JJ, Leslie RA, Patel S, Evans ML, Wattam TA, et al. (1999) Orexin A activates locus coeruleus cell firing and increases arousal in the rat. Proc Natl Acad Sci U S A 96: 10911–10916.
21. Horvath TL, Peyron C, Diano S, Ivanov A, Aston-Jones G, et al. (1999) Hypocretin (orexin) activation and synaptic innervations of the locus coeruleus noradrenergic system. J Comp Neurol 415: 145–159.
22. Sinton CM (2011) Orexin/hypocretin plays a role in response to physiological disequilibrium. Sleep Med Rev 15: 197–207.
23. Katayama S, Hamasu K, Shigemi K, Cline MA, Furuse M (2010) Intracerebroventricular injection of orexin-A, but not orexin-B, induces arousal of layer-type neonatal chicks. Comp Biochem Physiol A Mol Integr Physiol 157: 132–135.
24. Prober DA, Rihel J, Onah AA, Sung RJ, Schier AF (2006) Hypocretin/Orexin overexpression induces an insomnia-like phenotype in zebrafish. J Neurosci 26: 13400–13410.
25. Rigatto H, Moore M, Cates D (1986) Fetal breathing and behavior measured through a double-wall Plexiglass window in sheep. J Appl Physiol 61: 160–164.
26. van den Pol AN, Patrylo PR, Ghosh PK, Gao X-B (2001) Lateral hypothalamus: early developmental expression and response to hypocretin (orexin). J Comp Neurol 433: 349–363.
27. Steininger TL, Kilduff TS, Behan M, Benca RM, Landry CF (2004) Comparison of hypocretin/orexin and melanin-concentrating hormone neurons and axonal projections in the embryonic and postnatal rat brain. J Chem Neuroanat 27: 165–181.
28. Dickinson H, Walker DW, Castillo-Melendez M (2008) Onset of feeding at birth–Perinatal development of the hypothalamic mechanisms that induce appetite and feeding in the newborn. Neurosci Lett 436: 1–6.
29. Faraco JH, Appelbaum L, Marin W, Gaus SE, Mourrain P, et al. (2006) Regulation of hypocretin (orexin) expression in embryonic zebrafish. J Biol Chem 281: 29753–29761.
30. Yan A, Zhang L, Tang Z, Zhang T, Qin C, et al. (2011) Orange-spotted grouper (*Epinephelus coioides*) orexin: molecular cloning, tissue expression, ontogeny, daily rhythm and regulation of NPY expression. Peptides 32: 1363–1370.
31. Xu M, Volkoff H (2007) Molecular characterization of prepro-orexin in Atlantic cod (Gadus morhua): cloning, localization, developmental profile and role in food intake regulation. Mol Cell Endocrinol 271: 28–37.
32. Panula P. (2010) Hypocretin/orexin in fish physiology with emphasis on zebrafish. Acta Physiol 198: 381–386.

33. Kaslin J, Nystedt JM, Östergård M, Oeirsaro N, Panula P (2004) The orexin/hypocretin system in zebrafish is connected to the aminergic and cholinergic systems. J Neurosci 24: 2678–2689.
34. Milewski N, Ivell R, Grossman R, Ellendorf F (1989) Embryonal development of Arginine Vasotocin/Mesotocin gene expression in the chicken brain. J Neuroendocrinol 1: 473–484.
35. Arnold-Aldea SA, Sterritt C (1996) Sites of origin and pattern of migration of vasotocin/mesotocin neurons in developing brain of the chick. J Neurobiol 31: 103–116.
36. De Groef B, Grommen SV, Darras VM (2008) The chicken embryo as a model for developmental endocrinology: development of the thyrotropic, corticotropic, and somatotropic axes. Mol Cell Endocrinol 293: 17–24.
37. Ellestad LE, Saliba J, Porter TE (2011) Ontogenetic characterization of gene expression in the developing neuroendocrine system of the chick. Gen Comp Endocrinol 171: 82–93.
38. Bellairs R, Osmond M. (2005) The atlas of chick development. Oxford: Elsevier. 470 p.
39. Charvet CJ, Strieder GF (2010) Bigger brains cycle faster before neurogenesis begins: a comparison of brain development between chickens and bobwhite quail. Proc Biol Sci 277: 3469–3475.
40. Gilthorpe JD, Papantoniou E-K, Chédotal A, Lumsden A, Wingate RJT (2002) The migration of cerebellar rhombic lip derivatives. Development 129: 4719–4728.
41. Siegel S, Castellan NJ (1988) Nonparametric statistics for the behavioral sciences, 2nd Edition. New York: McGraw-Hill.
42. Huesa G, van den Pol AN, Finger TE (2005) Differential distribution of hypocretin (orexin) and melanin-concentrating hormone in the Goldfish brain. J Comp Neurol 488: 476–491.
43. Russo F, Pavone LM, Tafuri S, Avallone L, Staiano N, et al. (2008) Expression of orexin A and its receptor 1 in the bovine urethroprostetic complex. Anat Rec 291: 169–174.
44. Wang Q-P, Koyama Y, Guan J-L, Takahashi K, Kayama Y, et al. (2005) The orexinergic synaptic innervation of serotonin- and orexin 1-receptors-containing neurons in the dorsal raphe nucleus. Regul Pept 126: 35–42.
45. Mäkelä KA, Wigren HK, Zant JC, Sakurai T, Alhonen L, et al. (2010) Characterization of sleep-wake patterns in a novel transgenic mouse line overexpressing human prepro-orexin/hypocretin. Acta Physiol 198: 237–249.
46. Saper CB (2005) An open letter to our readers on the use of antibodies. J Comp Neurol 493: 477–78.
47. Boratyn GM, Schäffer AA, Agarwala R, Altschul SF, Lipman DJ, et al. (2012) Domain enhanced lookup time accelerated BLAST. Biol Direct 7: 12.
48. Gray EG, Whittaker VP (1962) The isolation of nerve endings from brain: an electron-microscopic study of cell fragments derived by homogenization and centrifugation. J Anat 96: 79–88.
49. Schägger H, von Jagow G (1987) Tricine-sodium dodecyl sulfate-polyacrylamide gel electrophoresis for the separation of proteins in the range from 1 to 100 kDa. Anal Biochem 166: 368–379.
50. Porkka-Heiskanen T, Alanko L, Kalinchuk A, Heiskanen S, Stenberg D (2004) The effect of age on prepro-orexin gene expression and content of orexin A and B in the rat brain. Neurobiol Aging 25: 231–238.
51. Wechsler W, Miller K (1967) Electron microscopy of neuronal and glial differentiation in the developing brain of the chick. Prog Brain Res 26: 93–144.
52. Madarász E (2013) Diversity of neural stem/progenitor populations: varieties by age, regional origin and environment. In: Bonfanti L, editor. Neural stem cells – New perspectives. pp. 45–72. InTech, DOI: 10.5772/55678.
53. Yuan L, Ni Y, Barth S, Wang Y, Grossmann R, et al. (2009) Layer and broiler chicks exhibit similar hypothalamic expression of orexigenic neuropeptides but distinct expression of genes related to energy homeostasis and obesity. Brain Res 1273: 18–28.
54. Altman J, Bayer SA (1986) The development of the rat hypothalamus. Adv Anat Embryol Cell Biol 100: 1–178.
55. Szarek E, Cheah P-S, Schwartz J, Thomas P (2010) Molecular genetics of the developing neuroendocrine hypothalamus. Mol Cell Endocrinol 323: 115–123.
56. Golden JA, Zitz JC, McFadden K, Cepko CL (1997) Cell migration in the developing chick diencephalon. Development 124: 3525–3533.
57. Yamamoto Y, Ueta Y, Hara Y, Serino R, Nomura M, et al. (2000) Postnatal development of orexin/hypocretin in rats. Brain Res Mol Brain Res 78: 108–119.
58. McClennan KM, Parker KL, Tobet S (2006) Development of the ventromedial nucleus of the hypothalamus. Front Neuroendocrinol 27: 193–209.
59. Sawai N, Ueta Y, Nakazato M, Ozawa H (2010) Developmental and aging change of orexin-A and -B immunoreactive neurons in the male rat hypothalamus. Neurosci Lett 468: 51–55.
60. Modirrousta M, Mainville L, Jones BE (2005) Orexin and MCH neurons express c-Fos differently after sleep deprivation vs. recovery and bear different adrenergic receptors. Eur J Neurosci 21: 2807–2816.
61. Harrison TA, Chen C-T, Dun NJ, Chang J-K (1999) Hypothalamic orexin A-immunoreactive neurons project to the rat dorsal medulla. Neurosci Lett 273: 17–20.
62. Kilduff TS, Peyron C (2000) The hypocretin/orexin ligand-receptor system: implications for sleep and sleep disorders. Trends Neurosci 23: 359–365.
63. Mikrouli E, Wörtwein G, Soylu, Mathé AA, Petersén Å (2011) Increased numbers of orexin/hypocretin neurons in a genetic rat depression model. Neuropeptides 45: 401–406.
64. Amiot C, Brischoux F, Colard C, La Roche A, Fellmann D, et al. (2005) Hypocretin/orexin-containing neurons are produced in one sharp peak in the developing ventral diencephalon. Eur J Neurosci 22: 531–534.
65. Volkoff H (2012) Sleep and orexins in nonmammalian vertebrates. Vitam Horm 89: 315–339.
66. Fabris C, Cozzi B, Hay-Schmidt A, Naver B, Møller M (2004) Demonstration of an orexinergic innervation of the pineal gland of the pig. J Comp Neurol 471: 113–127.
67. Katayama S, Shigemi K, Cline MA, Furuse M (2010) Intracerebroventricular injection of orexin-A stimulates monoamine metabolism but not HPA axis in neonatal chicks. Neurosci Lett 484: 157–161.
68. Stoyanova II, Rutten WLC, le Feber J (2012) Orexin-A in cortical coltures: expression and effect on synaptogenesis during development. Cell Mol Neurobiol 32: 49–57.
69. Sokołowska P, Urbańska A, Namiecińska M, Biegańska K, Zawilska JB (2012) Orexins promote survival of cortical neurons. Neurosci Lett 506: 303–306.
70. Li Y, Xu Y, van den Pol AN (2013) Reversed synaptic effects of hypocretin and NPY mediated by excitatory GABA-dependent synaptic activity in developing MCH neurons. J Neurophysiol 109: 1571–1578.
71. Mellor DJ, Diesch TJ (2007) Birth and hatching: key events in the onset of awareness in the lamb and chick. N Z Vet J 55: 51–60.
72. Girault E, Yi C-X, Fliers E, Kalsbeek A (2012) Orexin, feeding, and energy balance. Prog Brain Res 198: 47–64.
73. Tsujino N, Sakurai T (2013) Role of orexin in modulating arousal, feeding, and motivation. Front Behav Neurosci 7: 28.
74. Heinonen MV, Purhonen AK, Mäkelä KA, Herzig KH (2008) Functions of orexins in peripheral tissues. Acta Physiol 192: 471–485.
75. Song Z, Everaert N, Wang Y, Decuypere E, Buyse J (2013) The endocrine control of energy homeostasis in chickens. Gen Comp Endocrinol 190: 112–117.
76. Kaminski T, Smolinska N (2012) Expression of orexin receptors in the pituitary. Vitam Horm 89: 61–73.
77. Ohkubo T, Tsukada A, Shamoto K (2003) cDNA cloning of chicken orexin receptor and tissue distribution: sexually dimorphic expression in chicken gonads. J Mol Endocrinol 31: 499–508.
78. Walter I, Hegarty B, Seebacher F (2010) AMP-activated kinase controls metabolism and heat production during embryonic development in birds. J Exp Biol 213: 3167–3176.
79. Darras VM, Van Herck SLJ, Geysens S, Reyns GE (2009) Involvement of thyroid hormones in chicken embryonic development. Gen Comp Endocrinol 163: 58–62.
80. Madden CJ, Tupone D, Morrrison SF (2012) Orexin modulates brown adipose tissue thermogenesis. Biomol Concepts 3: 381–386.
81. Landry JP, Hawkins C, Wiebe S, Balaban E, Pompeiano M (2014) Opposing effects of hypoxia on catecholaminergic locus coeruleus neurons and hypocretin/orexin neurons in chick embryos. Dev Neurobiol in press, doi: 10.1002/dneu.22182.

Mycoplasma gallisepticum Lipid Associated Membrane Proteins Up-regulate Inflammatory Genes in Chicken Tracheal Epithelial Cells via TLR-2 Ligation through an NF-κB Dependent Pathway

Sanjukta Majumder[1,3], Frank Zappulla[2], Lawrence K. Silbart[1,2,3,4*]

1 Department of Animal Science, The University of Connecticut, Storrs, Connecticut, United States of America, 2 Department of Pathobiology and Veterinary Sciences, The University of Connecticut, Storrs, Connecticut, United States of America, 3 Center of Excellence for Vaccine Research, The University of Connecticut, Storrs, Connecticut, United States of America, 4 Department of Allied Health Sciences, The University of Connecticut, Storrs, Connecticut, United States of America

Abstract

Mycoplasma gallisepticum-mediated respiratory inflammation in chickens is associated with accumulation of leukocytes in the tracheal submucosa. However the molecular mechanisms underpinning these changes have not been well described. We hypothesized that the initial inflammatory events are initiated upon ligation of mycoplasma lipid associated membrane proteins (LAMP) to TLRs expressed on chicken tracheal epithelial cells (TEC). To test this hypothesis, live bacteria or LAMPs isolated from a virulent (R_{low}) or a non-virulent (R_{high}) strain were incubated with primary TECs or chicken tracheae *ex vivo*. Microarray analysis identified up-regulation of several inflammatory and chemokine genes in TECs as early as 1.5 hours post-exposure. Kinetic analysis using RT-qPCR identified the peak of expression for most genes to be at either 1.5 or 6 hours. *Ex-vivo* exposure also showed up-regulation of inflammatory genes in epithelial cells by 1.5 hours. Among the commonly up-regulated genes were IL-1β, IL-6, IL-8, IL-12p40, CCL-20, and NOS-2, all of which are important immune-modulators and/or chemo-attractants of leukocytes. While these inflammatory genes were up-regulated in all four treatment groups, R_{low} exposed epithelial cells both *in vitro* and *ex vivo* showed the most dramatic up-regulation, inducing over 100 unique genes by 5-fold or more in TECs. Upon addition of a TLR-2 inhibitor, LAMP-mediated gene expression of IL-1β and CCL-20 was reduced by almost 5-fold while expression of IL-12p40, IL-6, IL-8 and NOS-2 mRNA was reduced by about 2–3 fold. Conversely, an NF-κB inhibitor abrogated the response entirely for all six genes. miRNA-146a, a negative regulator of TLR-2 signaling, was up-regulated in TECs in response to either R_{low} or R_{high} exposure. Taken together we conclude that LAMPs isolated from both R_{high} and R_{low} induced rapid, TLR-2 dependent but transient up-regulation of inflammatory genes in primary TECs through an NF-κB dependent pathway.

Editor: Mitchell F. Balish, Miami University, United States of America

Funding: Support was provided by the United States Department of Agriculture, National Institute of Food and Agriculture to LKS (Hatch project number CONS00930) [http://portal.nifa.usda.gov/web/crisprojectpages/0179772-the-role-of-membrane-associated-lipoproteins-and-hydrogen-peroxide-in-the-pathogenesis-of-mycoplasma-gallisepticum-in-chickens.html]. The funders had no role in study design, data collection and analysis, decision to publish, or preparation of the manuscript.

Competing Interests: The authors have declared that no competing interests exist.

* Email: Lawrence.Silbart@uconn.edu

Introduction

Mycoplasma gallisepticum (*M. gallisepticum*) is an avian respiratory pathogen causing severe inflammation of the trachea, air sacs and lungs, especially in the presence of a co-infection [1–3]. This pathogen is known to invade, survive and multiply inside a variety of non-phagocytic cells such as chicken RBCs, HeLa cells, and chicken fibroblasts, [4–9]. In addition, *M. gallisepticum* is known to colonize many extra-pulmonary tissues including blood, heart, spleen, liver and brain [4,5,7,8,10]. Indikova et al. (2013) suggested that invasion may occur at the air sac, where the mucosal barrier is quite thin [7]. However, there is yet no clear evidence that *M. gallisepticum* invades tracheal epithelial cells *in vivo* [unpublished observations], as it predominantly colonizes the mucosal surface and only rarely is found inside phagocytic vacuoles [11]. Nonetheless, the organism orchestrates immuno-pathological changes in the tracheal mucosa marked by infiltration of heterophils, macrophages and lymphocytes [2,12,13] soon after attachment and colonization of the respiratory surface.

A previous study from our laboratory reported up-regulation of several chemokines including lymphotactin, CXCL-13, RANTES and MIP-1β in chicken trachea isolated from live birds within 24 hours of experimental *M. gallisepticum* infection [12]. These chemokines are primarily produced by macrophages, lymphocytes and NK cells; cell types not found in large numbers in the uninfected tracheal mucosa [14–19]. However, chemokines and cytokines that are produced by epithelial cells upon infection are known for their ability to recruit phagocytic cells and lymphocytes into infected tissues [20]. Due to the protective layer of mucus, it is not clear if the initial interaction of mycoplasmas with the host epithelium is driven by viable organisms or microbial components such as lipoprotein-bearing membrane fragments or both, although substantial evidence supports the notion that the initial "pathogen perception" occurs upon interaction of various PAMPs with TLRs [20–24]. Previous studies conducted using other mycoplasma species suggest an important role for epithelial cells in inflammation. For example, A549 human lung epithelial cells increase their production of IL-8, TNF-α, IL-1β, and IL-6 following *Mycoplasma pneumoniae (M. pneumoniae)* exposure [25]. Similarly, cultured human endocervical epithelial cells exposed to *Mycoplasma genitalium (M. genitalium)* secreted several pro-inflammatory chemokines and cytokines including IL-6, IL-7, IL-8, MCP-1 and GM-CSF [26–28].

Due to the lack of a peptidoglycan cell wall or outer membrane, mycoplasmas do not possess lipopolysaccharides (LPS), lipotechoic acid or flagella. Even though certain mycoplasmas are known for production of exotoxins, like the *M. pneumoniae* CARDS toxin or *Mycoplasma arthritidis* mitogen MAM [29–32], the majority of mycoplasmas including *M. gallisepticum* are not known to produce or secrete any exotoxin. Their surface-exposed membranes are composed of a single lipid bi-layer with numerous embedded integral and peripheral proteins and membrane anchored lipoproteins [33–35]. Phase and antigenic variable expression of these membrane lipoproteins provides a mechanism of immune evasion [36–46], and the importance of these molecules is reflected by the percentage of the mycoplasma genome devoted to lipoproteins. For example, in *M. gallisepticum* about 10% of the genome is devoted to *vlhA*s (variable lipoprotein hemagglutinins) which includes 38 genes with signature *vlhA* features and 5 pseudogenes possessing *vlhA* sequence homology [47].

Mycoplasma lipoproteins are known to partition into the Triton X-114 detergent phase during phase partitioning. This detergent phase fraction may also contain other hydrophobic proteins besides lipoproteins [48], and therefore has been termed "lipid associated membrane proteins" (LAMPs) [48–51]. In other mycoplasma species, the detergent phase fraction containing these LAMPs was found to activate NF-κB via TLR-1, 2, 6 as well as CD-14 via a MyD88 pathway, and induce expression of pro-inflammatory cytokines in monocytes and macrophages [43,48,50–53]. Recently, it was also found that mycoplasma LAMPs are capable of activating the NLRP3 inflammasome resulting in the induction of IL-1β [54]. Several other studies found that lipoproteins purified from the TX-114 fraction induce inflammatory responses via TLR-2 or TLR-1/2 andTLR-2/6 heterodimers [28,34,48–50,55–59]. However, the vast majority of these *in-vitro* studies were performed using leukocytes even though the initial interactions between mycoplasma membrane components and host cells occur at the mucosal surface upon contact with epithelial cells [28,60,61]. Thus, we hypothesized that LAMPs of *M. gallisepticum* ligate TLR-2 on respiratory epithelial cells, resulting in the up-regulation of inflammatory chemokine and cytokine genes via an NF- κB dependent pathway. To test this hypothesis, *M. gallisepticum* LAMPs were incubated with primary chicken tracheal epithelial cells in culture (TEC) or tracheae *ex vivo* to examine differential gene expression and to determine if the response is mediated via TLR-2 ligation. Similar studies using viable organisms were conducted to assess the relative contribution of LAMPs to early inflammatory events, using the low passage, adherent and virulent *M. gallisepticum* strain R_{low} or a high passage, non-adherent and non-virulent strain, R_{high}.

Materials and Methods

Bacterial Strains and Culture Conditions

M. gallisepticum low passage virulent strain R_{low} (passage 17) and high passage non-virulent strain R_{high} (passage 167) were cultured at 37°C in modified Hayflicks medium supplemented with 10% horse serum and 5% yeast extract until mid-log phase as determined by acid-mediated shift of phenol red dye from red to orange, as previously described [2]. Cell density was measured and a mycoplasma concentration of 0.9×10^8 to1.6×10^8 cfu (colony forming unit) per milliliter, approximately mid-log phase, was used.

Isolation of TX-114 phase proteins

M. gallisepticum strains R_{low} and R_{high} were grown to mid-log phase as previously described and pelleted by centrifuging at 10,000×g for 20 minutes. Pellets were washed twice with PBS and suspended in 750 µl of TS buffer (10 mM Tris, 150 mM NaCl, pH 7.5) containing 1 mM PMSF and 1% TX-114 and rocked for 30 minutes at 4°C, followed by centrifugation at 10,000×g at 4°C for 5 minutes. The soluble phase was transferred to a new tube and incubated at 37°C with rocking for 10 minutes and then centrifuged for 5 minutes at room temperature to separate the aqueous and detergent phases. 500 µl of TS buffer containing 1 mM PMSF and 1% TX114 was added to the detergent phase obtained in the previous step and thoroughly mixed and incubated for 15 min at 4°C followed by 10 min at 37°C with rocking followed by centrifugation for 5 minutes (at 10,000×g) at room temperature. The detergent phase was collected and the previous step was repeated to obtain the final detergent phase. The LAMPs were precipitated overnight at −20°C with 2 volumes of methanol and centrifuged at 15,000×g for 20 minutes. Precipitated protein was suspended in PBS by sonication for 30 seconds at output 5 using Biosonik ultrasonic disintegrator (Bronwill Scientific; Rochester, NY). Protein concentration was determined by Quick Start Bradford protein assay kit (Bio Rad; Hercules, CA) according to manufacturer's instructions.

Cell culture and exposure/stimulation

A primary chicken tracheal epithelial cell culture was established based upon two previously described protocols [62,63]. Five-week-old female specific pathogen free chicken tracheae were obtained from SPAFAS (Charles River Laboratories; Mansfield, CT) in sterile PBS (phosphate-buffered saline) containing 1X penicillin-streptomycin to inhibit bacterial and fungal growth. The tracheae were rinsed twice in DMEM (Dulbecco's modified eagles medium) (Gibco, Life technologies; Grand Island, NY) under sterile conditions. After removal of the surrounding adipose and muscular tissues, tracheae were cut into 2 cm pieces and incised vertically. They were then twice rinsed for 5 minutes in PBS/DTT (Dithiothreitol) (Sigma Aldrich; St. Louis, Missouri) (0.0385 g DTT- in 50 ml 1X PBS) to remove non-adherent mucus. The pieces were then rinsed twice with PBS and DMEM. To dissociate the epithelial cells from the underlying connective tissue, about 3–4 tracheal pieces were placed in a T25 flask containing 25 ml dissociation solution [DMEM 50 ml, protease type XIV 0.14 g (Sigma Aldrich), DNAse 0.01 g (Sigma Aldrich) and antibiotic/antimycotic 1X (Gibco, Life technologies)]. The flasks were gently shaken for 15 minutes at 37°C to slightly loosen the cells. 10% FBS (Gibco, Life technologies) was added to block protease activity after incubation. The tracheae were washed twice with fresh DMEM. The luminal surface of tracheae was scraped gently with a sterile scalpel in a petri dish containing fresh DMEM to obtain the epithelial cells. Cells were centrifuged at 1,250 rpm for

5 minutes to remove media. The epithelial cells were placed in 10 ml dissociation solution for 10 minutes at 37°C and then pipetted up and down several times to dissociate clumped cells. 10% FBS was added to the dissociation solution to stop the reaction. Cells were centrifuged at 1,250 rpm for 5 min to remove residual enzymes and washed twice with PBS. Cells were suspended in DMEM supplemented with 10% FBS and plated in a T75 flask for 4 hours to allow adherent cells (primarily fibroblasts and macrophages) to attach. The unattached cells were collected and precipitated by centrifugation at 1,250 rpm for 5 minutes and suspended in ATE medium [DMEM F-12+ Glutamax, (Gibco, Life technologies) 10% FBS (Gibco, Life technologies), 10% chick embryo extract (US Biologicals; Salem, MA), 1X MEM non-essential amino acids (NEAA) (Gibco, Life technologies), 1X antibiotic/antimycotic (Gibco, Life technologies)], counted on a hemocytometer and plated on 5% matrigel (BD Biosciences; San Jose, CA) coated T12.5 flasks. Exposure studies were done at 96 hours post-plating when the flasks reached 70–80% confluence, at which time they were exposed to either 5×10^8 cfu (roughly equal to 500 multiplicity of infection (MOI) live strain R_{low}, R_{high} as previously described [64] or LAMPs isolated from each strain at a concentration of 5 µg/mL. This concentration was based on preliminary studies where 5 µg/mL and 50 µg/mL LAMPs showed comparable potency (based on changes in gene regulation) and roughly equivalent to 500 MOI (5×10^8 cfu) live mycoplasma. All experiments were done with 6 replicates each for 1.5, 6, and 24 hours.

Whole tracheal exposure

Tracheae from 5-week-old female specific-pathogen free white leghorn chickens were obtained from SPAFAS (Charles River Laboratories; Mansfied, CT) in sterile PBS containing 1X penicillin-streptomycin to inhibit bacterial and fungal growth. Surrounding adipose tissues were removed and tracheae were cut into 0.5 inch pieces by vertical incision and rinsed 3 times with PBS and DMEM under sterile conditions. The tracheae were exposed to either 10^9 cfu *M. gallisepticum* strains R_{low} and R_{high} or 10 µg/mL LAMPs from either strain for 1.5 or 6 hours in ATE medium at 37°C, 5% CO_2. After exposure, tracheae were digested in dissociation solution (described previously) for 15 minutes at 37°C and immediately placed on ice. Epithelial cells from the luminal surface of tracheal pieces were lightly scraped using a sterile scalpel. Epithelial cells were then preserved in RNA later (Ambion, Life Technologies; Grand Island, NY) at 4°C for future RNA isolation (detailed below). All exposures were done with 6 replicates each for 1.5, and 6 hours.

Immunocytostaining

Tracheal epithelial cells and DF-1(Chicken embryonic fibroblast) cells grown on coverslips were fixed with 10% formalin and permeablized with 0.25% Triton X-100. Immunocytochemistry was performed using primary monoclonal anti-vimentin antibody (Sigma-aldrich) and anti E-cadherin antibody (Millipore; Billerica, MA) at a concentration of 1:200. Fluorescence-tagged secondary antibodies used were goat anti mouse IgG FITC (Sigma-aldrich) for visualization of vimentin and Alexa Fluor 546 Goat Anti-Rabbit IgG (H+L) (Life Technologies; Grand Island, NY) for visualization of E-cadherin at a 1:250 dilution. Vectashied HardSet mounting medium containing DAPI (4′, 6-Diamidino-2-phenylindole) (Vector Laboratories; Burlingame, CA) was used to mount cells on a slide for imaging. Images of immunostaining were captured using a Nikon A1R Spectral Confocal Microscope (Nikon Instruments Inc.; Melville, NY).

Signaling inhibitors

Tracheal epithelial cells were incubated with either 3 µg/mL R_{low} LAMPs or 5 µg/mL R_{high} LAMPs in the presence or absence of signaling inhibitors. TLR-2/4 signaling inhibitor OxPAPC (oxidated 1-palmitoyl-2-arachidonyl-sn- glycero-3-phosphorylcholine), TLR-4 inhibitor CLI-095, and NF-κB inhibitor Celastrol were purchased from Invivogen (Invivogen; San Diego, CA). Cells were co-incubated with either 10 µg/mL or 30 µg/mL OxPAPC and LAMPs for 6 hours, in accordance with the manufacturer's instruction. Cells were pre-incubated with 1 µg/mL CLI-095 for 6 hours before exposure to LAMPs and then further incubated for 6 hours after LAMP exposure. Pre-incubation of cells with 5 µM Celastrol for 30 minutes was done before LAMP exposure for 6 hours. All experiments were performed with 6 replicates each.

RNA isolation and cDNA synthesis

Total RNA was extracted from cells using TRIzol reagent (Life Technologies) and purified using RNeasy mini columns according to the manufacturer's instructions (Qiagen; Valencia, CA). On-column DNase digestion was done using RNase free DNase (Qiagen;). RNA quality and quantity was assessed using the Agilent 2100 Bioanalyzer with the RNA pico kit (Agilent technologies; Mendon, MA). All RNA samples had a RNA integrity number of 8 or more. 500 ng of RNA from individual samples was reverse transcribed using iScript reverse transcription supermix for RT-qPCR (Bio Rad; Hercules, CA) according to the manufacturer's recommendation, and 2 µg RNA was reverse transcribed for PCR reaction to assess epithelial-specific gene expression.

Microarray

Agilent chicken gene expression microarray slides were utilized (Agilent technologies). Total RNA (50 ng) was utilized as starting material for microarray hybridization. Four biological replicates for each of five exposure conditions utilized were: R_{high}, R_{low}, R_{high} LAMPs, R_{low} LAMPs and media control. Dye swap technical replicates were created for each biological replicate totaling eight replicates for each exposure condition. The Agilent two-color microarray-based gene expression analysis protocol version 6.5 (http://www.genome.duke.edu/cores/microarray/services/agilent-microarrays/documents/LIQA_G4140-90050_GeneExpression_Two_Color_v6.5.pdf) was followed. All incubations were performed utilizing the Applied Biosystem Geneamp PCR system 9700 (Life Technologies). The Agilent two-color low-input quick amp labeling kit (Agilent technologies) was utilized for cDNA synthesis, *in-vitro* amplification and labeling of nucleic acids. Purification of labeled cRNA was performed with the Qiagen RNeasy mini kit). Purified cRNA was fragmented using the Agilent gene expression hybridization kit (Agilent technologies). Microarray slides and hybridization gasket were assembled in a hybridization chamber (Agilent technologies). Samples were placed in a rotating hybridization oven set to 10 rpm at 65°C for 17 hours. Microarray slides were scanned using a GenePix 4000B laser scanner (Molecular Devices; Sunnyvale, CA) following the instructions in the GenePixPro 7 user guide. Feature extraction was performed utilizing GenePixPro 7 software (Molecular Devices). Microarray images were visually inspected for quality control of features (spots on microarray slide that have spotted oligonucleotide probes). Background fluorescence of each feature was calculated as the mean of the five closest negative control features. Each channel's background-corrected median fluorescence value was used in an intensity-based analysis utilizing Agilent GeneSpring (v12.5) software (Agilent technologies). Quantile normalization was performed on all the background-corrected intensity values and samples were clustered according to their original exposure group. Features were removed if they were at saturating intensity or flagged "bad" in the aforementioned visual inspection. Genes were removed from downstream analysis if < 80% of the features representing a gene were already excluded following preprocessing of data. Genes with duplicate or triplicate features on the microarray were grouped and their mean values were used for a gene-level analysis. Quantile normalization was then performed on the gene-level *in-silico* experiment. All microarray datasets have been deposited into Gene Expression Omnibus database repository, accession number GSE61520 (http://www.ncbi.nlm.nih.gov/geo/query/acc.cgi?acc=GSE61520).

Polymerase Chain Reaction

PCR reactions were performed using cDNA to identify expression of epithelial cell-specific genes in tracheal epithelial cell cultures using GoTaq Green master mix (Promega; Madison, WI). Cycle conditions were as follows: 94°C for 3 minutes, 94°C for 30 seconds, 58°C for 30 seconds, 72°C for 1 minute. Step 2 to 4 was repeated 30 times. Final extension was performed at 72°C for 10 minutes. Primers for the epithelial cells specific genes are listed on **Table 1**.

Real time quantitative PCR (RT-qPCR)

Primers specific for chicken genes were designed using Primer 3 input version 0.4.0 (http://frodo.wi.mit.edu/) or as described in Mohammed et al [12] (**Table 2**). RT-qPCR was performed using 1 µl of cDNA from the reverse transcription reaction using iTaq universal SYBR green supermix (Bio Rad). Amplification was performed using an Applied Biosystem 7900 HT (Life Technologies) by incubating samples at 50°C for 2 minutes, 95°C for 1 min, followed by 40 cycles of 95°C for 15 seconds and 58–60°C (depending on Tm values of specific primers) for 60 seconds. Melt curve analysis was performed to confirm that a single, product-specific amplification had occurred. A stepwise temperature gradient was used (65–95°C) with 0.5°C increments and 2 sec/step. Amplicon sizes were confirmed by agarose gel electrophoresis. The reference gene for all real time reactions was GAPDH. Absolute fold change compared to the media controls were calculated using the Ct values based upon the following equation:

$$Fold\ change\left(\frac{Test}{Control}\right) = 2^{\Delta\Delta}Ct =$$

$$2^{[(Ct\ gene\ of\ interest - Ct\ GAPDH)\ Control - (Ct\ gene\ of\ interest - Ct\ GAPDH)\ Test]}$$

Gel electrophoresis was performed using a 0.8% agarose gel to determine the product size for each gene.

Statistical analysis

All statistical analyses were performed using the Statistical Analysis Software (SAS) program Version 9.2 (SAS Institute; Inc Cary, NC). Multiple pairwise comparisons of mRNA fold differences were analyzed using the mixed design analysis of variance (ANOVA) with repeated measures, with mRNA fold difference being the dependent variable and treatments or time being the independent variables. Post hoc mean comparison analyses were performed using least square means. Results were denoted as fold change ± SEM. Significant differences were denoted as * = $P<0.05$, ** = $P<0.01$, *** = $P<0.001$.

Results

Tracheal epithelial cell culture and immunocytostaining

Primary tracheal epithelial cell cultures were established based on published methods [62,63]. Confirmation was performed using PCR amplification of epithelial cell specific genes and morphological examination based on E-cadherin staining patterns. A chicken embryonic fibroblast cell line (DF-1) was used as a negative control. E-cadherin staining was observed only at the contact points between cells, which is typical of epithelial cell morphology. Very few cells in the TEC culture stained for vimentin, suggesting an extremely low level of fibroblast contamination. As a positive control, DF-1 chicken fibroblast cells stained positively for vimentin and not for E-cadherin (**Figure 1A–D, Figure S4**).

Microarray analysis – global gene expression profile

Microarray analysis of chicken tracheal epithelial cells at 1.5 hours post-exposure identified a total of 166, 43, 55 and 38 genes differentially regulated ≥5-fold ($p \leq 0.05$) after exposure to either live R_{low} and R_{high}, or to 5 µg/mL R_{low} or R_{high} LAMPs respectively (**Figure 2**). 23 genes were commonly up-regulated ≥ 5-fold in TECs in all four exposure groups, which included many inflammatory chemokine and cytokine genes (**Figure 2; indicated by the asterisk***). Gene ontology analysis of commonly up-regulated genes (≥2-fold) identified categories such as immune system processes, signal transduction, regulation of apoptosis and stress response (**Table 3, Figure S1 and Table S1**). Exposure to viable R_{low} resulted in differential expression of 110 unique genes by a factor of ≥5- fold ($p \leq 0.05$) (**Table S2**) whereas only six or fewer genes were unique in TECs exposed to R_{high}, R_{low} LAMPs or R_{high} LAMPs (**Figure 2**). Pathway analysis identified

Table 1. Epithelial gene specific primers.

Gene ID	Primer Name	Sequence 5′-3′
395209	Retinoic acid responder Forward	ACA TCA ACT CCC ACG AGG CGT CC
	Retinoic acid responder Reverse	ACT GCT GCC AAC AAT GGC CAA GC
408039	Keratin 14 Forward	CAC TGC CAG CCC GCT GTG CT
	Keratin 14 Reverse	ACC TTG TCC AGG TAG GCG GCC
407779	Keratin 5 Forward	TGC TGC TTT CCT GCT GCT CAG C
	Keratin 5 Reverse	ACG GTC ACT TCA TGG ATG CCA CC
414833	Cytochrome P-450 2C45 Forward	CCA CGT GGG AGA TGT TGC TCC TG
	Cytochrome P-450 2C45 Reverse	TGG CAG CAA ACT CAT CCG CAC G

Table 2. Gene specific primers for RT-qPCR.

Primer Name	Sequence 5′-3′
GAPDH Forward	ATT CTA CAC ACG GAC ACT TCA
GAPDH Reverse	CAC CAG TGG ACT CCA CAA CAT A
IL-12p40 Forward	TGAAGGAGTTCCCAGATGC
IL-12p40 Reverse	CGTCTTGCTTGGCTCTTTATA
IL-1β Forward	GCT GGA ACT GGG CAG AT
IL-1β Reverse	GGT AGA AGA TGA AGC GGG TC
IL-8 Forward	GTG CAT TAG CAC TCA TTC TAA GTT
IL-8 Reverse	GGC CAT AAG TGC CTT TAC G
IL-6 Forward	CCT GTT CGC CTT TCA GAC CTA
IL-6 Reverse	AGT CTG GGA TGA CCA CTT C
IL-10 Forward	AGAGATGCTGCGCTTCTACA
IL-10 Reverse	GCTTGATGGCTTTGCTCC
CCL-20 Forward	GCC AGA AGC TCA AGA GGA TG
CCL-20 Reverse	TCC AGA AGT TCA ACG GTT CC
NOS-2 Forward	TGA TCT TTG CTG CCA AAC AG
NOS-2 Reverse	TCC TCT GAG GGA AAA TGG TG
miRNA-146a Forward	GAGAACTGAATTCCATGGGTTG
miRNA-146a Reverse	TCCAAGCTGAAGAACTGAGC

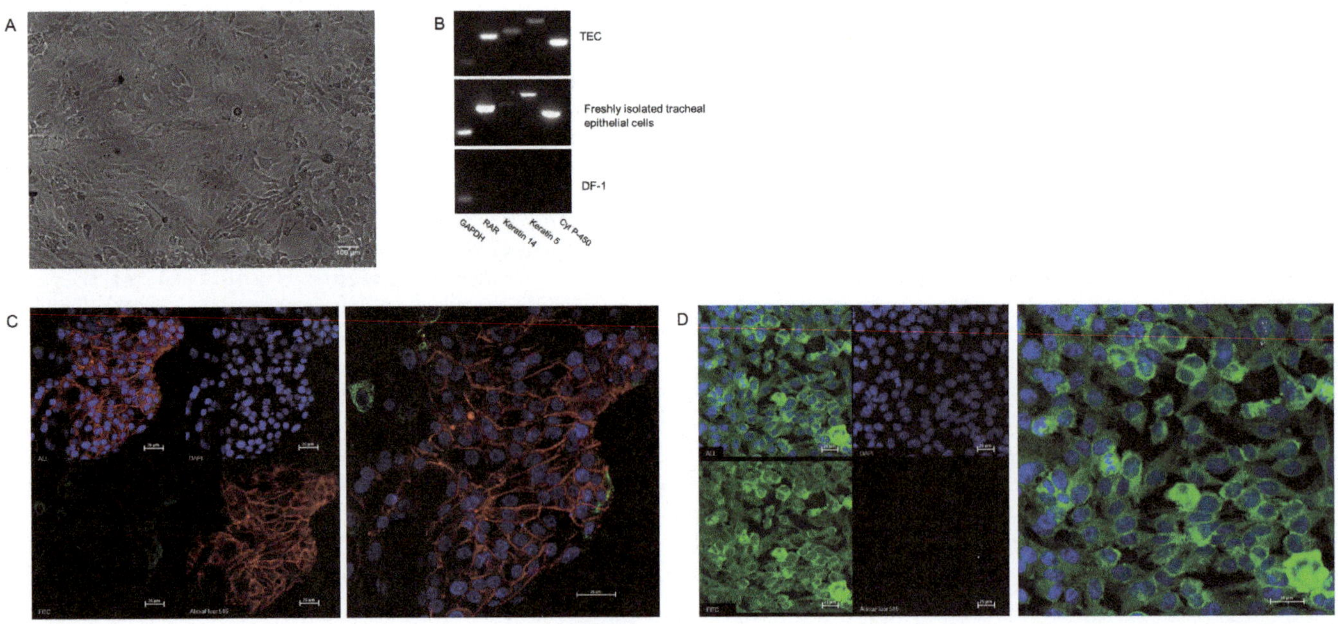

Figure 1. Primary chicken tracheal epithelial cell culture (TEC). Primary chicken tracheal epithelial cells were isolated and cultured as described in the Methods section. **1A:** Primary chicken tracheal epithelial cells at 100X magnification. **1B:** Confirmation of tracheal epithelial cell identity both *in vitro* and freshly isolated (*ex vivo*) from tracheae after *ex-vivo* exposure: PCR amplified epithelial cell specific genes from cDNA in agarose gel, compared to chicken embryonic fibroblast (DF-1) cells. **1C:** Tracheal epithelial cells stained for E-cadherin and Vimentin at (400X magnification). Left panel shows TECs at different filter setting Blue (DAPI) for nuclear staining, Green (FITC) for Vimentin and Red (AlexaFluor 546) for E-cadherin, right panel shows merged picture for all filters. **1D:** DF-1 fibroblast cells stained for E-cadherin and Vimentin at 400X magnification. Left panel shows DF-1 cells at different filter setting; Blue (DAPI) for nuclear staining, Green (FITC) for Vimentin and Red (AlexaFluor 546) for E-cadherin; right panel shows merged picture for all filters.

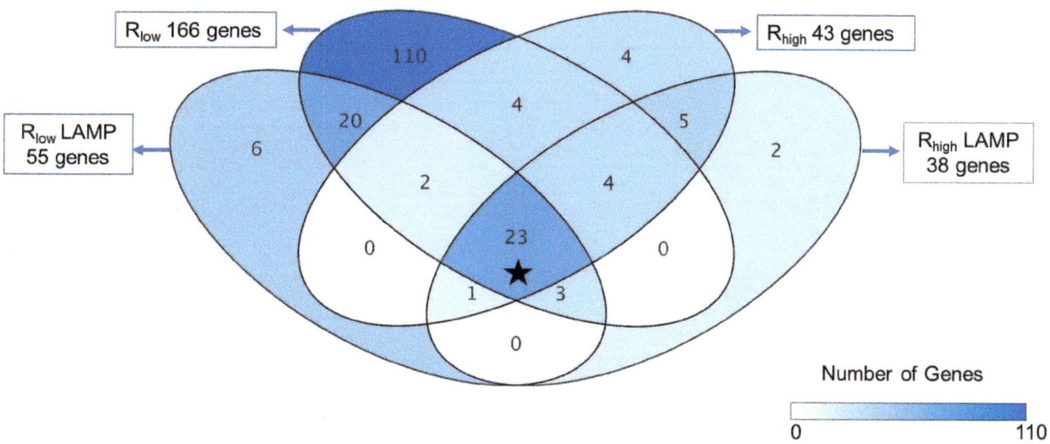

Figure 2. Distribution of differentially regulated genes in TECs. Differentially regulated genes (≥5 fold) in tracheal epithelial cell after exposure to live R_{low}, R_{high} or LAMPs isolated from either strain 1.5 hours after exposure. The star (*) in the figure represent commonly up-regulated genes upon all four exposures, from which six follow up genes were chosen. n = 8 (4 biological replicates x2 dye swap technical replicates) for all microarray experiments.

Table 3. Genes of significant interest from microarray analysis.

Entrez ID	Gene Name	mRNA Fold Change in TECs exposed to:			
		R_{low}	R_{high}	R_{low} LAMP	R_{high} LAMP
404671	Interleukin 12B	207.80	71.80	194.67	78.21
395196	Interleukin 1, beta	9.89	7.86	6.75	5.65
395082	Chemokine (C-C motif) ligand 20	55.34	11.67	43.92	12.98
395337	Interleukin 6	42.33	30.57	27.31	20.95
396495	Interleukin 8	22.92	20.72	17.87	19.44
395807	Nitric oxide synthase 2, inducible	10.53	3.68	8.41	3.94
396451	Prostaglandin-endoperoxide synthase 2	12.98	10.65	13.13	9.76
374012	Baculoviral IAP repeat-containing 2	5.42	4.07	5.45	3.48
396384	Interferon regulatory factor 1 (IRF1)	5.66	5.48	4.73	5.07
396424	Plasminogen activator, urokinase	7.15	16.65	7.95	14.86
396033	Nuclear factor of kappa light polypeptide gene enhancer in B-cells 1	2.55	2.08	2.58	2.02
418404	Nuclear factor of kappa light polypeptide gene enhancer in B-cells inhibitor, zeta	10.24	17.96	12.14	15.32
396093	Nuclear factor of kappa light polypeptide gene enhancer in B-cells inhibitor, alpha	5.00	4.15	5.00	3.62
417465	Chemokine (C-C motif) ligand 5	2.63	2.65	2.38	2.65
396330	Interferon regulatory factor 7	6.57	5.21	5.44	4.22
421219	Toll-like receptor 15	2.75	2.53	3.69	2.11
396093	Nuclear factor of kappa light polypeptide gene enhancer in B-cells inhibitor, alpha	5.00	4.15	5.00	3.62
417247	Similar to TL1A; tumor necrosis factor (ligand) superfamily, member 15	4.22	14.47	4.08	10.33
423471	TNF receptor-associated factor 3	3.68	5.35	4.39	5.46
408036	Epiregulin	4.01	2.02	2.80	2.66
422219	Interleukin 13 receptor, alpha 2	5.40	3.25	4.57	3.64
421686	Interleukin 20 receptor, alpha	5.01	3.73	3.72	3.97
424704	Interleukin 23 receptor	2.34	2.41	2.48	4.44
422884	TNFAIP3 interacting protein 2	10.95	4.77	7.09	7.01
768950	CD80 molecule	2.96	4.77	2.44	4.02

Representative list of Table S1: mRNA fold changes ≥2 (p-value ≤0.05) in TECs exposed to R_{low}, R_{high}, R_{low} LAMP and R_{high} LAMP compared to control.

Table 4. Pathway analysis of differentially regulated genes.

Pathway	No. of genes from different pathways up-regulated in TEC's exposed to:				Total no. of genes in pathway
	R_{low}	R_{high}	R_{low} LAMP	R_{high} LAMP	
Toll-like receptor signaling pathway	17	15	13	13	70
TNF-alpha NF-kB Signaling Pathway	10	9	11	10	157
Adipogenesis	14	7	4	4	100
Senescence and Autophagy	10	8	7	7	73
EGFR1 Signaling Pathway	8	4	5	2	148
MAPK signaling pathway	5	7	4	5	123
Apoptosis	5	6	5	6	65
Type II interferon signaling pathway	6	4	4	4	22

Analysis performed using GeneSpring (v12.5), within genes that are differentially expressed ≥2-fold (p-value ≤0.05).

differential expression of genes in the TLR signaling pathway, with 12 out of 70 genes commonly up-regulated in all four exposure groups. Other pathways of note included the TNF-α/NF-κB signaling, apoptosis, and type II interferon pathways (**Table 4 and Figure S3**).

Differential gene expression in R_{low}, R_{low} LAMP, R_{high} and R_{high} LAMP exposed TECs

A concentration of 5 μg/mL LAMPs optimally induced the expression of IL-1β and CCL-20, which was roughly comparable to the up-regulation induced by 500 MOI (5×10^8 cfu) live mycoplasma (data not shown). mRNA transcripts of six immune response associated genes up-regulated in TECs upon exposure to each of the four treatments were validated by RT-qPCR at 1.5, 6 and 24 hours. TECs' expression of IL-12p40, IL-1β and IL-6 peaked at 1.5 hours post-exposures in all four exposure groups and waned significantly thereafter in contrast to CCL-20 and nitric oxide synthase-2 (NOS-2) which peaked at 6 hours and returned to near baseline levels within 24 hours. IL-8 expression peaked at 6 hours in R_{low} exposed TECs, however R_{high} and R_{low} LAMP exposed TECs exhibited the highest level of IL-8 gene expression at 1.5 hours ($p\leq0.01$ and $p\leq0.001$) (**Figure S2A–D**). Five out of six genes (IL-6, IL-8, IL-12p40, CCL-20 and NOS-2) were expressed at significantly higher levels in R_{low} exposed TECs when compared to TECs exposed to R_{high} or LAMPs isolated from either strain, at one or more time point (**Figure 3A–E**). IL-1β gene expression in TECs did not significantly differ between any of the four exposures at any time point (**Figure 3F**). We also observed that R_{low} LAMP exposed TECs had a significantly higher level of the IL-12p40 gene expression when compared to TECs exposed to R_{high} LAMP at 1.5 hours ($p\leq0.05$) (**Figure 3A**) and CCL-20 when compared to TECs exposed to R_{high} or R_{high} LAMP at 1.5 and 6 hours ($p\leq0.01$ and $p\leq0.001$) (**Figure 3D**).

Differential gene expression in TECs by mycoplasma LAMPs in the presence of signaling inhibitors

OxPAPC, a TLR-2 and 4 signaling inhibitor, reduced expression of all 6 genes in a concentration dependent manner (**Figure 4A–F**). IL-12p40 gene expression was reduced by more than 2-fold in TECs exposed to LAMPs when incubated with OxPAPC at 30 μg/mL when compared to both R_{low} ($P<0.05$) and R_{high} LAMP ($P<0.01$) exposed TECs (**Figure 4A**). IL–1β and CCL-20 gene expression were reduced by more than 5-fold compared to TECs exposed to R_{low} ($P<0.001$) or R_{high} ($P<0.001$) LAMPs in the absence of the inhibitor (**Figure 4B, E**). IL-8 ($P<0.001$), IL-6 ($P<0.01$) and NOS-2 ($P<0.001$) gene expression was also significantly reduced by approximately 2–3 fold (**Figure 4C, D, and F**). No difference was observed upon exposure to CLI-095, a selective TLR-4 inhibitor, for any of the genes analyzed in this study, supporting the hypothesis that *M. gallisepticum* LAMPs signal via TLR-2 and not TLR-4 (**Figure 4A–F**). In the presence of Celastrol, an NF-κB inhibitor, cell signaling was abolished entirely (comparable to control levels) in TECs exposed to any of the four treatments ($P<0.001$ for all six genes analyzed) (**Figure 4A–F**).

Comparison of gene regulation in R_{low}, R_{low} LAMP, R_{high} and R_{high} LAMP exposed tracheal epithelial cells *ex vivo*

mRNA transcripts of all six genes were also up-regulated in tracheal epithelial cells isolated from whole tracheal tissues exposed *ex vivo* to live R_{low}, R_{high} or the LAMPs isolated therefrom. Most genes followed a similar pattern of expression as seen in the *in vitro* experiments. IL-12p40 was expressed at a significantly higher level in R_{low} exposed trachea at both time points compared to others, and CCL-20 was significantly higher in R_{low} exposed trachea than all others at 1.5 hours ($p\leq0.001$) (**Figure 5A, 5B**). IL-8 expression was higher in both R_{low} and R_{high} exposed trachea when compared to the LAMP exposed tracheae at both time points but IL-6 was found to be higher in the LAMP-exposed tissues ($p\leq0.001$) at 1.5 hours and lower at 6 hours ($p\leq0.01$, $p\leq0.05$) when compared to tracheae exposed to live R_{low} or R_{high}. Although IL–1β expression did not differ between any exposure groups at 1.5 hours, at 6 hours tracheae exposed to the live mycoplasma were found to express IL–1β at a higher level than either LAMP-exposed tracheae ($p\leq0.001$ for R_{low}, $p\leq0.05$ for R_{high}). NOS-2 expression did not differ between any exposure groups at any time point (**Figure 5A, 5B**).

Micro RNA and IL-10 gene expression

Expression analysis of four miRNA genes including mir-21, mir-146a, mir-146b, and mir-146c1, as well as IL-10 was assessed in TECs exposed to either LAMPs or live organisms. IL-10 gene expression in all TECs peaked at 1.5 hours, concomitant with the pro-inflammatory genes (**Figure 6A**). Expression analysis of miRNAs showed that miRNA146a increased over time in TECs exposed to live mycoplasmas; however in TECs exposed to the LAMPs from both strains, miRNA146a expression peaked at 6 hours (**Figure 6B**). Expression of miRNA21, miRNA146b and

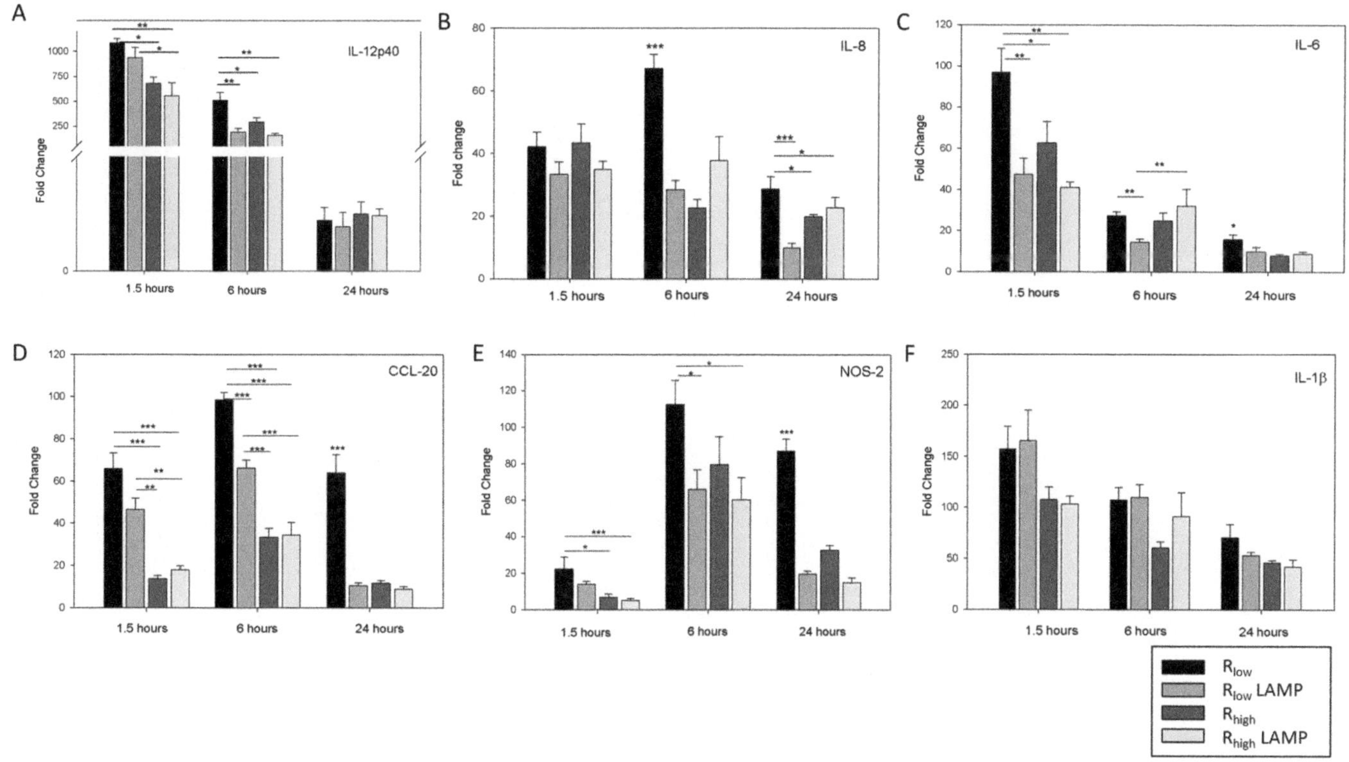

Figure 3. Differential gene expression in TECs post-exposure. mRNA fold difference in TECs exposed to R_{low}, R_{low} LAMP, R_{high} or R_{high} LAMP at 1.5, 6 and 24 hours respectively. Samples normalized to housekeeping gene GAPDH and un-exposed TECs as control. n = 6 for all experiments. Results are denoted as fold change ± SEM with all control values set at 1. Significant differences denoted as * = $P<0.05$, ** = $P<0.01$, *** = $P<0.001$. **A:** IL-12p40 mRNA. **B:** IL-8 mRNA. **C:** IL-6 mRNA. **D:** CCL-20 mRNA. **E:** NOS-2 mRNA. **F:** IL-1β mRNA.

miRNA146c1 did not differ from media controls at any time point in any exposure group (data not shown).

Discussion

Bacterial cell envelope components such as LPS, lipotechoic acid, peptidoglycan, flagella and lipoproteins are well characterized PAMPs that interact with host cell pattern recognition receptors such as TLRs, thereby contributing in part to the inflammation that ensues post-infection [20,43,65]. With the exception of lipoproteins, *M. gallisepticum* is devoid of these PAMPs, yet is able to initiate a robust inflammatory response marked by infiltration of leukocytes to the submucosa, often in absence of tissue invasion [2,12,13,66,67]. Mycoplasma lipoproteins are well known for their pro-inflammatory properties, initiated upon TLR ligation and NF-κB activation [34,48–51,55,56,68]. However, the vast majority of studies examining these effects have focused on monocytes/macrophages maintained in culture rather than epithelial cells, the primary site of mycoplasma attachment and colonization [11,69].

Previous studies from our laboratory in which live birds were exposed to *M. gallisepticum* intra-tracheally reported alterations in inflammatory gene expression in whole tracheal tissue [12]. The current study is novel in that it reports interaction of *M. gallisepticum* lipid associated membrane proteins, a mixture of lipoproteins, specifically with host airway epithelial cells.

A study by Walter et al (2001) reported that IL-12p40 was expressed by airway epithelial cells during viral tracheobronchitis [70,71]. We also observed IL-12p40 mRNA to be significantly up-regulated both in TECs and epithelial cells from tracheae upon exposure to live mycoplasma or LAMPs within 1.5 hours of exposure. But this signal waned rapidly thereafter, suggesting that IL-12p40 acts as an early, but not sustained, inflammatory event. IL-1β and IL-6 mRNA expression were also up-regulated and followed similar kinetics to that observed with IL-12p40. mRNA expression of two important chemokines, CCL-20 and IL-8 were also significantly up-regulated in epithelial cells *in-vitro* and *ex-vivo* after exposure to LAMPs or live organisms, as was NOS-2. These molecules are known for their ability to chemo-attract and activate leukocytes at the site of infection [72–77]. Several other inflammation associated genes, including TLR-15, were up-regulated to a lesser degree in TECs in all four exposure groups (**Table 3**, RT-qPCR data not shown). This cytokine and chemokine expression profile is in keeping with earlier studies that reported *M. pneumoniae* and *M. genitalium* mediated production of IL-8, TNF-α, IL-1β, IL-6 IL-7, MCP-1 and GM-CSF from epithelial cells [25–28].

A previously published study from our laboratory however, reported down-regulation of IL-12p40, IL-8, IL–1β, and CCL-20 mRNA in tracheal tissues at day-1 post-infection, whereas chemokines like MIP-1β, CXCL-13, RANTES and lymphotactin were found to be up-regulated [12]. As this later set of chemokines are known to be produced primarily by macrophages, lymphocytes and NK cells [14–19], types of cells not found in large numbers in normal tracheal mucosa, we believe transient but robust expression of chemokines and cytokines like IL-12p40, IL-8, IL-6, IL–1β, and CCL-20 by tracheal epithelial cells may be responsible for initially attracting the inflammatory cells into the tracheal submucosa. However these signals appear to be transient and

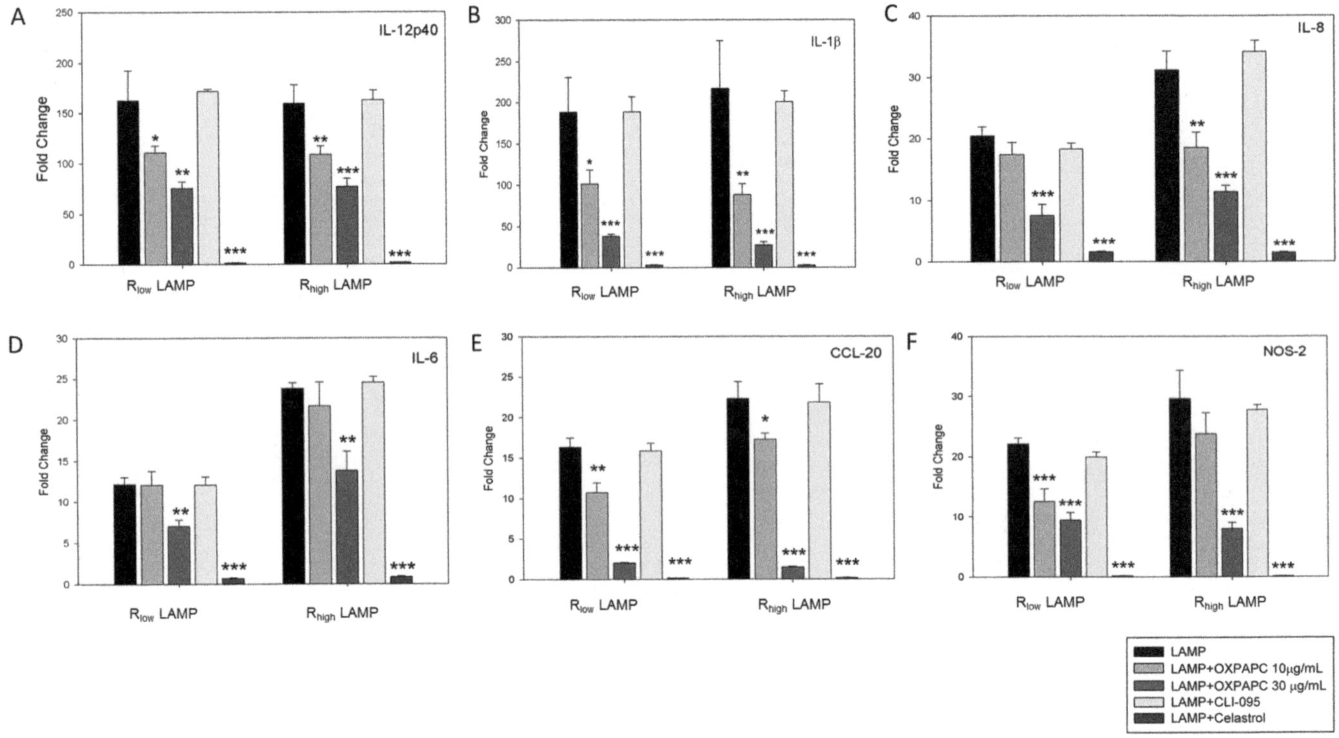

Figure 4. Differential gene expression in TECs exposed to LAMPs in the presence of signaling inhibitors. Epithelial cells were exposed to LAMPs isolated from R_{low} or R_{high} in the presence or absence of signaling inhibitors for 6 hours. Samples were normalized to the housekeeping gene GAPDH and un-exposed TECs served as control. n = 6 for all experiments. Results are denoted as fold change ± SEM with all control values set at 1. Significant differences denoted as * = P<0.05, ** = P<0.01, *** = P<0.001. **A.** IL-12p40. **B.** IL-1β. **C.** IL-8. **D.** IL-6. **E.** CCL-20. **F.** NOS-2.

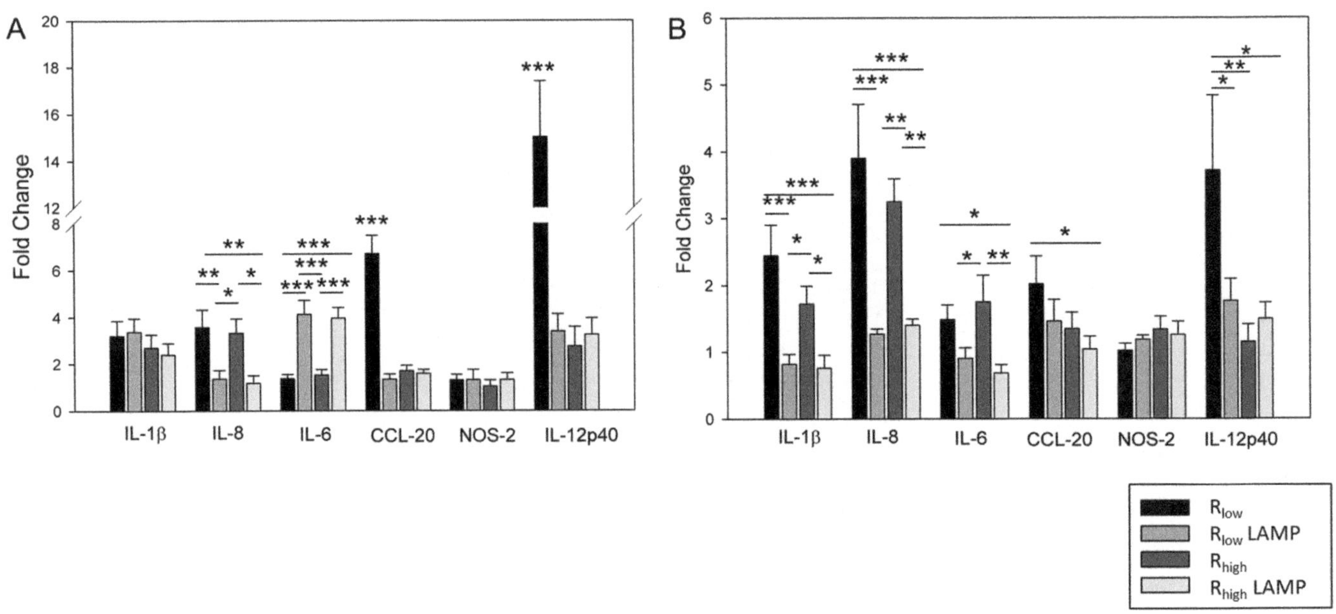

Figure 5. Differential gene expression in tracheal epithelial cells after *ex-vivo* exposure to LAMPs. Comparison of mRNA fold difference in tracheal epithelial cells from tracheal explant exposed to R_{low}, R_{low} LAMP, R_{high} or R_{high} LAMP at 1.5 and 6 hours respectively. Samples normalized to housekeeping gene GAPDH and un-exposed tracheae as control. n = 6 for all experiments. Results are denoted as fold change ± SEM with all control values set at 1. Significant differences denoted as * = P<0.05, ** = P<0.01, *** = P<0.001. **A:** mRNA fold difference of all genes at 1.5 hours. **B:** mRNA fold difference of all genes at 6 hours.

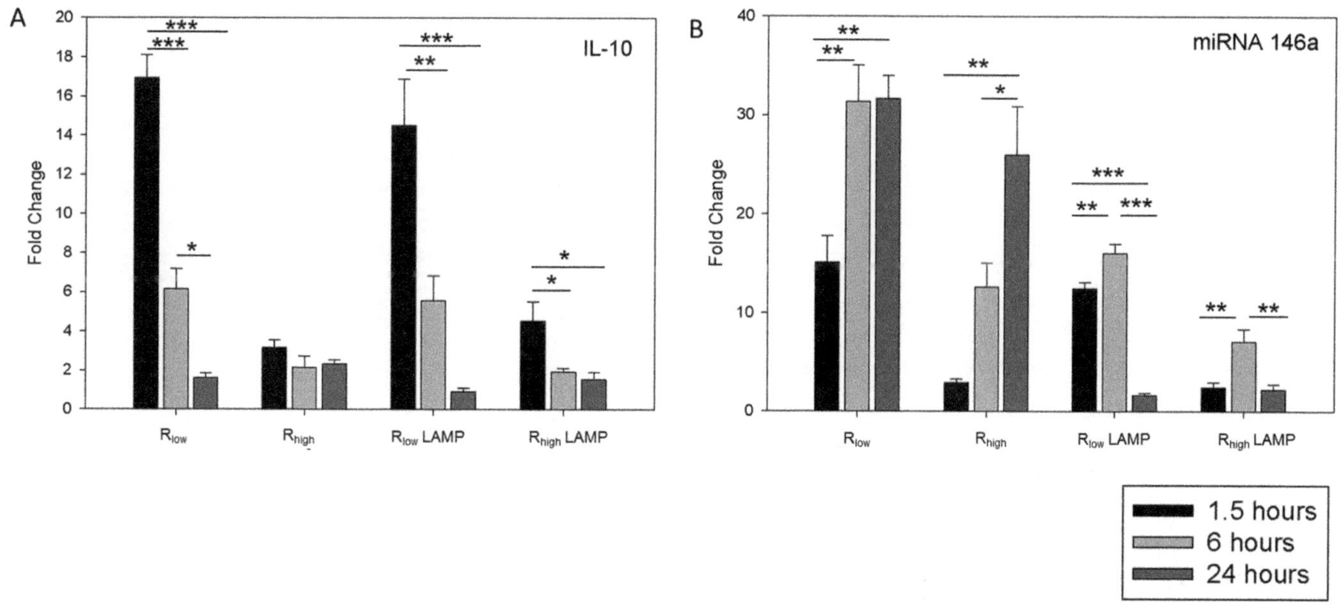

Figure 6. RT-qPCR analysis of miRNA and IL-10 differential expression in TECs. Epithelial cells were exposed to R_{low}, R_{low} LAMP, R_{high} or R_{high} LAMP at 1.5, 6 and 24 hours respectively. Samples were normalized to housekeeping gene GAPDH and un-exposed TECs as control. n = 6 for all experiments. Results are denoted as fold change ± SEM with all control values set at 1. Significant differences denoted as * = $P<0.05$, ** = $P<0.01$, *** = $P<0.001$. **A:** mRNA fold difference of IL-10 in TECs at all three time points post exposure. **B:** mRNA fold difference of miRNA-146a in TECs at all three time points post exposure.

subsequent signaling events appear to involve a unique set of inflammatory genes not observed in epithelial cells.

In the current study we also observed that R_{low} was by far the most potent stimulus for initiating differential gene expression by epithelial cells when compared to live R_{high} or LAMPs from either strain. TECs exposed to R_{low} not only up-regulated inflammatory genes to a significantly higher extent, but up-regulated more than a hundred additional unique genes by ≥5 fold. The R_{high} strain is non-virulent as it lacks several virulence determinant proteins of R_{low}, *especially* GapA and CrmA [7,78] two significant cytadhesion-associated proteins homologous to P1 and P40/P90 of *M. pneumoniae* [78–84]. The significantly diminished cytadhesion capability of R_{high} [7,82,85,86], may explain the reduced differential gene expression induced by this strain. Subtle differences in gene expression observed between the LAMPs prepared from R_{low} and R_{high} may also be explained by the differences identified by Szczepanek et al. involving 29 mutations in the variable GAA repeat region associated with phase variable expression of vlhA genes between these two strains [86].

When TECs were exposed to LAMPs in the presence of OxPAPC, a competitive inhibitor of lipoprotein and LPS mediated signaling via TLR-2 and TLR-4 respectively [87], expression of all six genes was significantly reduced. However in the presence of CLI-095, a selective TLR-4 inhibitor, no changes in gene expression were observed. When TECs were exposed to Celastrol, an NF-κB inhibitor [88], LAMP-mediated gene expression was completely abrogated. This observation is in keeping with previous studies from other mycoplasma species in which LAMP-induced inflammation was mediated upon TLR-2 ligation and activation of NF-κB [28,34,49–51,53,55,56]. Moreover, these observations apply to early time-points post-exposure, in a highly relevant cell population.

The kinetics of inflammatory gene expression in the current study was found to be rapid, peaking at either 1.5 hours or 6 hours, and then waning by 24 hours. As modulation of host responses is often accompanied by concurrent pro- and anti-inflammatory mechanisms [89], we hypothesized that a compensatory, homeostatic mechanism may be working in concert with the inflammatory response. Upon NF-κB activation, certain anti-inflammatory genes and micro RNA's are expressed that participate in the homeostatic regulation of inflammatory responses. For example, miRNA-146a, which is induced by LPS via NF-κB activation, down-regulates IRAK-1 and TRAF-6 and in turn suppresses further activation of NF-κB [90]. miRNA146a also negatively regulate TLR-2 signaling [91]. miRNA-21, on the other hand can promote IL-10 production by regulating PDCD4 (programmed cell death 4), an inhibitor of IL-10 production [90]. We observed miRNA-146a expression to be increasingly up-regulated until 24 hours in TECs exposed to either R_{low} or R_{high} in contrast to the pattern observed upon exposure to LAMPs, which peaked at 6 hours and waned thereafter, likely due to the lack of LAMP re-stimulation [91]. No difference in expression was observed for miRNA146b, miRNA146c1 or miRNA21. Conversely, the anti-inflammatory cytokine IL-10 showed no reciprocal relationship to pro-inflammatory gene expression, but was significantly up-regulated by the epithelial cells initially upon exposure to live R_{low} and the LAMPs (but not R_{high}). IL-10 is known to selectively inhibit nuclear localization of NF-κB by blocking IκB kinase activity and inducing nuclear translocation and DNA-binding of the repressive p50–p50 homodimer [92,93]. Therefore, miRNA-146a and in part IL-10 may play a role in regulating the over-exuberant pro-inflammatory response observed during *M.gallisepticum* infection.

Taken together our data suggest that *M. gallisepticum* LAMPs have potent inflammatory properties and can mediate changes in gene expression in chicken tracheal epithelial cells almost immediately upon exposure. However, the response appears to be transient in nature likely due to host compensatory mechanisms. Thus, continuous LAMP-mediated stimulation by adherent, replicating mycoplasma may be necessary to sustain the response. Studies using chemical inhibitors of specific signaling pathways indicated that mycoplasma LAMPs ligate TLR2 on TECs and activate NF-κB resulting in downstream expression of several pro-inflammatory chemokines and cytokines. Among the up-regulated genes are chemokines and cytokines known for leukocyte chemo-attraction and activation, consistent with the immunopathology associated with infection. Our data also support the notion that the virulent R_{low} strain possesses additional mechanisms of initiating inflammatory responses in tracheal epithelial cells beyond that mediated by LAMPs alone.

Supporting Information

Figure S1 Distribution of differentially regulated genes in TECs. Differentially regulated genes (≥2 fold) in tracheal epithelial cells after exposure to live R_{low}, R_{high} or LAMPs isolated from either strain for 1.5 hours. n = 8 (4 biological replicates x2 dye swap technical replicates) for all microarray experiments.

Figure S2 Kinetic analysis of differentially regulated genes encoding inflammatory chemokines and cytokines. Differential gene expression in TECs exposed to R_{low}, R_{low} LAMP, R_{high} or R_{high} LAMP at 1.5, 6 and 24 hours respectively. Samples normalized to housekeeping gene GAPDH and un-exposed TECs as control. n = 6 for all experiments. Results are denoted as fold change ± SEM with all control values set at 1. Significant differences denoted as * = $P<0.05$, ** = $P<0.01$, *** = $P<0.001$. **A**: mRNA fold difference in R_{low} exposed cells **B**: mRNA fold difference in R_{high} exposed cells. **C**: mRNA fold difference in R_{low} LAMP exposed cells. **D**: mRNA fold difference in R_{high} LAMP exposed cells.

Figure S3 TLR- Signaling pathway. Toll like receptor signaling network: Common genes up-regulated in TECs exposed to R_{low}, R_{high}, R_{low} LAMP or R_{high} LAMP are depicted in yellow boxes.

Figure S4 Original agarose gels photos of amplified products of epithelial cell specific genes. 1A: Confirmation of tracheal epithelial cells in culture *in vitro* using amplification of epithelial cell specific genes compared to chicken embryonic fibroblast (DF-1) cells. **1B:** Confirmation of epithelial cell specific genes in freshly isolated epithelial cells from tracheae after *ex-vivo* exposure.

Table S1 Differentially expressed genes (≥2-fold, p-value ≤0.05). Genes commonly up-regulated in TECs exposed to R_{low}, R_{high}, R_{low} lipoprotein and R_{high} lipoprotein: analyzed for gene ontology hierarchal clustering (Excludes unknown genes listed as finished cDNA clones).

Table S2 Differentially expressed unique genes in R_{low} exposed TECs (≥5-fold, p-value ≤0.05) (Excludes unknown genes listed as finished cDNA clones).

Acknowledgments

We acknowledge Dr. Steven J. Geary for providing us with the *Mycoplasma gallisepticum* strains and for his critical review of the manuscript; Dr. Steven M. Szczepanek for his helpful inputs during the early stages of project development and critical review of the manuscript. We acknowledge Dr. Tania B. Huedo-Medina for her assistance with the statistical analyses. We also thank Ms. Xiaofen Liao for her help during isolation of mycoplasma LAMPs and Ms. Debra Rood for her maintenance of the laboratory.

Author Contributions

Conceived and designed the experiments: LKS SM. Performed the experiments: SM FZ. Analyzed the data: SM FZ. Wrote the paper: LKS SM FZ.

References

1. Sato S, Nonomura I, Shimizu F, Shoya S, Horiuchi T (1970) Mixed infection with *Mycoplasma gallisepticum* and the B1 strain of Newcastle disease virus in chickens. Natl Inst Anim Health Q (Tokyo) 10: 58–65.
2. Gaunson JE, Philip CJ, Whithear KG, Browning GF (2000) Lymphocytic infiltration in the chicken trachea in response to *Mycoplasma gallisepticum* infection. Microbiology 146 (Pt5): 1223–1229.
3. Stipkovits L, Egyed L, Palfi V, Beres A, Pitlik E, et al. (2012) Effect of low-pathogenicity influenza virus H3N8 infection on *Mycoplasma gallisepticum* infection of chickens. Avian Pathol 41: 51–57.
4. Winner F, Rosengarten R, Citti C (2000) In vitro cell invasion of *Mycoplasma gallisepticum*. Infect Immun 68: 4238–4244.
5. Vogl G, Plaickner A, Szathmary S, Stipkovits L, Rosengarten R, et al. (2008) *Mycoplasma gallisepticum* invades chicken erythrocytes during infection. Infect Immun 76: 71–77.
6. Furnkranz U, Siebert-Gulle K, Rosengarten R, Szostak MP (2013) Factors influencing the cell adhesion and invasion capacity of *Mycoplasma gallisepticum*. Acta Vet Scand 55: 63.
7. Indikova I, Much P, Stipkovits L, Siebert-Gulle K, Szostak MP, et al. (2013) Role of the GapA and CrmA cytadhesins of *Mycoplasma gallisepticum* in promoting virulence and host colonization. Infect Immun.
8. Much P, Winner F, Stipkovits L, Rosengarten R, Citti C (2002) *Mycoplasma gallisepticum*: Influence of cell invasiveness on the outcome of experimental infection in chickens. FEMS Immunol Med Microbiol 34: 181–186.
9. Jenkins C, Geary SJ, Gladd M, Djordjevic SP (2007) The *Mycoplasma gallisepticum* OsmC-like protein MG1142 resides on the cell surface and binds heparin. Microbiology 153: 1455–1463.
10. Grodio JL, Dhondt KV, O'Connell PH, Schat KA (2008) Detection and quantification of *Mycoplasma gallisepticum* genome load in conjunctival samples of experimentally infected house finches (Carpodacus mexicanus) using real-time polymerase chain reaction. Avian Pathol 37: 385–391.
11. Tajima M, Nunoya T, Yagihashi T (1979) An ultrastructural study on the interaction of *Mycoplasma gallisepticum* with the chicken tracheal epithelium. Am J Vet Res 40: 1009–1014.
12. Mohammed J, Frasca S Jr, Cecchini K, Rood D, Nyaoke AC, et al. (2007) Chemokine and cytokine gene expression profiles in chickens inoculated with *Mycoplasma gallisepticum* strains Rlow or GT5. Vaccine 25: 8611–8621.
13. Gaunson JE, Philip CJ, Whithear KG, Browning GF (2006) The cellular immune response in the tracheal mucosa to *Mycoplasma gallisepticum* in vaccinated and unvaccinated chickens in the acute and chronic stages of disease. Vaccine 24: 2627–2633.
14. Bystry RS, Aluvihare V, Welch KA, Kallikourdis M, Betz AG (2001) B cells and professional APCs recruit regulatory T cells via CCL4. Nat Immunol 2: 1126–1132.
15. Sherry B, Tekamp-Olson P, Gallegos C, Bauer D, Davatelis G, et al. (1988) Resolution of the two components of macrophage inflammatory protein 1, and cloning and characterization of one of those components, macrophage inflammatory protein 1 beta. J Exp Med 168: 2251–2259.
16. Legler DF, Loetscher M, Roos RS, Clark-Lewis I, Baggiolini M, et al. (1998) B cell-attracting chemokine 1, a human CXC chemokine expressed in lymphoid tissues, selectively attracts B lymphocytes via BLR1/CXCR5. J Exp Med 187: 655–660.
17. Gunn MD, Ngo VN, Ansel KM, Ekland EH, Cyster JG, et al. (1998) A B-cell-homing chemokine made in lymphoid follicles activates Burkitt's lymphoma receptor-1. Nature 391: 799–803.
18. Kelner GS, Kennedy J, Bacon KB, Kleyensteuber S, Largaespada DA, et al. (1994) Lymphotactin: a cytokine that represents a new class of chemokine. Science 266: 1395–1399.
19. Schall TJ, Jongstra J, Dyer BJ, Jorgensen J, Clayberger C, et al. (1988) A human T cell-specific molecule is a member of a new gene family. J Immunol 141: 1018–1025.

20. Gomez MI, Prince A (2008) Airway epithelial cell signaling in response to bacterial pathogens. Pediatr Pulmonol 43: 11–19.
21. Fournier B, Philpott DJ (2005) Recognition of *Staphylococcus aureus* by the innate immune system. Clin Microbiol Rev 18: 521–540.
22. Prince A (2006) Flagellar activation of epithelial signaling. Am J Respir Cell Mol Biol 34: 548–551.
23. Liu X, Wetzler LM, Nascimento LO, Massari P (2010) Human airway epithelial cell responses to *Neisseria lactamica* and purified porin via Toll-like receptor 2-dependent signaling. Infect Immun 78: 5314–5323.
24. Roussel L, Martel G, Berube J, Rousseau S (2011) *P. aeruginosa* drives CXCL8 synthesis via redundant toll-like receptors and NADPH oxidase in CFTRF508 airway epithelial cells. J Cyst Fibros 10: 107–113.
25. Yang J, Hooper WC, Phillips DJ, Talkington DF (2002) Regulation of proinflammatory cytokines in human lung epithelial cells infected with *Mycoplasma pneumoniae*. Infect Immun 70: 3649–3655.
26. McGowin CL, Annan RS, Quayle AJ, Greene SJ, Ma L, et al. (2012) Persistent *Mycoplasma genitalium* infection of human endocervical epithelial cells elicits chronic inflammatory cytokine secretion. Infect Immun 80: 3842–3849.
27. McGowin CL, Popov VL, Pyles RB (2009) Intracellular *Mycoplasma genitalium* infection of human vaginal and cervical epithelial cells elicits distinct patterns of inflammatory cytokine secretion and provides a possible survival niche against macrophage-mediated killing. BMC Microbiol 9: 139.
28. McGowin CL, Ma L, Martin DH, Pyles RB (2009) *Mycoplasma genitalium*-encoded MG309 activates NF-kappaB via Toll-like receptors 2 and 6 to elicit proinflammatory cytokine secretion from human genital epithelial cells. Infect Immun 77: 1175–1181.
29. Krishnan M, Kannan TR, Baseman JB (2013) *Mycoplasma pneumoniae* CARDS toxin is internalized via clathrin-mediated endocytosis. PLoS One 8: e62706.
30. Medina JL, Coalson JJ, Brooks EG, Winter VT, Chaparro A, et al. (2012) *Mycoplasma pneumoniae* CARDS toxin induces pulmonary eosinophilic and lymphocytic inflammation. Am J Respir Cell Mol Biol 46: 815–822.
31. Cole BC (1991) The immunobiology of *Mycoplasma arthritidis* and its superantigen MAM. Curr Top Microbiol Immunol 174: 107–119.
32. Cole BC, Aldridge KE, Ward JR (1977) Mycoplasma-dependent activation of normal lymphocytes: mitogenic potential of mycoplasmas for mouse lymphocytes. Infect Immun 18: 393–399.
33. Zuo LL, Wu YM, You XX (2009) Mycoplasma lipoproteins and Toll-like receptors. J Zhejiang Univ Sci B 10: 67–76.
34. Shimizu T, Kida Y, Kuwano K (2008) A triacylated lipoprotein from *Mycoplasma genitalium* activates NF-kappaB through Toll-like receptor 1 (TLR1) and TLR2. Infect Immun 76: 3672–3678.
35. Chambaud I, Wroblewski H, Blanchard A (1999) Interactions between mycoplasma lipoproteins and the host immune system. Trends Microbiol 7: 493–499.
36. Tulman ER, Liao X, Szczepanek SM, Ley DH, Kutish GF, et al. (2012) Extensive variation in surface lipoprotein gene content and genomic changes associated with virulence during evolution of a novel North American house finch epizootic strain of *Mycoplasma gallisepticum*. Microbiology 158: 2073–2088.
37. Xu CG, Hao YQ, Zhang L, Hao RX, Liu XL, et al. (2014) Molecular cloning and immune response analysis of putative variable lipoproteins from *Mycoplasma mycoides* subsp capri. Genet Mol Res 13: 1527–1539.
38. Noormohammadi AH, Markham PF, Kanci A, Whithear KG, Browning GF (2000) A novel mechanism for control of antigenic variation in the haemagglutinin gene family of *Mycoplasma synoviae*. Mol Microbiol 35: 911–923.
39. Yogev D, Menaker D, Strutzberg K, Levisohn S, Kirchhoff H, et al. (1994) A surface epitope undergoing high-frequency phase variation is shared by *Mycoplasma gallisepticum* and Mycoplasma bovis. Infect Immun 62: 4962–4968.
40. Chopra-Dewasthaly R, Baumgartner M, Gamper E, Innerebner C, Zimmermann M, et al. (2012) Role of Vpma phase variation in *Mycoplasma agalactiae* pathogenesis. FEMS Immunol Med Microbiol 66: 307–322.
41. Wu HN, Kawaguchi C, Nakane D, Miyata M (2012) "Mycoplasmal antigen modulation," a novel surface variation suggested for a lipoprotein specifically localized on *Mycoplasma mobile*. Curr Microbiol 64: 433–440.
42. Nouvel LX, Marenda M, Sirand-Pugnet P, Sagne E, Glew M, et al. (2009) Occurrence, plasticity, and evolution of the vpma gene family, a genetic system devoted to high-frequency surface variation in *Mycoplasma agalactiae*. J Bacteriol 191: 4111–4121.
43. You XX, Zeng YH, Wu YM (2006) Interactions between mycoplasma lipid-associated membrane proteins and the host cells. J Zhejiang Univ Sci B 7: 342–350.
44. Behrens A, Heller M, Kirchhoff H, Yogev D, Rosengarten R (1994) A family of phase- and size-variant membrane surface lipoprotein antigens (Vsps) of *Mycoplasma bovis*. Infect Immun 62: 5075–5084.
45. Calcutt MJ, Kim MF, Karpas AB, Muhlradt PF, Wise KS (1999) Differential posttranslational processing confers intraspecies variation of a major surface lipoprotein and a macrophage-activating lipopeptide of *Mycoplasma fermentans*. Infect Immun 67: 760–771.
46. Citti C, Wise KS (1995) *Mycoplasma hyorhinis* vlp gene transcription: critical role in phase variation and expression of surface lipoproteins. Mol Microbiol 18: 649–660.
47. Papazisi L, Gorton TS, Kutish G, Markham PF, Browning GF, et al. (2003) The complete genome sequence of the avian pathogen *Mycoplasma gallisepticum* strain R(low). Microbiology 149: 2307–2316.
48. Liu YC, Lin IH, Chung WJ, Hu WS, Ng WV, et al. (2012) Proteomics characterization of cytoplasmic and lipid-associated membrane proteins of human pathogen *Mycoplasma fermentans* M64. PLoS One 7: e35304.
49. He J, Wang S, Zeng Y, You X, Ma X, et al. (2014) Binding of CD14 to *Mycoplasma genitalium*-Derived Lipid-Associated Membrane Proteins Upregulates TNF-alpha. Inflammation 37: 322–330.
50. He J, You X, Zeng Y, Yu M, Zuo L, et al. (2009) *Mycoplasma genitalium*-derived lipid-associated membrane proteins activate NF-kappaB through toll-like receptors 1, 2, and 6 and CD14 in a MyD88-dependent pathway. Clin Vaccine Immunol 16: 1750–1757.
51. Logunov D, Shchebliakov DV, Zubkova OV, Shmarov MM, Rakovskaia IV, et al. (2009) [Lipid-associated membrane lipopeptides of *M. arginini* activate NF-kB by interacting with TLR2/1, TLR2/6, and TLR2/CD14]. Mol Gen Mikrobiol Virusol: 25–28.
52. You X, Wu Y, Zeng Y, Deng Z, Qiu H, et al. (2008) *Mycoplasma genitalium*-derived lipid-associated membrane proteins induce activation of MAPKs, NF-kappaB and AP-1 in THP-1 cells. FEMS Immunol Med Microbiol 52: 228–236.
53. Qiu H, Wu YM, You XX, Yu MJ, Zeng YH (2007) [*Mycoplasma genitalium* lipid-associated membrane proteins induce human monocytic cell express proinflammatory cytokines and apoptosis by activating nuclear factor kappaB]. Wei Sheng Wu Xue Bao 47: 899–904.
54. Xu Y, Li H, Chen W, Yao X, Xing Y, et al. (2013) *Mycoplasma hyorhinis* activates the NLRP3 inflammasome and promotes migration and invasion of gastric cancer cells. PLoS One 8: e77955.
55. Shimizu T, Kida Y, Kuwano K (2005) A dipalmitoylated lipoprotein from *Mycoplasma pneumoniae* activates NF-kappa B through TLR1, TLR2, and TLR6. J Immunol 175: 4641–4646.
56. Shimizu T, Kida Y, Kuwano K (2007) Triacylated lipoproteins derived from *Mycoplasma pneumoniae* activate nuclear factor-kappaB through toll-like receptors 1 and 2. Immunology 121: 473–483.
57. Seya T, Matsumoto M (2002) A lipoprotein family from *Mycoplasma fermentans* confers host immune activation through Toll-like receptor 2. Int J Biochem Cell Biol 34: 901–906.
58. Deiters U, Muhlradt PF (1999) Mycoplasmal lipopeptide MALP-2 induces the chemoattractant proteins macrophage inflammatory protein 1alpha (MIP-1alpha), monocyte chemoattractant protein 1, and MIP-2 and promotes leukocyte infiltration in mice. Infect Immun 67: 3390–3398.
59. Into T, Kiura K, Yasuda M, Kataoka H, Inoue N, et al. (2004) Stimulation of human Toll-like receptor (TLR) 2 and TLR6 with membrane lipoproteins of *Mycoplasma fermentans* induces apoptotic cell death after NF-kappa B activation. Cell Microbiol 6: 187–199.
60. Fichorova RN, Cronin AO, Lien E, Anderson DJ, Ingalls RR (2002) Response to *Neisseria gonorrhoeae* by cervicovaginal epithelial cells occurs in the absence of toll-like receptor 4-mediated signaling. J Immunol 168: 2424–2432.
61. Choi SY, Lim JW, Shimizu T, Kuwano K, Kim JM, et al. (2012) Reactive oxygen species mediate Jak2/Stat3 activation and IL-8 expression in pulmonary epithelial cells stimulated with lipid-associated membrane proteins from *Mycoplasma pneumoniae*. Inflammation Research 61: 493–501.
62. Zaffuto KM, Estevez CN, Afonso CL (2008) Primary chicken tracheal cell culture system for the study of infection with avian respiratory viruses. Avian Pathol 37: 25–31.
63. Shen CI, Wang CH, Liao JW, Hsu TW, Kuo SM, et al. The infection of primary avian tracheal epithelial cells with infectious bronchitis virus. Vet Res 41: 6.
64. Bischof DF, Janis C, Vilei EM, Bertoni G, Frey J (2008) Cytotoxicity of *Mycoplasma mycoides* subsp. mycoides small colony type to bovine epithelial cells. Infect Immun 76: 263–269.
65. Love W, Dobbs N, Tabor L, Simecka JW (2010) Toll-like receptor 2 (TLR2) plays a major role in innate resistance in the lung against murine Mycoplasma. PLoS One 5: e10739.
66. Razin S, Yogev D, Naot Y (1998) Molecular biology and pathogenicity of mycoplasmas. Microbiol Mol Biol Rev 62: 1094–1156.
67. Javed MA, Frasca S Jr, Rood D, Cecchini K, Gladd M, et al. (2005) Correlates of immune protection in chickens vaccinated with *Mycoplasma gallisepticum* strain GT5 following challenge with pathogenic M. gallisepticum strain R(low). Infect Immun 73: 5410–5419.
68. Rawadi G (2000) *Mycoplasma fermentans* interaction with monocytes/macrophages: molecular basis. Microbes Infect 2: 955–964.
69. Rottem S (2003) Interaction of mycoplasmas with host cells. Physiol Rev 83: 417–432.
70. Walter MJ, Kajiwara N, Karanja P, Castro M, Holtzman MJ (2001) Interleukin 12 p40 production by barrier epithelial cells during airway inflammation. J Exp Med 193: 339–351.
71. Oppmann B, Lesley R, Blom B, Timans JC, Xu Y, et al. (2000) Novel p19 protein engages IL-12p40 to form a cytokine, IL-23, with biological activities similar as well as distinct from IL-12. Immunity 13: 715–725.
72. Hieshima K, Imai T, Opdenakker G, Van Damme J, Kusuda J, et al. (1997) Molecular cloning of a novel human CC chemokine liver and activation-regulated chemokine (LARC) expressed in liver. Chemotactic activity for lymphocytes and gene localization on chromosome 2. J Biol Chem 272: 5846–5853.

73. Baggiolini M, Clark-Lewis I (1992) Interleukin-8, a chemotactic and inflammatory cytokine. FEBS Lett 307: 97–101.
74. Zamora R, Vodovotz Y, Billiar TR (2000) Inducible nitric oxide synthase and inflammatory diseases. Mol Med 6: 347–373.
75. Medina S, Del Rio M, Hernanz A, Guaza C, De la Fuente M (2005) Nitric oxide released by accessory cells mediates the gastrin-releasing peptide effect on murine lymphocyte chemotaxis. Regul Pept 131: 46–53.
76. Hsieh CS, Macatonia SE, Tripp CS, Wolf SF, O'Garra A, et al. (1993) Development of TH1 CD4+ T cells through IL-12 produced by Listeria-induced macrophages. Science 260: 547–549.
77. Xing Z, Zganiacz A, Santosuosso M (2000) Role of IL-12 in macrophage activation during intracellular infection: IL-12 and mycobacteria synergistically release TNF-alpha and nitric oxide from macrophages via IFN-gamma induction. J Leukoc Biol 68: 897–902.
78. Papazisi L, Frasca S Jr, Gladd M, Liao X, Yogev D, et al. (2002) GapA and CrmA coexpression is essential for *Mycoplasma gallisepticum* cytadherence and virulence. Infect Immun 70: 6839–6845.
79. Dallo SF, Chavoya A, Baseman JB (1990) Characterization of the gene for a 30-kilodalton adhesion-related protein of *Mycoplasma pneumoniae*. Infect Immun 58: 4163–4165.
80. Krause DC, Balish MF (2001) Structure, function, and assembly of the terminal organelle of *Mycoplasma pneumoniae*. FEMS Microbiol Lett 198: 1–7.
81. Kahane I, Tucker S, Leith DK, Morrison-Plummer J, Baseman JB (1985) Detection of the major adhesin P1 in triton shells of virulent *Mycoplasma pneumoniae*. Infect Immun 50: 944–946.
82. Papazisi L, Troy KE, Gorton TS, Liao X, Geary SJ (2000) Analysis of cytadherence-deficient, GapA-negative *Mycoplasma gallisepticum* strain R. Infect Immun 68: 6643–6649.
83. Krause DC, Balish MF (2004) Cellular engineering in a minimal microbe: structure and assembly of the terminal organelle of *Mycoplasma pneumoniae*. Mol Microbiol 51: 917–924.
84. Krause DC (1996) *Mycoplasma pneumoniae* cytadherence: unravelling the tie that binds. Mol Microbiol 20: 247–253.
85. May M, Papazisi L, Gorton TS, Geary SJ (2006) Identification of fibronectin-binding proteins in *Mycoplasma gallisepticum* strain R. Infect Immun 74: 1777–1785.
86. Szczepanek SM, Tulman ER, Gorton TS, Liao X, Lu Z, et al. (2010) Comparative genomic analyses of attenuated strains of *Mycoplasma gallisepticum*. Infect Immun 78: 1760–1771.
87. Erridge C, Kennedy S, Spickett CM, Webb DJ (2008) Oxidized phospholipid inhibition of toll-like receptor (TLR) signaling is restricted to TLR2 and TLR4: roles for CD14, LPS-binding protein, and MD2 as targets for specificity of inhibition. J Biol Chem 283: 24748–24759.
88. Sethi G, Ahn KS, Pandey MK, Aggarwal BB (2007) Celastrol, a novel triterpene, potentiates TNF-induced apoptosis and suppresses invasion of tumor cells by inhibiting NF-kappaB-regulated gene products and TAK1-mediated NF-kappaB activation. Blood 109: 2727–2735.
89. Griesinger G, Saleh L, Bauer S, Husslein P, Knofler M (2001) Production of pro- and anti-inflammatory cytokines of human placental trophoblasts in response to pathogenic bacteria. J Soc Gynecol Investig 8: 334–340.
90. Alam MM, O'Neill LA (2011) MicroRNAs and the resolution phase of inflammation in macrophages. Eur J Immunol 41: 2482–2485.
91. Quinn EM, Wang JH, O'Callaghan G, Redmond HP (2013) MicroRNA-146a is upregulated by and negatively regulates TLR2 signaling. PLoS One 8: e62232.
92. Wang P, Wu P, Siegel MI, Egan RW, Billah MM (1995) Interleukin (IL)-10 inhibits nuclear factor kappa B (NF kappa B) activation in human monocytes. IL-10 and IL-4 suppress cytokine synthesis by different mechanisms. J Biol Chem 270: 9558–9563.
93. Driessler F, Venstrom K, Sabat R, Asadullah K, Schottelius AJ (2004) Molecular mechanisms of interleukin-10-mediated inhibition of NF-kappaB activity: a role for p50. Clin Exp Immunol 135: 64–73.

14

Endothelin Receptor B2 (*EDNRB2*) Is Responsible for the Tyrosinase-Independent Recessive White (mo^w) and Mottled (*mo*) Plumage Phenotypes in the Chicken

Keiji Kinoshita[1], Toyoko Akiyama[2], Makoto Mizutani[1], Ai Shinomiya[2], Akira Ishikawa[3], Hassan Hassan Younis[3,4], Masaoki Tsudzuki[5,6], Takao Namikawa[1], Yoichi Matsuda[1,3]*

1 Avian Bioscience Research Center, Graduate School of Bioagricultural Sciences, Nagoya University, Nagoya, Japan, **2** Department of Biology, Keio University, Yokohama, Japan, **3** Laboratory of Animal Genetics, Department of Applied Molecular Biosciences, Graduate School of Bioagricultural Sciences, Nagoya University, Nagoya, Japan, **4** Department of Poultry Production, Faculty of Agriculture, Kafr El-Sheikh University, Kafr El-Sheikh, Egypt, **5** Laboratory of Animal Breeding and Genetics, Graduate School of Biosphere Science, Hiroshima University, Higashi-Hiroshima, Japan, **6** Japanese Avian Bioresource Project Research Center, Hiroshima University, Higashi-Hiroshima, Japan

Abstract

A mutation that confers white plumage with black eyes was identified in the Minohiki breed of Japanese native chicken (*Gallus gallus domesticus*). The white plumage, with a few partially pigmented feathers, was not associated with the tyrosinase gene, and displayed an autosomal recessive mode of inheritance against the pigmented phenotype. All F_1 offspring derived from crosses with mottled chickens (*mo/mo*), which show characteristic pigmented feathers with white tips, had plumage with a mottled-like pattern. This result indicates that the white plumage mutation is a novel allele at the *mo* locus; we propose the gene symbol mo^w for this mutant allele. Furthermore, the F_1 hybrid between the mo^w/mo^w chicken and the *panda* (*s/s*) mutant of Japanese quail (*Coturnix japonica*), whose causative gene is the *endothelin receptor B2* (*EDNRB2*) gene, showed a mo^w/mo^w chicken-like plumage, suggesting the possibility that the mutations in parental species are alleles of the same gene, *EDNRB2*. Nucleotide sequencing of the entire coding region of *EDNRB2* revealed a non-synonymous G1008T substitution, which causes Cys244Phe amino acid substitution in exon 5 (which is part of the extracellular loop between the putative fourth and fifth transmembrane domains of EDNRB2) in the mutant chicken. This Cys244Phe mutation was also present in individuals of four Japanese breeds with white plumage. We also identified a non-synonymous substitution leading to Arg332His substitution that was responsible for the mottled (*mo/mo*) plumage phenotype. These results suggest that the EDN3 (*endothelin 3*)–EDNRB2 signaling is essential for normal pigmentation in birds, and that the mutations of *EDNRB2* may cause defective binding of the protein with endothelins, which interferes with melanocyte differentiation, proliferation, and migration.

Editor: Alexandre Roulin, University of Lausanne, Switzerland

Funding: This research was supported by the National BioResource Project (NBRP) Chicken/Quail and Grants-in-Aid for Scientific Research on Innovative Areas (no. 23113004) and Scientific Research (B) (no. 20310143) from the Ministry of Education, Culture, Sports, Science and Technology, Japan, and grants from Keio University. The funders had no role in study design, data collection and analysis, decision to publish, or preparation of the manuscript.

Competing Interests: The authors have declared that no competing interests exist.

* E-mail: yoimatsu@agr.nagoya-u.ac.jp

Introduction

Animals with pigment disorders are easily distinguishable from other individuals by virtue of their different body colours. Such disorders have been well analysed at the molecular level, with more than 200 genes associated with pigmentation are known in mammals [1,2], and the genes associated with plumage colour mutations have also been increasingly identified in birds [3]. Some of these genes or pigments play important roles not only in integumental pigmentation but also in the senses of vision or hearing [1,4,5,6]. The occurrence of novel pigment-disorder mutants provides the opportunity to understand the functions and network of pigmentation-related genes, and to establish whether they might exhibit the same function in multiple species. In this study, we detected white-plumage mutants in a line of Minohiki (MH), a Japanese native breed of chicken (*Gallus gallus domesticus*), and investigated the gene responsible for the pigmentation phenotype.

In the chicken, two autosomal loci associated with white plumage colour are well known. One is an autosomal "dominant white" locus (*I*) that comprises a multiple-allelic series of the gene: dominant white (*I*), smoky (I^S), dun (I^D), and wild type (i^+) [7,8]. The dominant white plumage phenotype is often expressed in commercial chicken breeds, as represented by White Leghorn, and *I* is incompletely dominant to the other *I* alleles. Genetic linkage mapping and nucleotide sequencing revealed that the responsible gene for the dominant white plumage is *PMEL17*, which encodes a matrix protein of pre-melanosomes [9]. The other locus is an autosomal "recessive white" locus (*c*), which comprises recessive white (*c*), albino (c^a), red-eyed white (c^{re}), and wild-type (C^+) alleles [8,10]. The former three allelic genes (*c*, c^a, and c^{re}) are associated with exclusively white plumage, whereas the wild type (C^+) has pigmented plumage. These pigmentation phenotypes at the *c* locus are caused by multiple alleles of the tyrosinase (*TYR*) gene, which encodes a key enzyme required for melanin synthesis [11,12,13,14]. White plumage in chickens is considered to be mostly controlled by these two loci, although allelism between different breeds with white plumage has not been sufficiently tested to confirm the identity of the locus responsible for white plumage.

On the other hand, the molecular basis of white spotting coat phenotypes, in which the ability of cells on particular parts of the skin to make pigment is impaired and the skin becomes pink and the fur white, have been well characterised in rat and mouse. This pattern is caused by abnormalities in the differentiation, survival, and migration of melanocytes derived from neural crest cells [15,16,17,18]. Abnormality of the *endothelin* (*EDN*) and *endothelin receptor B* (*EDNRB*) genes are well known to cause the white spotting phenotype. Endothelins (EDNs), which exists as the isotypes EDN1, EDN2, and EDN3, are the 21-amino-acid ligands of endothelin receptors EDNRs, which are G protein-coupled receptors. Endothelins were first reported to be vasoconstricting peptides but now are known to have important roles in the proliferation and differentiation of pigment cells not only in the integument but also in internal organs [19,20,21,22,23,24,25,26]. Endothelins affect the development of neural crest-derived pigment cells in the melanocyte population in a dose-dependent manner *in vitro* in mouse and quail embryos [27,28,29,30,31].

The two subtypes of EDNRs in human and mouse are EDNRA and EDNRB [18,20,32,33,34,35]. EDNRB contains seven transmembrane domains, and is required for the development of melanocytes and enteric neurons [36,37,38]. Spontaneous mutations in *EDN3* and *EDNRB* in mouse are designated *lethal spotting* (*ls*) and *piebald lethal* (s^l), respectively. Both homozygous mutants display similar phenotypes of hypopigmentation and aganglionic megacolon [36,39]. The hypopigmented phenotype is caused by a decrease in the number of melanoblasts and abnormal cell migration [40,41].

Birds also have the *EDNRB2* gene, a paralog of *EDNRB*, which is conserved in *Xenopus* and platypus but not in zebrafish and therians, such as human and mouse [42,43]. The avian EDNRB and EDNRB2 show similar affinities for EDN1, EDN2, and EDN3 with no clear pharmacological differences, and do not show differential inhibition by antagonists. The interaction between EDN3 and EDNRB2 is essential for development and migration of neural crest-derived cell lineages [36,39,44]. Whereas *EDN3* is expressed in the ectoderm and gut mesenchyme [45], *EDNRB2* is expressed throughout the melanocyte lineage [42]. In Aves, EDNRB2 is important for melanoblast migration along the dorsolateral pathway [46,47]. In Japanese quail (*Coturnix japonica*), mutation of *EDNRB2* is associated with the *panda* (*s*) and *dotted-white* (s^{dw}) plumage phenotypes. The *panda* mutant has white plumage with coloured patches on the head, back, tail, cheek, and wings, whereas the *dotted-white* mutant has a large area of white plumage more than the panda mutant, with only a few small coloured spots on the head and/or back and occasionally with no coloured spots [48,49,50]. These mutant plumage phenotypes of Japanese quail are similar to those of the mottled chicken and white MH lines that were the focus of the present study.

Minohiki is a Japanese long-tailed chicken breed, and was designated a national natural treasure of Japan in 1940. The MH breed has been maintained as a closed colony at Nagoya University, Japan, since 1988. Typically, MH individuals are covered with light brown plumage either with or without the Columbian (*Co*) plumage pattern, in which black pigment is restricted to the hackle, wing, foot and tail feathers, but often display a white plumage colour mutation with a few partially pigmented feathers on the hackle, shoulder, or tail. Neonatal chicks with the white plumage mutation have whitish yellow down and often exhibit a small brown spot on the head. In a preliminary crossing test of white MH with white Ukokkei (Japanese Silkie) that was homozygous for a recessive *c* allele, all F_1 hybrids had coloured (normally pigmented) plumage. This finding strongly suggests that the white plumage mutation of MH is controlled by a novel *TYR* (*c*)-independent autosomal recessive gene. Mottling (*mo*) is a common plumage colour-pattern mutation, in which pigmented feathers have white tips, in many chicken breeds worldwide. The chick down phenotype of the white MH mutant is similar to that of the mottled phenotype, although a mottled chicken develops pigmented feathers with a white tip in the adult. This "mottling" pattern is controlled by an autosomal recessive gene designated *mo* [51,52,53]. In addition, another allele at the *mo* locus, the pied plumage represented by Exchequer Leghorn, often exhibits mottled-like feathers and infrequently all black, all white, or mixed feathers [53]. In the current study, we performed allelism tests and linkage mapping to identify the candidate gene associated with the novel white plumage and mottled plumage, and determined nucleotide sequences of the candidate gene for the novel white and mottled plumage patterns in several other chicken breeds. We present strong evidence that *EDNRB2* is associated with these mutant plumage patterns in chickens.

Results

Characteristics of the white plumage mutant

The typical plumage of the MH line is light brown either with or without the Columbian plumage (*Co*) pattern (i^+/i^+, $e^{+/-}$ or e^y/e^y, $Co/-$ or co^+/co^+, C^+/C^+) (Figures 1A-1 and A-2). Mutant males and females exhibited white plumage over the whole body except for a few partially pigmented feathers on the head, hackle, shoulder, saddle, and tail along the dorsal region (Figures 1B-1 and 1B-2). This plumage pattern was prominent in adult males (Figures 1B-1 and 1C). In adult females, slightly pigmented feathers were located in the dorsal occipital area (Figure 1B-2). Newly hatched chicks of the wild type displayed exclusively brownish-yellow down feathers (Figure 1D), and the white mutant occasionally showed wholly whitish yellow down feathers with one or two small brown spots (Figure 1E) or no spots (Figure 1F) on the head. The pigmented head spot mostly disappeared as the chicks approached maturity. The white mutant individuals appeared healthy and displayed normal fertility and the existence of pigments in the iris pigment epithelium, and the visual and auditory senses were normal.

Mode of inheritance of the white plumage mutation

To examine the association of the white plumage mutation of the MH line with the dominant white (*I*) locus and/or recessive white (*c*) locus, white mutant MH females were mated with males of two tester lines: PNP/DO (the wild type with normally pigmented plumage, i^+/i^+, C^+/C^+) and CAL (autosomal recessive albino, i^+/i^+, c^a/c^a) (Table 1). In the cross with the PNP/DO line, 26 F_1 individuals all exhibited wild-type plumage, and 26 F_2 progeny were segregated into 20 of the wild type and six of the black-eyed white type with a ratio close to 3:1 ($0.80>P>0.70$). In the cross with the CAL, 15 F_1 individuals all exhibited wild-type plumage, and the 307 F_2 progeny were segregated into 184 wild type, 58 black-eyed white, and 65 red-eyed white (albino) phenotypes with a ratio approaching 9:3:4 ($0.30>P>0.20$). These results collectively indicated that the white plumage mutation in the MH line was controlled by a *PMEL17* (at *I* locus)- and *TYR* (at *c* locus)-independent autosomal recessive gene.

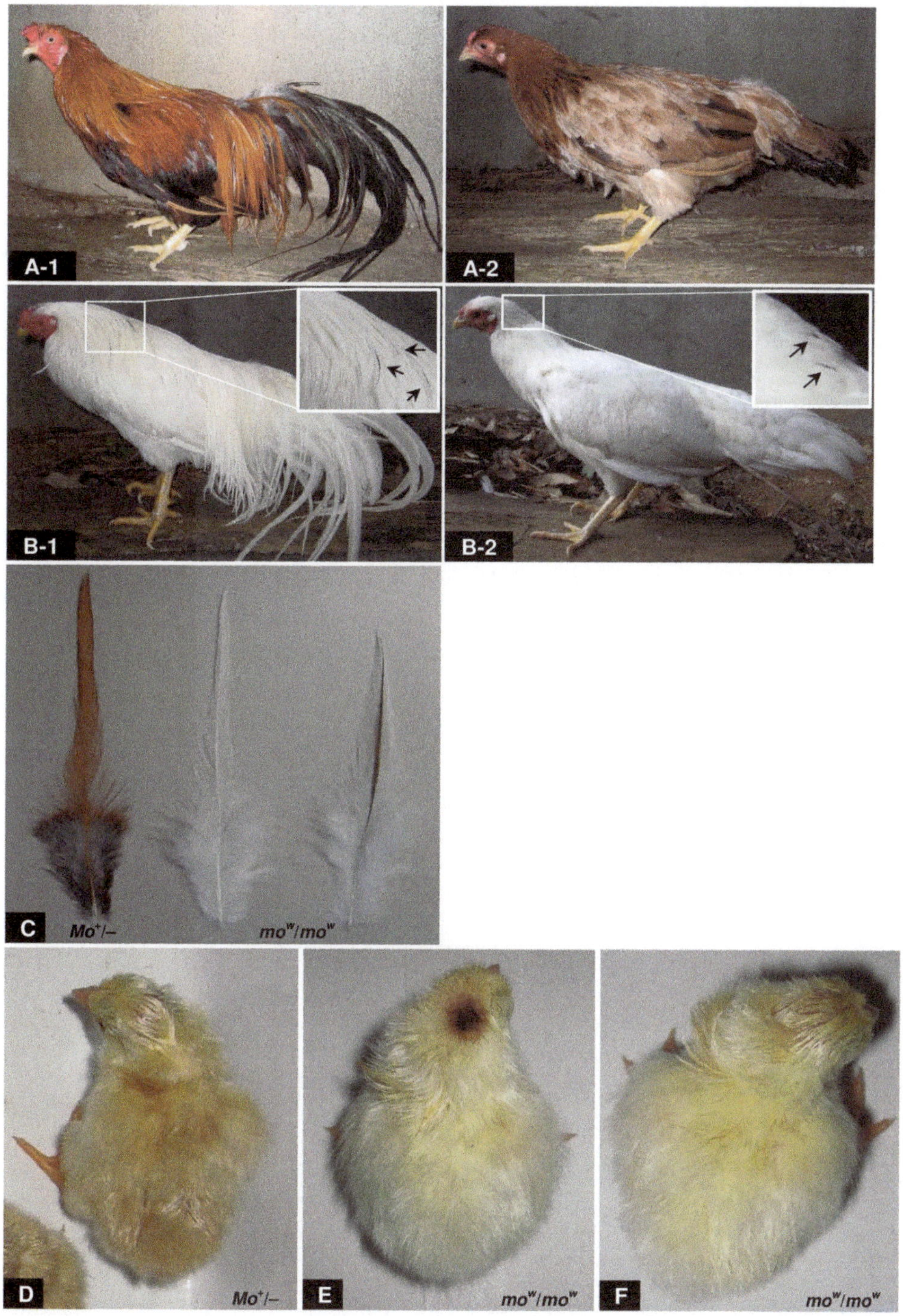

Figure 1. Plumage phenotypes in the Minohiki (MH) line. (A, B) Plumage colours in adult MH chickens with wild-type plumage (Mo^{+}) (i^{+}/i^{+}, $Co/-$ or co^{+}/co^{+}, C^{+}/C^{+}) (A-1, A-2) and white plumage (mo^{w}/mo^{w}) (B-1, B-2). Males are shown in A-1 and B-1, and females are shown in A-2 and B-2. The white mutant shows exclusively white plumage, with the exception of a few partially pigmented feathers at the back of the head, neck, and/or saddle hackle. Squares show magnified areas. Arrows indicate partially pigmented feathers. (C) Feathers of the neck hackle from a wild-type MH adult male ($Mo^{+/-}$) (left) and white MH adult male (mo^{w}/mo^{w}) (middle and right). (D–F) Down colours of newly hatched chicks of the wild type ($Mo^{+/-}$) (D) and white mutant (mo^{w}/mo^{w}) (E, F). The white mutant chick (mo^{w}/mo^{w}) has yellowish down with either a pigmented spot (E) or no spot (F) on the head.

Allelism of the white and mottled (*mo*) plumage phenotypes of chickens and the *panda* (*s*) plumage phenotype of Japanese quail

Females with the wild-type and mottled phenotypes are shown in Figures 2A-1 and 2A-2 in the CB line and in Figures 2B-1 and 2B-2 in the EJ line, respectively. The genotypes of the extended black (*E*) locus were E/E in CB and e^{+}/e^{+} in EJ. The mottled individuals commonly exhibited pigmented plumage with white markings at the tips of feathers (Figure 2C-1 right in CB; Figure 2C-2 right in EJ). The mottled chicks in both lines exhibited whitish yellow down with small brown-black spots on the head

(Figure 2D-1 right in CB; Figure 2D-2 right in EJ). To test whether the white plumage mutant in the MH line is an allelic variant at the mottled (*mo*) locus, mottled males of CB and EJ were mated with white mutant MH females (Table 1). In the mating with mottled CB, both F_1 males (Figure 3A-1) and females (Figure 3A-2) exhibited mottled-like plumage, which was intermediate between that of the white MH line and mottled CB. Following mating with mottled EJ, F_1 males and females exhibited similar plumage intermediate between that of the white MH line and mottled EJ (Figure 3A-3). Four F_1 chicks of mottled CB showed whitish yellow down with one or two black spots on the head as well as the mottled CB phenotype (Figure 3B; Table 1). The plumage of F_1 hybrids consisted of pure white or black feathers with white spots at the tips of feathers (Figure 3C). Nine F_1 chicks of mottled EJ also had whitish yellow down with one or two brown-black spots on the head (Table 1). Two female F_1 hybrids generated by crossing between mottled CB and the white MH mutant were backcrossed with a male white MH mutant, and 40 backcross progeny were obtained. Eighteen and 22 individuals showed the white mutant plumage and mottled-like plumage, respectively. This segregation ratio was close to the expected 1:1 ratio ($0.70>P>0.50$). These allelism tests confirmed that the mutations in the parental lines were allelic at the same *mo* locus; therefore, we proposed the new gene symbol mo^w for the white plumage mutation in the MH line.

The *panda* mutant of Japanese quail (*s/s*) has white plumage with small coloured patches, which is caused by a non-synonymous mutation in the *EDNRB2* gene. We therefore obtained a F_1 hybrid between the white mutant chicken (mo^w/mo^w) and the *panda* mutant of Japanese quail (*s/s*) by artificial insemination. The F_1 hybrid chick also showed yellowish down with one brown spot on the head as well as the white mutant chicken (Figures 4A-1 and A-2), and several small coloured patches were observed on the wing in the eight week-old bird (Figure 4B–4E, the same individual shown in Figures 4A-1 and A-2). These results show that the mutations in parental species are alleles of the same gene, *EDNRB2*.

Nucleotide sequences of *EDNRB2* in the mo^w mutant

Based on the results of allelism tests, we determined nucleotide sequences of the *EDNRB2* gene in the white MH mutant using the primers shown in Figure S1 and Table S1. Direct sequencing of *EDNRB2* cDNA revealed four single-nucleotide polymorphisms (SNPs) in the 1528 bp fragments between the wild type and the white MH mutant: three synonymous substitutions (C>G at nucleotide position 691, T>C at position 1,021, and T>C at position 1,159) and one non-synonymous G>T substitution at position 1,008. The non-synonymous substitution resulted in an amino acid substitution of cysteine (Cys) by phenylalanine (Phe) at position 244 (Cys244Phe) in EDNRB2 (Figure 5; Table 2). The *EDNRB2* cDNA sequences of the wild type (Mo^+/Mo^+) and the white mutant (mo^w/mo^w) were deposited with DDBJ (accession nos. AB697059 and AB697060, respectively). The G1008T substitution (Cys244Phe) was observed in other chicken breeds [Minohiki (Shizuoka), Uzurao, Shokoku, Onagadori, and Ohiki] that show white plumage with a few partially pigmented feathers (Table 3).

Complete association of G1008T substitution in *EDNRB2* with the mo^w mutation

To examine the association of *EDNRB2* with the white plumage mutation in the MH line, genotyping of *EDNRB2* was performed for F_2 progeny obtained from the mating between the white MH mutant and CAL line (Table 1), and their genotypes were compared with the segregation patterns of plumage. The G1008T substitution in exon 5 of *EDNRB2*, which was observed in the white MH mutant, destroyed a *Pae*I recognition site (G↑CATG↓C). Two sizes of fragments (354 bp and 159 bp) were produced by *Pae*I digestion from the wild-type allele (Mo^+) but not from the white mutant allele (mo^w) (Figure 6A, 6B). The linkage mapping using 93 F_2 progeny (50 wild-type and 43 white mutant individuals) showed that logarithm of odds (LOD) scores between the *mo* locus and the three markers *ADL0255*, *EDNRB2*, and *MCW0295* were 2.3, 27.2, and 17.1, respectively. No recombination was observed between the T/T genotype (513 bp) of *EDNRB2* and the mo^w allele for the examined 43 white mutant individuals (Figure S2). In the other 149 F_2 progeny excluding the albino white individuals ($n=65$), 15 white mutant individuals (mo^w/mo^w) showed the T/T genotype (513 bp), and the remaining 134 pigmented individuals (Mo^+/Mo^+ or Mo^+/mo^w) carried the G/G or G/T genotype (354 bp and 159 bp) (Figure 6B). This result confirmed complete association between the recessive white allele (mo^w) and the G1008T substitution in *EDNRB2*.

Cys244Phe mutation of *EDNRB2* in different chicken breeds

To confirm that the G1008T (Cys244Phe) substitution in exon 5 of *EDNRB2* causes the white plumage phenotype at the *mo* locus, we genotyped the genomic DNA fragment containing exon 5 of *EDNRB2* for 204 individuals from 22 different breeds, including Red jungle fowl (*Gallus gallus*), using the PCR-RFLP method (Figure 6A, 6B; Table S2). Twelve individuals from the breeds Minohiki (Shizuoka; $n=2$), Onagadori (Kanagawa; $n=4$), Ohiki (Hiroshima; $n=1$), Shokoku (Mie; $n=3$), and Uzurao (Ehime; $n=2$) had white plumage with a few pigmented feathers and were homozygous for the T/T allele (Phe/Phe) at position 1,008 (Phe244Phe) as well as the white mutant in MH line ($n=8$). On the other hand, six individuals with white plumage, two Shokoku (Ehime), four Uzurao (Ehime), which were not homozygous for the T/T allele (Phe/Phe) were confirmed to be homozygous for the recessive white (*c*) locus by a test cross with CAL (c^a/c^a) individuals (data not shown). In addition, the other 38 white-plumaged individuals of six breeds (Chabo, Chan, Koshamo, Japanese Silkie, CB, and White Leghorn) and 140 pigmented-feathered individuals of 22 breeds, including Red jungle fowl, were homozygous for the G allele at position 1,008 with only eight exceptions (six wild-type Minohiki and two Uzurao), which were G/T heterozygotes. These results collectively suggested that the G>T substitution at 1,008 in exon 5, which is responsible for the Cys244Phe substitution, was closely associated with the novel recessive allele (mo^w) showing white plumage with a few pigmented feathers in Japanese native chickens.

EDNRB2 mutations at the *mo* locus in mottled chickens

We determined the nucleotide sequences of cDNA fragments of the entire coding region of *EDNRB2* for EJ chickens with the wild-type (Mo^+/Mo^+) and mottled (*mo/mo*) plumage (AB697061 and AB697062, respectively) (Table 2). Direct sequencing revealed seven SNPs that involved four synonymous substitutions (T508C, C691G, C835T, and T1021C) and three non-synonymous substitutions (C300T, A320G, and G1272A) between the two plumage types. These resulted in amino acid changes of Thr>Ile at position 8, Thr>Ala at position 15, and Arg>His at position 332, respectively (Figure 5; Table 2).

To confirm that the three missense mutations leading to amino acid substitutions (Thr8Ile, Thr15Ala and Arg332His) in *EDNRB2* are associated with the mottled plumage phenotype, we examined the presence of the three mutations in three additional chicken

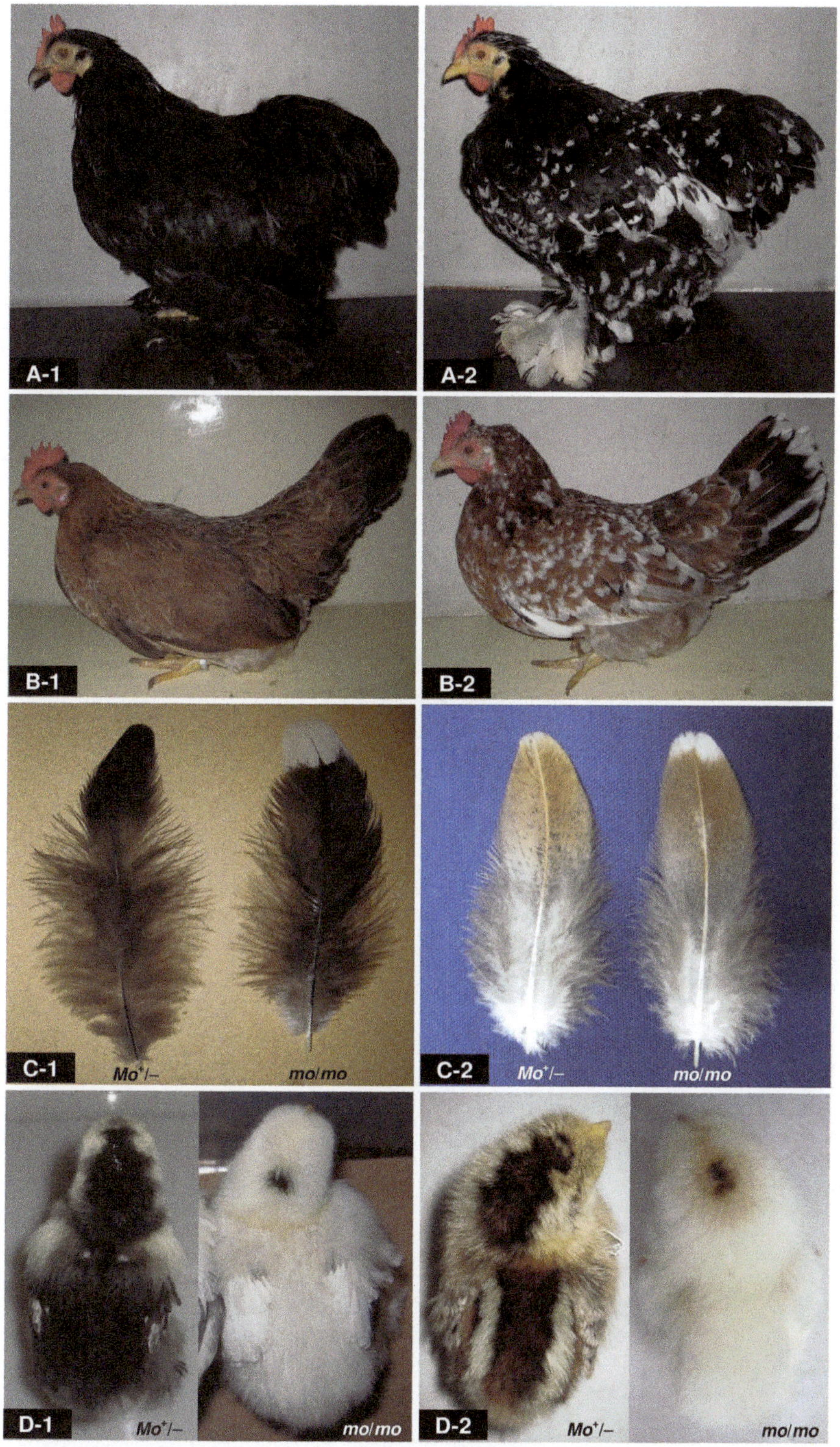

Figure 2. Wild-type and mottled plumage phenotypes with two different *extended black* (*E*) backgrounds in Cochin bantam (CB) and Ehime-jidori (EJ). (A) The wild-type ($Mo^{+/-}$) (A-1) and mottled plumage (*mo/mo*) (A-2) in adult CB females with an *E/E* genetic background. (B) The wild-type ($Mo^{+/-}$) (B-1) and mottled plumage (*mo/mo*) (B-2) in adult EJ females with an e^{+}/e^{+} genetic background. (C-1) Feathers of the saddle from the wild-type CB female ($Mo^{+/-}$) (left) and the mottled CB female (*mo/mo*) (right). (C-2) Feathers of the saddle from the wild-type EJ female ($Mo^{+/-}$) (left) and the mottled EJ female (*mo/mo*) (right). (D) Down colour of newly hatched chicks of the wild type ($Mo^{+/-}$) (D-1, left) and the mottled type (*mo/mo*) (D-1, right) in CB, and the wild type ($Mo^{+/-}$) (D-2, left) and the mottled type (*mo/mo*) in EJ (D-2, right). These mottled-type chicks (*mo/mo*) have white yellowish down with pigmented spots on the head.

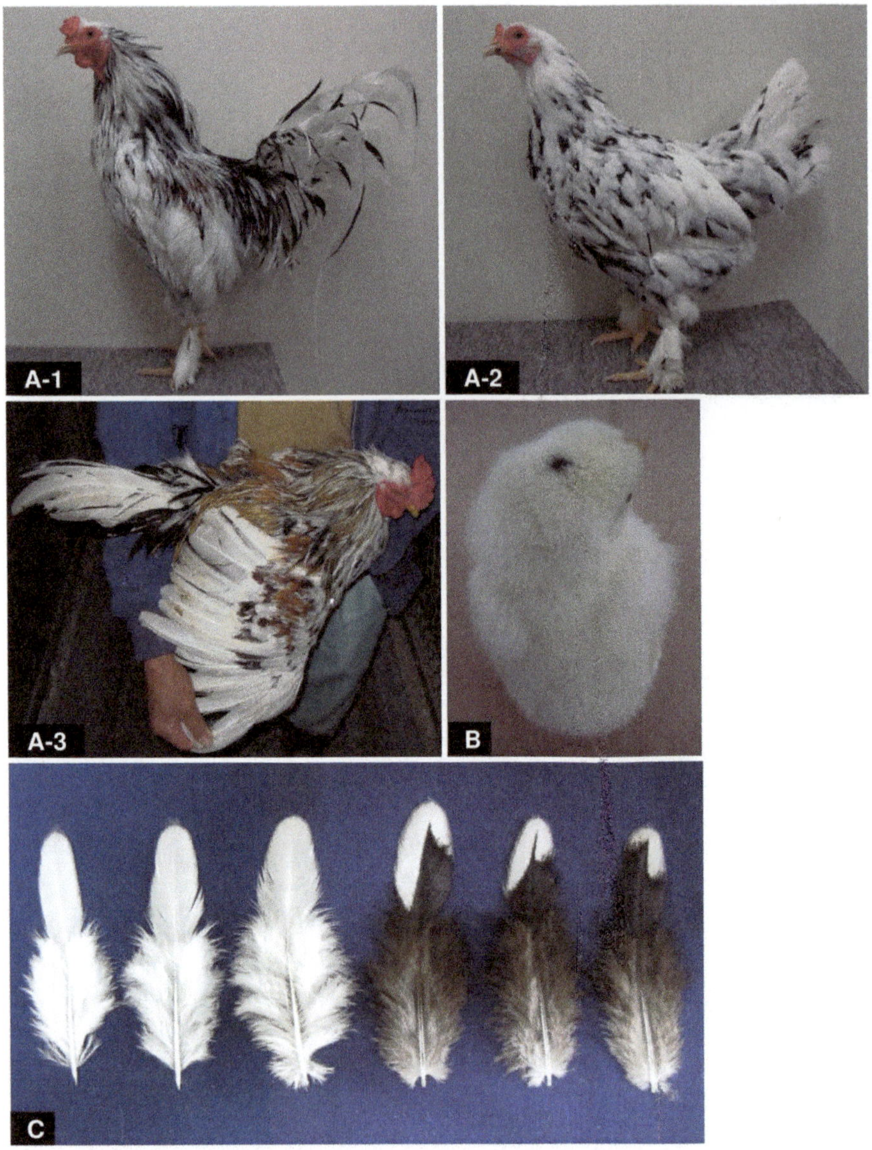

Figure 3. Allelism of mottled (*mo*) and white (mo^w) plumage. (A-1, A-2) An F_1 adult male (A-1) and an F_1 adult female (A-2) that were obtained from a mating of a mottled CB male with a white MH female. (A-3) F_1 adult male that was obtained from mating a mottled EJ male with a white female. All F_1 adult chickens derived from the two matings exhibited mottled-like plumage. (B) A newly hatched chick obtained from the mating of a mottled CB male with a white MH female, which has whitish down with a pigmented spot on the head. (C) Feathers of the saddle from a F_1 female (A-2) obtained from the mating of a mottled CB male with a white MH female. In the F_1 progeny, pure white feathers (left) and black feathers with non-pigmentation at the tips (right) were mixed.

breeds with mottled plumage (CB, Chabo and Uzurao) by genomic sequencing of exons 3 to 9 (Table 3). The three missense mutations were homozygous specifically in the breeds with mottled plumage (EJ, CB, Chabo, and Uzurao). This result indicates that the three non-synonymous nucleotide substitutions are specific for mottled plumage (*mo*/*mo*) and are not associated with white plumage (mo^w/mo^w), although the mottled and white plumage phenotypes resulted from mutations that occurred in the same causative gene. The non-mottled breeds were all homozygous for Thr at position 8, Thr at position 15 and Arg at position 332 except for the Rhode Island Red (RIR-Y8/NU), Sebright bantam and Large Cochin, which had the Thr8Ile and Thr15Ala substitutions. The individuals in RIR-Y8/NU (n = 15) that were homozygous for Thr8Ile and Thr15Ala both showed similar plumage to that of the other non-mottled individuals (n = 3) with Thr at position 8 and Thr at position 15. This suggested that the Arg332His substitution was essential for the mottled plumage phenotype, whereas the two non-synonymous mutations in exon 3 (Thr8Ile and Thr15Ala) might have little effect on plumage colour.

Arg332His mutation of *EDNRB2* in other chicken breeds

The G1272A (Arg332His) substitution in exon 7 of *EDNRB2* was surveyed for 98 individuals of 14 breeds including Red jungle fowl with a variety of plumage patterns using the PCR-RFLP method (Table S3). Digestion of the 646-bp PCR product with *Sfa*NI produced two fragments (241 bp and 405 bp) for the wild-type allele (Mo^+) and one uncut fragment (646 bp) for the mottled allele (*mo*) (Figure 6). The 24 individuals of Chabo (Gunma,

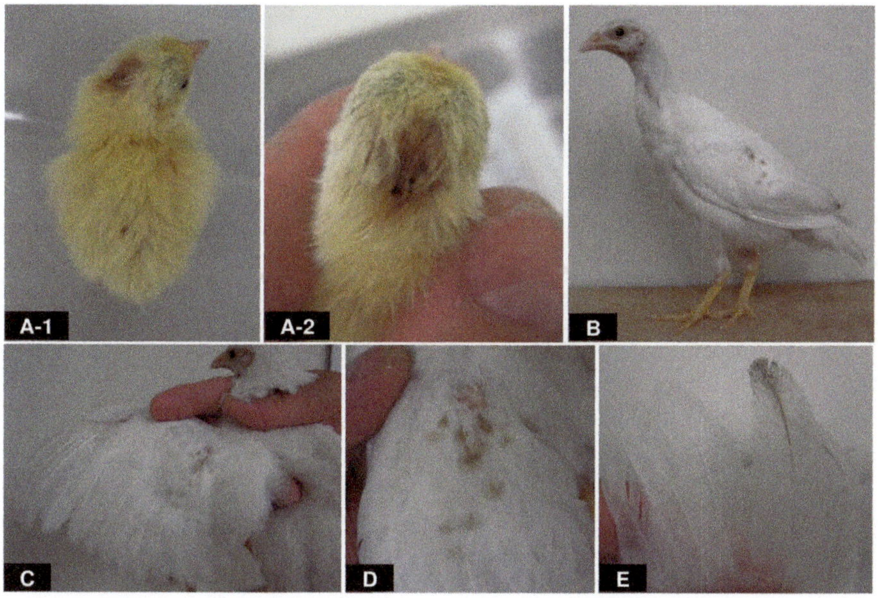

Figure 4. Allelism of white (*mo^w*) plumage of chicken and panda (*s*) plumage of Japanese quail. (A-1, A-2) A newly hatched F_1 hybrid chick between the white mutant male of chicken (*mo^w/mo^w*) and the *panda* mutant female of Japanese quail (*s/s*). It has whitish yellow down with one brown spot on the head. (B) The phenotype of 8 week-old young bird of the same individual shown in A-1 and A-2. It has the white plumage with several small coloured patches observed in wings. (C, D) Coloured patches in the wing. (E) Pigmented tip of feather from the wing.

Hiroshima University, and Hiroshima; $n = 16$) and Koshamo (Kagoshima and Hiroshima University; $n = 8$) with mottled plumage were all homozygous for the A/A allele (His/His) at position 1,272 (His332His), as were mottled EJ ($n = 8$) and CB ($n = 3$) chickens. The other 60 non-mottled individuals of 14 breeds were homozygous for the G allele at position 1,272 except for three non-mottled EJ individuals with heterozygous G/A (Table S3). These results suggested that the G>A substitution at 1,272 in exon 7, leading to the Arg332His substitution, was completely associated with the mottled allele (*mo*) in Japanese native chickens.

Genomic DNA sequences of *EDNRB2* at the *mo* locus

Nucleotide sequences of the genomic DNA fragments containing the open reading frame from exons 3–9 and introns 3–8 of *EDNRB2* were determined for the wild-type MH, white MH mutant, and mottled EJ chickens using the primers shown in Figure S1, and then compared with the reference genomic sequence on chromosome 4 in the UCSC chicken genome (May 2006 assembly). Seventy-five SNPs were identified among the sequences of the three chicken types compared with the genome database (Table S4). In addition, an 8-bp insertion in intron 3 of MH with the pigmented wild-type plumage (Mo^+/Mo^+) and a 4-bp deletion in intron 7 of the white MH mutant (mo^w/mo^w) were observed. The 432-bp LTR/ERVK sequence was located at positions 11,261,544–11,261,975 of intron 5 on the basis of the chicken reference genomic sequence (Type I) (Figure S3), whereas this 432 bp LTR/ERVK sequence was absent from intron 5 in the MH line (Mo^+/Mo^+, mo^w/mo^w) and mottled EJ (*mo/mo*) (Type II), in which an unrelated 295 bp sequence was present at the same position instead of the 432 bp LTR/ERVK. A homologous sequence was shared with Japanese quail (*Coturnix japonica*) (GenBank accession no. AY360822), which showed 91% nucleotide sequence identity (267/295 bp) (data not shown). This result suggested that the Type II sequence was the ancestral type present in the common ancestor of chicken and Japanese quail, and that this 295 bp sequence element was replaced with the 432-bp LTR/ERVK sequence in an evolutionary lineage of chicken after its divergence.

Expression of the *mo^w* and *mo* allelic genes

The expression levels of *EDNRB2* mRNA in the head skin and liver tissues were examined for three-day-old chicks with the white (mo^w/mo^w) and mottled (*mo/mo*) genotypes, and compared with those of the wild type (Figure 7). PCR amplification efficiencies were checked by preparing standard curves using target-specific primers (*EDNRB2*) and control primers (*GAPDH*). PCR amplification efficiencies and correlation coefficient (R^2) were 90.256% and 0.997 for *EDNRB2* and 92.525% and 0.996 for *GAPDH* (data not shown). The relative expression level of *EDNRB2* in pigmented skin of the white mutant (mo^w/mo^w) was not different from that of the wild-type (Mo^+/Mo^+) skin ($p>0.05$); however, the relative expression level in non-pigmented skin of the mo^w/mo^w chicks was significantly lower than those in pigmented skin of the same mo^w/mo^w individuals and the wild-type skin (1/4 decrease for the non-pigmented skin) ($p<0.05$) (Figure 7A). In the mottled type (*mo/mo*), the *EDNRB2* expression in pigmented skin was significantly lower than the wild-type (Mo^+/Mo^+) ($p<0.05$). The expression was also lower in non-pigmented skin than that in pigmented skin of the same individuals (approximately 1/2 decrease for the non-pigmented skin) ($p<0.05$) (Figure 7A). However, the expression levels in liver tissues of the mo^w/mo^w and *mo/mo* chicks were similar to those of the wild type (Figure 7B).

Discussion

In the present study, we identified a novel recessive mutation associated with white plumage in Minohiki and several other Japanese chicken breeds. Complementation tests revealed that the novel white plumage mutation was controlled by a *TYR* (*c*)-independent autosomal recessive gene at the mottled (*mo*) locus. This new mutant allele is designated mo^w and is an allelic variant for *mo* of mottled chickens. Furthermore, the intergeneric hybrid

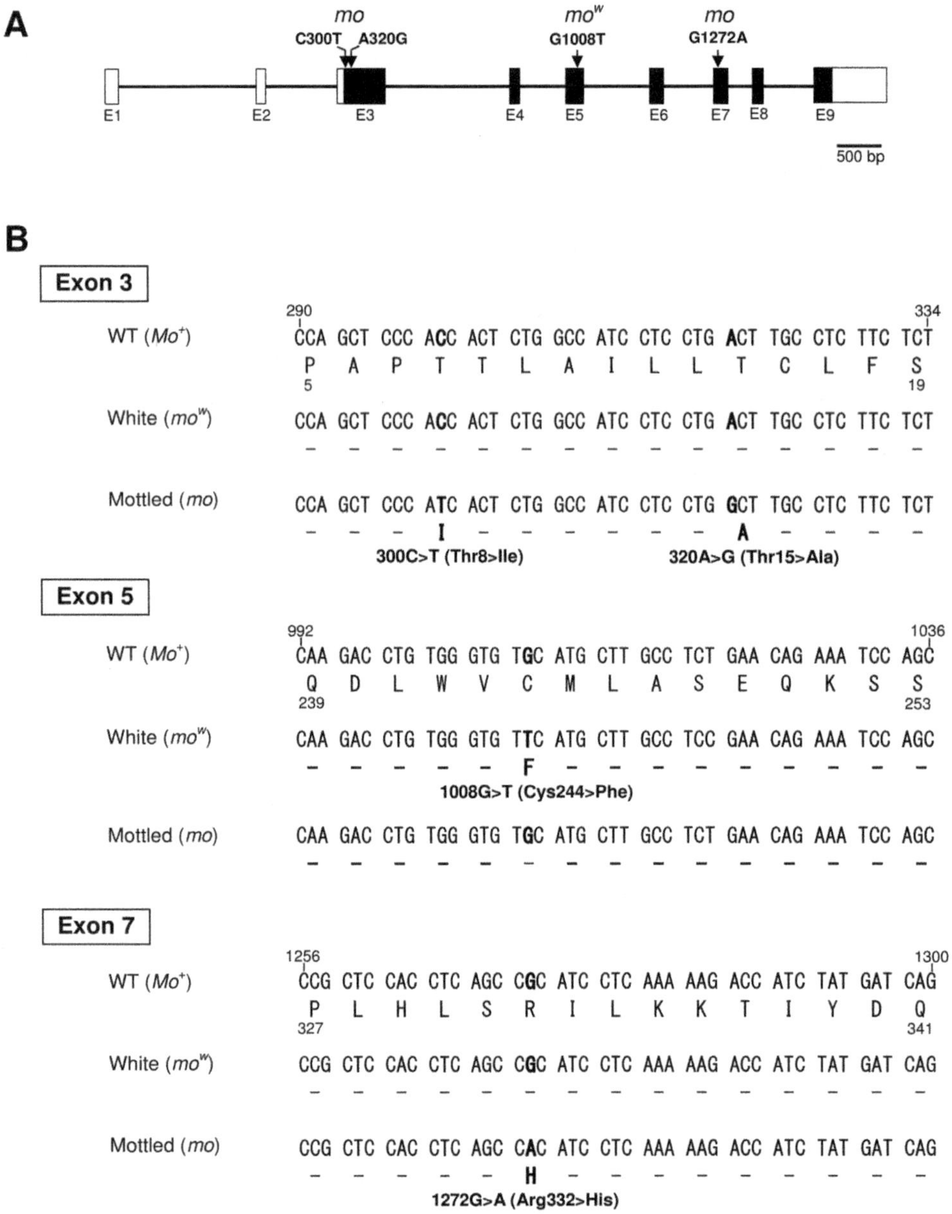

Figure 5. Comparison of *EDNRB2* nucleotide sequences among the wild-type (*Mo*$^+$), white (*mo*^{w}), and mottled (*mo*) alleles. (A) A schematic illustration of the genomic structure of chicken *EDNRB2*. Arrows indicate the positions of non-synonymous nucleotide substitutions found in the white mutant (*mo*^{w}) and mottled (*mo*) alleles. White boxes indicate untranslated exons at 5′ and 3′ ends, and black boxes indicate the coding exons. (B) Partial DNA sequences of exons 3, 5 and 7 of the wild-type (*Mo*$^+$/*Mo*$^+$), white mutant (*mo*^{w}/*mo*^{w}) and mottled (*mo*/*mo*) alleles. One non-synonymous substitution (G1008T/Cys244Phe) and three non-synonymous substitutions (C300T/Thr8Ile, A320G/Thr15Ala, and G1272A/Arg332His) are specific to the white mutant (*mo*^{w}) and mottled (*mo*) alleles, respectively.

between the white mutant chicken (*mo*^{w}/*mo*^{w}) and the *panda* mutant of Japanese quail (*s*/*s*) showed a *mo*^{w}/*mo*^{w} chicken-like plumage. This result showed that the mutations in parental species are alleles of the same gene, *EDNRB2*, which is the causative gene of the *panda* plumage of quail. Nucleotide sequencing revealed a non-synonymous nucleotide substitution from G to T at position 1,008 in exon 5 of *EDNRB2* in the white mutant chicken, which leads to the Cys244Phe amino acid substitution in EDNRB2. The association of this missense mutation (G1008T) with the white plumage phenotype was confirmed by genotyping of F_2 progeny and several other Japanese chicken breeds with white plumage.

EDNRB2 is one of the receptors for EDNs, which are strong mitogens for melanoblasts [19,20,22,23,24]. Several types of EDNs and EDNRs are reported in a wide variety of vertebrates [32,54,55], which show molecular diversity in terms of gene duplication, mutation and chromosomal translocation during evolution [43]. *EDNRB2* is a paralog of *EDNRB* identified in birds, *Xenopus*, and platypus [24,42,43]. The avian EDNRB and EDNRB2 show similar pharmacological properties to EDN1, EDN2, and EDN3 [54]. The EDN3 and EDNRB signal transduction system is reported to be indispensable for the development of neural crest-derived melanocytes or enteric neurons [36,37,38]. Kawasaki-Nishihara et al. [24] suggested that

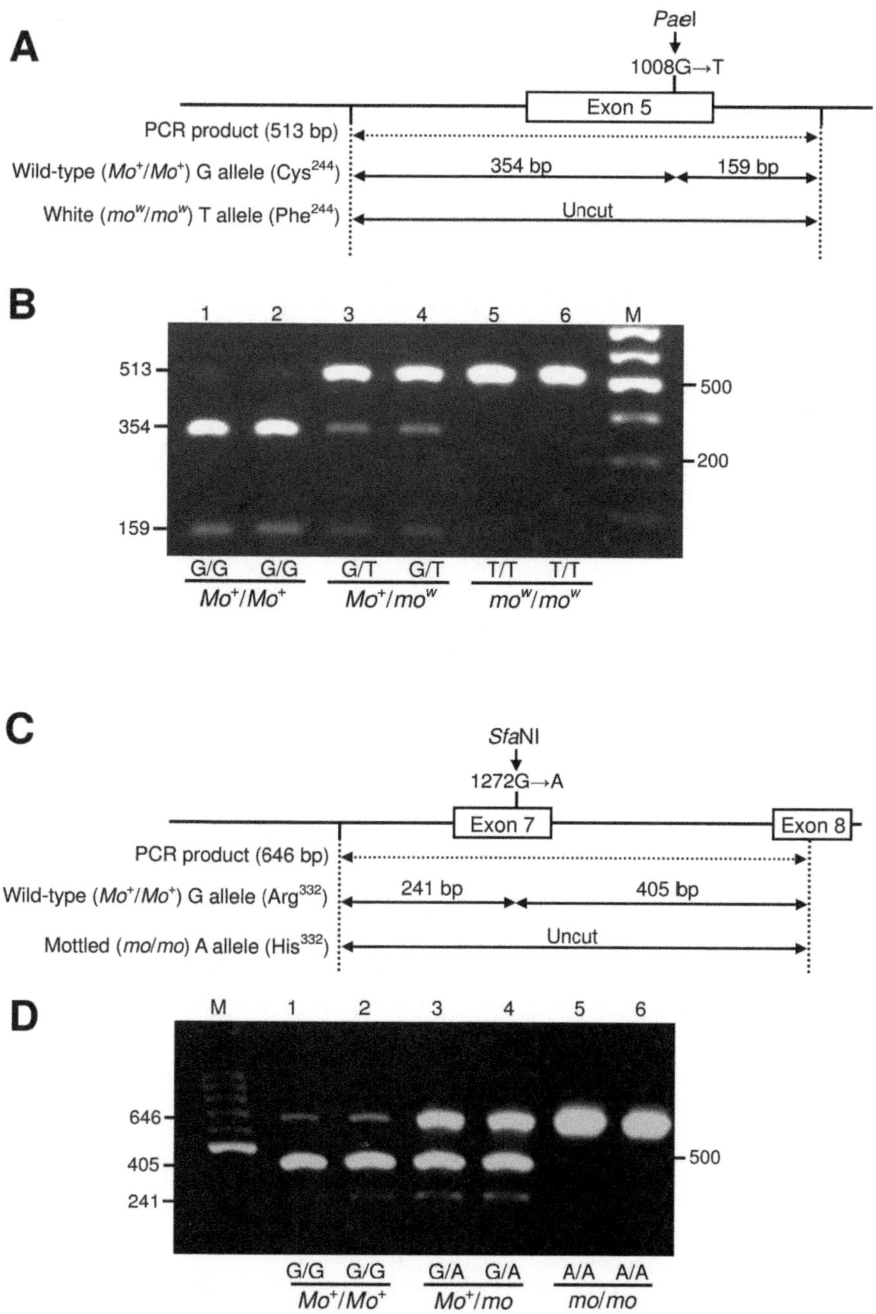

Figure 6. Genotyping of the G1008T (Cys244Phe) mutation in *mo*^{w} allele and the G1272A (Arg332His) mutation in *mo* allele. (A) Schematic representation of the *Pae*I-RFLP in the genomic DNA fragment of exon 5 of chicken *EDNRB2*, which was PCR-amplified using the primers EDNRB2_Int4F and EDNRB2_Int5R1 (Figure S1; Table S1) and was used for genotyping of the Cys244Phe mutation. Digestion with *Pae*I (G ↑ CATG ↓ C) produces two DNA fragments (354 bp and 159 bp) in the wild-type *Mo*$^+$ allele, whereas the DNA fragments derived from the *mo*^{w} allele were not digested with *Pae*I. (B) Genotyping of the F_2 progeny that were obtained by crossing a CAL male with a white MH female. The genotypes were determined by agarose gel electrophoresis after digestion of the PCR products (513 bp) with *Pae*I. The nucleotides at position 1,008 in six individuals, genotypes, and plumage colour phenotypes are indicated below the lanes. M, Gene Ladder 100 (0.1–2 kbp) (Wako, Japan) was used as a molecular size marker. (C) Schematic diagram of the *Sfa*NI-RFLP in the genomic DNA fragment of exon 7, which was PCR-amplified using the primer set EDNRB2_Int6F and EDNRB2_Ex8R (Figure S1; Table S1) and used for genotyping of the Arg332His mutation. (D) Agarose gel electrophoresis of the PCR products (646 bp) after *Sfa*NI-digestion. Two DNA fragments (241 bp + 405 bp) are produced in the wild-type *Mo*$^+$ allele, whereas the DNA fragments derived from the *mo* allele were not digested with *Sfa*NI. The nucleotides at position 1,272 in six individuals, genotypes, and plumage colour phenotypes are indicated below the lanes. M, Gene Ladder 100 (0.1–2 kbp) (Wako, Japan) was used as a molecular size marker.

EDN3–EDNRB2 signaling is required for normal melanoblast migration in *Xenopus* embryos on the basis of *in vivo* experiments. The present results indicated that the aberrant EDNRB2 causes hypopigmentation in feathers and suggested that normal EDNRB2 is essential for normal pigmentation in chickens, as in *Xenopus* or platypus [43].

The *mo*^{w} mutation is located in the extracellular loop between the putative fourth and fifth transmembrane domains of EDNRB2

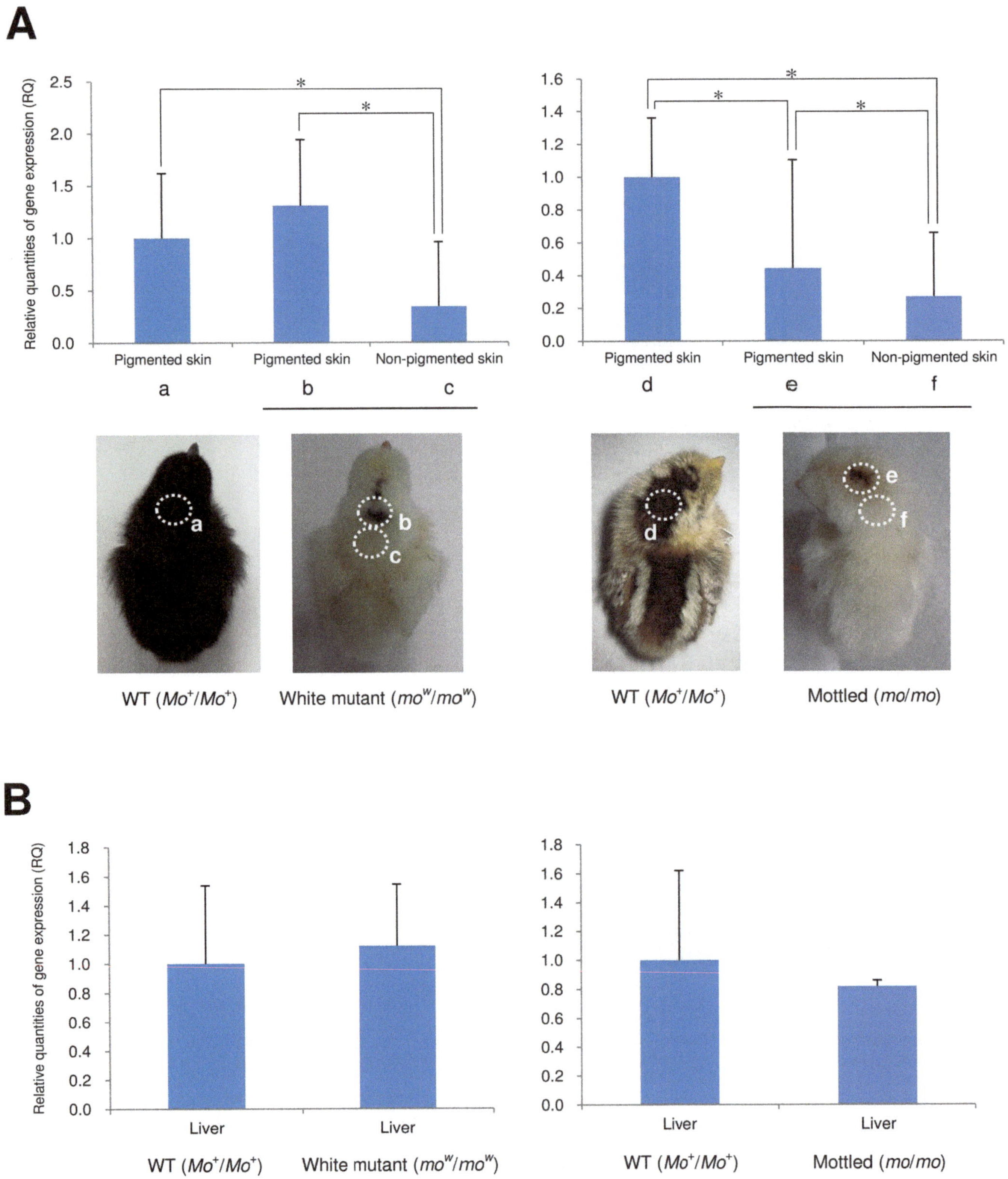

Figure 7. Expression analysis of *EDNRB2* by quantitative real-time RT-PCR in three-day-old chicks with the wild-type (*Mo*$^{+}$), white (*mo*^{W}) and mottled (*mo*) plumage. (A) Relative expression levels in skin tissues of chicks with the wild-type (*Mo*$^{+}$/*Mo*$^{+}$) (n = 9) (a) and white mutant (*mo*^{W}/*mo*^{W}) plumage (n = 6) (b, c) in the F_2 progeny that were obtained from the mating of a white Shokoku male (*mo*^{W}/*mo*^{W}) with a GSP female (*Mo*$^{+}$/*Mo*$^{+}$); and chicks with the wild-type (*Mo*$^{+}$/*Mo*$^{+}$) (n = 3) (d) and mottled type (*mo*/*mo*) plumage (n = 2) (e, f) in EJ line. Dotted circles indicate the regions from which skins were collected for analysis. Each bar shows the average expression level, which is presented as the quantity of gene expression relative to that of the wild type. (B) Expression level in liver tissues of the same individuals which were used for expression analysis of skins: the wild-type (*Mo*$^{+}$/*Mo*$^{+}$) (n = 9) and white mutant (*mo*^{W}/*mo*^{W}) chicks (n = 6) in the F_2 progeny between GSP and white Shokoku; and the wild-type (*Mo*$^{+}$/*Mo*$^{+}$) (n = 3) and mottled (*mo*/*mo*) plumage (n = 2) in EJ. Asterisks indicate a statistically significant difference at $P < 0.05$ (one-way ANOVA followed by Tukey HSD test). The vertical bars indicate standard deviations.

(Figure 8), which is considered to play an important role in the interaction with EDN3 [54]. Amino acid alignment of EDNRB and EDNRB2 shows that Cys-244 is evolutionally highly conserved in six species from four classes (Mammalia, Aves, Amphibia, and Osteichthyes) (Table 4). This result strongly suggests that the presence of Cys at position 244 is crucial for the basic function of EDNRB2. On the other hand, the Cys244Phe substitution was identified in five Japanese native breeds [Minohiki (Shizuoka), Onagadori, Ohiki, Shokoku, and Uzurao]. Except for Uzurao (a rumpless breed), all of these breeds have a long tail, and are considered to have a close genetic relationship [56,57,58]. This finding suggests that the mo^{w} mutation may have originated from a common ancestor of a Japanese or Asian population of the long-tailed native chicken breeds. Therefore, the genetic analysis of plumage inheritance provides valuable information not only about the genetic and molecular basis of plumage colour but also the phylogenetic relationships and histories of chicken breeds.

We identified three mottled plumage-specific non-synonymous substitutions in the coding region of *EDNRB2* for four breeds (EJ, Chabo, CB, and Koshamo): two non-synonymous substitutions, Thr8Ile and Thr15Ala in the N-terminal putative signal peptide (1–23 residues) and Arg332His in the sixth transmembrane domain (SOSUIsignal, http://bp.nuap.nagoya-u.ac.jp/sosui/sosuisignal/) (Figure 8). These three mutations were found in all *mo* chickens that we analysed. Of the three mutation sites, Arg-332 is evolutionally highly conserved in *EDNRB* and *EDNRB2* of vertebrates. The Arg332His substitution was also identified in the *panda* plumage (*s/s*) mutant of Japanese quail [59]; however, the other mutations (Thr8Ile and Thr15Ala) were not found in the *panda* mutant quail. Interestingly, Thr8Ile and Thr15Ala mutations are also present in non-mottled chicken breeds (RIR, Large Cochin, and Sebright bantam). These results suggest that the Arg332His substitution is a primary cause of the mottled plumage pattern, although Thr8Ile and Thr15Ala are located in the region of the putative signal sequence (amino acids 1–23) of EDNRB2,

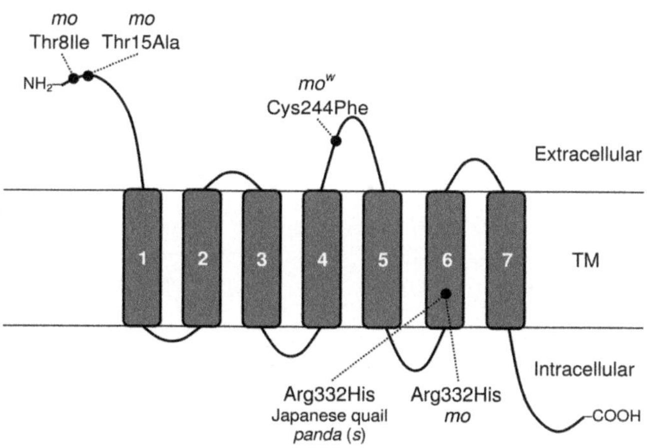

Figure 8. Schematic diagram of the structure of the EDNRB2 protein. Black circles indicate the positions of amino acid substitution in the mo^{w} and *mo* alleles. The Cys244Phe substitution in the mo^{w} allele was located in the extracellular loop between the putative fourth and fifth transmembrane (TM) domains of EDNRB2. The other three substitutions were identified at the *mo* locus: Thr8Ile and Thr15Ala in the N-terminal amino acids that constitute the cleaved peptide signal, and Arg332His in the sixth TM domain. The Arg332His substitution of EDNRB2 was previously reported in the *panda* (*s/s*) plumage mutant of Japanese quail (Miwa *et al.*, 2007). The grey-shaded rectangles represent the TM domains.

which is generally considered to mediate the post-translational transport of the protein, these mutations may have little influence on binding to the ligand. However, these two non-synonymous mutations (Thr8Ile and Thr15Ala) may cause the difference in plumage pattern between the white mutant chicken and the *panda* quail, although the amino acid sequence homology of EDNRB2 is 97.7% (426/436 amino acids) between the wild-type chicken and Japanese quail. The phenotype of the mo^{w} mutant chicken is similar to that of the *dotted-white* (s^{dw}) mutant at the *s* (*EDNRB2*) locus in Japanese quail [49,59]. No mutations were identified in the coding region of *EDNRB2* in this mutant quail; however, the expression level of the gene was reported to be remarkably declined compared with that of the wild type. This result suggests that the s^{dw} mutation probably occurred in the regulatory region of the gene, thus leading to the lower quantity of EDNRB2. Chickens homozygous for the mo^{w} allele showed much lower levels of pigmentation than those homozygous for the *mo* allele; nevertheless the *EDNRB2* expression level in liver tissue of mo^{w} homozygotes was similar to that of the wild type. This result suggests that the Cys244Phe mutation in the mo^{w} allele may not cause down-regulation of *EDNRB2* but may cause defective functioning of EDNRB2 with respect to binding with EDN ligands, thus resulting in interference with melanocyte differentiation, proliferation, and migration [32,33,34,35]. To verify this function, we are now examining the gene expression in the developmental stage of embryos and in skins collected from all the shades of each feather color between the wild-type (Mo^{+}/Mo^{+}) and the mutant types (*mo/mo* and mo^{w}/mo^{w}).

Several outstanding questions remain to be addressed. Why did Aves acquire *EDNRB2* in addition to *EDNRB*? Do these receptors share other functions besides controlling pigmentation? Do these receptors show any differences in function or role in pigmentation? The functional divergence of these receptors and their molecular evolution are also interesting topics for future research. Mutation of *EDNRB* in mouse causes white coat colour and megacolon in the homologous condition, and these results in lethality within five weeks after birth [36,39]. These abnormalities are considered to be caused by incomplete development of nerve ganglia because of abnormality of the EDN–EDNRB signal transduction system (reviewed in [60]). Given that such disorders are not observed in the chicken mutants, the EDN–EDNRB system appears to function normally in mo^{w} and *mo* chickens. However, the dramatic effects of the *EDNRB2* mutation on pigment production in chickens and quails suggest that *EDNRB2* is required for avian melanoblasts to promote melanocyte differentiation and to enter the migration pathway from the neural crest. The EDN–EDNRB signal transduction system in mammals is understood to control the migration of nerve or bowel precursor cells by a dorsoventral route, and the migration of pigment cells mainly by a dorsolateral route. The avian *EDNRB* and *EDNRE2* genes may have evolved at partially different functions after the gene duplication; therefore, the EDN–EDNRB2 system in Aves is considered to play a part of the role of the EDN–EDNRB system, such as the differentiation of pigment cells. Fibromelanosis (*Fm*) of the Silkie chicken is a mutant phenotype of pigmentation, which exhibits extensive pigmentation of dermal layer of skin and internal connective tissues. This phenotype is caused by a duplication of a genomic region containing *EDN3*, which is a ligand of the EDN–EDNRB system and has a major role in melanocyte proliferation [25,26]. To generate the birds with mo^{w}/mo^{w} and *Fm*/− genotype and to examine their phenotypes provide us a clue for understanding the function and molecular mechanism of the EDN–EDNRB2 signaling system in Aves. The mo^{w} allele appears to be a malfunctional or loss-of-function mutation; therefore, the pigmentation is predicted to be modified or suppressed in the mo^w/mo^w background. We are now advancing this experiment. *EDNRB2*-mutated chickens with a variety of plumage patterns are an effective tool to elucidate the EDNRB2 function in the proliferation and differentiation of melanocytes and neural crest cells. In addition, such mutants are particularly important in order to analyse the molecular diversity of *EDNRB* in vertebrates and the origin of the *EDNRB2* mutation that occurred in Asian chicken breeds.

Methods

Allelism and progeny tests

For the allelism test of the white plumage mutant identified in the MH line, white MH females were mated with males of four tester lines: the Fayoumi (PNP/DO) (i^+/i^+, Mo^+/Mo^+, C^+/C^+); autosomal albino (CAL) (i^+/i^+, Mo^+/Mo^+, c^a/c^a); mottled Cochin bantam (CB) (i^+/i^+, mo/mo, C^+/C^+); and mottled Ehime-jidori (EJ) (i^+/i^+, mo/mo, C^+/C^+) lines (Table 1). We examined the colours of the chick down and adult plumage in F_1, F_2, and/or backcross progeny obtained from the four test matings. Following the mating of CAL with white MH, we examined the phenotypes and genotypes of the F_2 progeny to determine the mode of inheritance for white plumage in the MH line, and performed linkage mapping of the white plumage locus. The segregation data of the F_2 progeny were analysed with the chi-square test. Furthermore, To test the allelism of the white plumage (mo^w/mo^w) of chicken and the *panda* plumage (s/s) of Japanese quail whose causative gene is the *endothelin receptor B2* (*EDNRB2*) gene, an intergeneric F_1 hybrid was obtained from artificially inseminated female *panda* quails with semen of the white chicken male. Animal care and all experimental procedures were approved by the Animal Experiment Committee, Graduate School of Bioagricultural Sciences, Nagoya University (approval nos 2012031206 and 2012050102), and the experiments were conducted according to Regulations on Animal Experiments at Nagoya University.

cDNA sequencing of *EDNRB2*

We determined cDNA sequences of the entire coding region of *EDNRB2* for four individuals from MH and EJ lines (Table 2), which exhibited three different types of plumage: the wild-type (MH and EJ), white (MH), and mottled (EJ) plumage. Dorsal skin tissue (2.5 mm^2) that contained developing feathers was dissected from one individual of each line and stored in RNAlater (Ambion, Austin, TX, USA). Total RNA was extracted using the TRIzol reagent (Invitrogen, Carlsbad, CA, USA) and 1.5 μg RNA was reverse-transcribed using the PrimeScript RT-PCR Kit (Takara, Otsu, Japan). The cDNA fragments including the entire coding region of *EDNRB2* were amplified using the primer pair EDNRB2_F1/EDNRB2_R1 (Figure S1; Table S1). Internal sequencing primers were used for direct sequencing, which were designed based on the cDNA sequence of chicken *EDNRB2* (GenBank accession no. NM_204120). PCR was carried out in a 50-μl reaction volume containing 50 ng cDNA, 1× KOD FX buffer, 200 μM dNTPs, 1.5 μl of 10 μM solution for each of the forward and reverse primers, and 1 unit KOD FX DNA polymerase (TOYOBO, Osaka, Japan). Each PCR reaction involved initial denaturation of 2 min at 94°C; 35 cycles of 98°C for 10 s, 64°C for 30 s, and 68°C for 2 min; and a final extension at 68°C for 7 min. The PCR products were purified from the gel using the Gel-M gel extraction kit (Viogene, Umeå, Sweden). Cycle-sequencing reactions used the Big Dye Terminator v3.1 Cycle Sequencing Kit (Applied Biosystems, Foster City, CA, USA) and nucleotide sequences were determined using an ABI PRISM 3130 DNA Analyser (Applied Biosystems).

Linkage mapping

To confirm the association of the candidate gene (*EDNRB2*) with the white plumage mutation in MH line, we constructed a resource family by crossing a CAL male with a white MH female, as described above. Intercrossing of an F_1 male with four F_1 females generated 307 F_2 progeny. Two microsatellite markers (*MCW0295* and *ADL0255*) on chromosome 4 were genotyped for the two grandparents, five F_1 parents, and 93 F_2 offspring. The PCR products of the markers were electrophoresed on either a 3.5% agarose gel or a 10% or 12% polyacrylamide gel. The genotyping of *EDNRB2* was performed 58 mutant individuals with white plumage and 184 individuals with the wild-type pigmented plumage excluding recessive albino individuals (n = 65). Linkage analysis between genotypes of microsatellite markers and *EDNRB2* and the plumage phenotypes was conducted using the Map Manager QTX software program [61]. Map units in centiMorgan (cM) were computed by applying the Kosambi function [62].

Genomic DNA sequencing of *EDNRB2*

Genomic DNA sequences of exons 3 to 9 of the *EDNRB2* gene were determined for 18 chicken breeds including Red jungle fowl, which exhibited three different types of plumage (the wild-type, white and mottled plumage) (Table 3). Additionally, nucleotide sequences of genomic DNA fragments containing the open reading frame from exons 3 to 9 and their introns were determined for the wild-type MH, white MH mutant, and mottled EJ chickens. Blood samples were collected, and genomic DNA was extracted using DNAzol solution (Molecular Research Center, Cincinnati, OH, USA). The genomic fragment (5,914 bp) was amplified from 50 ng template genomic DNA using the primer pair EDNRB2_F1 and EDNRB2_R1 (Figure S1; Table S1). The internal primers were designed based on a reference genomic sequence on chromosome 4 in the UCSC chicken genome (May 2006 assembly). The PCR, which was carried out with KOD FX DNA polymerase (TOYOBO), involved initial denaturation of 2 min at 94°C; 35 cycles of 98°C for 10 s, 64°C for 30 s and 68°C for 6 min; and a final extension at 68°C for 7 min. The DNA sequence data sets were analysed using ATGC ver.5 sequence assembly software (Genetyx, Tokyo, Japan).

Quantitative real-time RT-PCR

Expression of *EDNRB2* was analysed using quantitative real-time RT-PCR (qRT-PCR) for three-day-chicks with three different plumage phenotypes in three different genotypes: the wild type and white mutant chicks in the F_2 progeny obtained from the mating of a white Shokoku male (mo^w/mo^w) with a GSP female (Mo^+/Mo^+); and the wild-type (Mo^+/Mo^+) and mottled (mo/mo) chicks in Ehime-jidori (EJ). Pigmented skin tissue of the wild-type chicks was collected from the back of the head, and pigmented and non-pigmented skin tissues were collected from the white mutant and mottled chicks. Total RNA was extracted from the head skin tissues including the pigmented and non-pigmented down feathers and liver tissues using the TRIzol reagent (Invitrogen), and complementary DNA was synthesised using the PrimeScript RT-PCR Kit (Takara). Quantitative real-time PCR was performed using SYBR *Premix Ex Taq*II (Takara) and the expressed dose was quantified with the StepOnePlus realtime PCR system (Applied Biosystems). The sequences of the primers were 5′-GCTTGCTTCATCCCGTTCAGA-3′ (sense) and 5′-ATGGCCAATGGCAAGCAGA-3′ (antisense). The following program conditions were applied for qRT-PCR analyses:

95°C for 30 s followed by 40 cycles that each comprised 95°C for 5 s followed by 60°C for 30 s following manufacturer's instruction. The expression levels were normalised against glyceraldehyde-3-phosphate dehydrogenase (*GAPDH*), which was amplified in the same run following the same procedure described above. The sequences of the *GAPDH* primers used were 5′-GGAGAAAC-CAGCCAAGTATGATG-3′ (sense) and 5′-AAAGGTGGAG-GAATGGCTGTCA-3′ (antisense). Each quantitative PCR was performed in triplicate to verify the results, and the mean mRNA expression was used for data analysis. Gene expression level was analysed using the $2^{-\Delta\Delta CT}$ method. Expression levels in skin and liver tissues were statistically compared among experimental groups by one-way ANOVA (analysis of variance) followed by Tukey HSD (honestly significant difference) test of the statistical discovery software JMP version 10.0.2 (SAS Institute, Cary, NC).

Supporting Information

Figure S1 Genomic structure of *EDNRB2*. Arrows indicate the PCR primers that were used for nucleotide sequencing. The primers with asterisks were used for genotyping of the G1008T (Cys244Phe) and G1272A (Arg322His) mutations. White boxes indicate untranslated exons at 5′ and 3′ ends, and black boxes indicate the coding exons.

Figure S2 Genetic linkage map of the mo^w mutation on chicken chromosome 4. The linkage map was constructed using a population of 93 F_2 progeny (50 wild-type and 43 white mutant individuals) obtained from the mating of a CAL male with a white MH female. Two microsatellite markers (*ADL0255* and *MCW0295*) and *EDNRB2* on chromosome 4 were genotyped for the F_2 progeny, and their genotypes were compared with the segregation patterns of plumage.

Figure S3 Partial sequences in intron 5 of *EDNRB2* in the Minohiki (MH) line and the mottled Ehime-jidori (EJ) line. (A) The 432-bp LTR/ERVK sequence is located at positions 11,261,544–11, 261,975 of intron 5 on the basis of the chicken reference genomic sequence (Type I). This LTR/ERVK sequence is absent in intron 5 of *EDNRB2* in the MH line (Mo^+/Mo^+, mo^w/mo^w) and the mottled EJ line (Mo^+/Mo^+, mo/mo) (Type II), in which the unrelated 295-bp sequence replaced the LTR/ERVK at the same position. (B) Comparison of partial sequences in intron 5 of Type I and II sequences.

Table S1 List of primers used for amplifying DNA fragments of chicken.

Table S2 Distribution of the G1008T nucleotide substitution leading to Cys244Phe in *EDNRB2* in 22 chicken breeds including Red jungle fowl.

Table S3 Distribution of the G1272A nucleotide substitution leading to Arg332His in *EDNRB2* in 14 chicken breeds including Red jungle fowl.

Table S4 DNA sequence polymorphism in *EDNRB2* among three alleles (*Mo^+*, *mo^w* and *mo*).

Author Contributions

Conceived and designed the experiments: KK TA MM AS YM. Performed the experiments: KK MM HHY. Analyzed the data: KK MM YM. Contributed reagents/materials/analysis tools: KK MM AI MT TN YM. Wrote the paper: KK TA YM.

References

1. Nordlund JJ, Boissy RE, Hearing VJ, King CY, Oetting WS, et al. (2006) The pigmentary system: physiology and pathophysiology. MaldenOxford, Victoria: Blackwell Publishing Ltd. 1229 p.
2. Borovanský J, Riley PA (2011) Melanins and melanosomes. London: Wiley-Blackwell, 407 p.
3. Roulin A, Ducrest A-L (2013) Genetics of colouration in birds. Seminars Cell Dev Biol 24: 594–608.
4. Tachibana M, Perez-Jurado LA, Nakayama A, Hodgkinson CA, Li X, et al. (1994) Cloning of MITF, the human homolog of the mouse *microphthalmia* gene and assignment to chromosome 3p14.1-p12.3. Hum Mol Genet 3: 553–557.
5. Nobukuni Y, Watanabe A, Takeda K, Skarka H, Tachibana M (1996) Analyses of loss-of-function mutations of the *MITF* gene suggest that haploinsufficiency is a cause of Waardenburg syndrome type 2A. Am J Hum Genet 59: 76–83.
6. Uehara S, Izumi Y, Kubo Y, Wang CC, Mineta K, et al. (2009) Specific expression of *Gsta4* in mouse cochlear melanocytes: a novel role for hearing and melanocyte differentiation. Pigment Cell Melanoma Res 22: 111–119.
7. Ziehl MA, Hollander WF (1987) Dun, a new plumage-color mutant at the *I*-locus in the fowl (*Gallus gallus*). Iowa State J Res 62: 337–342.
8. Smyth JR Jr (1990) Genetics of plumage, skin and eye pigmentation in chickens. In: Crawford RD, editor. Poultry breeding and genetics. AmsterdamNewYork: Elsevier. pp. 109–167.
9. Kerje S, Sharma P, Gunnarsson U, Kim H, Bagchi S, et al. (2004) The *Dominant white*, *Dun* and *Smoky* color variants in chicken are associated with insertion/deletion polymorphisms in the *PMEL17* gene. Genetics 168: 1507–1518.
10. Brumbaugh JA, Barger TW, Oetting WS (1983) A "new" allele at the *C* pigment locus in the fowl. J Hered 74: 331–336.
11. Smyth JR Jr, Ring NM, Brumbaugh JA (1986) A fourth allele at the *C*-locus of the chicken. Poultry Sci 65 (Suppl. 1): 129.
12. Tobita-Teramoto T, Jang GY, Kino K, Salter DW, Brumbaugh JA, et al. (2000) Autosomal albino chicken mutation (c^a/c^a) deletes hexanucleotide (-delta-GACTGG817) at a copper-binding site of the tyrosinase gene. Poult Sci 79: 46–50.
13. Chang CM, Coville JL, Coquerelle G, Gourichon D, Oulmouden A, et al. (2006) Complete association between a retroviral insertion in the tyrosinase gene and the recessive white mutation in chickens. BMC Genomics 7: 19.
14. Sato S, Otake T, Suzuki C, Saburi J, Kobayashi E (2007) Mapping of the recessive white locus and analysis of the tyrosinase gene in chickens. Poult Sci 86: 2126–2133.
15. Gariepy CE, Cass DT, Yanagisawa M (1996) Null mutation of endothelin receptor type B gene in spotting lethal rats causes aganglionic megacolon and white coat color. Proc Natl Acad Sci U S A. 23: 867–872.
16. Yoshida H, Kunisada T, Grimm T, Nishimura EK, Nishioka E, et al. (2001) Melanocyte migration and survival controlled by SCF/c-kit expression. J Investig Dermatol Symp Proc 6: 1–5.
17. Bennett DC, Lamoreux ML (2003) The color loci of mice – a genetic century. Pigment Cell Res 16: 333–344.
18. Lamoureux ML, Delmas V, Larue L, Bennett DC (2010) The color of mice: A model genetic network. West Sussex: Wiley-Blackwell. 297 p.
19. Yanagisawa M, Kurihara H, Kimura S, Tomobe Y, Kobayashi M, et al. (1988) A novel potent vasoconstrictor peptide produced by vascular endothelial cells. Nature 332: 411–415.
20. Imokawa G, Yada Y, Miyagishi M (1992) Endothelins secreted from human keratinocytes are intrinsic mitogens for human melanocytes. J Biol Chem 267: 24675–24680.
21. Hirai M, Miyabo S, Ooya E, Miyanaga K, Aoyagi N, et al. (1991) Endothelin-3 stimulates the hypothalamic-pituitary-adrenal axis. Life Sci 48: 2359–2363.
22. Aoki H, Yamada Y, Kunisada T (2009) Two distinct types of mouse melanocyte: differential signaling requirement for the maintenance of noncutaneous and dermal versus epidermal melanocytes. Development 136: 2511–2521.
23. Saldana-Caboverde A, Kos L (2010) Roles of endothelin signaling in melanocyte development and melanoma. Pigment Cell Melanoma Res 23: 160–170.
24. Kawasaki-Nishihara A, Nishihara D, Nakamura H, Yamamoto H (2011) ET3/Ednrb2 signaling is critically involved in regulating melanophore migration in *Xenopus*. Dev Dyn 240: 1454–1466.
25. Shinomiya A, Kayashima Y, Kinoshita K, Mizutani M, Namikawa T, et al. (2012) Duplication of the *endothelin 3* gene is closely correlated with *Fibromelanosis* (*Fm*), the hypermelanization of the internal organs of Silky chickens. Genetics 190: 627–638.
26. Dorshorst B, Molin AM, Rubin CJ, Johansson AM, Strömstedt L, et al. (2011) A complex genomic rearrangement involving the endothelin 3 locus causes dermal hyperpigmentation in the chicken. PLoS Genet 7: e1002412.

27. Lahav R, Ziller C, Dupin E, Le Douarin NM (1996) Endothelin 3 promotes neural crest cell proliferation and mediates a vast increase in melanocyte number in culture. Proc Natl Acad Sci USA 93: 3892–3897.
28. Lahav R, Dupin E, Lecoin L, Glavieux C, Champeval D, et al. (1998) Endothelin 3 selectively promotes survival and proliferation of neural crest-derived glial and melanocytic precursors in vitro. Proc Natl Acad Sci USA 95:14214–14219.
29. Reid K, Turnley AM, Maxwell GD, Kurihara Y, Kurihara H, et al. (1996) Multiple roles for endothelin in melanocyte development: regulation of progenitor number and stimulation of differentiation. Development 122: 3911–3919.
30. Opdecamp K, Kos L, Arnheiter H, Pavan WJ (1998) Endothelin signalling in the development of neural crest-derived melanocytes. Biochem Cell Biol 76: 1093–1099.
31. Dupin E, Glavieux C, Vaigot P, Le Douarin NM (2000) Endothelin 3 induces the reversion of melanocytes to glia through a neural crest-derived glial-melanocytic progenitor. Proc Natl Acad Sci USA 97: 7882–7887.
32. Arai H, Hori S, Aramori I, Ohkubo H, Nakanishi S (1990) Cloning and expression of cDNA encoding an endothelin receptor. Nature 348: 730–732.
33. Sakurai T, Yanagisawa M, Takuwa Y, Miyazaki H, Kimura S, et al. (1990) Cloning of a cDNA encoding a non-isopeptide-selective subtype of the endothelin receptor. Nature 348: 732–735.
34. Sakurai T, Yanagisawa M, Masaki T (1992) Molecular characterization of endothelin receptors. Trends Pharmacol Sci 13: 103–108.
35. Kusserow H, Unger T (2004) Vasoactive peptides, their receptors and drug development. Basic Clin Pharmacol Toxicol 94: 5–12.
36. Hosoda K, Hammer RE, Richardson JA, Baynash AG, Cheung JC, et al. (1994) Targeted and natural (piebald-lethal) mutations of endothelin-B receptor gene produce megacolon associated with spotted coat color in mice. Cell 79: 1267–1276.
37. Metallinos DL, Bowling AT, Rine J (1998) A missense mutation in the endothelin-B receptor gene is associated with lethal white foal syndrome: an equine version of Hirschsprung disease. Mamm Genome 9: 426–431.
38. Opgenorth TJ (1995) Endothelin receptor antagonism. Adv Pharmacol 33: 1–65.
39. Baynash AG, Hosoda K, Giaid A, Richardson JA, Emoto N, et al. (1994) Interaction of endothelin-3 with endothelin-B receptor is essential for development of epidermal melanocytes and enteric neurons. Cell 79: 1277–1285.
40. Pavan WJ, Tilghman SM (1994) Piebald lethal (*s^l*) acts early to disrupt the development of neural crest-derived melanocytes. Proc Natl Acad Sci USA 91: 7159–7163.
41. Lee H, Levorse JM, Shin MK (2003) The endothelin receptor-B is required for the migration of neural crest-derived melanocyte and enteric neuron precursors. Dev Biol 259: 162–175.
42. Lecoin L, Sakurai T, Ngo M, Abe Y, Yanagisawa M, et al. (1998) Cloning and characterization of a novel endothelin receptor subtype in the avian class. Proc Natl Acad Sci USA 95: 3024–3029.
43. Braasch I, Volff JN, Schartl M (2009) The endothelin system: evolution of vertebrate-specific ligand-receptor interactions by three rounds of genome duplication. Mol Biol Evol 26: 783–799.
44. Le Douarin NM, Kalcheim C (2009) The neural crest. Second editionCam-Cambridge: Cambridge University press. 445 p.
45. Nataf V, Amemiya A, Yanagisawa M, Le Douarin NM (1998) The expression pattern of endothelin 3 in the avian embryo. Mech Dev 73: 217–220.
46. Pla P, Alberti C, Solov'eva O, Pasdar M, Kunisada T, et al. (2005) Ednrb2 orients cell migration towards the dorsolateral neural crest pathway and promotes melanocyte differentiation. Pigment Cell Res 18: 181–187.
47. Harris ML, Hall R, Erickson CA (2008) Directing pathfinding along the dorsolateral path—the role of EDNRB2 and EphB2 in overcoming inhibition. Development 135: 4113–4122.
48. Mizutani M, Chiho K, Umezawa H, Kuramasu S (1974) Genetic analysis of a new plumage—panda in Japanese quail (in Japanese with English summary). Exp Anim 23: 59–61.
49. Tsudzuki M, Nakane Y, Wakasugi N, Mizutani M (1993) Allelism of panda and dotted white plumage genes in Japanese quail. J Hered 84: 225–229.
50. Miwa M, Inoue-Murayama M, Kobayashi N, Kayang BB, Mizutani M, et al. (2006) Mapping of panda plumage color locus on the microsatellite linkage map of the Japanese quail. BMC Genet 7: 2.
51. Hutt FB (1949) Genetics of the fowl. New York, McGraw-Hill Book Company, Inc, 590 p.
52. Somes RG Jr (1980) The mottling gene, the basis of six plumage color patterns in the domestic fowl. Poult Sci 59: 1370–1374.
53. Carefoot WC (1987) Evidence that the mottled (*mo*) and pied (*pi*) plumage genes of the domestic fowl are identical. Br Poult Sci 28: 753–754.
54. Rubanyli GM, Polokoff MA (1994) Endothelins: molecular biology, biochemistry, pharmacology, physiology, and pathophysiology. Pharmacological Reviews 46: 325–415.
55. Hirata Y (1996) Endothelin peptides. Curr Opin Nephrol Hypertens 5: 12–15.
56. Oana H (1951) The histories of native Japanese chickens. Nihonkei-Kenkyusha, Tokyo, Japan. (in Japanese) 293 p.
57. Osman SAM, Sekino M, Nishibori M, Yamamoto Y, Tsudzuki M (2005) Genetic variability and relationships of native Japanese chickens assessed by microsatellite DNA profiling—Focusing on the breeds established in Kochi Prefecture, Japan. Asian-Australas J Anim Sci 18: 755–761.
58. Tadano R, Sekino M, Nishibori M, Tsudzuki M (2007) Microsatellite marker analysis for the genetic relationships among Japanese long-tailed chicken breeds. Poult Sci 86: 460–469.
59. Miwa M, Inoue-Murayama M, Aoki H, Kunisada T, Hiragaki T, et al. (2007) *Endothelin receptor B2 (EDNRB2)* is associated with the *panda* plumage colour mutation in Japanese quail. Anim Genet 38: 103–108.
60. McCallion AS, Chakravarti A (2001) EDNRB/EDN3 and Hirschsprung disease type II. Pigment Cell Res 14: 161–169.
61. Manly KF, Cudmore RH Jr, Meer JM (2001) Map Manager QTX, cross-platform software for genetic mapping. Mamm Genome 12: 930–932.
62. Kosambi D (1944) The estimation of map distances from recombination values. Ann Eugen 12: 172–175.

15

Large Sex Differences in Chicken Behavior and Brain Gene Expression Coincide with Few Differences in Promoter DNA-Methylation

Daniel Nätt[1,2]*, Beatrix Agnvall[1], Per Jensen[1]

1 IFM Biology, AVIAN Behaviour and Genomics group, Linköping University, Linköping, Sweden, 2 Department of Clinical and Experimental Medicine, Laboratory of Integrative and Behavioral Neuroscience, Linköping University, Linköping, Sweden

Abstract

While behavioral sex differences have repeatedly been reported across taxa, the underlying epigenetic mechanisms in the brain are mostly lacking. Birds have previously shown to have only limited dosage compensation, leading to high sex bias of Z-chromosome gene expression. In chickens, a male hyper-methylated region (MHM) on the Z-chromosome has been associated with a local type of dosage compensation, but a more detailed characterization of the avian methylome is limiting our interpretations. Here we report an analysis of genome wide sex differences in promoter DNA-methylation and gene expression in the brain of three weeks old chickens, and associated sex differences in behavior of Red Junglefowl (ancestor of domestic chickens). Combining DNA-methylation tiling arrays with gene expression microarrays we show that a specific locus of the MHM region, together with the promoter for the *zinc finger RNA binding protein* (*ZFR*) gene on chromosome 1, is strongly associated with sex dimorphism in gene expression. Except for this, we found few differences in promoter DNA-methylation, even though hundreds of genes were robustly differentially expressed across distantly related breeds. Several of the differentially expressed genes are known to affect behavior, and as suggested from their functional annotation, we found that female Red Junglefowl are more explorative and fearful in a range of tests performed throughout their lives. This paper identifies new sites and, with increased resolution, confirms known sites where DNA-methylation seems to affect sexually dimorphic gene expression, but the general lack of this association is noticeable and strengthens the view that birds do not have dosage compensation.

Editor: Wei Yan, University of Nevada School of Medicine, United States of America

Funding: Grant support came from The Swedish Research Council (2008-14496-59340-36), The Swedish Research Council for Environment, Agricultural Sciences and Spatial Planning FORMAS (221-2007-838), and the European Research Council (ERC grant 322206 GENEWELL). The funders had no role in study design, data collection and analysis, decision to publish, or preparation of the manuscript.

Competing Interests: The authors have declared that no competing interests exist.

* E-mail: daniel.natt@liu.se

Background

A wide range of strategies for reproduction and social behavior exists among animals. Depending on whether the species lives solitary or in groups, in matriarchates or patriarchates, and in polyandry, polygyny or polygamy, the roles of the two sexes may differ dramatically [1] [2]. This may lead to the evolution of distinctly different behavioral roles of the sexes, shaping behavioral differences of various kinds [1]. Although there are many accounts of such sex specific behavioral roles, very little is known about the genetic mechanisms behind them. As the genomes of males and females of the same species are highly similar (except for the sex chromosomes), we would expect gene expression and epigenetic factors to be important in shaping the phenotypic differences.

Sex specific gene expression has been observed in many taxa such as insects, nematodes, birds and mammals [3]. For instance, approximately 80% of the gene expression which differs between *Drosophila simulans* and *melanogaster* is attributable to sexually dimorphic genes [4]. While few cases have directly linked gene expression with unique behavioral traits, at least in rodents, plenty of genetic and epigenetic differences have been identified in brain regions critical for behavioral control (reviewed in [5]). In mice, sexual dimorphisms in brain gene expression are present even before embryonic hormonal secretion, which suggests functional differences in the brain that are independent of embryonic hormones [6]. However, there is still limited knowledge of the relationship between sex differences in gene expression and epigenetic factors on one hand and the corresponding behavioral differences on the other.

Studies on sex specific epigenetic mechanism often address the concept of dosage compensation. Organisms with heteromorphic sex chromosomes, such as mammals (female:XX, male: XY) and birds (female:ZW, male:ZZ), face a genetic problem since the heterogametic sex (males in mammals and females in birds) only get half the dosage of the dominant sex chromosome, potentially leading to lower expression from genes on this chromosome. In mammals, this loss of dosage is compensated by a general silencing of one of the female X-chromosomes [7]. The *Xist* gene, which transcribes a long non-coding RNA and is expressed only from the silenced chromosome [8], seems to initiate this by mediating histone modifications and promoter methylation of cytosine residues all over the affected chromosome [9] [10]. Unlike mammals, birds seem to lack global mechanisms for dosage compensation leading to highly biased expression of genes on the

Z-chromosome (reviewed in [11]). Surprisingly, even though the Z-chromosome contains about 10% of all known genes in the chicken genome, this apparently does not lead to any functional failure of biological systems. Recently it has been suggested that birds partially use mammalian-type dosage compensation to circumvent some of the problems [12] [13]. In this context, a so called male hypermethylated region (MHM) on the Z-chromosome has been identified [14], and just like *Xist* it transcribes a large noncoding RNA that is thought to mediate DNA-methylation locally around itself. Interestingly, it has been suggested that the MHM region may cause down-regulation of the closely linked *DMRT1* gene, which previously was shown to be important for sex determination in species of many taxa including birds [15,16].

The overall aim of this experiment was to identify epigenetic targets possibly involved in regulating sexually dimorphic behaviors. Specifically, we studied sex differences in gene expression and DNA-methylation on a genome wide scale in the brains of three weeks old chickens and characterized sex differences in behavior. By sampling brains early in adolescence, just prior to when most sexually dimorphic behaviors emerge in the chicken, we hoped to identify key regulators that initiate the sexual differentiation of the brain during this period. By focusing the genetic analysis on thalamus/hypothalamus we primarily aimed to identify gene targets involved in stress regulation and therefore focused on behaviors relevant to stress and fear. To evaluate the generality of our findings, we used two genetically distinct breeds with unique selection histories over several thousand years; the Red Junglefowl (*Gallus gallus*), ancestor of domestic chickens, and the domesticated White Leghorn (*Gallus gallus domesticus*). Both breeds are highly sexually dimorphic, with an excessively ornamented male of about double the size of the more cryptic female [17]. Both sexes are sexually promiscuous, but sexual coercion by the male is often necessary for copulation to occur [18] [19]. While the domesticated breed still expresses most of its natural behaviors, commercial selection for certain sexually relevant characteristics (egg laying frequency, egg size, body mass), has changed the expression level of sexual characters, leading for example to larger but less colorful sex ornaments.

Results and Discussion

Gene expression: Limited dosage compensation

To examine epigenetic differences between the sexes, we extracted DNA and mRNA from the same samples, each comprising a part of the brain enriched for hypothalamus and thalamus. Samples were collected from 12 Red Junglefowl (RJF) of each sex when they were 21 days old, and were pooled into two pools per sex for gene expression microarray and DNA-methylation tiling array analysis. An identical sample set was also collected for domesticated White Leghorn chicks (WL). The total number of animals was therefore 24, pooled and hybridized onto eight arrays, four arrays of each sex and breed.

For gene expression, the mRNA was hybridized to Affymetrix GeneChip Chicken Genome Arrays. Consistent with previous findings reporting limited dosage compensation in the homogametic avian male, the total proportion of genes on the Z-chromosome that showed lower expression in females was highly significant in both RJF (Figure 1; 87% was lower in females, $\chi^2 = 275.8$, $p<0.0001$) and WL (90% was lower in females, $\chi^2 = 312.2$ $p<0.0001$) compared to a 50/50 distribution. Significantly differentially expressed (DE) probesets (Table S1) were mainly located on the Z-chromosome and over-represented by lower expression in females in both the RJF (Figure 2A) and WL (Figure 2B). However, most Z linked genes were not significantly DE and, more interestingly, some were strongly up-regulated in females, suggesting active mechanisms against dosage (Figure 3A). Even though three of these genes overlapped with the dosage compensated region surrounding MHM between 25–35 Mb previously identified by Melamed and Arnold [12], most probesets within this region did not reach significant DE. On the contrary, like the rest of the Z chromosome, most probesets within this 10 Mb region had a significantly lower expression in females than in males (RJF: 77% lower in females, $\chi^2 = 15.2$, $p<0.001$; WL: 83% lower in females, $\chi^2 = 24.4$, $p<0.0001$, compared to a 50/50 distribution) indicating a more complicated control mechanism focused on individual genes than general silencing through mammalian type dosage compensation in the region. One transcript from a novel gene (ENSGALG00000018479) in the periphery of the MHM region on the Z chromosome showed a particularly strong compensational signal (overexpression in females) (Figure 3A). The *DMRT1* gene was not significantly DE between sexes, while the *DMRT3* gene, which is located very close downstream, was so, but only in RJF. To verify and further characterize our results from the MHM region, we performed qPCR on an independent set of RJF brains. This showed that the predicted exonic region of the novel gene in MHM, was strongly DE between sexes, while an intronic EST and a flanking EST region closer to the DMRT1/3 cluster showed much more variation (Figure 4A).

Gene expression: Autosomal sex dimorphic gene expression

Although the autosomes had fewer significantly DE genes in total, most were up-regulated in females (Table S1). Using cluster analysis, we identified three larger clades with unique sex differences in gene expression, consisting of: 1) W chromosome genes, 2) Z chromosome genes and 3) autosomal genes (cluster analysis is represented by the heat maps of Figure 2A, B and D). There was a large overlap of the significantly DE genes between the breeds (Figure 2C), but most autosomal genes were only DE in one of the two breeds (Figure 2A, B and D), leaving only one autosomal gene verified in the overlap: the *zinc finger RNA binding protein* (*ZFR*) on chromosome 1 (Figure 3D). Two highly similar paralogs to the *ZFR* gene are present in the chicken genome; one on chromosome 1 and the other on Z. To find out which of the two paralogs that was responsible for the observed signals, we compared the genomic sequence of each of them to the sequences of the expression array probeset family GgaAffx.25782.x, as well as the Gga.19912.1.S1_at and the Gga.15339.1.S1_s_at probesets; all of which hybridize to both or either of the two paralogs. Significant DE was only found on the four (out of six) probesets most similar to the chromosome 1 paralog, which strongly indicates that the signal came from the *ZFR* on chromosome 1 (Figure S1). To clarify this further we performed qPCR on our independent set of RJF brains, which showed that the *ZRF* on chromosome 1 was strongly up-regulated in females, while the chromosome Z paralog was instead modestly up-regulated in males, as could be expected under no dosage compensation (Figure 4B).

DNA-methylation: No mammalian type dosage compensation

The DNA extracted from the same brain samples as the mRNA was analyzed for methylation differences, using a custom-made tiling array together with methylated DNA immunoprecipitation (MeDIP), which allowed us to analyze 3623 promoter regions (defined as 7.5 kb upstream and 3.5 kb downstream from gene

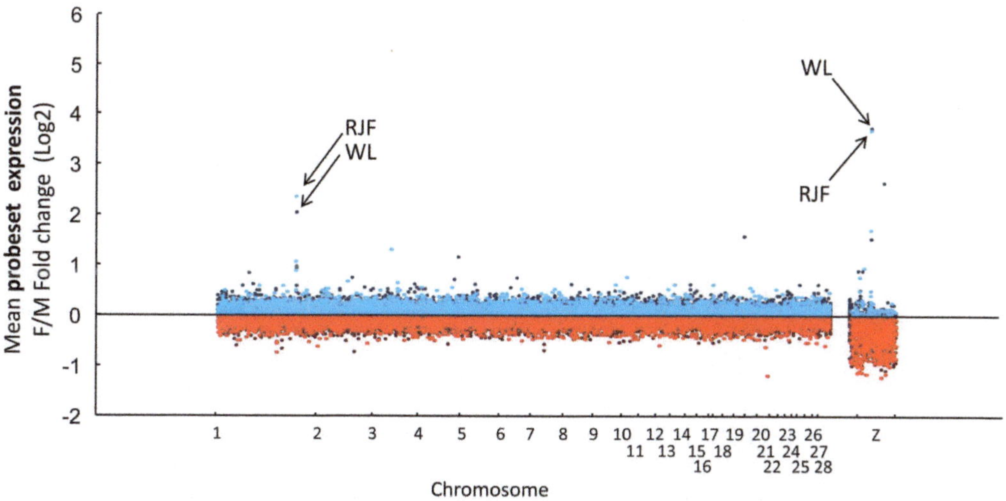

Figure 1. Differential expression of genes in females (F) compared to males (M) in Red Junglefowl (RJF) and White Leghorn (WL) respectively. Each dot represents the mean fold change difference (log 2) of one microarray probeset. Red dots indicate down-regulation in females, and blue dots up-regulation. Clear dots indicate RJF and dark colored dots indicate WL. Arrows indicate the two probesets on chromosome 1 and Z with the strongest fold change signals across breeds within the whole experiment. Genebuild: WASHUC2.

start site) covering about 385K probes simultaneously. Twelve gene promoters in the RJF (Figure 5A) and 31 in WL (Figure 5B) contained significantly differentially methylated (DM) probes between sexes (for details see Table S2). After considering just the overlap between breeds (Figure 5C) four gene promoters remained (Figure 5D).

The most differentially methylated region was found in the putative promoter of the novel gene in MHM that also showed the greatest differential expression on the Z chromosome (Figure 3B). There were 37 significantly DM probes hypermethylated in males and all were specifically associated with the promoter of the novel gene within the MHM, while the neighboring genes were unaffected (Figure 3C). Together with the gene expression data, this strongly suggests that sex specific regulation within the MHM region is localized to specific transcripts. To further explore this we performed bisulfite sequencing on our independent set of RJF brains. Interestingly, while a repeat region up-stream of the transcription start site was verified as strongly methylated in males and lacking methylation in females, CpGs within the predicted second exon of the novel gene were methylated in both sexes (Figure 6A).

DNA-methylation: Autosomal genes and the Zinc finger RNA binding protein

Since *ZFR* was the only autosomal gene verified as significantly DE in both breeds, differential regulation of autosomal genes may mainly contribute to breed specific sex differences, and not sex differences present in both breeds. In line with this, even though plenty of autosomal promoters were significantly DM within breeds (Figure 5A and B), only the promoter to the *ZFR* gene was DM in both breeds (Figure 5D). While male promoter hyper-methylation of the novel gene in MHM (Figure 3C) was associated with lower gene expression compared to females (Figure 3B), the opposite relationship was seen on *ZFR* (Figure 3D and E). Notably, the strongly differentially methylated MHM promoter on Z (Figure 3C) contained a CpG island, which the *ZFR* promoter lacked (Figure 3F).

To confidently assign the DM signal to the chromosome 1 paralog of *ZFR* (see previous discussion), we blasted the oligonucleotide sequences of the four strongest DM probes to the chicken genome. While all four perfectly aligned to the promoter region near the chromosome 1 paralog, none aligned to the Z counterpart. We also verified this by bisulfite sequencing on our independent set of RJF brains, using PCR primers specific for the DM region on chromosome 1 after bisulfite conversion. Surprisingly, very little PCR product was generated from female bisulfite treated DNA compared to male DNA (Figure 6B). Since the PCR-primers were designed to not overlap CG-dinucleotides, female cytosine residues at the primer annealing sites might have been protected against bisulfite conversion by another type of DNA-modification than CpG-methylation.

Functions of differentially expressed or methylated genes

Since our study focused on gene expression and DNA-methylation differences in the brain, we specifically looked for gene candidates with functions in behavioral control. We therefore combined manual annotation with gene ontology analysis, and produced a list of possible "behavioral" genes (Table 1). While none of the genes were both significantly differentially expressed and methylated, many of them were verified between breeds, even though more were present in RJF than in WL. One interesting example was seen in the Tyrosine hydroxylase pathway, which involves dopamine and norepinephrine synthesis, where three key enzymes (*DBH*, *MOXD1*, *TH*) had genes with hypomethylated promoters in RJF females compared to males, while such a relationship was absent in WL. The tyrosine hydroxylase pathway and dopaminergic reward system has repeatedly been associated with different aspects of social and exploratory behavior (for examples see [20,21] [22]).Furthermore, the two receptor genes *GABRA2* (a GABA receptor subunit) and *NTRK2* (coding for the BDNF TrkB receptor) also showed differential expression/ methylation, and both have previously been associated with the reward system [23] [24].

Another interesting Z-linked gene, which was less expressed in females of both breeds, was the highly conserved *CRHBP* (*corticotrophin releasing hormone binding protein*). In vertebrates, CRH (corticotropin-releasing hormone) is one of the main controllers of the HPA-axis. CRHBP binds CRH and inhibits its interaction

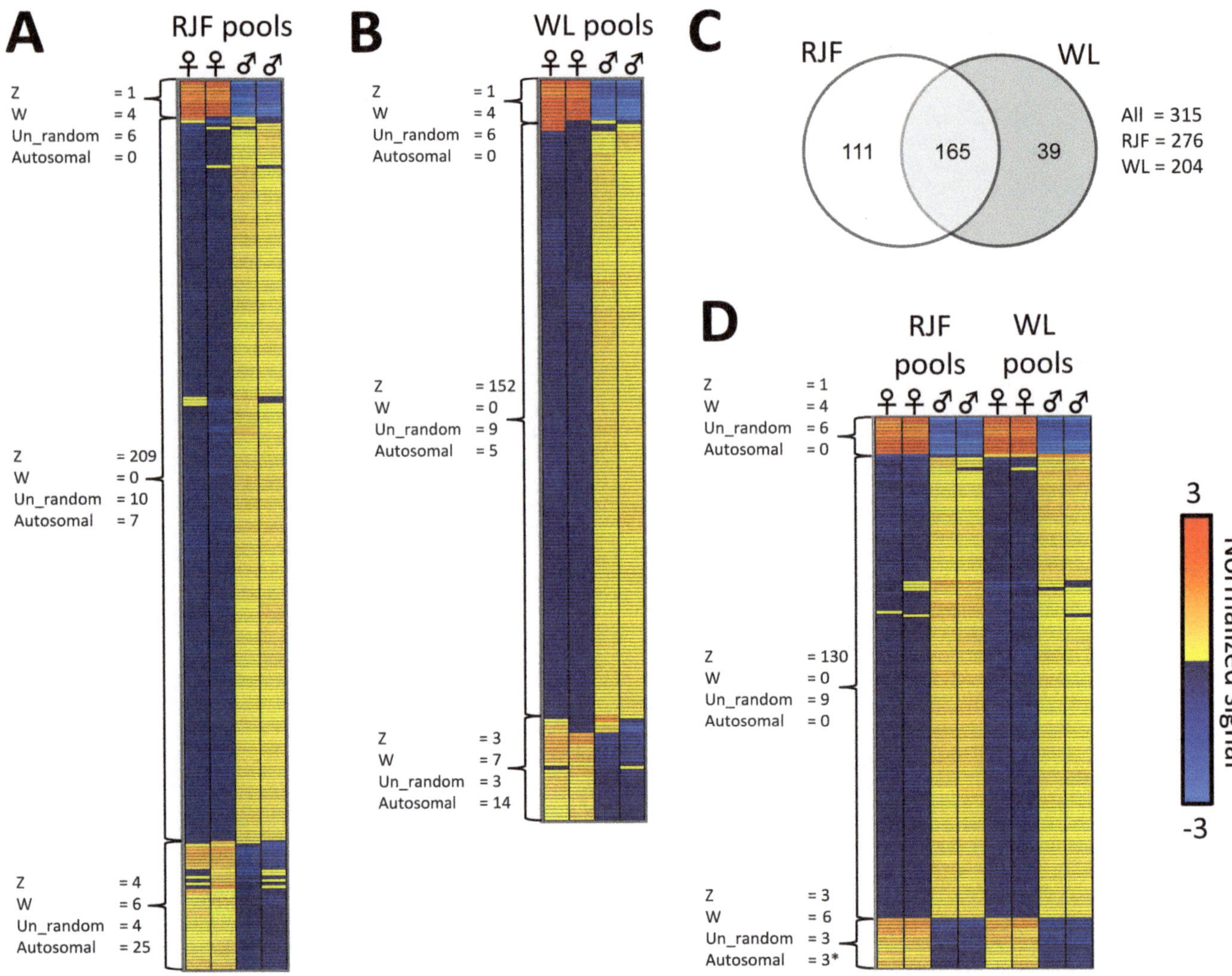

Figure 2. Significant gene expression differences between sexes within and across breeds. Heat map columns represent individual microarrays, while rows represent significantly differentially expressed (DE) probesets adjusted for false discovery rate. Heat maps are organized using hierarchical cluster analysis (average linkage) identifying three major clades both within and across breeds (clades are represented by brackets). **A)** Probesets DE within the Red Junglefowl (RJF pools). **B)** Probesets DE within the White Leghorn (WL pools). **C)** Venn-diagram showing numbers of DE probesets within breeds that are also DE in the other breed. **D)** Probesets DE across breeds. *Note that DE probesets annotated to autosomes are common within breed, but only three probesets remain in the across breed comparison, all annotated to the same gene: *ZFR* on chromosome 1. Each microarray was hybridized with a pool of six birds.

with the CRH receptors, thereby working as an anxiolytic agent [25]. Hypothetically, the lower dosage of *CRHBP* expression in female birds would suggest that females may have a stronger stress response. While *CRHBP* is conserved on the Z chromosome in chicken, turkey and zebra finch, but found on many different autosomes in other vertebrates, it may play a particularly important role in behavioral sex differences of birds.

When considering all significant DE genes, GO analysis (Table S3) did not reveal significant terms associated with the biological functions of reproduction and sex development. When only considering the genes up-regulated, in females terms like "sex differentiation" and "external genitalia morphogenesis" were significant. This was mainly due to two paralogs of the *Nipped-B* (*NIPL*) gene on the Z and W chromosomes respectively which were up-regulated in females of both breeds. Similarly, when considering all significant DM promoters (Table S4), no significant terms associated with biological function of reproduction or sex development were found. Nevertheless, disregarding correction for multiple testing (FDR), some interesting terms were high ranked on the lists when looking at WL separately, such as "male, female gonadal development" and "gamete generation", which was associated mainly with four significantly DM genes: *WNT4*, *SGPL1*, *CRTAP*, *BCL2*. Interestingly, even though *WNT4* and *CRTAP* were not significantly DM in the RJF, they were still high ranked (531 and 85 out of 383385 probes).

Behavioral sex differences in Red Junglefowl

Since most of our behavioral gene candidates were identified within the RJF, we subjected 158 males and 141 females of this breed to a battery of standardized behavioral tests designed mainly to phenotype different aspects of fear, exploration and sociality applied at different ages. We hypothesized that females should express more fear related behaviors than males based on a higher expression of *CRHBP* in males, and that the sexes should differ in

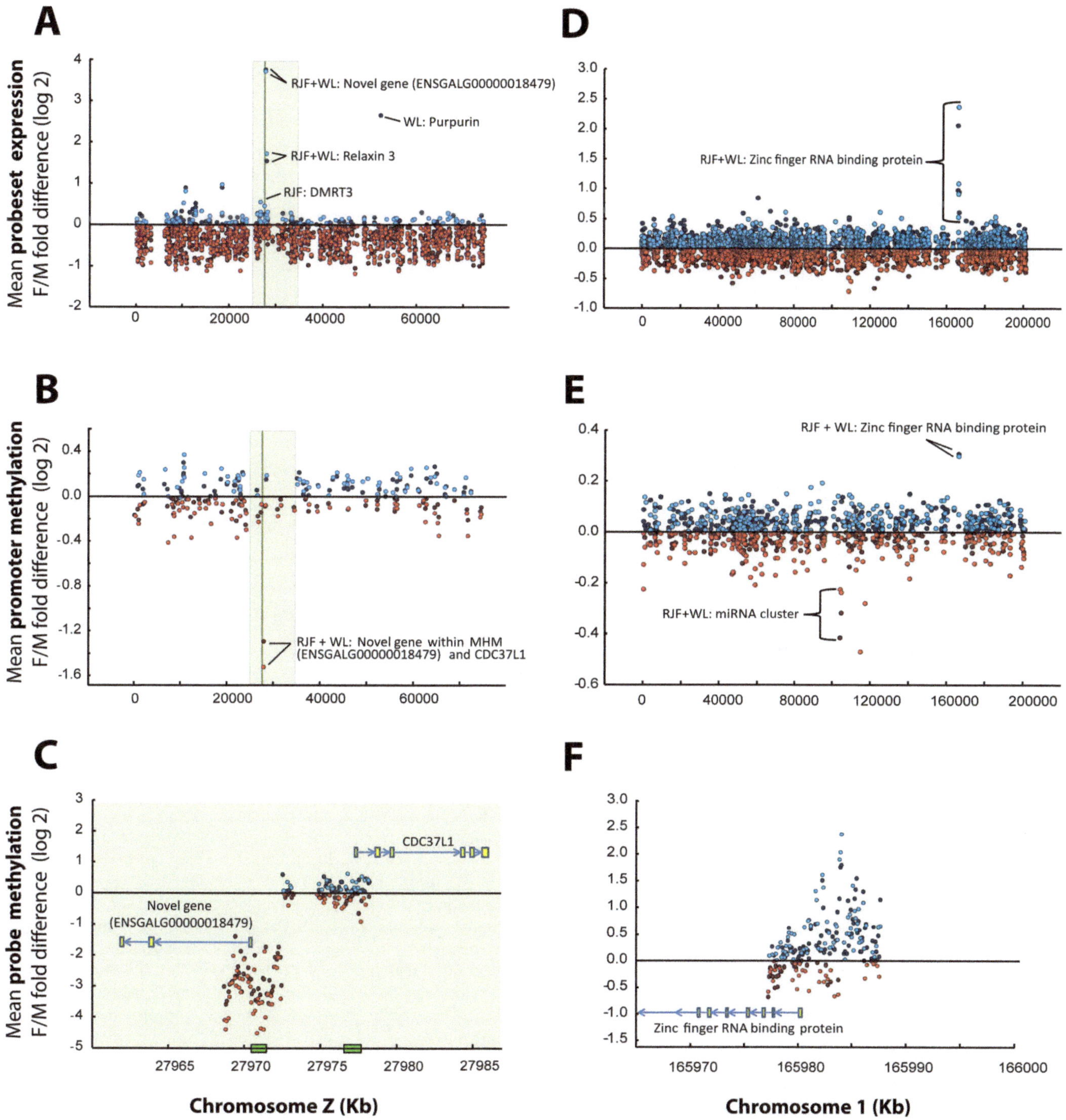

Figure 3. Gene expression and DNA-methylation differences between females (F) and males (M) on chromosome Z and 1 respectively. Dots represent fold change differences (log 2) within three categories: A) and D) = Expression microarray probesets; B) and E) = DNA-methylation tiling array probes averaged within promoter; C) and F) = Individual DNA-methylation tiling array probes. A) shows gene expression differences on the Z chromosome. B) shows promoter methylation differences on the Z-chromosome. C) shows individual probe differences in the promoters of a novel gene close to MHM and *CDC37L1*. D) shows gene expression differences on chromosome 1. E) shows promoter methylation differences on chromosome 1. F) shows individual probe differences in the promoter to *ZFR* on chromosome 1. Red dots signify down-regulation in females, and blue dots up-regulation. Clear dots indicate Red Junglefowl (RJF) and dark colored dots White Leghorn (WL). The clear green shaded area represents the dosage compensated region reported by [12], and the dark green line represent the location of the male hyper methylated region reported by [14]. Genebuild: WASHUC2.

novelty exploration and sociality, since this previously was shown to be affected by the tyrosine hydroxylase pathway and dopamine release (see previous discussion).

The behavioral test results are all summarized in Table S5. Social affiliation and companion propensity was tested in a social reinstatement test at three weeks of age, but did not detect any

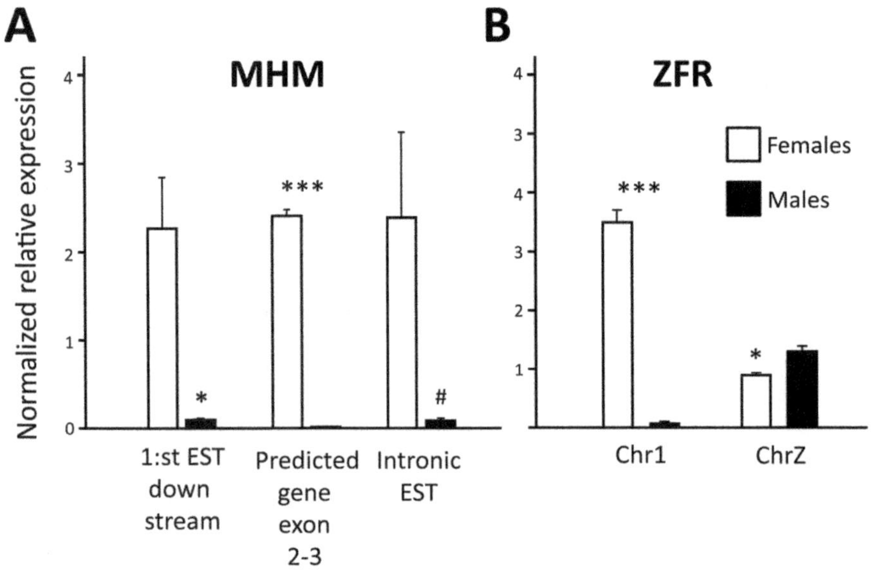

Figure 4. Independent verification of gene expression using qPCR. Gene expression was analyzed on an independent set of RJF brains (females: n = 4, males: n = 7). **A**) The exonic region of the novel gene within MHM was more strongly expressed compared to EST region downstream and within intronic region. **B**) The *ZFR* paralog on chromosome 1 was highly up-regulated in females, while the *ZFR* paralog on chromosome Z showed an expected none dosage compensated male bias. Independent t-test adjusted for unequal variance, ***p<0.0001, *p<0.01, #p<0.1.

significant differences between the sexes. In an open field test one week later, males entered the center zone quicker and more often than females, and spent less time in the corners of the arena, which all indicates less fear in males. No differences were detected when we repeated the test at 16 weeks of age. At 13 weeks a foraging and exploration test was conducted where males were significantly less prone to explore the arena and to exploit novel and hidden food. To further measure fearfulness, we used two different tests, where the first measured the reactions to a simulated aerial predator attack, and the second was the widely used tonic immobility (TI) test. These tests were applied when the birds were 15 and 17 weeks old respectively. Females preened less, vocalized more and made more escape attempts in predator test, while they required more induction attempts and remained longer in TI; all indicates more fear in females. At 27 weeks, undisturbed behavior was recorded while groups of birds were roaming freely in an enriched pen. Here, females explored more and were more active, while males performed more perching, comfort and jump/flight behavior.

In general, the tests suggest that females were more explorative and prone to forage, but also more fearful in their reactions to various stressful stimuli. To derive more general reaction patterns that may differ between the sexes, we used a two-step principal component analysis (PCA). First, we entered all behavioral variables from all the tests (see Table S5) in a PCA, which generated four factors with an eigenvalue over one. From this first solution, we selected one variable from each test (the one with the highest communality in the four-factor solution) and performed a second PCA based on these seven variables. The results of the second PCA, rendering four factors that explained 71% of the variation, are shown in Table 2. The first factor mainly spanned SR-social and UB-explore, and was tentatively named "Social/Exploration". The second factor was named "Fear" since TI-first had the highest loading. The interpretation of the third factor was more elusive, but based on the observed loadings was tentatively labeled "Activity". The last factor was labeled "Foraging/Exploration".

We then calculated factor scores for all individuals on each of the four factors, and tested for sex differences. As seen in Table 3, there were significant sex differences on the three first factors. Females scored higher on all of them, indicating higher exploration, fear and general activity, which supports the findings from the genetic and epigenetic analysis discussed above.

General discussion

Our data show consistent differences in behavior and genome wide gene expression, and to a smaller extent, DNA-methylation between sexes in chickens. As previously reported, it is clear that the juvenile chicken brain has very limited mammalian type dosage compensation, and we show that this also account for DNA-methylation on the Z-chromosome. In fact, few sites are strongly differentially methylated in promoter regions between sexes in chickens. One of these sites, the so called male hyper-methylated region (MHM) [14] on the Z-chromosome, is linked to a large methylated sequence, which selectively suppresses expression of a specific transcript in males. We also found a highly methylated site associated with female up-regulation of the *zinc finger RNA binding protein* gene on chromosome 1, which still is functionally uncharacterized. Seemingly, this site was also associated with non-CpG-methylation (see further discussion below). Additionally, we identified several differentially expressed genes known to affect behavior, and as suggested from their functional annotation, we showed that female Red Junglefowl are more explorative and fearful.

Teranishi *et al.* showed that a cloned 2.2 kb repetitive sequence on the short arm of the Z chromosomes is strongly hypermethylated in male chickens (the MHM region) and mainly transcribes a long non-coding RNA in females [14]. We are aware that the DE/DM signal in the MHM region in the present study could originate from the same ncRNA. Nevertheless, the MHM contains several open reading frames which could potentially translate into proteins [26]. In addition, within the MHM region there is a predicted gene with three possible exons, where the two last is located within a region with no repeats (Ensembl genebuild). Since the DE signal

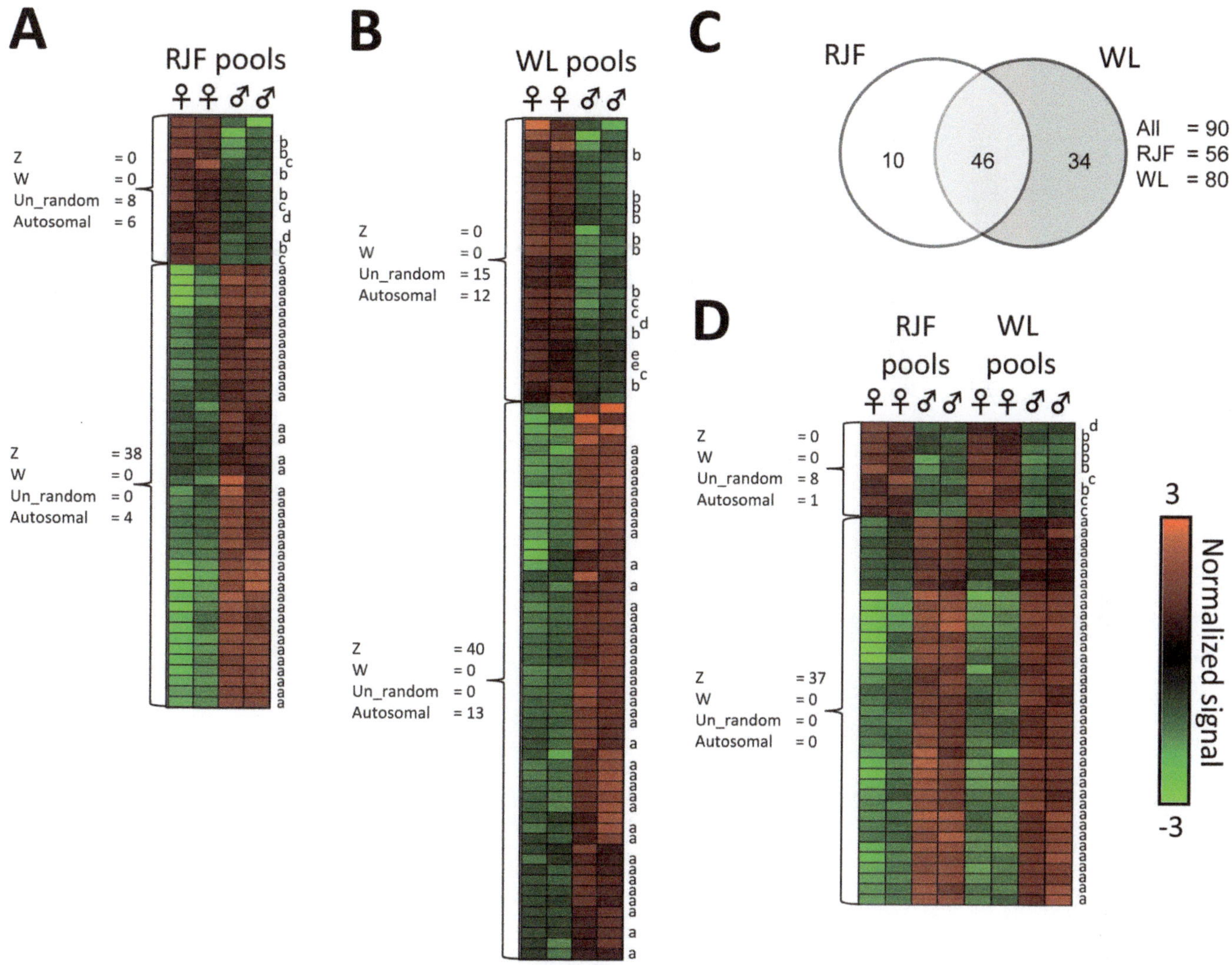

Figure 5. Significant promoter DNA-methylation differences between sexes within and across breeds. Heat map columns represent individual tiling arrays, while rows represent significantly differentially methylated (DM) probes adjusted for false discovery rate. Heat maps are organized using hierarchical cluster analysis (average linkage) identifying two major clades both within and across breeds (represented by brackets). **A**) Probes DM within Red Junglefowl (RJF pools). **B**) Probes DM within White Leghorn (WL pools). **C**) Venn-diagram showing how many of the DM probes within breeds that are present across, in both, breeds. **D**) Probes DM across breeds. Lower case letters next to heat map rows indicate that multiple probes are significantly DM in the same promoter; the same letter indicates the same promoter. Note that "d" and "a" represent probes in the promoters of *ZFR* and the novel gene in MHM respectively. Each tiling array was hybridized with a pool of six birds.

is associated only with the 1.8 kb probeset covering these exons and not the neighboring probesets, spanning other parts of the 9.5 kb ncRNA [14], our signal could still come from a protein coding gene or a splice variant of the ncRNA. Furthermore, while Teranishi *et al.* [14] originally found MHM and its associated long ncRNA in various tissues and developmental stages, analysis of chicken embryos using the Affymetrix's GeneChip Chicken Genome array has in some cases failed to detected differential expression of this probeset [27,28]. Since other studies, including our own, report very strong female bias using the same platform but at other developmental stages, tissues and genetic backgrounds [13,29], it suggests dynamic regulation of the MHM region.

Manks and Ellegren [13] have concluded that dosage compensation in chickens is regulated on a gene-by-gene level. Our qPCR and bisulfite sequencing analysis adds another level of complexity to the regulation of the MHM region by showing that the exonic part of the novel MHM gene shows much less variation between sexes than surrounding regions. The impact of this regional difference is still unknown, but it is tempting to speculate that the region may harbor a dynamic transcription pattern, involving both non-coding and coding RNA important for sex differentiation. Interestingly, Bisoni *et al.* have also associated the MHM region with female histone H4 hyper-acetylation [30], an epigenetic mark usually associated with activation of transcription. It remains to be investigated how specific this histone modification is targeted to the exonic region of novel gene in MHM, but since Bisoni *et al.* did not find differential H4 acetylation on the adjacent *DMRT1* gene, there may be a relationship between female H4 acetylation and female DNA(hypo)-methylation at this very specific site.

In humans, the loss of one copy of *DMRT1* can cause phenotypic sex reversal [16], and has been implicated as important also in bird sex determination [15]. Notably, *DMRT1* is located very close to the MHM region. In our study, *DMRT1* transcripts were not significantly DE between sexes, as they are in

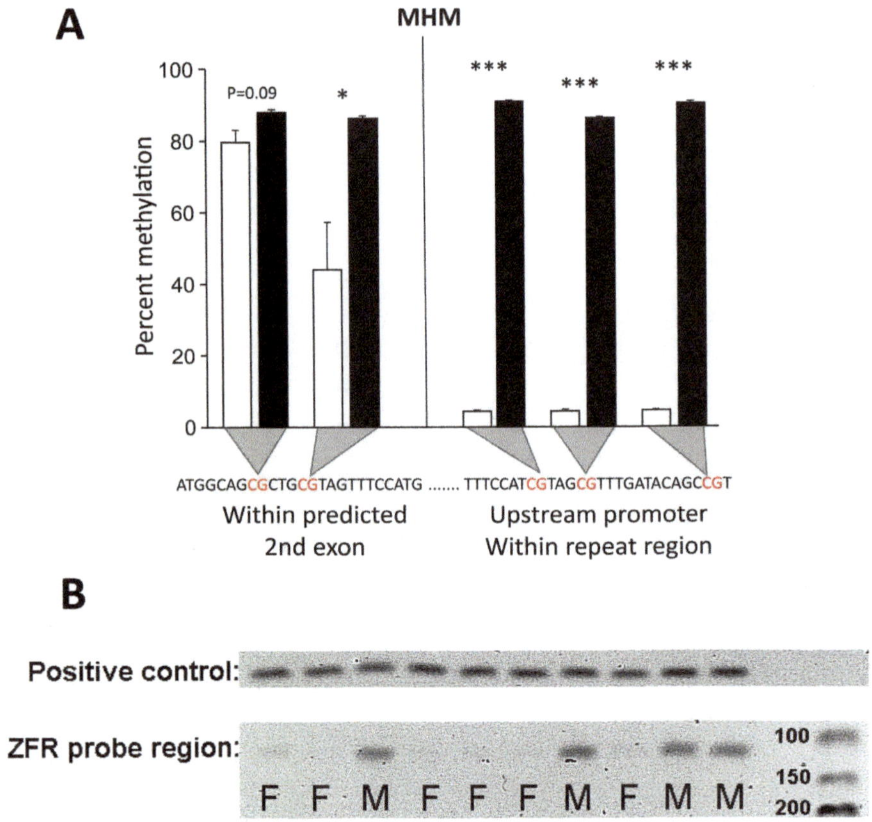

Figure 6. Independent verification of DNA-methylation using bisulfite sequencing. A) Bisulfite sequencing of the novel gene within the MHM region shows that the predicted second exon and the repeat region in the promoter have different DNA-methylation patterns. **B**) Agarose gel electrophoresis shows that PCR using bisulfite converted primers annealing in regions with no CG-dinucleotides, failed to amplify in females, but not in males. Independent t-test adjusted for unequal variance, ***p<0.0001, *p<0.01, #p<0.1.

Table 1. Top candidate genes related to sexually dimorphic behavior in chickens (Red Junglefowl).

Ensemble ID	*Name*	*Function*	*Behavioral keywords*	*Female vs. Male*
Differentially expressed				
ENSGALG00000002289	*CHAT*	Cholinergic regulation	Sexual, Learning, Locomotion	Up-regulated
ENSGALG00000004364	*ABR*	Synaptic plasticity	Stress, Learning	Up-regulated
ENSGALG00000016554	*ACE2*	Angiotensin regulation	Feeding, Drinking, Stress	Up-regulated
ENSGALG00000012594	*NTRK2*	Brain neurotrophic factor signaling, Dopamine interaction	Cognition, Learning, Feeding, Fear	Down-regulated
ENSGALG00000014994	*CRHBP*	Regulation of HPA-axis, Dopamine and Glutamate interaction	Stress, Learning, Memory	Down-regulated [a]
ENSGALG00000015147	*ALDH1A1*	Interaction with Dopamine and Norephrenaphrine pathways	Reward, Learning	Down-regulated [a]
Differentially methylated				
ENSGALG00000014206	*GABRA2*	GABA regulation	Behavior, Reward	Hyper-methylated [a]
ENSGALG00000007839	*NCAM1*	Synaptic plasticity	Brain development, Learning	Hyper-methylated [ab]
ENSGALG00000002020	*GLUD2*	Glutamate regulation	Fear, Learning, Memory	Hypo-methylated [ab]
ENSGALG00000002911	*DBH*	Tyrosine metabolism, Dopamine and Norepinephrine regulation	Reward, Learning, Maternal, Social	Hypo-methylated [b]
ENSGALG00000002926	*MOXD1*	Tyrosine metabolism, Dopamine and Norepinephrine regulation	Reward, Learning, Maternal, Social	Hypo-methylated [b]
ENSGALG00000006551	*TH*	Tyrosine metabolism, Dopamine and Norepinephrine regulation	Reward, Learning, Sexual, Social	Hypo-methylated [b]
ENSGALG00000008875	*PLCB1*	Long term potentiation	Sexual, Cognition, Learning	Hypo-methylated [ab]
ENSGALG00000015177	*GNA11*	Dopaminergic, Colinergic and Glutamatergic receptor signaling	Reward, Fear, Learning	Hypo-methylated [a]

[a]Validated as significant or top ranked differentially expressed or methylated in the White Leghorn breed.
[b]Not significant, but top ranked among the 225 (of 3623) most differentially methylated promoters.

Table 2. Factor scores from principal component analysis (PCA) of behavioral variables with the highest communality measured in a series of tests on Red Junglefowls.*

	Factors			
Variables	**1**	**2**	**3**	**4**
SR duration social zone (s)	−0.81	0.07	0.31	−0.12
OF4 frequency center	−0.35	−0.33	−0.65	0.33
FE Hidden food	0.26	0.50	0.26	0.59
AP Explore	0.43	−0.38	0.40	−0.34
OF16 crossed zones	−0.19	−0.50	0.45	0.56
TI First movement	−0.10	0.70	0.00	−0.03
UB Explore	0.85	−0.07	−0.15	0.13

Test abbreviation: SR= Social reinstatement, OF4= Openfield at 4 weeks of age, FE= Foraging and exploration, AP= Aerial predator, OF16=Openfield at 16 weeks of age, TI= Tonic immobility, UB= Undisturbed behavior.
*For all behavior test results see Table S3.

chicken embryos [26,27]. Instead we found that the first exon of *DMRT3*, a paralog located only 4.5 kb downstream from *DMRT1*, was strongly down-regulated in RJF males. Perhaps *DMRT1* and *DMRT3* play different roles in sexual development at different ages and tissues. Interestingly, we found no down-regulation of *DMRT3* in the WL breed. Due to commercial selection, the WL breed becomes sexually mature weeks before the RJF, which again may suggest that *DMRT1/3* expression is age dependent.

A few probesets of the *ZFR* gene on chromosome 1 have previously been found to have a female expression bias in chickens [29] [28]. While little is known about the function of this *ZFR* paralog, from its RNA binding properties it seems plausible that it plays an important role in RNA regulation during sexual development. Future experiments should therefore investigate if there are interactions between ZFR and the long non-coding RNA in the MHM region. The *ZFR* promoter is relatively CG poor and our results suggest that it contains non-CG-dinucleotide DNA-modifications. Methylation at CHG and CHH (where H can be either A, T or G) is commonly seen in plants, but does not occur widely in mammals [31]. To our knowledge this is the first time an indication of such a modification has been reported in an avian species, but it is clear that it needs further investigation. We also see an unexpected up-regulation of *ZFR* despite hypermethylation in females, which may indicate that a novel kind of epigenetic regulatory mechanism that are CG independent, or depend on both CG- and non-CG-sequence combinations, might be present in the region. Furthermore, we have previously demonstrated that a QTL covering the region around *ZFR* explains about 23% and 15% of the two fold differences in body weight between RJF and WL, in males and females respectively [32]. This QTL has also been associated with differences in fearfulness as measured by the tonic immobility test [33]. The *ZRF* gene has recently been suggested to be one of the most promising causal candidates within this QTL [34], but its precise functions remain to be investigated.

A large part of significantly DE and DM genes/promoters was associated with the un_random chromosome, which is a collection of unlinked sequences still awaiting alignment to real chromosomes. Since these genes lie randomly in relation to each other we decided to disregard them in many of our downstream analyses. However, after careful examination of our cluster analysis it seems likely that many of the significant un_random genes are in fact located on the sex chromosomes.

We initially designed our DNA-methylation tiling array to detect differences generated during chicken domestication, which might have biased the regions under analysis towards those important for this biological process. Nevertheless, making a gene ontology analysis of the 3623 gene promoters on the array did not show a significant enrichment of specific biological processes, which suggests an unbiased representation.

Many previous studies have explored sex differences in behavior, in many different species. For example, differences in foraging and social behavior, as well as stress and anxiety levels has widely been demonstrated in the wild [35] [36] [37] and under experimental conditions [38] [39]. Genetic findings of the present study suggest that sex behavioral differences are ubiquitous also in chickens. The battery of tests applied on the Red Junglefowl verified this, and across tests, females were more explorative, fearful and active. In the wild, Red Junglefowl form small harem-

Table 3. Mean factor scores for the four factors obtained in the between-test PCA, and the P-value obtained from a t-test of the difference between the sexes.

		Females		Males		
PCA Factor	**Interpretation**	**Mean**	**SEM**	**Mean**	**SEM**	**p-value**
1	Social/Exploration	0.19	±0.09	−0.20	±0.09	0.002
2	Fear	0.23	±0.09	−0.24	±0.09	0.0002
3	Activity	0.15	±0.09	−0.16	±0.08	0.02
4	Foraging/Exploration	−0.01	±0.09	0.01	±0.09	0.9

groups with one dominant male, a few subdominant males and a couple of females [18]. In such a group, the sexes have different roles and behaviors, where male reproductive success is more related to dominance and female success depends on maternal care. For example, high-ranked males have more access to females, provides females with resources such as food (courtship feeding) [40] [41] and defends the territory more vigilantly than low ranked males [42]. Females on the other hand incubate eggs, raise offspring without help from the males and do not participate in territory defense [43] [44]. Hence, one might expect that selection has favored different traits in the two sexes. Our results confirm these expected behavioral differences, and provide, for the first time a list of genomic sites associated with variation in gene expression and DNA-methylation that may be important for their development.

Conclusion

We have identified hundreds of genes genome wide with differential expression between sexes, but few differences in promoter DNA-methylation. After probing hundreds of promoters on the Z-chromosome, we can now for the first time be confident in saying that juvenile chicken lack mammalian type dosage compensation associated with large scale promoter DNA-methylation differences between sexes. On the other hand, our results indicate another type of cytosine-modification independent of CpG-methylation, which may play an important role in avian gene regulation and therefore stresses further investigation. Our results are important not only to understand the fundamental differences in how birds and mammals cope with a sexually unbalanced gene dosage, but also to understand how epigenetic factors may shape morphological, physiological as well as behavioral sex differences. Although the present results do not allow us to infer causal relationships between the epigenetic variation and the specific behavioral differences, the strong correlations call for further studies to reveal such connections.

Methods

Ethics statement

The experiments were approved by the "Regional Committee for Ethical Approval of Animal Experiments" in Linköping, Sweden (permit no 122-10). During all experiments, animals were handled carefully and in such a way that unnecessary stress was avoided. Animals were moved and transported in darkness, which reduces the stress responses of chickens, and were never exposed to any physical harmful stimuli. Killing was done by rapid dislocation of the necks, according to prevailing welfare standards and the ethical permit.

Breeding and housing

All birds in the experiment were pedigree bred and hatched. The eggs were incubated at 37.5°C and 55% relative humidity, with egg rotation every hour in a Marsalles 25 DIGIT incubator. At day 17 the temperature was increased to 37.8°C, the humidity to 65% and rotation turned off. The first day after hatching, birds were wing-tagged, weighed and vaccinated against Marek's disease. In the hatchery unit ("Kruijt") at Linköping University, the animals were held in small pens (0.75x0.75 m) in mixed-sex groups of about 30 birds with feed/water ad libitum and wood chip flooring. Pens were enlarged to double the size after two weeks and furnished with perches. Room temperature was about 27°C.

At five weeks of age animals were moved to a chicken research facility ("Wood-Gush") situated 10 km from the university, where they were kept in pens measuring 3x3x3 m and in sex separated groups of about 40 birds. The pens had a three-floor system with perches, nest boxes, and wood chips on the floor. Food and water was provided *ad libitum*.

Gene expression and DNA-methylation microarrays

Since the DNA-methylation tiling array was originally designed using WASHUC2 all results are presented using this genebuild's coordinates. For conversion to GalGal4 visit http://www.ensembl.org/Gallus_gallus/Info/Index.

Animal material, tissue sampling, preprocessing and micro/tiling array hybridization have been described in detail elsewhere [45]. In brief, breeds used for the gene expression and DNA methylation analysis originated out of 1) an outbreed zoo population of Red Junglefowl (RJF) kept as an experimental line for ten generations, and 2) a domesticated White Leghorn (WL) egg layer used as an experimental line since the 1970's.

In both breeds, brain samples were taken from 21 days old chicks (12 birds of each sex). From each brain, a region containing thalamus and hypothalamus was dissected out, immediately frozen and later homogenized in TRI reagents. RNA was isolated using the TRI manufacturer protocol with additional RNeasy (Qiagen) clean up, while DNA was isolated from the same TRI homogenate by ethanol precipitation followed by DNeasy (Qiagen) clean up. Before further processing, both RNA and DNA samples were separately mixed in eight pools with six brains per pool (two replicates of each sex within breed, in total 24 brains of each sex). For gene expression analysis, the RNA-pools were labeled and hybridized to the GeneChip Chicken Genome Array (Affymetrix) capable of analyzing 33457 transcripts. For DNA-methylation analysis, the DNA-pools were split, enriched using methylated DNA immunoprecipitation (MeDIP) and later co-hybridized with the original sample to a custom made DNA-methylation tiling array (Roche-NimbleGen) containing tiled 385K probes from 3623 promoters (defined as 7.5 kb upstream and 3.5 kb downstream from gene start site). The array data has been deposited at ArrayExpress and can be accessed with the following accession numbers: Gene expression arrays [E-MTAB644]; DNA-methylation [EMTAB-649].

Verification of microarray data

Hypothalamus tissue was collected and RNA/DNA extraction was done in same way as for the microarray experiment, but taken from three weeks old Red Junglefowls of an independent experimental population maintained in our lab. For gene expression verification, 1 µg RNA was reversely transcribed to cDNA using the RevertAid First Strand cDNA synthesis kit (Fermentas/Thermo Scientific) with oligo-dT primers and qPCR was performed with transcript specific primers seen in Table S6 using a 55°C annealing temperature. For DNA-methylation verification, 600 ng DNA was bisulfite converted using the EpiTect Fast Bisulfite Conversion Kit (Qiagen), amplified through PCR using the PyroMark PCR kit (Qiagen) and sequenced on a PyroMark 96 MD pyrosequencer. Prior to sequencing, a single PCR product was verified by 2% agarose gel electrophoresis. Bisulfite converted PCR and sequencing primers were designed using the PyroMark Assay Design software (Qiagen) and can be found in Table S6. PCR was performed at 94°C for 30 sec, 56°C for 30 sec and 72°C for 30 sec, through 45 cycles. All procedures followed manufactures recommendations.

Behavioral tests

Behavior was recorded in a Red Junglefowl population described previously by [46] and the behavioral tests used, except the undisturbed behaviors, were described comprehensively in the same publication. All behavioral variables used in the analysis are presented in Table S5. In brief, we studied 299 birds (158 males and 141 females) from three successive generations, originating from a cross between two captive zoo populations (the Gotala and Copenhagen population; the former being the RJF population used in the micro/tiling array experiments). Sociality was tested at three weeks of age by measuring duration in the social zone closest to a companion bird and distance moved in a standardized social reinstatement (SR) test (arena = 20×120×40 cm, social zone = 20×40 cm, test duration = 5 min, test variables were averaged between two duplicative trails for each animal). Fear/anxiety levels was tested at four (OF4) and sixteen (OF16) weeks of age by measuring frequency in center zone and duration in the peripheral part of an open field arena (arena = 4 weeks: 80×120×40 cm: 16 weeks: 190×190×100 cm, center zone = 4 weeks: 40×80 cm; 16 weeks: 100×100×100 cm, test duration: 5 min, test variables were averaged between two duplicative trails for each animal and age). Foraging and explorative behaviors were recorded at 13 weeks of age by measuring number of pecks directed at a bowl with hidden food (meal worms in wood shavings) in a choice between two other potential food resources (only wood shavings and familiar food pellets) and the frequency of changing between four identical clusters of food bowls, each containing all three food resources (arena: 95×95 cm, food deprivation: 1 h before trial, habituation to arena: 10 min before trail, test duration: 5 min) Anti-predator reaction (AP) was recorded at 15 weeks of age by measuring preening, vocalization, freezing and escape attempts after a brief exposure to an aerial predator model (hawk silhouette)(arena: 50×150×50 cm, baseline pre-test before predator: 5 min, test duration after predator: 5 min). General fearfulness, as measured by the tonic immobility reaction (TI), was recorded at 17 weeks of age by measuring number of induction attempts until the birds entered tonic immobility, as well as the time to first head movement and the duration of immobility (test duration: 10 min; if birds were immobile for more, a maximum value of 600 sec was given).

Undisturbed behaviors (UB) were recorded at 27 weeks of age in a pen similar to the home pen, measuring 2.5x3.0x3.0 m and furnished with a perch, wood chip flooring and *ad libitum* food and water. Habituation took place in groups of 7–11 familiar individuals (same sex) from 3 p.m. the day before observations began. At 9 a.m. behavioral observations started, using one-zero sampling with 10 seconds intervals and rotating focal animal sampling with five minutes for each individual. Recordings were repeated twice between 9-12 a.m. and twice between 2–5 p.m. Each animal was observed for a total of 20 minutes and percentage of exploration, activity, perching, jump/flight and comfort behavior was recorded.

Statistical analyses

Gene expression microarrays were normalized, filtered and analyzed with R/Bioconductor (www.bioconductor.org) using the affyPLM, geneFilter and limma packages as in [47]. DNA-methylation tiling arrays were analyzed using the Ringo, geneFilter and limma packages as in [45]. All array results were adjusted for multiple testing using false discovery rate (FDR, BH) algorithms [48]. The gene expression dataset was filtered to remove the non-variable and least variable probesets (IQR, cut off at 0.5; [49]). A low number of significantly differentially methylated probes suggested a high number of false negatives in DNA-methylation dataset, filtering up to 80% of the probes did not change the results significantly, hence the data was left unfiltered for downstream analysis. Gene ontology analysis was performed using human ortholog conversion with the Manteia web tool (manteia.igbmc.fr). The Ensembl's genome browser, BLASTN and BioMart tools were used for alignment and annotation analysis using the WASHUC2 genebuild. The Genesis and Statistica software were used for general statistical analysis.

For behavioral variables, qPCR and bisulfite sequencing means and SEM were calculated within sex. Bisulfite sequencing and qPCR data was normally distributed (determined by Shapiro-Wilk test) and analyzed using t-test adjusted for unequal variance (determined by Levene's test). Due to lack of normality the effects of sex on behaviors were assessed through a non-parametric Mann-Whitney U-test. Principal component analysis (PCA) was conducted in order to find patterns of behavior across the different tests. By first entering all variables into the PCA, and from that, choosing the variable from each test with highest communality on a four-factor solution (with eigenvalues over 1.0), we ended up with seven variables which were again entered into a "restricted" PCA. The resulting four factors explained 71% of the variance and the effects of sex on each factor score were then tested using a t-test.

Supporting Information

Figure S1 Fold change expression differences between females and males in probesets annotated to both or either of the two ZFR paralogs on chromomse 1 and Z respectively. Percentages on top of the columns indicate the sequence similarities of each probeset to the chromosome 1 and Z gene paralogs respectively. Note that only the probesets more similar to the chromosome 1 paralogs are significant. ***$p<0.001$, *$p<0.05$, #$p<0.1$ (adjusted for false discovery rate).

Table S1 Significantly differentially expressed probesets in females related to males.

Table S2 Significantly differentially methylated probes in females related to males.

Table S3 Gene ontology analysis of significantly differentially expressed (DE) genes in females related to males.

Table S4 Gene ontology analysis of significantly differentially methylated (DM) promoters in females related to males.

Table S5 Mean values of the behavior variables recorded in each of the behavioral test.

Table S6 Primers used in qPCR and bisulfite sequencing.

Acknowledgments

We like to thank the members of the AVIAN group, and especially Ida Gustafson, Lejla Bektić and Johan Bélteky for their help with sample collection and maintenance of the birds, and Petros Batakis for help with qPCR verifications. Markus Jöngren helped in developing and performing the behavioral tests. The work was carried out within the framework of the Linköping University strategic initiative LiU-Neuro, and the Swedish Center of Excellence in Animal Welfare Science.

Author Contributions

Conceived and designed the experiments: DN BA PJ. Performed the experiments: DN BA. Analyzed the data: DN BA PJ. Contributed reagents/materials/analysis tools: PJ. Wrote the paper: DN PJ BA.

References

1. Alverdes F (1927)(reprint version 1999)) Social Life in the Animal World. London: Routledge.
2. Taborsky M, Grantner A (1998) Behavioural time–energy budgets of cooperatively breeding Neolamprologus pulcher (Pisces: Cichlidae). Animal Behaviour 56: 1375–1382.
3. Ellegren H, Parsch J (2007) The evolution of sex-biased genes and sex-biased gene expression. Nat Rev Genet 8: 689–698.
4. Ranz JM, Castillo-Davis CI, Meiklejohn CD, Hartl DL (2003) Sex-Dependent Gene Expression and Evolution of the Drosophila Transcriptome. Science 300: 1742–1745.
5. Lenz KM, Nugent BM, McCarthy MM (2012) Sexual differentiation of the rodent brain: Dogma and beyond. Frontiers in Neuroscience.
6. Dewing P, Shi T, Horvath S, Vilain E (2003) Sexually dimorphic gene expression in mouse brain precedes gonadal differentiation. Molecular Brain Research 118: 82–90.
7. Lyon MF (1961) Gene Action in the X-chromosome of the Mouse (Mus musculus L.). Nature 190: 372–373.
8. Augui S, Nora EP, Heard E (2011) Regulation of X-chromosome inactivation by the X-inactivation centre. Nat Rev Genet 12: 429–442.
9. Basu R, Zhang L-F (2011) X chromosome inactivation: A silence that needs to be broken. genesis 49: 821–834.
10. Yasukochi Y, Maruyama O, Mahajan MC, Padden C, Euskirchen GM, et al. (2010) X chromosome-wide analyses of genomic DNA methylation states and gene expression in male and female neutrophils. Proceedings of the National Academy of Sciences 107: 3704–3709.
11. Naurin S, Hansson B, Bensch S, Hasselquist D (2010) Why does dosage compensation differ between XY and ZW taxa? Trends in Genetics 26: 15–20.
12. Melamed E, Arnold A (2007) Regional differences in dosage compensation on the chicken Z chromosome. Genome Biology 8: R202.
13. Mank JE, Ellegren H (2008) All dosage compensation is local: Gene-by-gene regulation of sex-biased expression on the chicken Z chromosome. Heredity 102: 312–320.
14. Teranishi M, Shimada Y, Hori T, Nakabayashi O, Kikuchi T, et al. (2001) Transcripts of the MHM region on the chicken Z chromosome accumulate as non-coding RNA in the nucleus of female cells adjacent to the DMRT1 locus. Chromosome Research 9: 147–165.
15. Raymond CS, Kettlewell JR, Hirsch B, Bardwell VJ, Zarkower D (1999) Expression of Dmrt1 in the Genital Ridge of Mouse and Chicken Embryos Suggests a Role in Vertebrate Sexual Development. Developmental Biology 215: 208–220.
16. Raymond CS, Shamu CE, Shen MM, Seifert KJ, Hirsch B, et al. (1998) Evidence for evolutionary conservation of sex-determining genes. Nature 391: 691–695.
17. Borowicz VA, Graves HB (1986) Social preferences of domestic hens for domestic vs. red junglefowl males and females. Behavioural Processes 12: 125–134.
18. Collias NE, Collias EC (1996) Social organization of a red junglefowl, Gallus gallus, population related to evolution theory. Animal Behaviour 51: 1337–1354.
19. McBride G, Parer IP, Foenander F (1969) The social organization and behaviour of the feral domestic fowl. Animal Behaviour Monographs 2: 127–181.
20. Cavanaugh BL, Lonstein JS (2010) Social novelty increases tyrosine hydroxylase immunoreactivity in the extended olfactory amygdala of female prairie voles. Physiology and Behavior 100: 381–386.
21. Tochigi M, Otowa T, Hibino H, Kato C, Otani T, et al. (2006) Combined analysis of association between personality traits and three functional polymorphisms in the tyrosine hydroxylase, monoamine oxidase A, and catechol-O-methyltransferase genes. Neuroscience Research 54: 180–185.
22. Pawlak CR, Ho Y-J, Schwarting RKW (2008) Animal models of human psychopathology based on individual differences in novelty-seeking and anxiety. Neuroscience & Biobehavioral Reviews 32: 1544–1568.
23. Enoch M-A (2008) The role of GABAA receptors in the development of alcoholism. Pharmacology Biochemistry and Behavior 90: 95–104.
24. Lobo MK, Covington HE III, Chaudhury D, Friedman AK, Sun H, et al. (2010) Cell Type-Specific Loss of BDNF Signaling Mimics Optogenetic Control of Cocaine Reward. Science 330: 385–390.
25. Westphal NJ, Seasholtz AF (2006) CRH-BP: the regulation and function of a phylogenetically conserved binding protein. Front Biosci 11: 1878–1891.
26. Roeszler KN, Itman C, Sinclair AH, Smith CA (2012) The long non-coding RNA, MHM, plays a role in chicken embryonic development, including gonadogenesis. Developmental Biology 366: 317–326.
27. Itoh Y, Melamed E, Yang X, Kampf K, Wang S, et al. (2007) Dosage compensation is less effective in birds than in mammals. Journal of Biology 6: 2.
28. Zhang S, Mathur S, Hattem G, Tassy O, Pourquie O (2010) Sex-dimorphic gene expression and ineffective dosage compensation of Z-linked genes in gastrulating chicken embryos. BMC genomics 11: 13.
29. Lee SI, Lee WK, Shin JH, Han BK, Moon S, et al. (2009) Sexually dimorphic gene expression in the chick brain before gonadal differentiation. Poultry science 88: 1003–1015.
30. Bisoni L, Batlle-Morera L, Bird AP, Suzuki M, McQueen HA (2005) Female-specific hyperacetylation of histone H4 in the chicken Z chromosome. Chromosome Research 13: 205–214.
31. He X-J, Chen T, Zhu J-K (2011) Regulation and function of DNA methylation in plants and animals. Cell Res 21: 442–465.
32. Kerje S, Carlborg Ö, Jacobsson L, Schütz K, Hartmann C, et al. (2003) The twofold difference in adult size between the red junglefowl and White Leghorn chickens is largely explained by a limited number of QTLs. Animal Genetics 34: 264–274.
33. Schütz KE, Kerje S, Jacobsson L, Forkman B, Carlborg Ö, et al. (2004) Major Growth QTLs in Fowl Are Related to Fearful Behavior: Possible Genetic Links between Fear Responses and Production Traits in a Red Junglefowl x White Leghorn Intercross. Behavior Genetics 34: 121–130.
34. Crooks L, Carlborg Ö, Marklund S, Johansson AM (2013) Identification of Null Alleles and Deletions from SNP Genotypes for an Intercross Between Domestic and Wild Chickens. G3: Genes|Genomes|Genetics.
35. Boyd LE (1988) Time budgets of adult Przewalski horses: Effects of sex, reproductive status and enclosure. Applied Animal Behaviour Science 21: 19–39.
36. Hoffman SG (1983) Sex-related foraging behavior in sequentially hermaphroditic hogfishes (Bodianus spp.). Ecology 64: 798–808.
37. McKeegan DEF, Deeming DC (1997) Effects of gender and group size on the time-activity budgets of adult breeding ostriches (Struthio camelus) in a farming environment. Applied Animal Behaviour Science 51: 159–177.
38. Johnston AL, File SE (1991) Sex differences in animal tests of anxiety. Physiology and Behavior 49: 245–250.
39. Palanza P, Gioiosa L, Parmigiani S (2001) Social stress in mice: Gender differences and effects of estrous cycle and social dominance. Physiology and Behavior 73: 411–420.
40. Evans CS, Evans L (1999) Chicken food calls are functionally referential. Animal Behaviour 58: 307–319.
41. Kruijt JP (1966) The Development of Ritualized Displays in Junglefowl. Philosophical Transactions of the Royal Society of London Series B, Biological Sciences 251: 479–484.
42. Johnson RA (1963) Habitat Preference and Behavior of Breeding Jungle Fowl in Central Western Thailand. The Wilson Bulletin 75: 270–272.
43. Collias NE, Collias EC (1967) A Field Study of the Red Jungle Fowl in North-Central India. The Condor 69: 360–386.
44. Sullivan MS (1991) Flock structure in red junglefowl. Applied Animal Behaviour Science 30: 381–386.
45. Natt D, Rubin C-J, Wright D, Johnsson M, Belteky J, et al. (2012) Heritable genome-wide variation of gene expression and promoter methylation between wild and domesticated chickens. BMC genomics 13: 59.
46. Agnvall B, Jöngren M, Strandberg E, Jensen P (2012) Heritability and Genetic Correlations of Fear-Related Behaviour in Red Junglefowl–Possible Implications for Early Domestication. PLoS One 7: e35162.
47. Goerlich VC, Nätt D, Elfwing M, Macdonald B, Jensen P (2012) Transgenerational effects of early experience on behavioral, hormonal and gene expression responses to acute stress in the precocial chicken. Hormones and behavior 61: 711–718.
48. Benjamini Y, Hochberg Y (1995) Controlling the False Discovery Rate: A Practical and Powerful Approach to Multiple Testing. Journal of the Royal Statistical Society Series B (Methodological) 57: 289–300.
49. Bourgon R, Gentleman R, Huber W (2010) Independent filtering increases detection power for high-throughput experiments. Proceedings of the National Academy of Sciences 107: 9546–9551.

16

Functional Variability of Snake Venom Metalloproteinases: Adaptive Advantages in Targeting Different Prey and Implications for Human Envenomation

Juliana L. Bernardoni[1], Leijiane F. Sousa[1], Luciana S. Wermelinger[2,5], Aline S. Lopes[3,6], Benedito C. Prezoto[4], Solange M. T. Serrano[3,6], Russolina B. Zingali[2], Ana M. Moura-da-Silva[1]*

1 Laboratório de Imunopatologia, Instituto Butantan, São Paulo, SP, Brazil, **2** Laboratório de Hemostasia e Venenos, Instituto de Bioquímica Médica, Universidade Federal do Rio de Janeiro, Rio do Janeiro, RJ, Brazil, **3** Laboratório Especial de Toxinologia Aplicada, Instituto Butantan, São Paulo, SP, Brazil, **4** Laboratório de Farmacologia, Instituto Butantan, São Paulo, SP, Brazil, **5** Laboratório de Fisiopatologia da Trombose, Faculdade de Farmácia, Universidade Federal do Rio de Janeiro, Rio do Janeiro, RJ, Brazil, **6** Center of Toxins, Immune-Response and Cell Signaling (CeTICS), FAPESP, São Paulo, SP, Brazil

Abstract

Snake venom metalloproteinases (SVMPs) are major components in most viperid venoms that induce disturbances in the hemostatic system and tissues of animals envenomated by snakes. These disturbances are involved in human pathology of snake bites and appear to be essential for the capture and digestion of snake's prey and avoidance of predators. SVMPs are a versatile family of venom toxins acting on different hemostatic targets which are present in venoms in distinct structural forms. However, the reason why a large number of different SVMPs are expressed in some venoms is still unclear. In this study, we evaluated the interference of five isolated SVMPs in blood coagulation of humans, birds and small rodents. P-III class SVMPs (fractions Ic, IIb and IIc) possess gelatinolytic and hemorrhagic activities, and, of these, two also show fibrinolytic activity. P-I class SVMPs (fractions IVa and IVb) are only fibrinolytic. P-III class SVMPs reduced clotting time of human plasma. Fraction IIc was characterized as prothrombin activator and fraction Ic as factor X activator. In the absence of Ca^{2+}, a firm clot was observed in chicken blood samples with fractions Ic, IIb and partially with fraction IIc. In contrast, without Ca^{2+}, only fraction IIc was able to induce a firm clot in rat blood. In conclusion, functionally distinct forms of SVMPs were found in *B. neuwiedi* venom that affect distinct mechanisms in the coagulation system of humans, birds and small rodents. Distinct SVMPs appear to be more specialized to rat or chicken blood, strengthening the current hypothesis that toxin diversity enhances the possibilities of the snakes for hunting different prey or evading different predators. This functional diversity also impacts the complexity of human envenoming since different hemostatic mechanisms will be targeted by SVMPs accounting for the complexity of the response of humans to venoms.

Editor: Eugene A. Permyakov, Russian Academy of Sciences, Institute for Biological Instrumentation, Russian Federation

Funding: This study was supported by FAPESP (2012/16277-9; 2012/23018-0; 2013-07467-1), CAPES (Edict 063/2010 1519/2011, Toxinology), FAPERJ (E-26/110.319/2010) and CNPq (grant numbers 483642/2012-6 and 569312010-7). The funders had no role in study design, data collection and analysis, decision to publish, or preparation of the manuscript.

Competing Interests: The authors have declared that no competing interests exist.

* Email: ana.moura@butantan.gov.br

Introduction

Venoms are trophic adaptations which allow venomous snakes to use potent toxins as a chemical means to subdue their prey [1]. This efficient predation mechanism evolved in venomous snakes by recruitment of genes coding for physiological functions to the venom system in which they underwent duplications followed by neofunctionalization of the new copies under accelerated evolution [2–5]. Under these mechanisms of evolution, gene copies that encode venom components usually conserve non-synonymous mutations and result in protein sequences with high degree of variability. It has also becoming evident that gene expression patterns of the different copies may also be variable representing an additional source of diversity in the final venom composition that may be responsible for inter- or intraspecific differences in toxins [6].

In snakes, it is reasonable to assume that the major protein families recruited to the venom apparatus have been selected by their efficiency to subdue prey [7]. In this regard, venoms of elapid snakes and from certain viperid species are very efficient in prey paralysis and killing due to potent neurotoxins enclosed within three-finger toxins and phospholipases A_2 (PLA_2) protein families. The presence of proteolytic enzymes, especially snake venom metalloproteinases (SVMPs), is also noted in snake venoms and some authors suggest that they may be involved in predigestion of prey [8]. However, in viperid venoms, the three-finger proteins are rare and PLA_2s are not abundant while metalloproteinases, particularly P-III class SVMPs (for classification of SVMPs see

Fox & Serrano [9]), acquire an apparent evolutionary advantage since they are expressed in high levels in the venomes of most species of vipers [7].

The expression of SVMP or PLA_2 phenotypes has been recently discussed by Mackessy [10] in venoms of North American *Crotalus spp*. The authors classified *Crotalus* venoms as Type I (predominantly SVMPs) or Type II (predominantly PLA_2s). Amongst several examples, there was an inverse correlation in the amount of PLA_2 compared to SVMP depending on geographical distribution of Mojave rattlesnakes [11]. In *Crotalus spp*, phospholipase activity of type II venoms presented a correlation with neurotoxicity and lethality [10], but the exact function of SVMPs in type I venoms is poorly understood. This is particularly important in the case of *Bothrops* snakes in which PLA_2 molecules lost their neurotoxic activity and instead present a tissue-damaging myotoxic activity [12]. Perhaps, as a consequence, most species of *Bothrops* have type I venoms with high contents of SVMPs and it is plausible that these enzymes have acquired important functions for subduing prey or even evading predators in these snakes. In this aspect, the potent action of proteinases on hemostatic system has been correlated to prey immobilization and killing, besides their assumed digestive function [13]. Indeed, SVMPs, particularly from P-III class, are related to the hydrolysis of extracellular matrix components [14–16], coagulation factors [17], inhibition of platelet aggregation [18,19], apoptosis of endothelial cells [20,21] and up-regulation of pro-inflammatory mediators expression [22,23] leading to a massive disruption of hemostasis that results in hemorrhages and severe tissue lesions at the venom inoculation site [24]. These mechanisms enhance the action of snake venom serine proteinases, present in lower levels in both type I and type II venoms, that are thrombin-like enzymes with procoagulant, anticoagulant, platelet aggregating and fibrinolytic activities [25].

Besides the importance of venom variability for snake ecology, this topic also has relevance for a correct understanding of venom composition for treatment of snake bites. For example, in the case of the Mojave rattlesnake, human envenomings by type II venom specimens were more severe than by type I [11] due to their neurotoxic activity. In *Bothrops* snakes the envenomation scenario is the opposite. The classical symptoms of envenoming by *Bothrops spp* are hemostatic disturbances and inflammatory reaction with tissue damage extending from the site of the bite [26] mainly due to the SVMP effects. Thus, the variability among components of SVMP protein family could be implied in the complexity of the mechanisms of action leading to the local tissue damaging. Therefore, knowing the correlation between different structural homologs and their function is essential to guarantee the production of antivenoms able to neutralize toxins acting on different targets.

Although the polarization between type I and type II venoms is currently accepted, it has becoming evident that some venoms occupy intermediate state between types I and II, with a wider range of different toxins, indicating that their major toxin pattern might still be under selection. Therefore, these venoms serve as important models to understand functional variability of venom components and the major killing strategies of individual toxins. The proteome of *Bothrops neuwiedi* venom has been recently characterized by our group [27] as an intermediate composition between type I and type II venoms. In this analysis, SVMPs accounted for almost 50% of venom proteome, however, with predominance of P-I class SVMPs. In addition, PLA_2s were present in a considerable amount of almost 10% [27]. Similarly, the venome of *B. pauloensis* (initially classified as *B. neuwiedi pauloensis*) also showed an intermediate type of composition in which 38% consisted of SVMPs (26% of P-III class SVMPs) and 32% of PLA_2s [28]. Another interesting aspect of *B. neuwiedi* venom is that a substantial structural variability was detected within SVMPs. Analyzing the cDNA sequences obtained from the venom gland of one *B. neuwiedi* specimen, we described the transcription of at least eleven different SVMP sequences with distinct domain structures and variable degrees of domain identity [29]. These data confirmed the existence of a wide variety of SVMP toxins in *B. neuwiedi* venom, some not yet characterized, with structural differences that might be relevant from the point of view of venom functional variability. Working with different snake populations, Dagda and coworkers [30] demonstrated the genetic basis for intraspecies variation in metalloproteinase-associated functions of Mojave rattlesnake venom. The authors described four distinct genes coding for SVMPs and their level of expression in different individuals explained the potencies of caseinolytic, fibrinolytic, and hemorrhagic activities in the whole venom samples [30].

The diversity of SVMPs in the venoms highlight the importance of this class of toxins for the adaptation of *Bothrops* snakes and brings out the question of why venoms should contain such a number of distinct forms of toxins from the same functional/enzymatic group, presumably with similar activities. In this work we approached this question using several experimental models and our results strongly suggest that the variability between members of the same toxin family present adaptive advantages for the snake. The characterization of SVMPs isolated from *B. neuwiedi* venom showed a marked diversity against targets of mammalian hemostatic system and remarkable differences in their effects on rodent or bird blood coagulation systems, suggesting the presence of effective arsenals against different potential prey or even predators.

Material and Methods

Venom

A pool of venoms from snakes of *B. neuwiedi* complex was extracted from adult specimens of both sexes kept under captivity at Instituto Butantan herpetarium. This includes the subspecies *B. n. pauloensis, B. n. matogrossensis, B. n. neuwiedi, B. n. marmoratus* and *B. n. diporus* [31]. After extraction, the venom was lyophilized and kept frozen until use.

Animals

Adult female *Gallus domesticus (white leghorn* chickens - 1.0 to 1.7 kg, 10 to 15 weeks) were purchased from commercial source. Male *Rattus norvegicus* (Wistar rats - 250 to 300 g) and *Mus musculus* (Swiss mice - 18 to 20 g) were bred at the Instituto Butantan. The animals had free access to water and food, and were kept under a 12-h light/dark cycle.

Ethical statement

All experiments involving mice, rats and chickens were approved by the Ethical Committee for Animal Research of the Instituto Butantan (CEUAIB), São Paulo, Brazil, identification number 1028/13, who certified its agreement with the Ethical Principles in Animal Research adopted by the Brazilian Council of Animal Experimentation Control (CONCEA).

2-D Gel Electrophoresis

For two-dimensional gel electrophoresis, 150 μg of the venom proteins were dissolved in Milli-Q water and mixed with DeStreak rehydration solution containing 1% IPG (immobilized pH gradient) buffer (GE Healthcare, Uppsala, Sweden) to a final

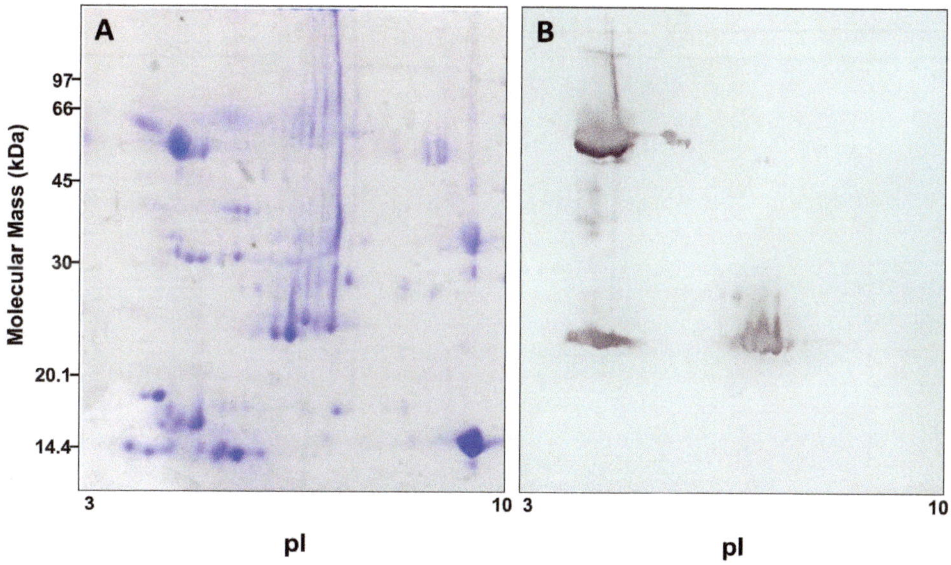

Figure 1. Characterization of different SVMPs *Bothrops neuwiedi* venom. Samples (150 μg) of *B. neuwiedi* venom were analyzed by 2-D gel electrophoresis in the pH range 3–10 and stained by Coomassie blue (A) or electrotransferred to nitrocellulose membranes and revealed with anti-jararhagin antibody followed by peroxidase labeled anti-rabbit IgG and enzyme substrate (B).

volume of 125 μL. The mixture was homogenized at room temperature and remained at rest for 30 min before centrifugation for 5 min at 12000 *g* and the supernatant was loaded on a 7 cm Immobiline DryStrip (pH 3–10, nonlinear, GE Healthcare) for equilibration for 18 h. First dimension IEF was carried out in an Ettan IPGphor Isoeletric Focusing System (GE Healthcare) at 20°C using a three-phase program: 500 V at 10 V/h; 4000 V at 3400 V/h; and 5000 V at 4600 V/h. After first dimension separation, the strip was placed in the rehydration tray and the proteins in the strip were washed, reduced and alkylated by sequential 20 min incubation steps in the following solutions: a) 50 mM Tris-HCl, pH 8.4, 2% (m/v) SDS (sodium dodecyl sulfate), 30% (v/v) glycerol, and 6 M urea (equilibration buffer, EB); b) 20 mg/mL dithiothreitol (DTT) in EB; and c) 30 mg/mL iodocetamide in EB. Then, the strip was directly applied to 12.5% polyacrylamide gel (10 cm×10 cm×1.0 mm) and submitted to electrophoresis at 170 V for the second dimension separation. The gels were stained with Coomassie blue or transferred to PVDF membranes. The blotted membranes were immersed in a blocking solution [5% non-fat milk in Tris-saline (20 mM Tris–HCl, 0.15 M NaCl, 0.05% v/v Tween 20, pH 7.4)] and then incubated with 1:1,000 diluted anti-class P-III SVMP (jararhagin) antibodies [32]. After washing with Tris-saline, the membranes were incubated with peroxidase labeled rabbit anti-horse IgG (1:1,000) and reactive bands detected by incubation with 4-chlor-α-naphtol and H_2O_2. The figures shown represent two independent runs.

Venom fractionation

Venom was fractionated by molecular exclusion and ion exchange chromatographies using the Äkta system (GE Healthcare). Samples of 50 mg crude lyophilized venom were dissolved in 200 μL of 20 mM Tris, 1 mM $CaCl_2$ and 150 mM NaCl, pH 7.8, and insoluble material was removed by centrifugation at 10,000 g for 10 min at room temperature. Proteins in the supernatant were applied to a Hiprep 16/60 S-200 column (GE Healthcare) in the same buffer and subjected to isocratic elution at a flow rate of 0.5 mL/min. The fractions containing metalloproteinase activities (hemorrhagic and fibrinolytic) were pooled according to major peaks and dialyzed against 20 mM Tris, 1 mM $CaCl_2$, pH 7.8 and applied to a Mono-Q HR 5/5 column (GE Healthcare) using the same buffer. Proteins from size exclusion peaks 1 and 2 were eluted by a 40 mL gradient from 0 to 0.25 M NaCl and 5 mL gradient from 0.25 to 1 M NaCl, at a flow rate of 1 mL/min in the same buffer. Proteins of size exclusion peak 4 were eluted by a 20 mL gradient from 0 to 0.4 M NaCl and an extra 5 mL gradient from 0.4 to 1 M NaCl, at a flow rate of 1 mL/min in the same buffer. All steps were carried out at room temperature and monitored at 280 nm. Purity of toxins was evaluated by SDS-PAGE 12.5%, under non-reducing conditions. Samples containing 10 μg of protein were dissolved in sample buffer (0.125 M Tris-HCl, pH 6.8 containing 10% glycerol, 2% SDS, and 0.001% bromophenol blue), boiled for 5 min and applied to the gel. Electrophoresis was performed at a current of 35 mA until the bromophenol blue indicator reaches the end of the gel. The gels were Coomassie or silver stained using standard protocols. Molecular weight markers: phosphorylase b (97 kDa), bovine serum albumin (66 kDa), ovalbumin (45 kDa), bovine carbonic anhydrase (30 kDa), trypsin inhibitor (20.1 kDa), and lactalbumin (14.4 kDa).

Protein identification by mass spectrometry

Protein bands of interest were excised from polyacrylamide gels and submitted to in gel digestion using trypsin according to Hanna *et al.* (2000). After the digestion procedure, the samples were reconstituted in 15 μL of 0.1% (v/v) formic acid and an aliquot (4.5 μL) of the resulting peptide mixture was injected on nanoAcquity UPLC Symmet C18 precolunm (180 μm i.d.×20 mm) (Waters, Milford, MA) and fractionated on a nanoAcquity UPLC BEH130 C18 column (75 μm i.d.×100 mm) (Waters, Milford, MA) at 35°C using a UPLC-ESI-Q-TOF system (Waters, Milford, MA, USA). Chromatography was performed with solvent A (0.1% formic acid in deionized water) and B (0.1% formic acid in acetonitrile) at a flow rate of 600 nL/min using the following gradient: 7% B in 1 min; to 45% B in 15 min; to 80% B in 2.5 min; hold at 80% B for 1 min; then

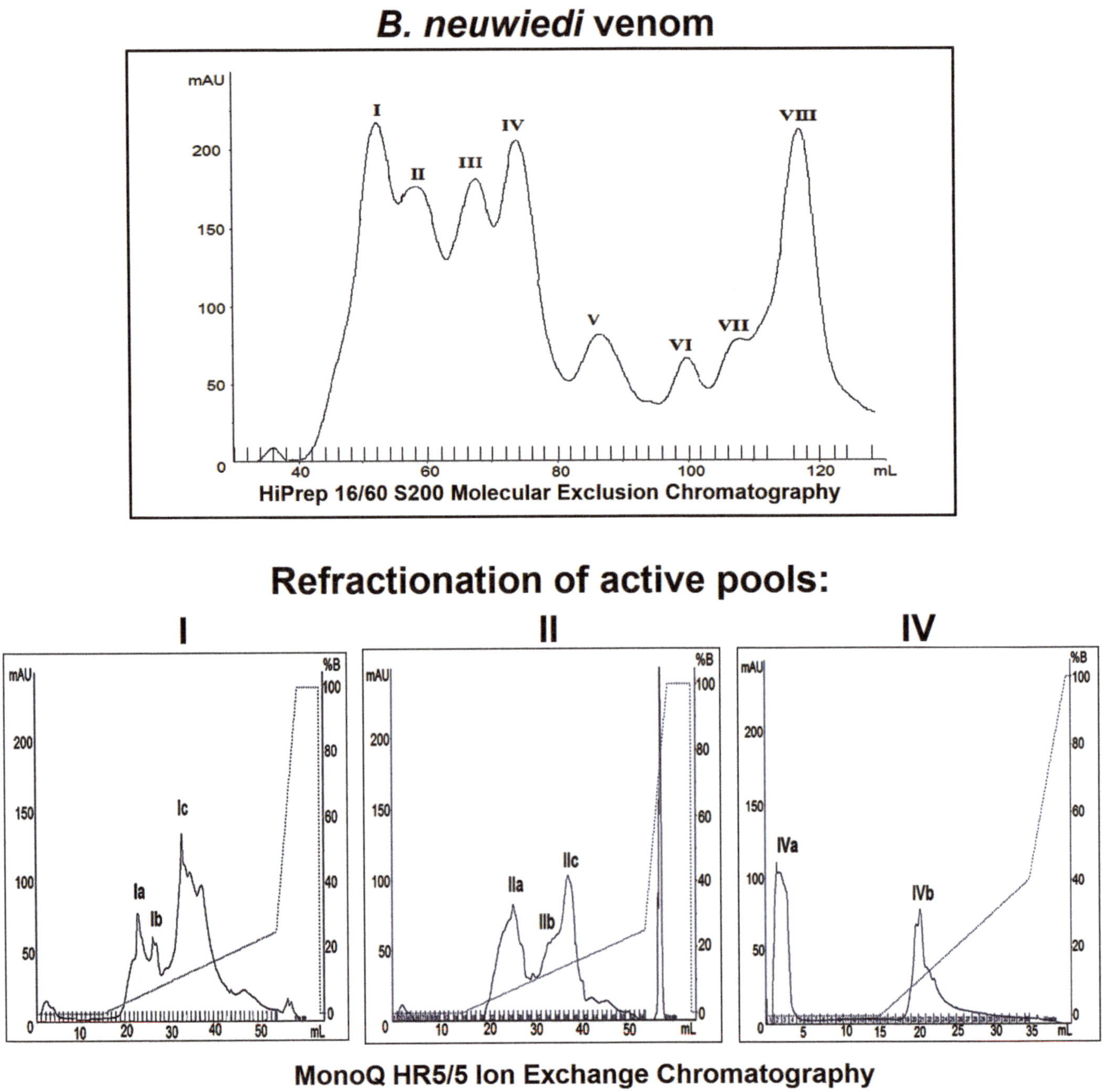

Figure 2. Isolation of *Bothrops neuwiedi* venom fractions enriched in SVMPs. (A) Samples of 50 mg of *B. neuwiedi* venom were applied on Hiprep 16/60 S200 column, equilibrated with 20 mM Tris, 150 mM NaCl and 1 mM $CaCl_2$ pH 7.8. Fractions of 2.0 mL were collected at a flow rate of 0.5 mL/min, monitored at A280 (nm). (B,C and D) Fractions I, II and IV of size exclusion chromatography were applied to a Mono-Q HR 5/5, equilibrated with 20 mM Tris pH 7.8 plus 1 mM CaCl2. Fractions of 1.0 mL were collected at a flow rate of 1.0 mL/min, monitored at A280 (nm).

back to 7% B in 1.5 min. The MS instrument was operated in data dependent mode, in which one full MS scan was acquired in the *m/z* range of 200–2000 Da followed by MS/MS acquisition using collision induced dissociation. The resulting fragment spectra were searched using MASCOT search engine (Matrix Science, UK) using serpentes (25210 sequences) database download from the Uniprot website (http://www.uniprot.org/) with a parent and fragment tolerance of 1.2 and 0.6 Da, respectively. Iodoacetamide derivative of cysteine and oxidation of methionine were specified in MASCOT as fixed and variable modifications, respectively.

Hemorrhagic activity

Hemorrhagic activity was assessed using samples of 10 μg of proteins diluted in 50 μL PBS, and injected *i.d.* into the dorsal skin of Swiss mice. Control mice received only 50 μL PBS. After 3 h, the animals were sacrificed by CO_2 inhalation, the dorsal skin removed and the extent of hemorrhagic lesion was calculated as the longest diameter multiplied by the diameter perpendicular to

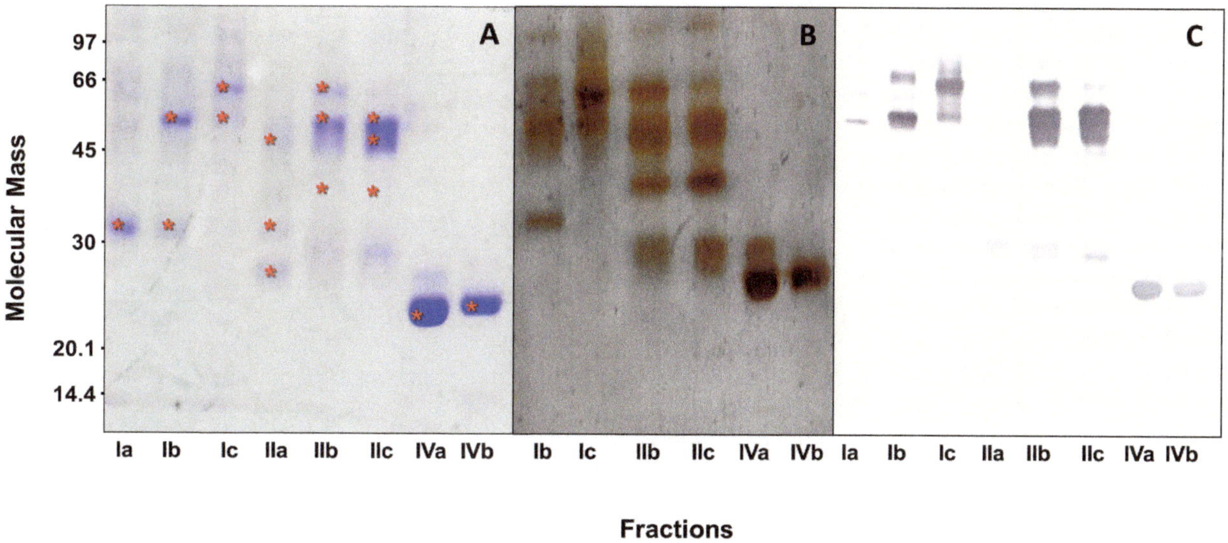

Figure 3. SDS-PAGE and Western blotting of the isolated fractions. Isolated fractions enriched with SVMPs (10 µg) were subjected to SDS-PAGE under non-reducing conditions and stained by Coomassie blue (A), silver stained (B) or electrotransferred to nitrocellulose membranes and revealed with anti-jararhagin antibody followed by peroxidase labeled anti-rabbit IgG and enzyme substrate (C). The bands with asterisks were cut and analyzed by mass spectrometry.

it. Results are expressed as mean ±SD of three mice in each group.

Fibrinolytic activity

Fibrinolytic activity was assayed by the fibrin-plate method, as previously described [33]. Briefly, a fibrin-agarose gel was prepared by mixing 3 mg/mL human fibrinogen (Calbiochem) with a pre-heated solution of 2% agarose in 50 mM Tris–HCl buffer pH 7.3 containing 200 mM NaCl, 50 mM $CaCl_2$ and 1 U/mL thrombin. Samples (10 µg) were applied to wells of the solidified gel and incubated at 37°C for 18 h, and then the area of the hydrolysis halo was measured and expressed as mean ±SD of three independent experiments.

Recalcification time

Samples (50 µL) of isolated SVMPs (0.1; 0.5; 1; 5 e 10 µg/mL) or TBS (used as negative control) were incubated for 1 minute with platelet poor plasma (PPP 50 µL). The reaction was initiated by addition of 100 µL of 0.025 M $CaCl_2$, and the clotting time (in seconds) was measured in a Coagulometer (KC 4 Delta - Tcoag version: v2.35). Results are expressed as mean ±SD of three independent experiments.

Thrombin and FXa generation assay

Samples (50 µL) of isolated SVMPs (1 µg/mL) diluted in Hepes-BSA buffer pH 7.5 (50 mM Hepes, 100 mM NaCl, 5 mM $CaCl_2$ and 1 mg/mL BSA) were coated in microplates. Reaction was started by addition of 50 µL/well prothrombin or factor X (2 µM and 0,4 µM, respectively) and aliquots of 10 µL were removed after incubation for 1, 5, 10, 15 and 20 min at 37°C and loaded into microplate wells containing 40 µL of stop buffer (50 mM Tris, 150 mM NaCl, 0.1% PEG 6000 and 20 mM EDTA, pH 7.5). After the addition of 50 µL of 200 µM S-2238 (D-Phe-Pip-Arg-pNA) or S-2765 D-Arg-Gly-Arg-pNA) (), the absorbance at 405 nm was recorded at 37°C for 20 min at 9s intervals using a Thermomax Microplate Reader (Molecular Devices). Thrombin and factor Xa were used as control samples. Results are expressed as mean ±SD of three independent experiments.

Collection of citrated rat and chicken whole blood samples

Male Wistar rats (250 to 300 g) were anesthetized with sodium pentobarbital (60 mg kg^{-1}; intraperitoneally). Blood samples (3 mL) drawn from the carotid arteries were collected into syringes containing 1:10 (v/v) 3.8% trisodium citrate. Chickens were restrained on their backs with wings spread. Feathers were removed and, after using xylocaine spray as a local anesthetic agent, small incisions were made around the brachial wing vein and blood samples (5 mL) carefully collected into syringes containing 1:10 (v/v) 3.8% trisodium citrate.

Thromboelastometric assays

Thrombelastometric assays using the ROTEM four-channel system (Pentapharm) were performed according to the manufacturer's instructions. Volumes (300 µL) of citrated chicken or rat whole blood samples were preloaded with 40 µL containing: Group 1 – only PBS (control, n = 3); Group 2–10 µg of crude venom (n = 3) and Group 3–10 µg of isolated SVMPs (n = 3). The final mixture of 340 µL was placed into the ROTEM cups and incubated up to 60 min for evaluating the following parameters of the ROTEM profile: clotting time (CT [s], the time from the start of the assay until formation of a clot with an amplitude of 2 mm - green); clot formation time (CFT [s], time from the end of CT [amplitude of 2 mm] until a clot firmness of 20 mm is achieved - pink); maximum clot firmness (MCF [mm], the peak strength of the clot, resulting from the interaction of fibrin, activated platelets and factor XIII [FXIII] - blue); and maximum lysis (ML [%], the maximum reduction in clot firmness observed after MCF has been reached, given as a percentage of the MCF value).

Results

The structural diversity of SVMPs was first confirmed in a pool of venoms collected from *B. neuwiedi* snakes kept under captivity

Table 1. Assignment of the proteins isolated from the SDS-PAGE bands of B. neuwiedi venom fractions to protein families by MS/MS and MASCOT.

Fractions	M. Mass	Peptides	Identified Proteins	Species	*gi* number	Score
		DXMXXR				
Ia	34 kDa	FXAFXYPGR	BthaT1	*B. alternatus*	gil48093528I	375
		SVPNDDEEXR	serine proteinase			
		VXGGDECDXNEHR				
		NNGNLDEIR				
		NPCCDATTCK				
Ib	57 kDa	ENVIITPCAQEDVK	BnMPIIIb - SVMP	*B. neuwiedi*	gil308212498I	427
		KENVIITPCAQEDVK				
		SECDIAESCTGQSAQCPTDDFHK				
	34 kDa	SVPNDDEEXR	BthaT1 - serine proteinase	*B. alternatus*	gil48093528I	120
		NNGNLDEIR				
Ic	67 kDa	IALVGIEIWSNR	BnMPIIIc - SVMP	*B. neuwiedi*	gil308212500I	218
		IYEIVNFLNEIFR				
	57 kDa	-	No Hit			
	53 kDa	TXCAGVXBGGK	Serine proteinase	*B. insularis*	gil20069139I	124
		SVANDDEVXR				
IIa	34 kDa	SVPNDDEEXR	BthTa1 - serine proteinase	*B. alternatus*	gil48093528I	69
		MYEXANXVNEXXR*				
	27 kDa	NNGDXDKXK	Bothropasin-SVMP	*B. jararaca*	gil4895110I	373
		MYEXANXVNEXFR**	Jararhagin-SVMP		gil62468I	166
		XTVKPDVDYTXNSFAEWR				
		NNGNLDEIR				
		GDEYFYCR				
		YPCCDAATCK				
	67 kDa	IALVGIEIWSNR	BnMPIIIc - SVMP	*B. neuwiedi*	gil308212500I	792
		IYEIVNFLNEIFR				
		YINVYKPQCILNEPLR				
		SECDIAESCTGQSAECPIDDFKR				
		NNGDXDKXK				
IIb		XPCAPEDVK	Bothropasin - SVMP		gil4895110I	551
		KXPCAPEDVK				
	57 kDa	DNSPGBNNPCK		*B. jararaca*		
		MYEXANXVNEXXR*				
		MYEXANXVNEXFR**	Jararhagin - SVMP		gil62468I	298
		XTVKPDVDYTXNSFAEWR				
		XPCAPEDVK				
	51 kDa	KXPCAPEDVK	Jararhagin - SVMP	*B. jararaca*	gil62468I	110
		DNSPGBNNPCK				
		NNGDXDKXK				
		XPCAPEDVK				
	57 kDa	KXPCAPEDVK	Bothropasin - SVMP	*B. jararaca*	gil4895110I	561
		DNSPGBNNPCK				
		MYELANXVNEXXR				

Table 1. Cont.

Fractions	M. Mass	Peptides	Identified Proteins	Species	*gi* number	Score
		XTVKPDVDYTXNSFAEWR				
		NNGDXDKXK				
		XPCAPEDVK	Bothropasin - SVMP		**gi|4895110|**	**508**
		KXPCAPEDVK				
	53 kDa	DNSPGBNNPCK		*B. jararaca*		
IIc		MYEXANXVNEXXR*	Jararhagin - SVMP		**gi|62468|**	**353**
		MYEXANXVNEXFR**				
		XTVKPDVDYTXNSFAEWR				
		ASMSECDPAEHCTGBSSECPADVFHK				
		XPCAPEDVK				
	51 kDa	KXPCAPEDVK	Jararhagin - SVMP	*B. jararaca*	**gi|62468|**	**173**
		DNSPGBNNPCK				
		ASMSECDPAEHCTGBSSECPADVFHK				
		DLIKVEK				
		YNSNVNTIR				
		TLTSFGEWR				
IVa	**22 kDa**	SCIMASTISK	BnMPIb - SVMP	*B. neuwiedi*	**gi|308212504|**	**1956**
		YIELAVVADHGMFTK				
		TWVHEMVNSLNGFFR				
		SMNVDASLVNLEVWSK				
		VAVTMAHELGHNLGMDHDDTCTCGAK				
		DLIKVEK				
		ERDLLPR				
		KDLIKVEK				
		YNSNLNTIR				
IVb	**23 kDa**	TLTSFGEWR	BnMPIa - SVMP	*B. neuwiedi*	**gi|308212516|**	**1820**
		VHEMVNTVNGFFR				
		YVELAVVADNGMFTK				
		SMNVDASLANLEVWSK				
		SMNVDASLANLEVWSKK				
		ISHDHAQLLTTIVFDNYVIGITK				

X= Leucine or Isoleucine, B= Lysine or Glutamine,
*Found only in Bothropasin sequence,
**Found only in Jararhagin sequence. C- or N-terminal peptides are underlined.

at the herpetarium of Instituto Butantan. When subjected to 2-D electrophoresis, the venom was fractionated in several spots distributed between p*I* 3 to 10 and apparent molecular masses between 10 kDa and 97 kDa (Figure 1A). Proteins transferred to PVDF membranes were then treated with antibodies against a P-III class SVMP (jararhagin), and the resulting molecular masses of the stained spots corresponded to the two major classes of SVMPs: a major group of around 60 kDa and acidic p*I*, compatible to the P-III class, and two spots of approximately 25 kDa revealed in acidic and neutral regions of the gel, which are characteristic of the P-I class (Figure 1B). These results confirm the presence of different SVMPs in *B. neuwiedi* venom.

To assess the functional diversity of the distinct structural forms, *B. neuwiedi* venom was subjected to a series of preparative chromatographies and fractions enriched with the SVMPs that were obtained. Size exclusion chromatography resolved *B. neuwiedi* venom in eight major fractions enumerated I to VIII (Figure 2A). The SVMPs main activities (hemorrhagic, fibrinolytic and reactivity to anti-SVMP antibodies) were concentrated in the fractions I, II and IV (data not shown) that were selected for the next anion-exchange chromatographic step. When submitted to anion-exchange chromatography at pH 7.8, fraction I was resolved into three peaks denominated Ia, Ib and Ic (Figure 2B) and peaks Ib and Ic showed hemorrhagic activity and were selected for further analysis. Fraction II was also resolved into three peaks denominated IIa, IIb and IIc (Figure 2C) and two of them (IIb and IIc) were selected since they presented hemorrhagic and fibrinolytic activities. Fraction IV was resolved into two peaks denominated IVa and IVb (Figure 2D) with fibrinolytic activity that were also selected. All selected fractions reacted with anti-

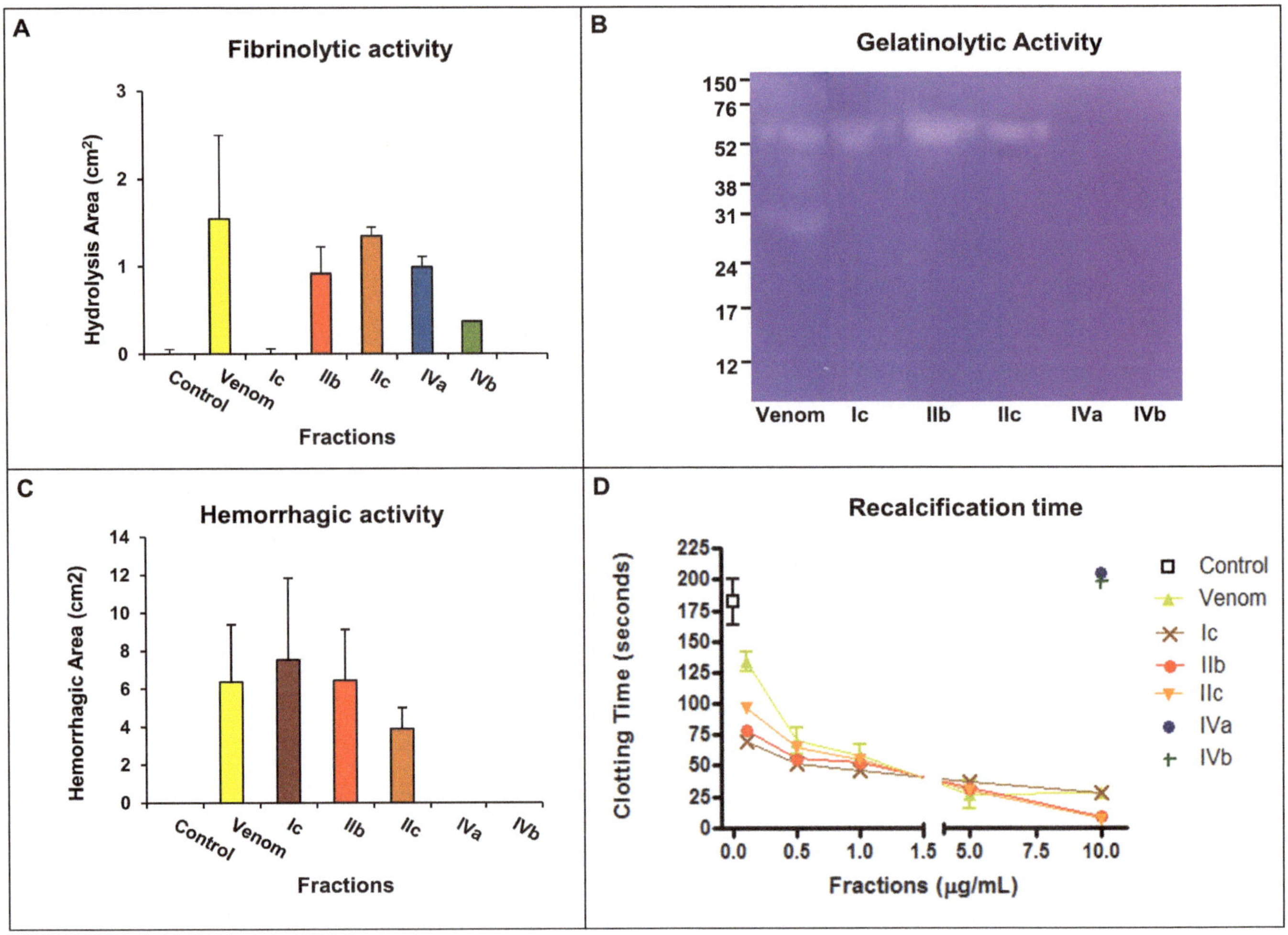

Figure 4. Fibrinolytic, Gelatinolytic, Hemorrhagic activity and Recalcification time of SVMPs. (A) Samples of 10 μg of each fraction was applied to the fibrin-agarose plate and the halos of lysis were measured. (B) Gelatinolytic activity of SVMPs (5 μg) on a 12.5% polyacrylamide gel copolymerized with gelatin. (C) Samples of 10 μg of each fraction were injected (i.d.) on the dorsum of mice followed by measuring of the hemorrhagic halo. (D) Samples with 0.1; 0.5; 1; 5 and 10 μg/mL SVMPs were incubated with platelet poor plasma. The reaction was initiated by addition of 0.025 M $CaCl_2$ and the time to clot formation was measured.

jararhagin antibodies, confirming their immunological identity with SVMPs (Figure 3C). Figure 3A shows the SDS-PAGE profile of selected fractions. Except for fractions Ia and IIa, the fractions contained major bands of molecular masses between 50–60 kDa and around 25 kDa, corresponding to SVMPs of the P-III and P-I classes, respectively. The major bands of each fraction were cut off the gel and subjected to mass spectrometry for protein identification. The fractions containing bands with SVMP molecular masses were run in another gel subjected to silver staining (Figure 3B).

As shown in Table 1, the fraction Ia major band showed only peptides characteristic of serine proteinases and fraction IIa showed three bands, two of them characterized as serine proteinases, therefore, these fractions were not selected for the functional tests. Fraction Ib showed two major bands, the band of 34 kDa was characterized as a serine proteinase and the 57 kDa band was identified as a *B. neuwiedi* SVMP class P-III (BnMPIIIb). However, due to the contamination with serine proteinases, this fraction was also rejected for the next step. Fraction Ic presented two bands, and the band of 67 kDa was identified as a *Bothrops neuwiedi* SVMP class P-III (BnMPIIIc). The three bands of fraction IIb included peptides of SVMPs class P-III (BnMPIIIc, bothropasin and jararhagin) and the three bands of fraction IIc were identified as bothropasin or jararhagin, indicating that the bands correspond to similar SVMPs class P-III probably at different processing stages due to autolysis of these toxins generating 30 kDa fragments corresponding to the disintegrin-cysteine-rich domains, as previously reported [32]. The bands of fractions IVa and IVb showed molecular masses characteristic SVMPs of class P-I and were identified as *B. neuwiedi* SVMPs (BnMPIb and BnMPIa, respectively), which are very similar in their protein sequence but differ in the isoeletric point and binding to the anion exchange columns [34].

Selected fractions were then subjected to a comparison of their functional activities under the same conditions. As shown in Figure 4, the proteolytic activity of each fraction on macromolecular substrates was variable: fraction Ic did not hydrolyze fibrin, and instead, it was efficient in the hydrolysis of gelatin. The opposite was observed with fractions IVa and IVb, which were fibrinolytic but not gelatinolytic. Fractions IIb and IIc hydrolyzed both, gelatin and fibrin (Figure 4A–B). These differences were also detected in the biological activities of SVMPs. As expected, only class P-III SVMPs (fractions Ic, IIb and IIc) were hemorrhagic with distinct potencies (Figure 4C). When tested for procoagulant activity, the fractions Ic, IIb and IIc reduced significantly the

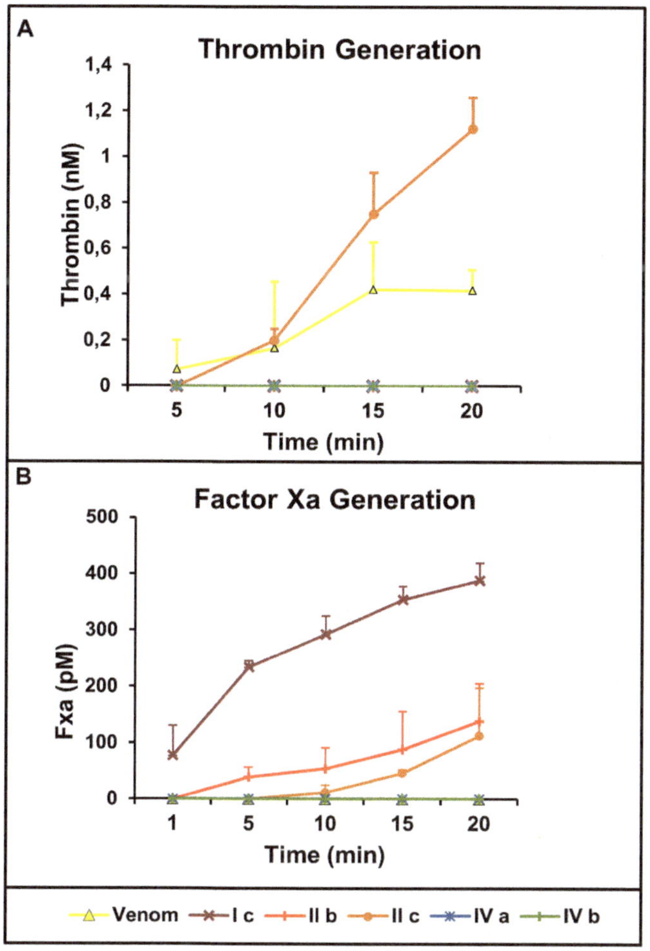

Figure 5. Prothrombin and Factor X activation by SVMPs fractions, as detected by S2238 and S2765 hydrolysis, respectively. Samples (1 µg/mL) of isolated SVMPs were incubated with 2 µM prothrombin (A) or 0.4 µM FX (B). Thrombin and FXa formed was determined after 1, 5, 10, 15 and 20 minutes of reaction. Assay conditions and quantification of thrombin and FXa are described in the Material and methods. Each point represents mean ±SD of three determinations.

plasma recalcification time compared to controls. The procoagulant effect occurred in a dose dependent manner and each fraction presented different potencies with IIb and IIc being the most active fractions. Fractions IVa and IVb, corresponding to class P-I SVMPs, showed neither hemorrhagic nor procoagulant activities (Figure 4C-D). The detection of only enzymatic activities in fractions IVa and IVb suggests that they may be involved mostly on prey digestion.

SVMPs have already been described as activators of factor II and factor X independently of the presence of calcium [35]. Therefore, in order to understand the mechanism of their procoagulant activity, we tested the selected fractions in the activation of coagulation factors *in vitro*, thereby identifying the differences of SVMPs in the clotting process. Only fraction IIc was able to generate thrombin faster than the whole venom (Figure 5A) pointing out its direct effect in prothrombin activation (factor II). Regarding the factor X activation, only the fraction Ic was able to generate factor Xa *in vitro*, which was detectable from 5 minutes of incubation (Figure 5B). The fractions IIb and IIc showed some activity on factor X, although the data did not show statistical significance. These results confirm the action of fraction IIc in activation of prothrombin while fraction Ic acts at the direct activation of factor X.

The next step was to verify if the different functional activities of SVMPs could play a role in their effectiveness to a broader spectrum of prey. For this purpose, we assessed the pro-coagulant activity of each fraction on citrated whole blood samples from rats and chickens, as representatives of mammalian and avian prey. Although the activation of coagulation factors is calcium dependent, most enzymes from viperid venoms can activate these factors even in the absence of divalent cations. Therefore we tested the coagulant activity of the fractions in the absence of calcium using rotational thromboelastometry. As shown in Figure 6, in the absence of calcium, the whole venom has a procoagulant action on both rat and chicken whole blood samples. The venom effect was faster on rat whole blood sample (green). Comparing the isolated fractions, only fraction IIc was effective in clotting rat whole blood sample, with the same clotting time (green) as the venom but resulting in a more stable clot (blue). On the other hand, fractions Ic, IIb and IIc were all able to clot chicken blood, but in a slower rate (green) than the whole venom. The most active on chicken blood was fraction IIb. Fractions IVa and IVb showed no activity on both systems, being similar to the PBS negative control. The fractions that showed pro-coagulant activity were treated with a metalloproteinase inhibitor (o-Phenanthroline) and after this treatment pro-coagulant activity was significantly inhibited in all fractions. Only a discrete and friable clot (pink) was observed in rat blood incubated with fraction IIc and in chicken blood incubated with fraction IIb after SVMP inhibition, confirming that metalloproteinases are the major enzymes responsible for the pro-coagulant activity presented in the fractions.

Table 2 summarizes the features of the SVMPs isolated in this study. Fraction Ic was identified as BnMPIIIc, a putative class P-III SVMP deduced from a cDNA sequence identified in the *B. neuwiedi* venom gland. Fraction Ic displayed high hemorrhagic activity and did not degrade fibrin. Fraction Ic was able to activate Factor X generating Factor Xa *in vitro*. In whole blood coagulation assays, fraction Ic was selective to clot chicken blood in the absence of calcium. Fraction IIb contained peptides identified in the class P-III SVMPs BnMPIIIc, jararhagin and bothropasin, from the venoms of *B. neuwiedi* and *B. jararaca*, respectively. Fraction IIb contained the usual characteristics of class P-III SVMPs with hemorrhagic, fibrinolytic and gelatinolytic activities and in whole blood assays, its action was observed only in chicken blood coagulation. Fraction IIc was also identified as a P-III class SVMP containing tryptic peptides identical to jararhagin or bothropasin but differed from the previous fractions by its remarkable prothrombin activation capacity and also by its higher clotting activity in rat blood samples compared to chicken. Except for a discrete fibrinolytic activity, fractions IVa and IVb, characterized as the class P-I SVMPs BnMPIb and BnMPIa, respectively, did not present any significant effect in the parameters related to the control of hemostasis evaluated in this study.

Discussion

There is increasing evidence that venom composition is significantly affected by post-genomic mechanisms (7) and that this plasticity is associated with diet [13,36,37]. One example is ontogenetic changes in venom that occur over the lifetimes of snakes in relation to changes in diet due to correlated changes in body size [38,39]. In this regard, *Bothrops* snakes are mostly generalists that nonetheless show significant changes in diet over

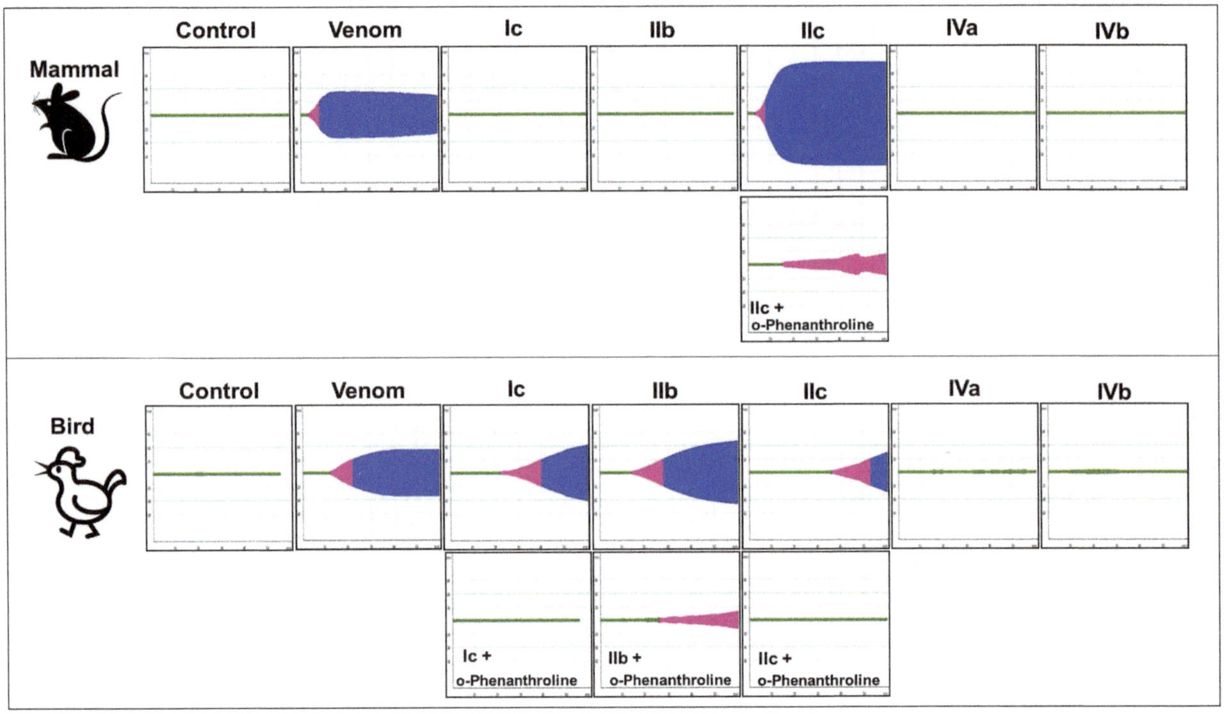

Figure 6. ROTEM profile of citrated rat or chicken whole blood samples treated with SVMPs fractions. Samples (40 μL) containing 10 μg SVMPs fractions were mixed with citrated rat or chicken whole blood samples (300 μL). ROTEM data are representative of three independent experiments and were acquired for 1 hour.

their lifetimes [38]. As such, to efficiently kill different prey, the toxin arsenal in these venoms must include toxins able to paralyze and kill different types of prey on which the snakes feed throughout their life cycle. To achieve such a toxin variety, a complex mechanism for modulation of gene expression has been described [6]. In venoms that disrupt hemostasis, the most variable toxin families (C-type lectins, serine proteinases and SVMPs) are encoded by multiple gene copies that undergo further selection and diversification at the post-transcriptional and post-translational levels [6]. As a result of this diversification process, it is hypothesized that toxins present in the snake venoms would act on distinct targets of coagulation and vascular systems of mammalian, avian, amphibian or invertebrate prey on which these animals feed. This assumption was first confirmed in this study in which the SVMPs isolated from *B. neuwiedi* venom were selective to different targets of the mammalian hemostatic system and acted with distinct potency on mammalian or bird blood.

Three distinct SVMPs P-III class were isolated and showed activity on different targets. Fractions Ic and IIc were unique in activating Factor X and Factor II of human coagulation system, respectively. Even the proteolysis profile of the SVMPs described in this study was different. Fraction Ic showed no action on fibrin but was effective in degrading gelatin, which is in agreement with its strong hemorrhagic activity associated with collagen digestion at the basement membrane of small vessels. Fraction IIb shows a broader spectrum of activities, with intermediate hemorrhagic, proteolytic and coagulant activity, but with no specific substrates. Acting together with the procoagulant serine proteinases, these enzymes would induce a rapid consumption of blood components and damage in blood vessels that would impair prey mobility and survival.

In parallel to the selectivity to different targets, we showed that SVMPs act distinctly on the coagulation system of different animals. Our initial tests were performed using the human coagulation system that is well adapted to the study of snake toxins. Further, we also tested the effects of isolated fractions on the coagulation of rat and chicken blood, which are more similar physiologically to snake prey. By using the thromboelastometric assay, only fraction IIc was effective in coagulation of the rat blood while fractions Ic and IIb were capable of clotting chicken blood. According to Martins et al. [38], *Bothrops* species are usually diet generalists, but the authors highlight that most subspecies of *B. neuwiedi* complex are mammal specialists. In this case, birds could represent an important predator of *B. neuwiedi* snakes explaining why the venom showed even more effectiveness against avian blood coagulation system. Thus, a dietary pattern between the species of *Bothrops* snakes is not likely to be the only factor modulating plasticity and venom composition could be affected also by other ecological parameters acting on the expression of different venom components.

The presence of isoforms of SVMPs and other venom proteins is a consequence of the evolutionary process of those protein families in snakes favoring diversification of their venom components. Besides the high mutation rates that follow gene duplication processes [4,5,40], alternative transcription [41] and recombination between the genes and primary mRNA transcripts have been demonstrated [29] for genes of snake venom serine proteinases and SVMPs, respectively. These mechanisms result in the production of structurally similar molecules in which the essential motifs, as catalytic sites, are conserved. These variable regions are often located in more flexible sites that may be involved in substrate binding and, therefore, driving the enzyme selectivity to distinct targets. The sequence variability in molecules with high structural similarity implies in several experimental problems encountered during this study. The complete purification of the different toxins belonging to the same class of SVMPs was

Table 2. Relative comparison of functional activities of isolated fractions.

Samples	Identified SVMPs - (Mass Spectrometry)	SVMP Class - (SDS-PAGE)	Biological Activities							
			Hemorr-hagic	Fibri-nolytic	Gelati-nolytic	Coagu-lant	FII Activa-tion	FX Activa-tion	Mam-mals	Birds
Venom			+++	+++	+++	+++	++	-	++	++
Ic	BnMPIIIc	P-III	+++	-	++	++	-	+++	-	++
IIb	BnMPIIIc/ jararhagin/bothropasin	P-III	+++	++	++	++	-	+	-	++
IIc	jararhagin/bothropasin	P-III	++	+++	++	++	+++	+	+++	+
IVa	BnMPIb	P-I	-	++	-	-	-	-	-	-
IVb	BnMPIIa	P-I	-	+	-	-	-	-	-	-

The biological activities shown above were classified as low (+), moderate (++), or high (+++) for graphical representation.

impossible in some cases. For this reason, we decided to carry on the study using fractions with predominance of SVMPs and devoid of serine proteinases. Other problem recurrent in the study concerned the precise characterization of the isolated bands by mass spectrometry. Some internal peptides are conserved in several members of the same SVMP class and are easily detected by mass spectrometry. Therefore, the identification of protein bands shown in Table 1 is only an indication of their SVMP nature. In this regard, the complete characterization of primary structures would be an essential requirement for depicting the structure/function relationships that would completely enlighten this first evidence of functional variability within the same toxin family.

Comparing the isolated *B. neuwiedi* SVMPs to already described toxins, two fractions containing class P-I SVMPs, identified in this study as BnMPIa and BnMPIb, showed only proteolytic action on fibrin and no activity on blood clotting. In previous studies, Modesto et al. [42] demonstrated that insularinase, a P-I class enzyme from the venom of *B. insularis*, which shows sequence identity with BnMPIa and BnMPIb higher than 90%, has pro-coagulant activity by activating coagulation Factor II, suggesting that targets and general function may differ even in closely related structures. Similarly, fraction IIc was identified in this study as jararhagin/bothropasin according to sequence of internal peptides identified by mass spectrometry. Jararhagin [43] and bothropasin [44] are isoforms of class P-III SVMPs from *B. jararaca* venom with sequence identity higher than 95% and only approximately 65% identity with BnMPIIb and BnMPIIc, indicated as a possible identification by mass spectrometry. Interestingly, neither jararhagin nor bothropasin show activation of human coagulant factors.

In contrast to the fractions containing P-III class SVMPs, those containing P-I class SVMPs showed little effects on the targets of hemostatic system accessed in this study. They presented only proteolytic activity on fibrin, which is consistent to previous data on the literature [34]. Thus, it is reasonable to expect that the major SVMP involved in prey killing or immobilization are those of the P-III class. In this scenario, P-I class SVMPs are more likely involved in the digestive function of snake venoms. Nevertheless, it is important to point out that a digestive activity of prey tissues may have a counterpart in the very deleterious effects of P-I class SVMPs in local lesions evoked in human victims of snake bite. Indeed, a strong pro-inflammatory action has already been reported for BaP1, a class P-I SVMP from *B. asper* venom [45,46] and neuwiedase, a P-I class SVMP from *B. neuwiedi* venom [47].

At this point, it is important to emphasize the relevance of the functional diversity of SVMPs for human victims of snake bites. Together with the digestive function of P-I class SVMPs, P-III class enzymes act in different targets of coagulation and fibrinolysis systems, endothelial cells and extracellular matrix components, accounting for most of systemic and local effects of snake bites. Fortunately, SVMPs are the predominant antigens recognized by commercial antivenoms [27]. However, it still has to be proven if the antibodies present in commercial antivenoms are able to recognize the distinct forms of SVMPs present in the venoms of *Bothrops* snakes and if they are able to neutralize the interaction of these SVMPs with their different targets. Therefore, understanding the diversity of this class of toxins is still very important to design antivenoms able to neutralize toxins responsible for the death and injury resulting from snake bites in humans.

Concluding Remarks

Many *Bothrops* snakes in South America have a paedomorphic venom in which the predominant phenotype is the abundance of P-III class SVMPs in venoms throughout their life cycles [48,49]. A striking feature of these enzymes is the versatility they show towards different biological systems [24,50] and this functional diversity may be due to their evolutionary origin in targeting different prey. The functional diversity of SVMPs shown in this study clarify the importance of this class of toxins for the feeding ecology of *Bothrops* snakes and suggest further directions for studies on the design of more efficient antivenoms.

Acknowledgments

The authors acknowledge the critical revision of the manuscript by Prof. H. L. Gibbs, from Ohio State University.

Author Contributions

Conceived and designed the experiments: JLB LSW BCP SMTS RBZ AMMS. Performed the experiments: JLB LFS LSW ASL. Analyzed the data: JLB LFS LSW ASL BCP SMTS RBZ AMMS. Contributed reagents/materials/analysis tools: LSW BCP SMTS RBZ AMMS. Wrote the paper: JLB LFS LSW ASL BCP SMTS RBZ AMMS.

References

1. Greene HW (1997) Snakes. The Evolution of Mistery in Nature. Berkeley: University of Califórnia Press.
2. Moura-da-Silva AM, Theakston RDG, Crampton JM (1996) Evolution of Disintegrin Cysteine-rich and mammalian Matrix-degrading Metalloproteinases: Gene duplication and divergence of a common ancestor rather than convergent evolution. Journal of Molecular Evolution 43: 263–269.
3. Calvete JJ, Marcinkiewicz C, Monleon D, Esteve V, Celda B, et al. (2005) Snake venom disintegrins: evolution of structure and function. Toxicon 45: 1063–1074.
4. Brust A, Sunagar K, Undheim EA, Vetter I, Yang DC, et al. (2013) Differential evolution and neofunctionalization of snake venom metalloprotease domains. Mol Cell Proteomics 12: 651–663.
5. Fry BG, Casewell NR, Wüster W, Vidal N, Young B, et al. (2012) The structural and functional diversification of the Toxicofera reptile venom system. Toxicon 60: 434–448.
6. Casewell NR, Wagstaff SC, Wüster W, Cook DA, Bolton FM, et al. (2014) Medically important differences in snake venom composition are dictated by distinct postgenomic mechanisms. Proc Natl Acad Sci U S A 111: 9205–9210.
7. Calvete JJ (2013) Snake venomics: From the inventory of toxins to biology. Toxicon.
8. Thomas RG, Pough FH (1979) The effect of rattlesnake venom on digestion of prey. Toxicon 17: 221–228.
9. Fox JW, Serrano SMT (2008) Insights into and speculations about snake venom metalloproteinase (SVMP) synthesis, folding and disulfide bond formation and their contribution to venom complexity. Febs Journal 275: 3016–3030.
10. Mackessy SP (2010) Evolutionary trends in venom composition in the western rattlesnakes (Crotalus viridis sensu lato): toxicity vs. tenderizers. Toxicon 55: 1463–1474.
11. Massey DJ, Calvete JJ, Sánchez EE, Sanz L, Richards K, et al. (2012) Venom variability and envenoming severity outcomes of the Crotalus scutulatus scutulatus (Mojave rattlesnake) from Southern Arizona. J Proteomics 75: 2576–2587.
12. Moura-da-Silva AM, Desmond H, Laing G, Theakston RDG (1991) Isolation and Comparison of Myotoxins Isolated From Venoms of Different Species of *Bothrops* Snakes. Toxicon 29: 713–723.
13. Andrade DV, Abe AS (1999) Relationship of venom ontogeny and diet in Bothrops. Herpetologica 55: 200–204.
14. Baramova EN, Shannon JD, Bjarnason JB, Fox JW (1989) Degradation of extracellular matrix proteins by hemorrhagic metalloproteinases. Archives of Biochemistry and Biophysics 275: 63–71.
15. Oliveira AK, Leme AFP, Asega AF, Camargo ACM, Fox JW, et al. (2010) New insights into the structural elements involved in the skin haemorrhage induced by snake venom metalloproteinases. Thrombosis and Haemostasis 104: 485–497.
16. Paes Leme AF, Sherman NE, Smalley DM, Sizukusa LO, Oliveira AK, et al. (2012) Hemorrhagic activity of HF3, a snake venom metalloproteinase: insights from the proteomic analysis of mouse skin and blood plasma. J Proteome Res 11: 279–291.
17. Kamiguti AS, Slupsky JR, Zuzel M, Hay CR (1994) Properties of fibrinogen cleaved by Jararhagin, a metalloproteinase from the venom of Bothrops jararaca. Thrombosis and Haemostasis 72: 244–249.
18. Kamiguti AS, Hay CRM, Zuzel M (1996) Inhibition of collagen-induced platelet aggregation as the result of cleavage of alpha(2)beta(1)-integrin by the snake venom metalloproteinase jararhagin. Biochemical Journal 320: 635–641.
19. Moura-da-Silva AM, Marcinkiewicz C, Marcinkiewicz M, Niewiarowski S (2001) Selective recognition of alpha(2)beta(1) integrin by Jararhagin, a metalloproteinase/disintegrin from Bothrops jararaca venom. Thrombosis Research 102: 153–159.
20. Tanjoni I, Weinlich R, Della-Casa M, Clissa PB, Saldanha-Gama RF, et al. (2005) Jararhagin, a snake venom metalloproteinase, induces a specialized form of apoptosis (anoikis) selective to endothelial cells. Apoptosis 10: 851–861.
21. Diaz C, Valverde L, Brenes O, Rucavado A, Gutierrez JM (2005) Characterization of events associated with Apoptosis/Anoikis induced by snake venom metalloproteinase BaP1 on human endothelial cells. Journal of Cellular Biochemistry 94: 520–528.
22. Clissa PB, Laing GD, Theakston RDG, Mota I, Taylor MJ, et al. (2001) The effect of jararhagin, a metalloproteinase from Bothrops jararaca venom, on pro-inflammatory cytokines released by murine peritoneal adherent cells. Toxicon 39: 1567–1573.
23. Lopes DS, Faquim-Mauro E, Magalhães GS, Lima IC, Baldo C, et al. (2012) Gene expression of inflammatory mediators induced by jararhagin on endothelial cells. Toxicon 60: 1072–1084.
24. Moura-da-Silva AM, Butera D, Tanjoni I (2007) Importance of snake venom metalloproteinases in cell biology: Effects on platelets, inflammatory and endothelial cells. Current Pharmaceutical Design 13: 2893–2905.
25. Kini RM (2005) Serine proteases affecting blood coagulation and fibrinolysis from snake venoms. Pathophysiol Haemost Thromb 34: 200–204.
26. Cardoso JL, Fan HW, França FO, Jorge MT, Leite RP, et al. (1993) Randomized comparative trial of three antivenoms in the treatment of envenoming by lance-headed vipers (Bothrops jararaca) in São Paulo, Brazil. Quarterly Journal of Medicine 86: 315–325.
27. Sousa LF, Nicolau CA, Peixoto PS, Bernardoni JL, Oliveira SS, et al. (2013) Comparison of phylogeny, venom composition and neutralization by antivenom in diverse species of bothrops complex. PLoS Negl Trop Dis 7: e2442.
28. Rodrigues RS, Boldrini-França J, Fonseca FP, de la Torre P, Henrique-Silva F, et al. (2012) Combined snake venomics and venom gland transcriptomic analysis of Bothropoides pauloensis. J Proteomics 75: 2707–2720.
29. Moura-da-Silva AM, Furlan MS, Caporrino MC, Grego KF, Portes-Junior JA, et al. (2011) Diversity of metalloproteinases in Bothrops neuwiedi snake venom transcripts: evidences for recombination between different classes of SVMPs. BMC Genet 12: 94.
30. Dagda RK, Gasanov S, De La Oiii Y, Rael ED, Lieb CS (2013) Genetic Basis for Variation of Metalloproteinase-Associated Biochemical Activity in Venom of the Mojave Rattlesnake (Crotalus scutulatus scutulatus). Biochem Res Int 2013: 251474.
31. Campbell JA, Lamar WW (2004) The Venomous Reptiles of the Western Hemisphere.
32. Moura-da-Silva AM, Della-Casa MS, David AS, Assakura MT, Butera D, et al. (2003) Evidence for heterogeneous forms of the snake venom metalloproteinase jararhagin: a factor contributing to snake venom variability. Archives of Biochemistry and Biophysics 409: 395–401.
33. Jespersen J, Astrup T (1983) A study of the fibrin plate assay of fibrinolytic agents. Optimal conditions, reproducibility and precision. Haemostasis 13: 301–315.
34. Baldo C, Tanjoni I, León IR, Batista IFC, Della-Casa MS, et al. (2008) BnP1, a novel P-I metalloproteinase from Bothrops neuwiedi venom: Biological effects benchmarking relatively to jararhagin, a P-IIISVMP. Toxicon 51: 54–65.
35. Kini RM, Rao VS, Joseph JS (2001) Procoagulant proteins from snake venoms. Haemostasis 31: 218–224.
36. Gibbs HL, Mackessy SP (2009) Functional basis of a molecular adaptation: prey-specific toxic effects of venom from Sistrurus rattlesnakes. Toxicon 53: 672–679.
37. Gibbs HL, Sanz L, Chiucchi JE, Farrell TM, Calvete JJ (2011) Proteomic analysis of ontogenetic and diet-related changes in venom composition of juvenile and adult Dusky Pigmy rattlesnakes (Sistrurus miliarius barbouri). J Proteomics 74: 2169–2179.
38. Martins M, Marques OAV, Sazima I (2002) Ecological andphylogenetic correlates of feeding habits in Neotropicalpitvipers of the genus *Bothrops*. In: Schuett G, Höggren M, Green HW, editors.Biology of the pit vipers.Indiana: Biological Science Press. pp.45–90.
39. Zelanis A, Tashima AK, Rocha MM, Furtado MF, Camargo AC, et al. (2010) Analysis of the ontogenetic variation in the venom proteome/peptidome of Bothrops jararaca reveals different strategies to deal with prey. J Proteome Res 9: 2278–2291.
40. Deshimaru M, Ogawa T, Nakashima K, Nobuhisa I, Chijiwa T, et al. (1996) Accelerated evolution of crotalinae snake venom gland serine proteases. FEBS Lett 397: 83–88.
41. Siigur E, Aaspõllu A, Siigur J (2001) Sequence diversity of Vipera lebetina snake venom gland serine proteinase homologs–result of alternative-splicing or genome alteration. Gene 263: 199–203.

42. Modesto JC, Junqueira-de-Azevedo IL, Neves-Ferreira AG, Fritzen M, Oliva ML, et al. (2005) Insularinase A, a prothrombin activator from Bothrops insularis venom, is a metalloprotease derived from a gene encoding protease and disintegrin domains. Biol Chem 386: 589–600.
43. Paine MJ, Desmond HP, Theakston RD, Crampton JM (1992) Purification, cloning, and molecular characterization of a high molecular weight hemorrhagic metalloprotease, jararhagin, from Bothrops jararaca venom. Insights into the disintegrin gene family. Journal of Biological Chemistry 267: 22869–22876.
44. Assakura MT, Silva CA, Mentele R, Camargo ACM, Serrano SMT (2003) Molecular cloning and expression of structural domains of bothropasin, a P-III metalloproteinase from the venom of Bothrops jararaca. Toxicon 41: 217–227.
45. Fernandes CM, Zamuner SR, Zuliani JP, Rucavado A, Gutierrez JM, et al. (2006) Inflammatory effects of BaP1 a metalloproteinase isolated from Bothrops asper snake venom: Leukocyte recruitment and release of cytokines. Toxicon 47: 549–559.
46. Gutierrez JM, Rucavado A, Chaves F, Diaz C, Escalante T (2009) Experimental pathology of local tissue damage induced by Bothrops asper snake venom. Toxicon 54: 958–975.
47. Lopes DS, Baldo C, Oliveira CF, Alcântara TM, Oliveira JDD, et al. (2009) Characterization of inflammatory reaction induced by neuwiedase, a P-I metalloproteinase isolated from Bothrops neuwiedi venom. Toxicon 54: 42–49.
48. Calvete JJ, Sanz L, Pérez A, Borges A, Vargas AM, et al. (2011) Snake population venomics and antivenomics of Bothrops atrox: Paedomorphism along its transamazonian dispersal and implications of geographic venom variability on snakebite management. J Proteomics 74: 510–527.
49. Calvete JJ (2010) Antivenomics and venom phenotyping: A marriage of convenience to address the performance and range of clinical use of antivenoms. Toxicon 56: 1284–1291.
50. Laing GD, Moura-da-Silva AM (2005) Jararhagin and its multiple effects on hemostasis. Toxicon 45: 987–996.

Growth Hormone-Regulated mRNAs and miRNAs in Chicken Hepatocytes

Xingguo Wang[1,2]◔, Lei Yang[1]◔, Huijuan Wang[1], Fang Shao[1], JianFeng Yu[1], Honglin Jiang[3], Yaoping Han[1], Daoqing Gong[2], Zhiliang Gu[1]*

1 Department of Life Science and Technology, Changshu Institute of Technology, Changshu, P R China, **2** College of Animal Science and Technology, Yangzhou University, Yangzhou, P R China, **3** Department of Animal and Poultry Sciences, Virginia Polytechnic Institute and State University, Blacksburg, Virginia, United States of America

Abstract

Growth hormone (GH) is a key regulatory factor in animal growth, development and metabolism. Based on the expression level of the GH receptor, the chicken liver is a major target organ of GH, but the biological effects of GH on the chicken liver are not fully understood. In this work we identified mRNAs and miRNAs that are regulated by GH in primary hepatocytes from female chickens through RNA-seq, and analyzed the functional relevance of these mRNAs and miRNAs through GO enrichment analysis and miRNA target prediction. A total of 164 mRNAs were found to be differentially expressed between GH-treated and control chicken hepatocytes, of which 112 were up-regulated and 52 were down-regulated by GH. A total of 225 chicken miRNAs were identified by the RNA-Seq analysis. Among these miRNAs 16 were up-regulated and 1 miRNA was down-regulated by GH. The GH-regulated mRNAs were mainly involved in growth and metabolism. Most of the GH-upregulated or GH-downregulated miRNAs were predicted to target the GH-downregulated or GH-upregulated mRNAs, respectively, involved in lipid metabolism. This study reveals that GH regulates the expression of many mRNAs involved in metabolism in female chicken hepatocytes, which suggests that GH plays an important role in regulating liver metabolism in female chickens. The results of this study also support the hypothesis that GH regulates lipid metabolism in chicken liver in part by regulating the expression of miRNAs that target the mRNAs involved in lipid metabolism.

Editor: Michael Schubert, Laboratoire de Biologie du Développement de Villefranche-sur-Mer, France

Funding: This research was supported by the National Natural Science Foundation of China (31072025, 31272438). The funders had no role in study design, data collection and analysis, decision to publish, or preparation of the manuscript.

Competing Interests: The authors have declared that no competing interests exist.

* Email: zhilianggu88@hotmail.com

◔ These authors contributed equally to this work.

Introduction

Growth hormone (GH) is a peptide hormone from the anterior pituitary gland [1,2]. It has many biological effects at both the whole body and tissue levels [3]. GH regulates animal growth, development and metabolism [3,4,5,6]. GH regulates the metabolism of not only protein but also that of lipid and carbohydrates [7]. GH initiates its function by binding to the GH receptor (GHR) [8,9,10]. Binding of GH to the GHR activates the receptor-associated tyrosine kinase JAK2 [11], and JAK2 then activates multiple proteins, including STAT1, STAT3, STAT5, MAPK, and PI3K [12]. These proteins in turn mediate GH-caused changes in gene expression or protein modification.

Liver is a key metabolic organ, and in chickens this is where most of the *de novo* synthesis of fatty acids occurs [13,14]. microRNAs (miRNAs) are a class of small non-coding RNAs about 22 nucleotides in length, and regulate gene expression by interacting with the 3′ untranslated regions (UTRs) of target mRNAs [15]. miRNAs have been shown to play important roles in many biological processes including liver metabolism. For example, miR-122, abundantly expressed in liver, modulates protein metabolism in liver by targeting cationic amino acid transporter 1 [16]; it regulates the synthesis of fatty acids and cholesterol by repressing the expression of aldolase-A, 3-hydroxy-3-methylglutaryl-coenzyme A reductase, and AMP-activated protein kinase [17,18]. miR-33 is another miRNA involved in liver metabolism: it regulates cholesterol efflux and high-density lipoprotein metabolism by targeting ATP-binding cassette, sub-family A (ABC1), member 1 and ATP-binding cassette, sub-family G (WHITE), member 1 [19], and it reduces fatty acid degradation by targeting multiple genes involved in fatty acid β-oxidation [20].

RNA sequencing (RNA-seq) is a novel gene expression profiling technology based on high-throughput DNA sequencing. The benefit of RNA-Seq over other large-scale gene expression profiling methods is its ability to measure mRNA expression in a single assay and, at the same time, reveal new genes and transcripts [21,22,23]. Similarly, RNA-seq can be also used to identify novel miRNAs and detect differentially expressed miRNAs between samples [24].

As in mammals [3,7,25,26], GH has metabolic effects in chickens: GH regulates lipid metabolism in chicken adipose tissue [27] and chicken liver [28]. However, it is unclear whether GH has the same growth-stimulating effect in chickens as in mammals because exogenous GH treatment to chickens causes no growth

Table 1. An overview of mRNA sequencing results.

Sample	Raw Reads	Clean Reads	Reads mapped to chicken genome	Reads mapped to chicken genes
chGH	16,474,842	13,638,494	10,669,529	8,812,163
PBS	10,662,250	7,473,018	5,652,712	4,656,574

responses and because plasma GH concentrations in chickens are in general not correlated with growth rates [29].

The mechanism by which GH regulates lipid metabolism in chicken liver is not clear. In this study, we determined the effects of GH on the expression levels of all mRNAs and miRNAs in primary hepatocytes from female chickens by RNA-seq. We analyzed the differentially expressed mRNAs or genes (DEG) and differentially expressed miRNAs (DEM) with multiple bioinformatics tools to correlate the DEG and the DEM to the physiological functions of GH. The main hypothesis to be tested in this study was that GH regulates liver metabolism in the chicken in part by regulating the expression of miRNAs that target mRNAs directly related to liver metabolism.

Materials and Methods

1. Culture of primary chicken hepatocytes

All procedures involving animals were approved by Changshu Institute of Technology Institutional Animal Care and Use Committee and conformed to the Guide for the Care and Use of Laboratory Animals of Jiangsu Province. All efforts were made to minimize suffering. Primary chicken hepatocytes were isolated from 4 female, 4-week-old Arbor Acres commercial chickens which were fasted 12 hours (h) before being anaesthetized by intraperitoneal injection of sodium thiopenthal (50 mg/kg) and anticoagulated by intraperitoneal injection of heparin (1750 U/kg). Livers were isolated and the chickens were sacrificed by removal of the hearts. Hepatocytes were isolated from the livers as previously described [30]. Hepatocytes from individual chickens were cultured separately. Hepatocytes were plated in 24-well plates or 10-cm dishes at a density of 1.3×10^6 cells/ml in Willam's E medium (Gibco, Grand Island, NY) supplemented with 5% chicken serum, 100 U/ml penicillin-streptomycin, 10 μg/ml insulin and 30 mmol/L NaCl in a humidified incubator at 37°C with 5% CO_2. Twenty-eight h later, hepatocytes were serum starved for 8 h, followed by 12 h of treatment with 500 ng/ml chicken GH (chGH) (Prospec, Ness-Ziona, Israel) or an equal volume of PBS. Cells were lysed and total RNA was isolated using TRIzol reagent (Invitrogen, Carlsbad, CA) following the manufacturer's directions.

Table 2. Top 10 GH up-regulated and top 10 GH down-regulated mRNA-encoding genes.

Name	PBS (RPKM)	chGH (RPKM)	fold change (RPKM (chGH/PBS))	P-value
up-regulated genes				
RPS28	0.52	21.63	40.74	0.0005
TTLL3	1.09	23.57	21.41	0.028
CISH	1.97	27.94	13.99	1.38E-10
SCN4A	1.87	20.79	10.95	5.29E-21
BLB1	0.74	7.13	9.53	0.009
TGM2	0.20	1.78	8.88	0.037
SS1R	0.68	5.33	8.75	0.015
SERPINA4	8.86	78.26	8.70	1.06E-18
GGA.45581	35.97	278.79	7.64	9.82E-31
CCK	3.23	24.44	7.46	5.05E-05
down-regulated genes				
AFP	38.74	0.10	0.0025	4.76E-40
RGS6	1.92	0.09	0.047	0.014
STAR	27.75	5.01	0.18	1.28E-08
CCKAR	5.57	1.01	0.18	0.013
KIAA0408	3.38	0.63	0.19	0.020
BCL6	19.86	4.26	0.21	8.27E-08
PDE10A	7.07	1.57	0.22	0.002
ENSGALG00000024377	26.06	6.18	0.23	0.044
NECAB1	7.12	1.74	0.24	0.010
TAGLN3	34.96	8.62	0.24	5.64E-06

Table 3. Real time RT-PCR validation of gene expression levels revealed by RNA-seq.

Gene	Real-time RT-PCR		RNA-seq	
	Fold change[1]	P-value	Fold change[2]	P-value
Group 1[3]				
FABP1	4.30	0.034	3.96	3.82E-07
FGFR3	2.37	3.93E-04	2.11	0.009
FURIN	1.71	0.012	2.30	2.82E-05
IRF8	2.68	0.005	2.50	1.69E-05
LPIN1	1.81	0.049	1.78	1.45E-04
MAPKAPK3	1.68	0.021	2.24	0.010
PHGDH	1.12	0.748	1.54	0.004
PKIG	1.47	0.094	1.67	0.046
THRSP	1.44	0.565	1.76	0.007
Group 2[4]				
ABCG8	0.28	0.048	0.33	2.14E-04
ALDH1A3	0.70	0.087	0.66	0.009
BCL6	0.18	0.003	0.21	8.27E-08
LPIG	0.33	5.69E-04	0.34	2.67E-07
NECAB1	0.43	0.447	0.24	0.010
PDE10A	0.30	0.042	0.22	0.002
PPAP2B	0.61	0.075	0.52	0.010
RGS6	0.49	0.218	0.05	0.014
STAR	0.17	0.024	0.18	1.28E-08
Group 3[5]				
FGF1	1.19	0.743	1.62	0.661
GPX7	1.15	0.760	3.66	0.552
MEF2A	0.90	0.665	6.79	0.461
NME1	0.90	0.800	7.83	0.384
PDGFB	0.78	0.350	1.72	0.694
PNPLA4	0.90	0.656	1.99	0.449
PRKAR2B	1.47	0.339	4.44	0.438
PTK2B	0.97	0.925	2.27	0.220
PTPRC	1.21	0.540	1.72	0.247
ROMO1	0.84	0.205	2.13	0.168
Group 4[6]				
ACER2	1.30	0.163	0.46	0.437
ADPGK	1.02	0.759	0.56	0.371
ATF7	1.14	0.602	0.31	0.445
BIRC5	0.93	0.753	0.26	0.685
CDK2AP1	1.23	0.613	0.28	0.384
DUSP28	0.90	0.628	0.17	0.471
FTO	1.33	0.159	0.39	0.472
HGF	1.87	0.463	0.49	0.470
MAFK	0.83	0.074	0.50	0.144
NT5M	1.30	0.497	0.45	0.488
RUNX2	0.98	0.939	0.157	0.272

[1]fold change by real-time RT-PCR is relative gene expression level (chGH/PBS).
[2]fold change by RNA-seq is RPKM (chGH/PBS).
[3]Group 1: fold change (RPKM (chGH/PBS)) >1.5 and P<0.05.
[4]Group 2: fold change (RPKM (chGH/PBS)) <2/3 and P<0.05.
[5]Group 3: fold change (RPKM (chGH/PBS)) >1.5 and P>0.05.
[6]Group 4: fold change (RPKM (chGH/PBS)) <2/3 and P>0.05.

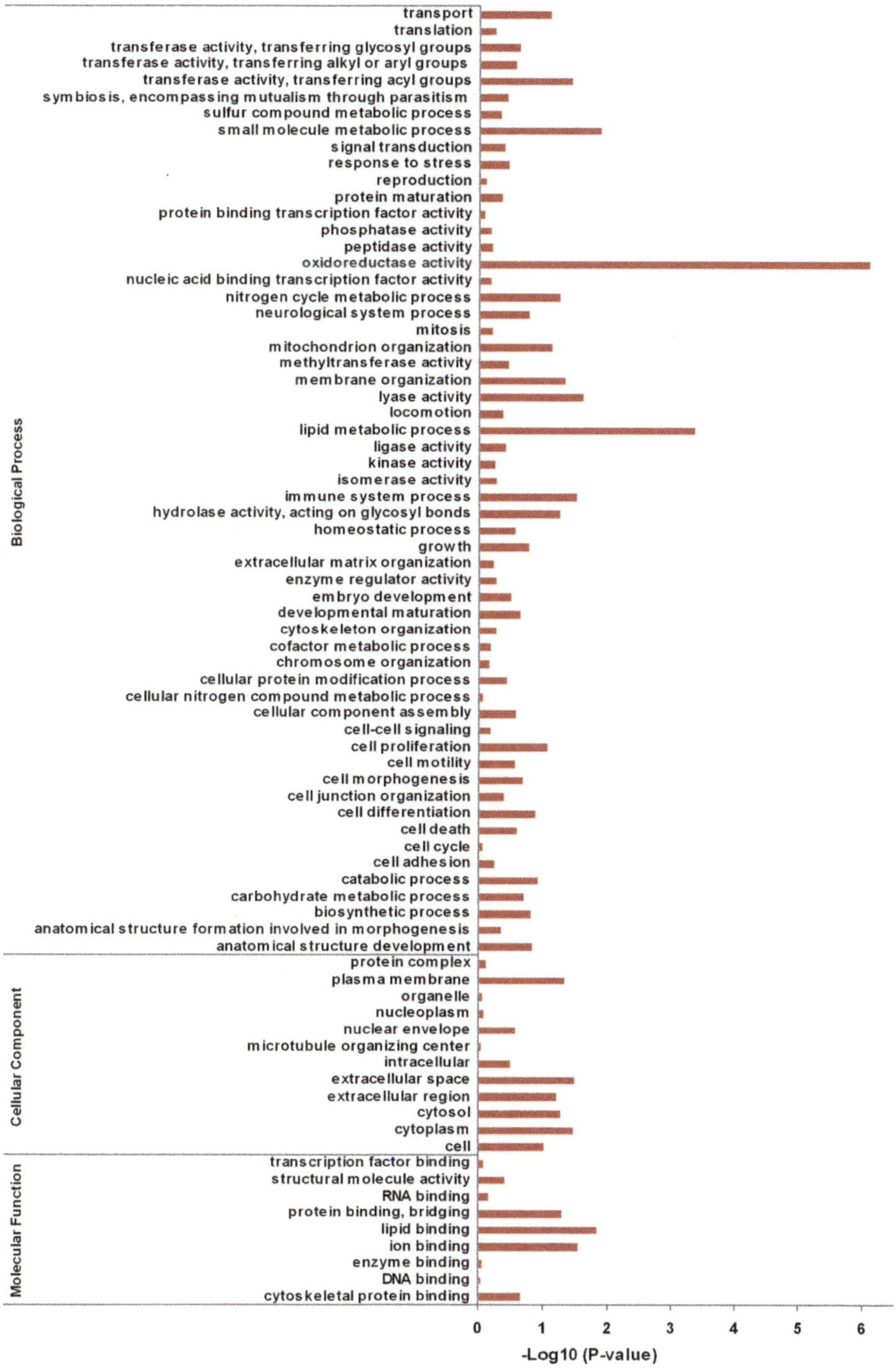

Figure 1. GO enrichment analysis of genes regulated by chGH in chicken hepatocytes. The GO terms are sorted by -Log10 of the enrichment P-value, which represents the enrichment significance of GO terms. The enrichment of GO terms is showed by comparing DEG with the whole genome from this figure.

2. Real time RT-PCR

Concentrations and quality of RNA samples were determined by NanoDrop ND2000 spectrophotometry (Thermo Scientific, Wilmington, DE) and formaldehyde-agarose gel electrophoresis. Five hundred ng of total RNA was reverse-transcribed to cDNA in a total volume of 10 μl using Takara PrimeScript RT reagent kit (Takara, Dalian, China). The relative expression levels of genes were quantified using SYBR Premix Ex Taq (Takara) on an Applied Biosystems 7500 Thermocycler (Applied Biosystems) according to the manufacturer's directions. In this analysis, GAPDH was used as an internal control. All reactions were run in duplicate. Data are means ± SEM of 4 independent cell culture experiments (i.e., 4 chickens) and analyzed by student's t-test. The primers for real time RT-PCR were presented in Table S1.

Table 4. List of growth-related mRNAs whose expression in chicken hepatocytes was regulated by chGH.

Name	PBS (RPKM)	chGH (RPKM)	fold change (RPKM (chGH/PBS))	P-value
BCL6	19.86	4.26	0.21	8.27E-08
CISH	1.97	27.94	13.99	1.38E-10
FOXP2	11.40	19.73	1.71	0.026
IRF8	25.75	65.31	2.50	1.69E-05
ROBO1	11.86	7.27	0.60	0.038
ULK2	23.90	70.81	2.92	2.97E-09

RPKM was denoted as a formula: $\text{RPKM} = \frac{\text{Total exon reads}}{\text{Mapped Reads (millions} \times \text{exon lenth (KB))}}$.

3. mRNA sequencing

RNA samples for mRNA sequencing were prepared using Illumina TrueSeq RNA Sample Preparation Kit according to the manufacturer's directions. The liver RNA samples from 4 chGH-treated or PBS-treated chickens were pooled in equal volumes after their concentrations were adjusted to 10 nM. Sequencing of the cDNA was performed by Personalbio (Shanghai, China) using the Illumina Miseq system.

4. mRNA analysis

The reads obtained from sequencing were mapped to the chicken genome (WASHUC2.69) in Ensembl using Bowtie/Tophat (2.0.5) (http://tophat.cbcb.umd.edu), and the reads of each gene were normalized using reads per kilo bases per million reads (RPKM). The significance was determined by normalizing the raw reads and calculating the P-value using DESeq (http://bioconductor.org/packages/release/bioc/html/DESeq.html). Genes with fold change (RPKM (chGH/PBS)) >1.5 or <2/3 and *P*-value <0.05 were identified as DEG.

Gene Ontology (GO) enrichment analysis was performed using GOslim (http://www.geneontology.org/page/go-slim-and-subset-guide). The data were presented as −log (P-value). $\text{P-value} = 1 - \sum_{i=0}^{m-1} \frac{\binom{M}{i}\binom{N-M}{n-i}}{\binom{N}{n}}$, where N is the total gene number in genome, n is the number of all DEG, M is the number of genes in genome that are involved in certain GO, and m is the number of DEG that are involved in certain GO. The signaling pathways were analyzed using the KEGG database.

5. Small RNA sequencing

The RNA samples used for small RNA sequencing were the same as for mRNA sequencing. Small RNA libraries for small RNA sequencing were constructed according to the Miseq small RNA sequencing protocol. Briefly, total RNA was ligated to the 3′ adapter. Then it was ligated to the 5′ adapter. The ligated RNA was reverse-transcribed to cDNA. The cDNA which had a 3′ adapter and a 5′ adapter was amplified by PCR. The PCR products with appropriate length were extracted from polyacrylamide gels to construct the small RNA libraries. The libraries of four samples were pooled in equal volumes after first being normalized to 10 nM. Sequencing of the small RNA libraries was performed by Personalbio using the Illumina Miseq system.

6. miRNA analysis

The raw reads from small RNA sequencing were treated by trimming the adapters and removing the low-quality sequences to obtain the clean reads. The clean reads with 15–30 nt were analyzed by counting and grouping identical sequences as unique reads. The unique reads were mapped to the chicken genome using Bowtie and BLAST searched against the ncRNA database Rfam (10.1) assess the quality of sequences and obtain ncRNA annotation. The sequence reads were first searched against the chicken miRNA database in miRBase (20.0) to identify known chicken miRNAs, then against the miRNA databases of other species in miRBase to identify chicken miRNAs homologous to known miRNAs in other species, and finally against the chicken genome to obtain their ~80 nt genomic sequences flanking the 5′ or 3′ end and analyzed using the program mireap (http://sourceforge.net/projects/mireap/) to predict potentially novel chicken miRNAs and their precursors according to the miRNA biogenesis principle [31].

The reads of miRNAs from control (PBS treated) samples and GH treated samples were normalized using reads per million (RPM). RPM = Actual miRNA count/Total count of clean reads*1000000. When the RPM of a certain miRNA in one type of samples was zero, it was revised to 0.01, and if the RPM of a certain miRNA in both types of samples was less than 1, the miRNA would not be used in further DEM analysis. Fold change and P-value were calculated from the RPM. Fold change = RPM (chGH)/RPM (PBS). P-value formula: $p(x|y) = \left(\frac{N_2}{N_1}\right)^y \frac{(x+y)!}{x!y!\left(1+\frac{N_2}{N_1}\right)^{(x+y+1)}}$ $\begin{matrix} C(y \le y_{min}|x) = \sum_{y=0}^{y \le y_{min}} p(y|x) \\ D(y \ge y_{max}|x) = \sum_{y \ge y_{max}}^{\infty} p(y|x) \end{matrix}$. The x and y represent normalized expression level, and the N1 and N2 represent total count of clean reads of a given miRNA in small RNA libraries of chGH and PBS groups, respectively. The miRNAs with fold change (RPM (chGH/PBS)) >1.5 or <2/3 and P-value <0.05 were identified as DEM [32].

Target genes of identified known chicken DEM were predicted in the DEG using miRanda with the TargetScan principle [30]. In brief, the target mRNAs of GH up-regulated miRNAs were predicted in GH down-regulated mRNAs; the target mRNAs of GH down-regulated miRNAs were predicted in the GH up-regulated mRNAs. Then GO enrichment analysis of GH-regulated mRNAs targeted by GH-regulated miRNAs was performed using the GOslim program.

Results

1. mRNA expression profiling by RNA-seq

The RNA-seq generated 16,474,842 and 10,662,250 paired end reads from chGH-treated group and PBS-treated group, respec-

Table 5. List of metabolism-related mRNAs whose expression in chicken hepatocytes was regulated by chGH.

Name	PBS (RPKM)	chGH (RPKM)	fold change (RPKM (chGH/PBS))	P-value
Protein metabolism				
AASS	35.18	53.89	1.51	0.029
ABCG5	15.51	7.35	0.47	0.018
ABCG8	20.88	6.94	0.33	2.14E-04
AKAP13	32.52	21.50	0.65	0.02311
BCL6	19.86	4.26	0.21	8.27E-08
CACNA1D	9.77	4.62	0.47	6.47E-04
CAMK1D	16.62	30.05	1.78	0.049
CEBPA	2.90	13.19	4.48	0.018
FGFR3	8.20	17.53	2.11	0.009
FOXP2	11.40	19.73	1.71	0.026
FZD5	22.61	46.43	2.02	0.021
F1NQS2	76.69	122.69	1.58	0.013
HAL	165.14	260.84	1.56	0.005
HistoneH4	12.98	36.83	2.79	0.0498
ICER	44.32	71.76	1.60	0.023
IRF8	25.75	65.31	2.50	1.69E-05
LPIN1	259.93	468.47	1.78	1.45E-04
MC5R	10.41	26.56	2.52	0.009
OXA1L	3.28	16.92	5.09	0.030
PHGDH	542.39	848.66	1.54	0.004
PKIG	163.59	277.14	1.67	0.046
PPAP2B	43.27	22.99	0.52	0.010
RAPGEF2	30.14	55.26	1.81	7.43E-04
RNL2	158.78	257.55	1.60	0.013
SLC7A2	19.42	30.91	1.57	0.048
UPP2	130.97	229.47	1.73	0.002
Carbohydrate metabolism				
CHIA	59.33	141.04	2.35	3.04E-06
E1BZP4	31.08	122.15	3.88	1.3E-10
MAN2A2	2.87	6.39	2.20	0.041
PCK2	51.79	102.40	1.95	0.003
ST6GAL1	33.42	54.46	1.61	0.018
Lipid metabolism				
ABHD5	23.45	47.53	2.00	8.61E-04
ACSL3	27.37	16.69	0.60	0.027
AKR1D1	0.85	4.83	5.57	0.043
ALDH1A3	148.38	99.67	0.66	0.009
ALDH8A1	108.87	174.87	1.58	0.008
CEBPA	2.90	13.19	4.48	0.018
ELOV6	196.41	117.72	0.59	0.005
ICER	44.32	71.76	1.60	0.023
LIPG	77.96	26.78	0.34	2.67E-07
LPIN1	259.93	468.47	1.78	1.45E-04
PLCD1	139.45	87.34	0.62	0.003
PPAP2B	43.27	22.99	0.52	0.010
RETSAT	18.49	37.63	2.01	0.024
STAR	27.75	5.01	0.18	1.28E-08
THRSP	74.53	133.21	1.76	0.007

Table 6. List of signal transduction-related mRNAs whose expression in chicken hepatocytes was regulated by chGH.

Name	PBS (RPKM)	chGH (RPKM)	fold change (RPKM (chGH/PBS))	P-value
Nucleic acid binding transcription factor				
BCL6	19.86	4.26	0.21	8.27E-08
CAMK1D	16.62	30.05	1.78	0.049
CEBPA	2.90	13.19	4.48	0.018
FOXP2	11.40	19.73	1.71	0.026017
ICER	44.32	71.76	1.60	0.023
IRF8	25.75	65.31	2.50	1.69E-05
PPAP2B	43.27	22.99	0.52	0.010
Signal transduction				
AKAP13	32.52	21.50	0.65	0.023
ALDH1A3	148.38	99.67	0.66	0.009
ARL5A	18.46	33.45	1.79	0.042
BCL6	19.86	4.26	0.21	8.27E-08
CACNA1D	9.77	4.62	0.47	6.47E-04
CBLB	5.26	2.37	0.44	0.046
CCKAR	5.57	1.01	0.18	0.013
CISH	1.97	27.94	13.99	1.38E-10
FGA	140.08	247.03	1.74	5.29E-04
FGFR3	8.20	17.53	2.11	0.009
FGG	111.03	176.06	1.56	0.009
FURIN	21.31	49.79	2.30	2.82E-05
FZD5	22.61	46.43	2.02	0.021
GPR1	49.72	24.24	0.48	0.005
SS1R	0.68	5.33	8.75	0.015
MAPKAPK3	7.28	16.57	2.24	0.010
MC5R	10.41	26.56	2.52	0.009
NCAM1	6.36	3.17	0.49	0.043
PDE10A	7.07	1.57	0.22	0.002
PLCD1	139.45	87.34	0.62	0.003
PPAP2B	43.27	22.99	0.52	0.010
RAPGEF2	30.14	55.26	1.81	7.43E-04
RGS6	1.92	0.09	0.047	0.014
SPTBN1	151.29	101.93	0.66	0.007

tively, with an average length of 151 bp. After filtering with Q30, 13,638,494 and 7,473,018 useful reads were obtained from the treated group and control group, respectively. We mapped the useful reads to the chicken genome using bowite/tophat software, and found that 75.64% and 78.23% of reads in the treated group and control group mapped to the chicken genome, respectively. Of them, 82.59% in the treated group and 82.38% in the control group can be mapped to genes (Table 1). A total of 16,736 genes were identified.

Among the identified 16,736 genes, 164 genes with fold change >1.5 and p-value <0.05 were identified as DEG, of which 112 were up-regulated and 52 were down-regulated by chGH treatment (Table S2). Table 2 shows the top 10 up-regulated DEG and the top 10 down-regulated DEG.

To confirm the result of RNA-seq, we classified the genes into four groups: 1) fold change (RPKM (chGH/PBS)) >1.5 and P< 0.05, 2) fold change (RPKM (chGH/PBS)) <2/3 and P<0.05, 3) fold change (RPKM (chGH/PBS))>1.5 and P>0.05, 4) fold change (RPKM (chGH/PBS)) <2/3 and P>0.05. And real-time RT-PCR was performed on a total of 39 genes that were randomly selected from four groups. Among them, 21 genes that were not differentially expressed between chGH and PBS based on RNA-seq were also found to be not differentially expressed by real-time RT-PCR, and 11 of 18 genes that were found to be differentially expressed by RNA-seq were also confirmed to be differentially expressed by real time RT-PCR (Table 3). Thus, our RNA-seq results were in general confirmed by real-time RT-PCR.

2. Functional analysis of differentially expressed mRNAs

To correlate the differentially expressed mRNAs with biological functions, we analyzed the functional bias of the DEG according to Gene Ontology enrichment. The analysis showed that the DEG included many genes involved in lipid binding, ion binding, transferase activity, oxidoreductase activity, immune system

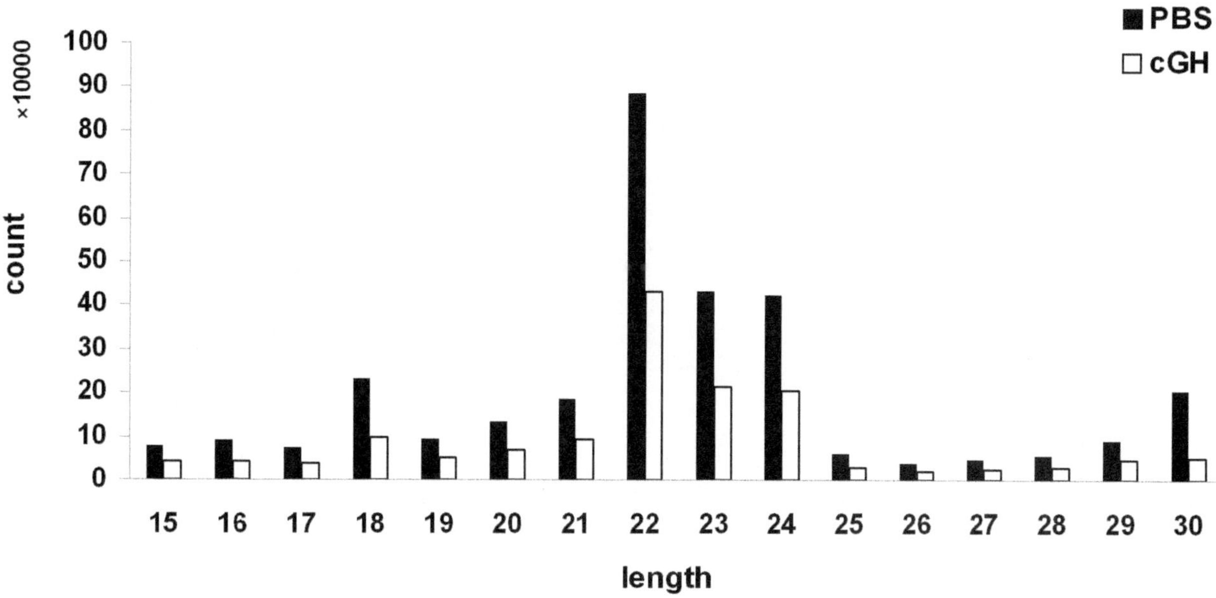

Figure 2. Length distributions of small RNA sequences.

process, lyase activity, and lipid metabolic process. Other enriched GO terms included growth, cellular nitrogen compound metabolic process, carbohydrate metabolic process, and biosynthetic process (Figure 1). Most of the KEGG Orthology (KO) terms were related to lipid metabolism (Table S3). Among the GH up-regulated genes, three were involved in the pathways controlling lipid metabolism: *AKR1D1* was involved in primary bile acid biosynthesis and steroid hormone biosynthesis pathway, *FABP1* was involved in PPAR and fat digestion and absorption pathway, and *LPIN1* was involved in glycerolipid metabolism pathway. Among the GH down-regulated genes, only one was involved in the pathway related to lipid metabolism: *PPAP2B* was involved in glycerolipid metabolism and fat digestion and absorption pathway.

2.1. Differentially expressed mRNAs involved in growth. We found that there were 6 GH-regulated genes involved in animal growth. Of them, *CISH*, *ULK2*, *IRF8*, and *FOXP2* were up-regulated by chGH, and *Bcl6* and *ROBO1* were down-regulated by chGH (Table 4). Both *Bcl6* and *ROBO1* are negative regulators of cell growth [33,34]. This indicates that chGH may regulate chicken growth by both increasing the expression of genes that positively regulate growth and reducing the expression of genes that negatively regulate growth.

2.2. Differentially expressed mRNAs related to metabolism. A total of 46 GH-regulated DEG were found to participate in protein, carbohydrate and lipid metabolism. Among them, 26 were related to protein metabolism as shown in Table 5, of which 20 were up-regulated and 6 were down-regulated by chGH, suggesting that GH plays an important role in protein metabolism in chicken hepatocytes. Further analysis showed that most of the 26 genes either promote protein synthesis or inhibit protein degradation, consistent with a previous study [7]. In addition to protein metabolism, 5 genes were related to carbohydrate metabolism, and all of them were up-regulated by chGH (Table 5). The specific functions of these genes include carbohydrate binding, transferase activity, and gluconeogenesis. As shown in Table 5, 15 DEG were related to lipid metabolism. Among these 15 genes, 8 showed increased expression after chGH treatment and all have oxidoreductase activity, suggesting that GH may promote lipid oxidation in chicken hepatocytes. Most of the 7 down-regulated genes were related to unsaturated fatty acid and long chain fatty acid biosynthesis, suggesting that GH may inhibit lipid synthesis in chicken hepatocytes.

2.3. Differentially expressed mRNAs related to signaling pathways. We also identified which GH-regulated genes might be involved in intracellular signaling. The analysis indicated that 7 GH-regulated genes have DNA binding activity, of which 5 were up-regulated and 2 were down-regulated by chGH, and 24 GH-regulated genes were components of signal transduction pathways, of which 11 were up-regulated and 13 were down-regulated by chGH (Table 6). These pathways include the STAT and MAPK pathways, which are known to be activated by GH [35,36] and pathways that are not known to be activated by GH.

3. miRNA profiling by RNA-seq

Small RNA libraries of chGH-treated and PBS-treated hepatocytes were deep sequenced, generating 8,248,771 raw reads from PBS-treated hepatocytes and 5,232,471 raw reads from chGH-treated cells. Of these sequences, 5,240,376 and 2,144,128 were clean reads. A total of 3,124,826 clean reads and a total of 1,487,885 clean reads from PBS-treated cells and chGH-treated cells, respectively, were found to be between 15 and 30 nt in length, and these reads were considered as potential miRNAs.

The majority of the 15–30 nt long reads ranged from 18 to 24 nt, and reads of 22 nt long were more abundant than reads of other lengths, indicating that the distribution of the small RNA sequences was consistent with the length range of miRNAs (Figure 2). In other words, most of the 15–30 nt long reads were likely miRNAs. A further analysis showed that most of the small RNAs could be mapped to the chicken genome. After the 15–30 nt reads were counted and grouped to generate unique reads, total reads or unique reads were compared to the sequences in Rfam database and classified. About 75% of total reads matched the sequences in Rfam. As shown in Figure 3, among the matched reads, ~80% of total reads represented miRNAs, and ~20% of unique reads represented miRNAs, indicating that the sequenced small RNA reads were enriched with miRNAs.

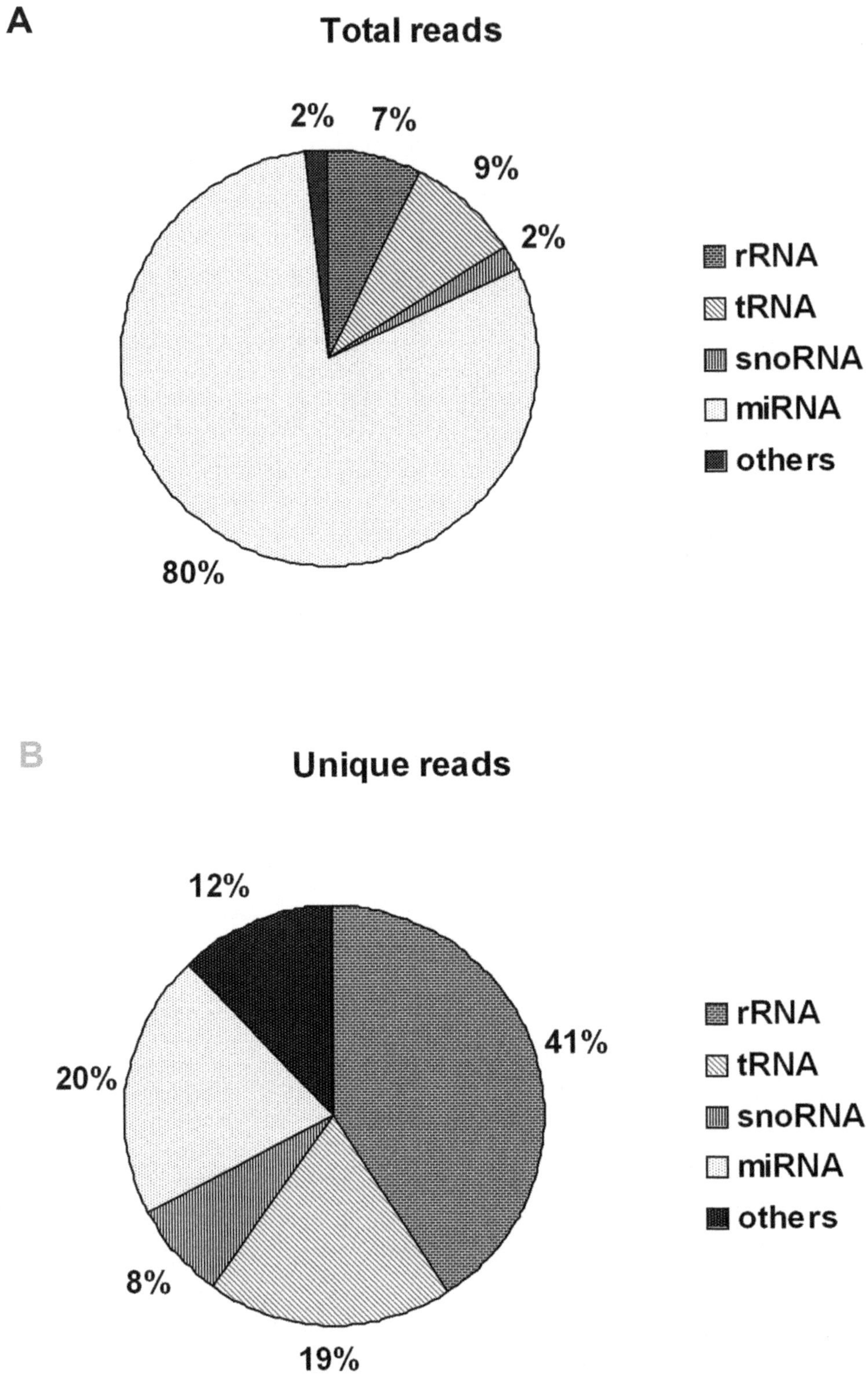

Figure 3. Annotation of small RNA sequences. (A) Annotation of total sequence reads. (B) Annotation of unique sequence reads.

The unique reads that matched miRNAs in Rfam were BLAST searched against chicken miRNAs in miRBase (20). Of 996 known chicken miRNAs in miRBase, 225 were identified in the present study. Among them, 219 known chicken miRNAs were identified from PBS-treated and 206 were identified from chGH-treated hepatocytes, which corresponded to 491 and 422 known chicken miRNA precursors, respectively (Tables 7 and S4). The remaining reads that did not match known chicken miRNAs were BLAST searched against all the miRNAs in other species, and 264 homologous miRNAs were identified. Of them, 259 were from PBS-treated cells and 234 were from chGH-treated cells (Table S5). The small RNA reads that had no matches in Rfam were

Table 7. Identification of known chicken miRNAs from chicken hepatocytes.

	miRNA	precursor	miRNA (unique)	miRNA (total)	precursor (unique)	precursor (total)
miRBase	996	734	-	-	-	-
PBS	219	491	5,010	1,552,789	8,447	1,958,885
chGH	206	422	4,240	751,527	6,927	948,397

analyzed to predict novel miRNAs and their precursors. A total of 95 sequences were predicted to be novel miRNAs, of which 93 were sequenced from PBS-treated cells and 73 from chGH-treated cells (Table S6). We estimated the potential of the precursor sequences for these miRNAs to form stable stem-loop hairpin structures (Figure S1). Interestingly, some of these sequences are related to known chicken miRNAs. For example, the predicted novel chicken miRNA gga-m0015-3p is complementary to the known chicken miRNA gga-miR-126-5p, the 3′ portion of gga-m0016-5p overlaps with the 5′ portion of gga-miR-219b, and the 5′ portion of gga-m0028-3p overlaps with the 3′ portion of gga-miR-3525 (Figure S2).

4. GH-regulated miRNAs

We estimated the expression levels of miRNAs based on their read numbers. The 10 most abundantly expressed miRNAs in chicken hepatocytes were listed in Table S7. Among the identified known chicken miRNAs, 17 were identified as DEM between PBS-treated and chGH-treated hepatocytes, of which 16 were up-regulated and 1 was down-regulated by chGH. Among the identified chicken miRNAs homologous to miRNAs in other species, 21 were DEM between PBS-treated and chGH-treated hepatocytes, of which 15 were up-regulated and 6 were down-regulated in chGH-treated cells. Among the predicted novel chicken miRNAs, 7 were DEM between PBS-treated and chGH-treated cells, of which 5 were up-regulated and 2 were down-regulated by chGH (Table 8).

5. Functional analysis of GH-regulated miRNAs

The major function of miRNAs is to down-regulate the expression of target mRNAs. To investigate the function of GH-regulated miRNAs, we determined which of the GH-regulated mRNAs could be targeted by the GH-regulated miRNAs. Among the GH down-regulated mRNAs, 32 were predicted as targets of GH up-regulated miRNAs. Among the GH up-regulated mRNAs, 12 were predicted as target genes of GH down-regulated miRNAs (Table 9). A GO enrichment analysis showed that these miRNA target genes were enriched in lipid metabolism, lipid binding, cell motility, and small molecule metabolic process (Figure 4). The most significant GO term was the lipid metabolic process. As shown in Table 10, the GH up-regulated miRNAs targeted 7 genes related to lipid metabolism and the GH down-regulated miRNAs were predicted to target one gene related to lipid metabolism. Among these GH-regulated miRNAs, miR-15b had more predicted target genes related to lipid metabolism than had any other miRs. Several GH-regulated miRNAs were predicted to target the same genes (Table 10).

Discussion

In this research through RNA-seq, we found a total of 164 DEG between chGH-treated and untreated chicken hepatocytes. Functional analyses showed most of the GH-regulated genes are involved in liver metabolism, indicating that GH regulates liver metabolism. Lipid metabolism is different between birds and mammals. In mammals lipogenesis occurs in liver, adipose tissue, and mammary gland, whereas in birds this occurs mostly in liver [37]. Lipid metabolic process was identified as a significant GO term among chGH-regulated genes, indicating that GH might play an important regulatory role in lipid metabolism in chicken hepatocytes. In the study of human adipose tissue, Zhao et al. (2011) found the GH-regulated DEG include those that stimulate triglyceride (TG)/ free fatty acid (FFA) cycle, and they also found a new TG hydrolase gene called patatin-like phospholipase domain containing 3 (*PNPLA3*), which could promote TG hydrolysis [38]. Comparing our DEG with those in the above report, we found there was little overlap, indicating the mechanism of GH regulation of lipid metabolism is different between birds and mammals, or between adipose tissue and liver. The chicken *PNPLA4* identified in our study is homologous to *PNPLA3* in mammals, suggesting this gene may play a role in regulating TG hydrolysis in the chicken liver.

In addition to genes that are involved in animal growth, many of the 164 DEG are involved in biosynthetic process (Table S8). This suggests that GH stimulates body growth in chickens not only by stimulating cell proliferation and hypertrophy but also by stimulating nutrient accumulation.

Recent research indicated that multiple signaling pathways are activated by GH, including the JAK2-STAT pathway, the MAPK-ERK1/2 pathway and the PI3K-AKT pathway [12]. In this study, 31 DEG are transcription factors or signaling molecules. Some of them belong to the pathways known to be activated by GH [35,36] while others belong to pathways that are not known to be activated by GH. Further study of the DEG showed that some of them, for example CAMK1D, had both DNA binding activity and tyrosine kinase activity. Another interesting GH-regulated transcription factor is BCL6. Studies showed that the expression of *BCL6* was controlled by GH through STAT5, and as a transcription factor BCL6 could mediate downstream gene expression [39,40]. We found that chicken *BCL6* gene has 11 potential STAT5 binding sites (data not shown), implying it could be regulated by chGH through STAT5.

The KEGG pathway analysis of GH-regulated DEG showed the KO terms were mainly related to metabolism, in particular, lipid metabolism. Two DEG were involved in fat digestion and absorption. One of them is *FABP1*, which is an important lipid-related gene [41] and has been shown to be up-regulated by GH in young chickens [42]. The other gene *PPAP2B* is involved in the glycerolipid metabolism pathway.

Among the identified miRNAs in this study, gga-miR-148a is the most abundant miRNA in chicken hepatocytes. This is consistent with the previous report, in which miR-148a was identified as the most abundant miRNA in porcine livers of different breeds [43]. This result indicated miR-148a might play important roles in liver. From many previous reports, miR-122

Table 8. chGH-regulated miRNAs among the identified known and predicted chicken miRNAs.

miRNA	RPM (PBS)	RPM (chGH)	fold change (RPM (chGH/PBS))	p-value
DEM among the identified known chicken miRNAs				
up-regulated miRNA				
gga-miR-15b	35.3	63.9	1.8	2.27E-07
gga-miR-19b	263.9	451.0	1.7	5.49E-36
gga-miR-29b	31.5	49.0	1.6	4.71E-04
gga-miR-99a-5p	9.2	15.4	1.7	0.022
gga-miR-146b-3p	3.8	7.5	2.0	0.043
gga-miR-181a-3p	45.0	68.6	1.5	7.91E-05
gga-miR-190	96.0	162.8	1.7	1.02E-13
gga-miR-193a	17.9	30.8	1.7	8.78E-04
gga-miR-194	15.6	23.8	1.5	0.019
gga-miR-223	55.7	94.2	1.7	1.71E-08
gga-miR-455-3p	15.5	24.7	1.6	0.008
gga-miR-1306	0.6	3.7	6.5	0.003
gga-miR-1618-5p	1.1	4.2	3.7	0.011
gga-miR-1628	0.4	2.3	6.1	0.019
gga-miR-1699	1.5	5.6	3.7	0.003
gga-miR-1731	35.9	56.0	1.6	1.72E-04
down-regulated miRNA				
gga-miR-1724	2.3	0.01	0.004	0.023
DEM among the miRNAs homologous to miRNAs in other species				
up-regulated miRNA				
aca-miR-16b-5p	3.2	7.9	2.4	0.009
aca-miR-30c-3p	11.1	19.6	1.8	0.005
ahy-miR-3512	21.4	52.7	2.5	2.30E-11
bta-miR-139	11.8	22.4	1.9	0.001
ccr-miR-92a	21.2	43.8	2.1	3.20E-07
ccr-miR-99	1.1	3.7	3.3	0.024
hsa-miR-34a-3p	1.7	4.7	2.7	0.027
hsa-miR-4792	852.8	1356.3	1.6	3.19E-81
mmu-miR-6238	0.8	2.8	3.7	0.036
oan-miR-1335	41.0	71.8	1.8	1.84E-07
ola-miR-122	19.3	30.3	1.6	0.005
ppt-miR-894	9.5	15.9	1.7	0.022
tca-miR-3885-5p	14.3	27.1	1.9	3.19E-04
xtr-miR-210	11.8	24.3	2.0	1.60E-04
xtr-miR-212	1.7	5.1	3.0	0.013
down-regulated miRNA				
ccr-miR-22b	12.2	5.1	0.4	0.005
ccr-miR-26a	75.8	29.4	0.4	9.45E-15
ccr-miR-130c	10.9	4.7	0.4	0.009
cgr-miR-425-5p	13.2	4.7	0.4	7.79E-04
ggo-let-7f	71.2	37.8	0.5	4.46E-08
ggo-miR-146a	34.34	11.2	0.3	4.96E-09
DEM among the predicted novel miRNAs				
up-regulated miRNA				
gga-m0060-3p	0.01	1.9	186.6	0.004
gga-m0006-5p	0.01	1.4	139.9	0.014
gga-m0072-3p	0.8	2.8	3.7	0.036
gga-m0085-3p	5.0	12.6	2.5	7.13E-04

Table 8. Cont.

miRNA	RPM (PBS)	RPM (chGH)	fold change (RPM (chGH/PBS))	p-value
gga-m0073-3p	6.9	14.0	2.0	0.004
down-regulated miRNA				
gga-m0018-5p	1.9	0.01	0.005	0.046
gga-m0011-5p	2.9	0.01	0.003	0.008

was known as the most abundant miRNA in liver. But in our study gga-miR-122-5p (previously named gga-miR-122) was identified as the fifth abundant miRNA in primary chicken hepatocytes, similar to the report by Li et al. which found miR-122 was the fourth abundant miRNA in porcine liver [43].

The differentially expressed miRNAs identified in this study might play various important roles in chGH regulation of growth, development and metabolism. miR-223 is expressed higher in the liver of Large White pig (lean type) than in the liver of Tongcheng pig (fatty type) [44]. In this study, we found gga-miR-223 was up-regulated by chGH, indicating it might play a role in lipid metabolism in chicken liver. miR-193a and -190 are expressed at higher levels in the liver of Erhualian pig than in the liver of Large White pig (The two breeds have different rate of lipid metabolism) [43]. In this study gga-miR-193a and 190 were also up-regulated by chGH, indicating they may play roles in lipid metabolism in chicken liver too. miR-15b was another up-regulated miRNA by the chGH treatment. This miRNA in pigs is expressed at a lower level in the liver of Erhualian pig than in the liver of Large White pig, opposite to miR-193a and -190 [43], implying it may play different roles between chickens and pigs. In male rat livers, miR-451 and miR-29b are down-regulated by GH [45]. gga-miR-451 was too down-regulated by GH in chicken hepatocytes in our study, indicating gga-miR-451 might mediate GH regulation of chicken liver metabolism but gga-miR-29b played different roles in GH regulation of liver metabolism comparing to miR-29b in rat. The expression of miR-122 is not changed by GH in male rat liver [45]. We found the same for gga-miR-122 in this study, indicating this miRNA might not be involved in GH regulation of liver metabolism. In this study we also found that some of GH-regulated DEG were potential targets of GH-regulated DEM. GO enrichment analysis showed that these DEG were enriched with genes involved in lipid metabolism, indicating that GH may regulate lipid metabolism through miRNAs. Among the GH-regulated DEM, miR-15b was predicted to target more GH-regulated DEG related to lipid metabolism than any other DEM, including ACSL3, LIPG, PLCD1, PPAP2B and STAR. miR-15b expression was increased in NAFLD models and it lead to inducing the storage of intracellular triglyceride [46]. When ACSL3 increases, triglycerides and free fatty acids reduce [47]. Knock down of ACSL3 decrease hepatic lipogenesis [48]. LIPG has substantial phospholipase activity, and it can reduce plasma concentrations of HDL cholesterol [49]. PLCD1 can catalyze the hydrolysis of membrane lipid phosphatidylinositol 4,5-bisphosphate into second messengers inositol 1,4,5-trisphosphate and diacylglycerol [50]. PPAP2B bioactive lysophospholipids, including lysophosphatidic acid and sphingosine-1-phosphate, and thereby terminates their signaling effects [51]. STAR plays a critical role in the rapid translocation of cholesterol across the outer and inner mitochondrial membranes [52]. It also plays a key role in steroidogenesis by enhancing the metabolism of cholesterol into pregnenolone [53]. This finding indicates miR-15b might be a

Table 9. GH-regulated chicken genes predicted to be targeted by GH-regulated chicken miRNAs.

miRNA	Target gene
gga-miR-15b	ABCG5, ABHD2, ACSL3, CBLB, ETNPPL, FAM3C, HEPHL1, HIVEP2, KIAA0408, KIAA1107, LIPG, MAST4, MYRIP, NCAM1, PANK1, PLCD1, PPAP2B, RGS6, STAR
gga-miR-19b	ABHD2, AKAP13, ALDH1A3, CBLB, LIPG, MYRIP, PPAP2B, SERPINB6
gga-miR-29b	ABCG5, ABCG8, AKAP13, LIPG, MAST4, PPAP2B, PRRG1, ROBO1, TSKU
gga-miR-146b-3p	ABHD2, ANXA13, PLCD1
gga-miR-190	CBLB, ELOVL6, MYRIP
gga-miR-193a	ABHD2, KIAA0408, MYRIP, PLCD1, PRRG1
gga-miR-194	ABHD2, AKAP13, CBLB, MAST4, MYRIP, PLCD1
gga-miR-223	ALDH1A3, CBLB, MAST4, PLCD1
gga-miR-455-3p	ABHD2, ELOVL6
gga-miR-1306	ABCG8, ANXA13, AKAP13, CCK1R
gga-miR-1618-5p	HEPHL1, MYRIP, SERPINB1
gga-miR-1628	ABHD2, CBLB, LIPG, PANK1, PLCD1, RGS6, SERPINB1, TPPP
gga-miR-1699	ABHD2, AKAP13, HEPHL1, MAST4, PLCD1, PPAP2B, PRRG1, TPPP
gga-miR-1724	AASS, CAMK1D, COQ4, DNAAF2, ECI1, EGLN3, FURIN, FZD5, PXDC1, RETSAT, TMEM229B, TOB2
gga-miR-1731	ABCG5, CCK1R, KIAA1107, PPAP2B, PRRG1, SPTBN1

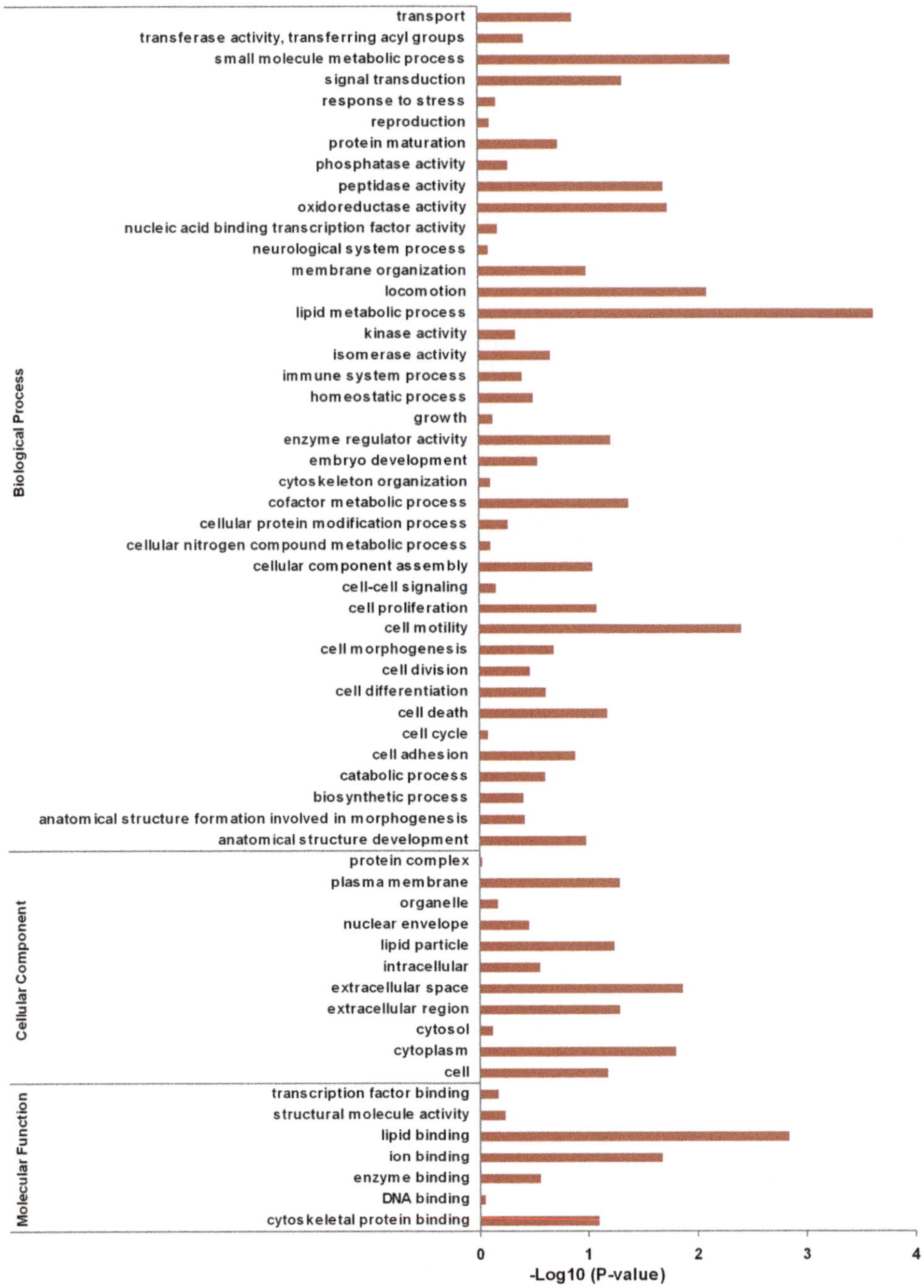

Figure 4. GO enrichment analysis of chGH-regulated mRNAs predicted to be targeted by GH-regulated miRNAs. The target mRNAs for GH up-regulated miRNAs were predicted in the GH down-regulated mRNAs; the target mRNAs for GH down-regulated miRNAs were predicted in the GH up-regulated mRNAs.

very important miRNA that mediates the effect of GH on lipid metabolism in chicken liver.

In mammals, the secretion of GH is characterized by an ultradian rhythm and sexual dimorphism. In the male rat, the major bursts of GH secretion occur at regular 3.3 h intervals separated by intervening trough periods with very low or undetectable basal GH levels [54,55]. GH is also secreted in a pulsatile manner in chickens [56,57]. In this study, hepatocytes from chickens were treated with one concentration of GH in culture. Therefore, a limitation of the study is that the observed GH-regulated mRNA and miRNA expression profiles may not represent those that occur in the chicken liver *in vivo*.

Conclusions

This study reveals that GH regulates the expression of many mRNAs involved in metabolism in female chicken hepatocytes, which suggests that GH plays an important role in regulating hepatic metabolism besides somatic growth. This study suggests that GH regulates lipid metabolism in female chicken liver in part

Table 10. Lipid metabolism-related genes predicted to be targeted by chGH-regulated miRNAs.

miRNA	Predicted target gene
up-regulated miRNA	
gga-miR-15b	ACSL3, LIPG, PLCD1, PPAP2B, STAR
gga-miR-19b	ALDH1A3, LIPG, PPAP2B
gga-miR-29b	LIPG, PPAP2B
gga-miR-146b-3p	PLCD1
gga-miR-190	ELOV6
gga-miR-193a	PLCD1
gga-miR-194	PLCD1
gga-miR-223	ALDH1A3, PLCD1
gga-miR-455-3p	ELOV6
gga-miR-1628	LIPG, PLCD1
gga-miR-1699	PLCD1, PPAP2B
gga-miR-1731	PPAP2B
down-regulated miRNA	
gga-miR-1724	RETSAT

by regulating the expression of miRNAs that target the mRNAs involved in lipid metabolism.

Supporting Information

Figure S1 Structures of predicted novel miRNAs. For each novel miRNA, the precursor name, position, strand, length and energy are shown in the first line. The sequence of precursor and total reads are described in the second line. The brackets in the third line denote the secondary structure. The sequence of major unique reads, novel miRNA name and the number of reads are shown below with '*'. Then the sequence of each unique reads and the number of reads are shown below with '−'.

Figure S2 Relationship between predicted novel miRNAs and known chicken miRNAs. For each novel miRNA, the name is listed in the first line. The sequence of known precursor and its name are described in the second line. The sequence of known miRNA and its name are shown below with '*'. Then the sequence of novel miRNA and its name are shown below with '−'. Note: The sequence of gga-m0015-3p is complementary to gga-miR-126-5p.

Table S1 Primers for real time RT-PCR.

Table S2 Differentially expressed genes by chGH treatment.

Table S3 KEGG of differentially expressed genes.

Table S4 Identified known chicken miRNAs.

Table S5 Identified miRNAs homologous to other species.

Table S6 Predicted novel miRNAs.

Table S7 Ten most abundant miRNAs.

Table S8 Differentially expressed genes related with biosynthetic process.

Author Contributions

Conceived and designed the experiments: HJ ZG. Performed the experiments: XW LY HW FS JY. Analyzed the data: XW LY ZG. Contributed to the writing of the manuscript: XW LY HJ YH DG ZG. Wrote the paper: XW LY HJ YH DG ZG.

References

1. Davidson MB (1987) Effect of growth hormone on carbohydrate and lipid metabolism. Endocr Rev 8: 115–131.
2. Press M (1988) Growth hormone and metabolism. Diabetes Metab Rev 4: 391–414.
3. Vijayakumar A, Novosyadlyy R, Wu Y, Yakar S, LeRoith D (2010) Biological effects of growth hormone on carbohydrate and lipid metabolism. Growth Horm IGF Res 20: 1–7.
4. Waters MJ, Brooks AJ (2012) Growth hormone and cell growth. Endocr Dev 23: 86–95.
5. Bartke A (2000) Effects of growth hormone on male reproductive functions. J Androl 21: 181–188.
6. Hull KL, Harvey S (2001) Growth hormone: roles in female reproduction. J Endocrinol 168: 1–23.
7. Moller N, Jorgensen JO (2009) Effects of growth hormone on glucose, lipid, and protein metabolism in human subjects. Endocr Rev 30: 152–177.
8. Wells JA (1996) Binding in the growth hormone receptor complex. Proc Natl Acad Sci U S A 93: 1–6.
9. Gent J, van Kerkhof P, Roza M, Bu G, Strous GJ (2002) Ligand-independent growth hormone receptor dimerization occurs in the endoplasmic reticulum and is required for ubiquitin system-dependent endocytosis. Proc Natl Acad Sci U S A 99: 9858–9863.
10. Brown RJ, Adams JJ, Pelekanos RA, Wan Y, McKinstry WJ, et al. (2005) Model for growth hormone receptor activation based on subunit rotation within a receptor dimer. Nat Struct Mol Biol 12: 814–821.
11. Argetsinger LS, Campbell GS, Yang X, Witthuhn BA, Silvennoinen O, et al. (1993) Identification of JAK2 as a growth hormone receptor-associated tyrosine kinase. Cell 74: 237–244.
12. Lanning NJ, Carter-Su C (2006) Recent advances in growth hormone signaling. Rev Endocr Metab Disord 7: 225–235.
13. O'Hea EK, Leveille GA (1968) Lipogenesis in isolated adipose tissue of the domestic chick (Gallus domesticus). Comp Biochem Physiol 26: 111–120.
14. Leveille GA, O'Hea EK, Chakbabarty K (1968) In vivo lipogenesis in the domestic chicken. Proc Soc Exp Biol Med 128: 398–401.
15. Bartel DP (2004) MicroRNAs: genomics, biogenesis, mechanism, and function. Cell 116: 281–297.
16. Chang J, Nicolas E, Marks D, Sander C, Lerro A, et al. (2004) miR-122, a mammalian liver-specific microRNA, is processed from hcr mRNA and may downregulate the high affinity cationic amino acid transporter CAT-1. RNA Biol 1: 106–113.
17. Krutzfeldt J, Rajewsky N, Braich R, Rajeev KG, Tuschl T, et al. (2005) Silencing of microRNAs in vivo with 'antagomirs'. Nature 438: 685–689.
18. Esau C, Davis S, Murray SF, Yu XX, Pandey SK, et al. (2006) miR-122 regulation of lipid metabolism revealed by in vivo antisense targeting. Cell Metab 3: 87–98.
19. Rayner KJ, Suarez Y, Davalos A, Parathath S, Fitzgerald ML, et al. (2010) MiR-33 contributes to the regulation of cholesterol homeostasis. Science 328: 1570–1573.
20. Gerin I, Clerbaux LA, Haumont O, Lanthier N, Das AK, et al. (2010) Expression of miR-33 from an SREBP2 intron inhibits cholesterol export and fatty acid oxidation. J Biol Chem 285: 33652–33661.
21. Mortazavi A, Williams BA, McCue K, Schaeffer L, Wold B (2008) Mapping and quantifying mammalian transcriptomes by RNA-Seq. Nat Methods 5: 621–628.
22. Cloonan N, Forrest AR, Kolle G, Gardiner BB, Faulkner GJ, et al. (2008) Stem cell transcriptome profiling via massive-scale mRNA sequencing. Nat Methods 5: 613–619.

23. Trapnell C, Roberts A, Goff L, Pertea G, Kim D, et al. (2012) Differential gene and transcript expression analysis of RNA-seq experiments with TopHat and Cufflinks. Nat Protoc 7: 562–578.
24. Creighton CJ, Reid JG, Gunaratne PH (2009) Expression profiling of microRNAs by deep sequencing. Brief Bioinform 10: 490–497.
25. Brooks AJ, Waters MJ (2010) The growth hormone receptor: mechanism of activation and clinical implications. Nat Rev Endocrinol 6: 515–525.
26. Ono M, Chia DJ, Merino-Martinez R, Flores-Morales A, Unterman TG, et al. (2007) Signal transducer and activator of transcription (Stat) 5b-mediated inhibition of insulin-like growth factor binding protein-1 gene transcription: a mechanism for repression of gene expression by growth hormone. Mol Endocrinol 21: 1443–1457.
27. Campbell RM, Scanes CG (1988) Pharmacological investigations on the lipolytic and antilipolytic effects of growth hormone (GH) in chicken adipose tissue in vitro: evidence for involvement of calcium and polyamines. Proc Soc Exp Biol Med 188: 177–184.
28. Cupo MA, Cartwright AL (1989) Lipid synthesis and lipoprotein secretion by chick liver cells in culture: influence of growth hormone and insulin-like growth factor-I. Comp Biochem Physiol B 94: 355–360.
29. Harvey S (2013) Growth hormone and growth? Gen Comp Endocrinol 190: 3–9.
30. Wang XG, Shao F, Wang HJ, Yang L, Yu JF, et al. (2013) MicroRNA-126 expression is decreased in cultured primary chicken hepatocytes and targets the sprouty-related EVH1 domain containing 1 mRNA. Poult Sci 92: 1888–1896.
31. Ambros V, Bartel B, Bartel DP, Burge CB, Carrington JC, et al. (2003) A uniform system for microRNA annotation. RNA 9: 277–279.
32. Chen C, Deng B, Qiao M, Zheng R, Chai J, et al. (2012) Solexa sequencing identification of conserved and novel microRNAs in backfat of Large White and Chinese Meishan pigs. PLoS One 7: e31426.
33. Albagli O, Lantoine D, Quief S, Quignon F, Englert C, et al. (1999) Overexpressed BCL6 (LAZ3) oncoprotein triggers apoptosis, delays S phase progression and associates with replication foci. Oncogene 18: 5063–5075.
34. Marlow R, Strickland P, Lee JS, Wu X, Pebenito M, et al. (2008) SLITs suppress tumor growth in vivo by silencing Sdf1/Cxcr4 within breast epithelium. Cancer Res 68: 7819–7827.
35. Herrington J, Smit LS, Schwartz J, Carter-Su C (2000) The role of STAT proteins in growth hormone signaling. Oncogene 19: 2585–2597.
36. Winston LA, Hunter T (1995) JAK2, Ras, and Raf are required for activation of extracellular signal-regulated kinase/mitogen-activated protein kinase by growth hormone. J Biol Chem 270: 30837–30840.
37. Bergen WG, Mersmann HJ (2005) Comparative aspects of lipid metabolism: impact on contemporary research and use of animal models. J Nutr 135: 2499–2502.
38. Zhao JT, Cowley MJ, Lee P, Birzniece V, Kaplan W, et al. (2011) Identification of novel GH-regulated pathway of lipid metabolism in adipose tissue: a gene expression study in hypopituitary men. J Clin Endocrinol Metab 96: E1188–1196.
39. Chen Y, Lin G, Huo JS, Barney D, Wang Z, et al. (2009) Computational and functional analysis of growth hormone (GH)-regulated genes identifies the transcriptional repressor B-cell lymphoma 6 (Bc16) as a participant in GH-regulated transcription. Endocrinology 150: 3645–3654.
40. Zhang Y, Laz EV, Waxman DJ (2012) Dynamic, sex-differential STAT5 and BCL6 binding to sex-biased, growth hormone-regulated genes in adult mouse liver. Mol Cell Biol 32: 880–896.
41. Musso G, Gambino R, Cassader M (2009) Recent insights into hepatic lipid metabolism in non-alcoholic fatty liver disease (NAFLD). Prog Lipid Res 48: 1–26.
42. Wang X, Carre W, Saxton AM, Cogburn LA (2007) Manipulation of thyroid status and/or GH injection alters hepatic gene expression in the juvenile chicken. Cytogenet Genome Res 117: 174–188.
43. Li R, Sun Q, Jia Y, Cong R, Ni Y, et al. (2012) Coordinated miRNA/mRNA expression profiles for understanding breed-specific metabolic characters of liver between Erhualian and large white pigs. PLoS One 7: e38716.
44. Xie SS, Li XY, Liu T, Cao JH, Zhong Q, et al. (2011) Discovery of porcine microRNAs in multiple tissues by a Solexa deep sequencing approach. PLoS One 6: e16235.
45. Cheung L, Gustavsson C, Norstedt G, Tollet-Egnell P (2009) Sex-different and growth hormone-regulated expression of microRNA in rat liver. BMC Mol Biol 10: 13.
46. Zhang Y, Cheng X, Lu Z, Wang J, Chen H, et al. (2013) Upregulation of miR-15b in NAFLD models and in the serum of patients with fatty liver disease. Diabetes Res Clin Pract 99: 327–334.
47. Wu M, Cao A, Dong B, Liu J (2011) Reduction of serum free fatty acids and triglycerides by liver-targeted expression of long chain acyl-CoA synthetase 3. Int J Mol Med 27: 655–662.
48. Bu SY, Mashek MT, Mashek DG (2009) Suppression of long chain acyl-CoA synthetase 3 decreases hepatic de novo fatty acid synthesis through decreased transcriptional activity. J Biol Chem 284: 30474–30483.
49. Jaye M, Lynch KJ, Krawiec J, Marchadier D, Maugeais C, et al. (1999) A novel endothelial-derived lipase that modulates HDL metabolism. Nat Genet 21: 424–428.
50. Sidhu RS, Clough RR, Bhullar RP (2005) Regulation of phospholipase C-delta1 through direct interactions with the small GTPase Ral and calmodulin. J Biol Chem 280: 21933–21941.
51. Ren H, Panchatcharam M, Mueller P, Escalante-Alcalde D, Morris AJ, et al. (2013) Lipid phosphate phosphatase (LPP3) and vascular development. Biochim Biophys Acta 1831: 126–132.
52. Estabrook RW, Rainey WE (1996) Twinkle, twinkle little StAR, how we wonder what you are. Proc Natl Acad Sci U S A 93: 13552–13554.
53. Sugawara T, Lin D, Holt JA, Martin KO, Javitt NB, et al. (1995) Structure of the human steroidogenic acute regulatory protein (StAR) gene: StAR stimulates mitochondrial cholesterol 27-hydroxylase activity. Biochemistry 34: 12506–12512.
54. Tannenbaum GS, Martin JB (1976) Evidence for an endogenous ultradian rhythm governing growth hormone secretion in the rat. Endocrinology 98: 562–570.
55. Stroh T, van Schouwenburg MR, Beaudet A, Tannenbaum GS (2009) Subcellular dynamics of somatostatin receptor subtype 1 in the rat arcuate nucleus: receptor localization and synaptic connectivity vary in parallel with the ultradian rhythm of growth hormone secretion. J Neurosci 29: 8198–8205.
56. Johnson RJ (1988) Diminution of pulsatile growth hormone secretion in the domestic fowl (Gallus domesticus): evidence of sexual dimorphism. J Endocrinol 119: 101–109.
57. Buonomo FC, Lauterio TJ, Scanes CG (1984) Episodic growth hormone secretion in the domestic fowl (Gallus domesticus): alpha adrenergic regulation. Comp Biochem Physiol C 78: 409–413.

18

Selected Lactic Acid-Producing Bacterial Isolates with the Capacity to Reduce *Salmonella* Translocation and Virulence Gene Expression in Chickens

Xiaojian Yang[1], Jennifer Brisbin[2], Hai Yu[1], Qi Wang[1], Fugui Yin[1], Yonggang Zhang[1], Parviz Sabour[1], Shayan Sharif[2], Joshua Gong[1]*

1 Guelph Food Research Centre, Agriculture and Agri-Food Canada, Guelph, Ontario, Canada, **2** Department of Pathobiology, University of Guelph, Guelph, Ontario, Canada

Abstract

Background: Probiotics have been used to control *Salmonella* colonization/infection in chickens. Yet the mechanisms of probiotic effects are not fully understood. This study has characterized our previously-selected lactic acid-producing bacterial (LAB) isolates for controlling *Salmonella* infection in chickens, particularly the mechanism underlying the control.

Methodology/Principal Findings: *In vitro* studies were conducted to characterize 14 LAB isolates for their tolerance to low pH (2.0) and high bile salt (0.3–1.5%) and susceptibility to antibiotics. Three chicken infection trials were subsequently carried out to evaluate four of the isolates for reducing the burden of *Salmonella enterica* serovar Typhimurium in the broiler cecum. Chicks were gavaged with LAB cultures (10^{6-7} CFU/chick) or phosphate-buffered saline (PBS) at 1 day of age followed by *Salmonella* challenge (10^4 CFU/chick) next day. Samples of cecal digesta, spleen, and liver were examined for *Salmonella* counts on days 1, 3, or 4 post-challenge. *Salmonella* in the cecum from Trial 3 was also assessed for the expression of ten virulence genes located in its pathogenicity island-1 (SPI-1). These genes play a role in *Salmonella* intestinal invasion. Tested LAB isolates (individuals or mixed cultures) were unable to lower *Salmonella* burden in the chicken cecum, but able to attenuate *Salmonella* infection in the spleen and liver. The LAB treatments also reduced almost all SPI-1 virulence gene expression (9 out of 10) in the chicken cecum, particularly at the low dose. *In vitro* treatment with the extracellular culture fluid from a LAB culture also down-regulated most SPI-1 virulence gene expression.

Conclusions/Significance: The possible correlation between attenuation of *Salmonella* infection in the chicken spleen and liver and reduction of *Salmonella* SPI-1 virulence gene expression in the chicken cecum by LAB isolates is a new observation. Suppression of *Salmonella* virulence gene expression *in vivo* can be one of the strategies for controlling *Salmonella* infection in chickens.

Editor: Mrutyunjay Suar, KIIT University, India

Funding: This research was supported by Agriculture & Agri-Food Canada and Ontario Ministry of Agriculture and Food Research - Food Safety Research Program. XY was a NSERC Visiting Fellows to the Canadian Federal Government Laboratories (NSERC-VF). The funders had no role in study design, data collection and analysis, decision to publish, or preparation of the manuscript.

Competing Interests: The authors have declared that no competing interests exist.

* E-mail: joshua.gong@agr.gc.ca

Introduction

Salmonella is a zoonotic pathogen. Its infection in human and domestic animals remains a serious and worldwide issue in public health, food safety, and livestock economies [1]. Consumption of *Salmonella*-contaminated livestock and their products, particularly poultry and poultry products, has often led to salmonellosis in humans. In addition, the increased level of antibiotic resistance in *Salmonella* recovered from animals potentially erodes the therapeutic effectiveness in antibiotic treatment of animal and human disease. Thus, control of *Salmonella* infection in animals is still urgently required.

Salmonella enterica serovar Typhimurium is one of three serotypes, sometimes responsible for 50% of the salmonellosis cases in humans [2]. The susceptibility of humans and animals to *Salmonella* infection is generally determined by both *Salmonella* virulence and host factors, such as age and genetics. The infection normally starts from the intestinal phase, through which *Salmonella* can enter the blood circulation and spread to various organs such as the liver and spleen, leading to systemic infection. There are two pathogenicity islands in *Salmonella* that are closely associated with virulence [3]. *Salmonella* pathogenicity island 1 (SPI-1) is critical in causing the intestinal phase of infection [3], while *Salmonella* pathogenicity island 2 (SPI-2) is essential for intracellular multiplication, which is necessary for systemic infection [4]. The SPI-1 is composed of a 40-kb DNA region coding for the type III secretion system (T3SS), including the structural, effector, and regulatory proteins.

It is important to control *Salmonella* infection at the farm level in order to reduce *Salmonella* contamination in poultry and poultry products. Attempts to control *Salmonella* infection and carriage by vaccination and antibiotic treatment of chickens have not yet produced significant results [5,6]. An alternative approach has been the use of competitive exclusion and probiotics [7]. Competitive exclusion of *Salmonella* is achieved by enhancing the establishment of normal intestinal microbiota in newly hatched chickens and thus inhibiting intestinal colonization of *Salmonella* [8]. Probiotics can have different modes of action to control the infection of enteric pathogens, such as secretion of antimicrobial substances (for example bacteriocins) [9], enhancement of digestive functions [10], and modulation of the mucosal and systemic immune responses [11,12]. Control of *Salmonella* burden and colonization has been one of the common strategies. Previous studies have shown that the expression of gene encoding virulence factors of *Salmonella* can be modulated by probiotics *in vitro* [13,14,15,16,17]. Recently, we identified several lactic acid-producing bacterial (LAB) isolates that were able to protect *Caenorhabditis elegans* from death caused by *S.* Typhimurium infection [18]. In the present study, we have investigated the probiotic properties of these isolates and, moreover, if they are able to reduce *Salmonella* infection in broilers and also modulate *Salmonella* SPI-1 virulence gene expression.

Results

Resistance of selected lactic acid-producing bacterial isolates to low pH, high bile salt, and antibiotics determined by *in vitro* studies

Among the 14 tested LAB isolates, eight (ALB2, ALB6, CL9, L3, LB1, LB2, LB4, and S64) have been reported previously to have antimicrobial activity towards *S.* Typhimurium DT104 [18]. The remaining six isolates (K16, K67, S8, S33, S66, and SG2) were also tested for their antimicrobial activity using the method of spot-on-the-lawn [19]. These isolates were able to inhibit the growth of *S.* Typhimurium DT104 with clear inhibition halos (diameter $\geq$16 mm).

Table 1 shows the tolerance of 14 selected LAB isolates to low pH pretreatment. Six isolates (ALB2, CL9, L3, LB1, LB4, and SG2) had similar optical densities at 600 nm (OD_{600}) after growth regardless if the cultures had been pretreated at pH 2 or 5.6, indicating their tolerance to low pH. However, the growth of seven out of eight remaining isolates (K16, K67, LB2, S8, S33, S64, and S66) was inhibited by the low pH pretreatment ($P<0.05$). In the test to examine tolerance to high bile salt, four (ALB2, CL9, K16, and S33) out of the 14 isolates showed poor growth ($OD_{600}<0.5$) after 24 h incubation at 37°C at most concentrations of bile salt above 0.3% (v/v), suggesting that they are sensitive to bile acid (Table 2). Eight isolates (K67, L3, LB1, LB2, LB4, S8, S66, and SG2) were able to grow with OD_{600} values greater than 1.0 at concentrations of bile salt from 0.3% to 1.5% (v/v), indicating good tolerance to bile salt. The remaining two isolates (ALB6 and S64) had a moderate growth with the OD_{600} values between 0.5 and 1.0 after 24 h incubation at bile salt concentrations above 0.3% (v/v).

Table 3 shows the susceptibility of the 14 tested LAB isolates to eight different antibiotics. The isolates varied in their susceptibility to the antibiotics. Three isolates (LB1, LB2, and LB4) were susceptible to all tested antibiotics within the concentrations examined. The majority of remaining isolates grew at the highest concentration of one or two antibiotics. Based on the microbiological cut-off values set by the European Food Safety Authority [20] and the European Commission [21], the majority of the 14 isolates could be categorized as susceptible to ampicillin and erythromycin and about half of the isolates were resistant to gentamicin, tetracycline, and ciprofloxacin.

Effect of selected lactic acid-producing bacterial isolates on *Salmonella* burden in the cecum of chickens

Isolates LB1 (*Lactobacillus zeae*), S8 (*Lactobacillus plantarum*), S64 (*Lactobacillus reuteri*), and S33 (*Pediococcus pentosaceus*) were selected for further *in vivo* studies after the *in vitro* characterization. The selection was based on their resistance to low pH, high bile salt, and antibiotics, their species identification, and previously reported ability to protect *C. elegans* from death caused by *Salmonella* infection [18]. In the *in vivo* studies, cecal digesta samples from all negative control groups of chickens (three chicken trials) had undetectable *Salmonella* counts that were below the detection limit of the plating method (2×10^2 Colony Forming Units (CFU)/g digesta) [22]. In Trial 1, *Salmonella* counts in the cecal digesta from the chickens in the positive control group (challenged with *Salmonella* only) on day 4 post-infection (PI) were 5.33±0.13 (Log_{10} CFU/g fresh digesta). LB1, S8, S33, or S64 treatment groups had 5.70±0.12, 5.38±0.12, 5.47±0.13, or 5.78±0.07 Log_{10}CFU of *Salmonella*/g fresh digesta in their ceca. No significant difference among these five treatments ($P>0.05$) was found.

Since the experimental design of Trials 2 and 3 was identical, data from these two trials were analyzed by a mixed model with trial as a fixed effect (Table 4). When the data from Trials 2 and 3 were pooled, among the four probiotic treatment groups, the low and high dose mixed culture groups and the high dose LB1 group had significantly higher *Salmonella* counts in the cecal digesta on days 3 and 4 PI than the positive control, indicating that the selected individual probiotic candidates (LB1, S8, and S64) or their combination at the tested level could not reduce the *Salmonella* burden in the cecum of chickens.

Effect of selected lactic acid-producing bacterial isolates on invasion of *Salmonella* in the spleen and liver of chickens

In Trial 1, eight and seven birds out of the 12 birds from the positive control group were found to be *Salmonella* positive in the spleen or liver, respectively, on day 4 PI after the tissue samples were enriched for *Salmonella*. This suggests a successful *Salmonella* challenge at the dose of 1×10^4 CFU/chick. As shown in Tables 5 and 6, the data on spleen and liver infection from Trials 2 and 3 were combined for analyses with trial as a fixed effect. No significant effect ($P>0.05$) of trial was observed. Compared with the positive control, the treatment with a low dose of mixed LAB cultures was able to attenuate *Salmonella* infection in the spleen (73% vs. 32%, $P=0.06$) and liver (74% vs. 44%, $P=0.07$) on days 3 and 4 PI. A similar result was also observed with the treatment of low dose LB1, which reduced *Salmonella* infection in the liver (74% vs. 47%, $P=0.09$).

Effect of selected lactic acid-producing bacterial isolates on the SPI-1 virulence gene expression of *Salmonella* in the cecum of chickens

In Trial 3, expression of 10 SPI-1 virulence genes (*hilA, hilC, hilD, sopB, sopD, sopE2, sipA, sipC, avrA,* and *sptP*) of *Salmonella* in the cecal digesta of chickens was investigated by RT-qPCR assays. Compared with the *Salmonella* cells from the chickens in the positive control group, application of LB1 or mixed LAB cultures did not significantly ($P>0.05$) affect expression levels of the 10 virulence genes on day 1 PI. Interestingly, expression of all the genes except *hilC* in the *Salmonella* cells from all the LAB treatment groups of chickens, regardless of dose and combinations, was down-regulated by 4 to 257 fold ($P<0.05$) on day 3 PI compared with the positive control group (Table 7). The low dose group

Table 1. Growth (OD_{600}) of selected lactic acid-producing bacterial isolateswith or without pretreatment of low pH*.

	Optical density at 600 nm (OD_{600})	
Isolate#	**pH 5.6**	**pH 2.0**
ALB2	0.99^{a}	0.98^{a}
ALB6	0.85^{b}	0.88^{a}
CL9	1.00^{a}	1.01^{a}
K16	0.97^{a}	0.87^{b}
K67	1.07^{a}	0.89^{b}
L3	1.05^{a}	1.03^{a}
LB1	1.01^{a}	1.03^{a}
LB2	1.02^{a}	0.58^{b}
LB4	1.01^{a}	1.02^{a}
S8	1.04^{a}	0.75^{b}
S33	1.12^{a}	0.95^{b}
S64	0.93^{a}	0.72^{b}
S66	1.06^{a}	0.73^{b}
SG2	0.73^{a}	0.74^{a}

*Tolerance to low pH was evaluated by incubating bacterial cells in simulated gastric fluid (pH 2.0 or 5.6) for 2 h prior to anaerobic incubation in the MRS broth at 37°C for 20 h.Values without common superscript in a row are significantly different ($P<0.05$). Values were average of triplicates.
#The 14 selected lactic acid-producing bacterial isolates belong to *Lactobacillus crispatus* (SG2), *Lactobacillus plantarum* (S8 and S66), *Lactobacillus salivarius* (ALB2 and ALB6), *Lactobacillus reuteri* (CL9, K67, and S64), *Lactobacillus rhamnosus* (L3, LB2, and LB4), *Lactobacillus zeae* (LB1), and *Pediococcus pentosaceus*(K16 and S33), based on the sequence analysis of 16S rRNA genes. While isolates ALB2, ALB6, L3, LB1, LB2, LB4, and SG2are from chickens, isolates CL9, K16, K67, S8, S33, S64, and S66 have the pig origin.

treated with mixed LAB cultures had the most dramatic decrease (18 to 257 fold) for all the genes, followed by the low dose LB1 group. Nevertheless, there was no significant ($P>0.05$) difference in the gene expression of *Salmonella* from these four groups of chickens that had been treated with LAB isolates. *In vitro* expression of SPI-1 virulence genes was also examined. Nine out of the 10 virulence genes in *Salmonella* were down-regulated when co-cultured with the extracellular culture fluid (ECF) from isolate LB1 cultures (Table 7). Only *sipC* was up-regulated.

Discussion

This study was to characterize our recently identified LAB isolates for controlling *Salmonella* infection in broilers, including

Table 2. Growth (OD_{600}) of selected lactic acid-producing bacterial isolates at different concentrations of bile salt*.

	Bile salt concentrations (%)				
	0	**0.3**	**0.6**	**1.0**	**1.5**
ALB2	1.96^{a}	0.90^{b}	0.43^{c}	0.31^{c}	0.31^{c}
ALB6	1.93^{a}	1.16^{b}	0.59^{c}	0.65^{bc}	0.65^{bc}
CL9	1.86^{a}	0.08^{b}	0.04^{b}	0.09^{b}	0.21^{b}
K16	1.86^{a}	0.21^{b}	0.05^{b}	0.16^{b}	0.19^{b}
K67	2.02^{a}	1.03^{b}	1.13^{ab}	1.33^{ab}	1.53^{ab}
L3	2.10^{a}	1.97^{a}	2.07^{a}	2.13^{a}	2.06^{a}
LB1	2.06^{a}	1.83^{a}	1.97^{a}	1.94^{a}	1.95^{a}
LB2	1.96^{a}	1.70^{b}	1.30^{c}	1.21^{d}	1.17^{d}
LB4	1.97^{a}	1.68^{b}	1.28^{c}	1.25^{cd}	1.20^{d}
S8	1.98^{a}	1.14^{a}	1.24^{a}	0.87^{a}	1.40^{a}
S33	1.92^{a}	0.28^{b}	0.15^{b}	0.49^{b}	0.86^{ab}
S64	1.82^{a}	1.12^{b}	0.58^{b}	0.79^{b}	0.98^{b}
S66	2.04^{a}	1.73^{b}	1.99^{a}	2.13^{a}	2.12^{a}
SG2	1.93^{a}	1.20^{a}	1.16^{a}	1.52^{a}	1.57^{a}

*Optical density at 600 nm (OD_{600}) was measured after incubation in the MRS broth at 37°C for 24 h under anaerobic atmosphere. The level of each inoculum was 1%. Values were average of triplicates. Values without common superscript in a row are significantly different ($P<0.05$).

Table 3. Susceptibility of selected lactic acid-producing bacterial isolates to various antibiotics.

Antibiotic	MIC (µg/ml) or inhibitory zone (mm)*													
	ALB2	ALB6	CL9	K16	K67	L3	LB1	LB2	LB4	S8	S33	S64	S66	SG2
Penicillin G (0–256 µg/ml)	0.3	0.3	2	2	0.5	0.8	1	1.3	0.8	21.3	0.2	1.7	0.8	1
Ciprofloxacin# (0–32 µg/ml)	13.3^{R}	4^{S}	$>32^{R}$	$>32^{R}$	$>32^{R}$	1^{S}	4^{S}	2^{S}	2^{S}	$>32^{R}$	$>32^{R}$	5.3^{R}	$>32^{R}$	$>32^{R}$
Tetracycline# (0–256 µg/ml)	$>256^{R}$	$>256^{R}$	$>256^{R}$	64^{R}	42.7^{R}	0.5^{S}	0.5^{S}	1.7^{S}	0.7^{S}	16^{S}	16^{S}	32^{R}	16^{S}	$>256^{R}$
Erythromycin# (0–256 µg/ml)	0.5^{S}	0.7^{S}	1^{S}	1^{S}	$>256^{R}$	0.2^{S}	0.5^{S}	0.3^{S}	0.3^{S}	1^{S}	0.5^{S}	$>256^{R}$	0.7^{S}	32^{R}
Ampicillin# (0–256 µg/ml)	0.5^{S}	0.5^{S}	1^{S}	4^{S}	0.3^{S}	12^{R}	2^{S}	4^{S}	2^{S}	1.5^{S}	0.3^{S}	1^{S}	0.3^{S}	1^{S}
Gentamicin# (0–256 µg/ml)	32^{R}	21.3^{R}	16^{S}	64^{R}	16^{R}	10.7^{S}	13.3^{S}	16^{S}	8^{S}	32^{R}	16^{S}	13.3^{R}	8^{S}	32^{R}
Chloramphenicol (30 µg/ml)	22	26.4	15.3	20.5	23.7	22.7	21.3	20	21.8	14. 7	22.8	25	22.5	14.2
Lincomycin (2 µg/ml)	0	0	0.6	0	0	11.8	15	13.9	10.7	0	0	0	15	10

*MIC (Minimum Inhibitory Concentration, µg/ml) for penicillin G, ciprofloxacin, tetracycline, erythromycin, ampicillin, and gentamicin was evaluated on the MRSagar with MIC Evaluator Strips (Oxoid) through gradient diffusion tests. The inhibitory zone (mm) for chloramphenicol and lincomycin was determined on the MRS agar using Oxoid Antimicrobial Discs with the concentrations indicated in the table. Values were average of triplicates.

#S, susceptible; R, resistant. Resistance is based on European Food Safety Authority [20] and European Commission [21].

Table 4. *Salmonella* counts in the cecal digesta on days 3 and 4 post-infection in Trials 2 and 3*.

Treatment	Log_{10}CFU/g digesta (mean ± standard error)			*P* value#		
	Trial 2 (n = 14)	Trial 3 (n = 8)	Combined (n = 22)	Trial 2	Trial 3	Combined
Negative control	0	0	0	NA	NA	NA
Positive control	5.36±0.14	6.58±0.23	5.80±0.17	NA	NA	NA
Low dose LB1	5.18±0.45	5.82±0.41	5.41±0.32	0.95	0.08	0.18
High dose LB1	6.43±0.16	7.04±0.07	6.65±0.12	<0.01	0.44	<0.01
Low dose mixture	6.98±0.06	6.77±0.12	6.90±0.06	< 0.01	0.94	< 0.01
High dose mixture	6.94±0.05	6.86±0.17	6.91±0.07	<0.01	0.84	<0.01

*Aftera series of 1:10 dilution, cecal digesta samples were incubated at 37°C for 24 h on Brilliant Green Sulfa Agar (BGS) supplemented with 200 μg/ml nalidixic acid.
#Individual trial was analyzed by SAS GLIMMIX procedure and Dunnett's method was used for adjustment of multiple comparisons with the positive control group as the control. The negative control group was not included for multiple comparison analysis. SAS GLIMMIX procedure was used for analysis of the two trials simultaneously (combination of the two trials) with trial as a fixed effect. NA, not applicable; *P* value for trial effect <0.01.

determination of the mechanism for the control in particular. We have demonstrated that orally administered LAB isolates at a low dose (10^6 CFU/strain/chick) could attenuate *Salmonella* infection in the spleen and liver of broilers, which coincided with down-regulation of *Salmonella* SPI-1 virulence gene expression in the chicken cecum. In addition, our data on *in vitro* expression of *Salmonella* SPI-1 virulence genes also support our *in vivo* observations, suggesting a possible correlation between the attenuation of organ infection and down regulation of SPI-1 virulence gene expression. The LAB treatments were unable to lower cecal *Salmonella* burden in the present study. The reduction of *Salmonella* burden in the gastrointestinal tract by probiotics is subjected to multiple factors, among which antimicrobial substances (*e.g.* bacteriocins) produced by probiotic bacteria can have a direct impact [9]. In this regards, we speculate that the LAB isolates tested in the present study may not have produced antimicrobial substances. Further studies are required to determine the underlying reason.

S. Typhimurium harbours more than 80 virulence genes. The ten genes examined in the present study are located in SPI-1 and have important roles in the intestinal invasion of *Salmonella* [4]. Expression of SPI-1 genes is controlled by 5 regulators (HilA, HilC, HilD, InvF, and SprB) with HilA being a master regulator [4]. In addition, these SPI-1 regulators can modulate SPI-2 gene expression that is essential for intracellular multiplication and lead to systemic infections. For instance, HilD is required for activating

Table 5. *Salmonella* invasion to the spleen on days 3 and 4 post-infection*.

Treatment	Infected birds/total birds (infection percentage, %)			*P* value#		
	Trial 2	Trial 3	Combined	Trial 2	Trial 3	Combined
Negative control	0/8	0/14	0/22	0.03	<0.01	<0.01
	(0)	(0)	(0)			
Positive control	5/8	11/14	16/22	NA	NA	NA
	(63)	(79)	(73)			
Low dose LB1	3/8	7/14	10/22	0.62	0.24	0.14
	(38)	(50)	(45)			
High dose LB1	3/8	9/14	12/22	0.62	0.68	0.28
	(38)	(64)	(55)			
Low dose mixture	1/8	6/14	7/22	0.12	0.12	0.06
	(13)	(43)	(32)			
High dose mixture	7/8	10/14	17/22	0.57	1.00	0.74
	(88)	(71)	(77)			

*Samples were enriched overnight at 37°C in Selenite Brilliant Green Sulfa Enrichment (Difco) broth, followed by plating onto Brilliant Green Sulfa Agar (BGS) supplemented with 200 μg/ml nalidixic acid to determine the presence or absence of *Salmonella* colonies.
#Individual trial was analyzed by exact logistic regression via SAS LOGISTIC procedure. SAS GLIMMIX procedure was used for analysis of the two trials simultaneously (combination of the two trials) with trial as a fixed effect, except that, for groups with zero (*i.e.* the negative control), exact logistic regression was used with trial as stratum via SAS LOGISTIC procedure. NA, not applicable; *P* value for trial effect = 0.21.

Table 6. *Salmonella* invasion to the liver on days 3 and 4 post-infection*.

Treatment	Infected birds/total birds (infection percentage, %)			*P* value[#]		
	Trial 2	Trial 3	Combined	Trial 2	Trial 3	Combined
Negative control	0/14	0/20	0/34	<0.01	<0.01	<0.01
	(0)	(0)	(0)			
Positive control	8/14	17/20	25/34	NA	NA	NA
	(57)	(85)	(74)			
Low dose LB1	5/14	11/20	16/34	0.45	0.08	0.09
	(36)	(55)	(47)			
High dose LB1	9/14	14/20	23/34	1.00	0.45	0.62
	(64)	(70)	(68)			
Low dose mixture	3/14	12/20	15/34	0.12	0.16	0.07
	(21)	(60)	(44)			
High dose mixture	13/14	16/20	29/34	0.08	1.00	0.30
	(93)	(80)	(85)			

*Samples were enriched overnight at 37°C in Selenite Brilliant Green Sulfa Enrichment (Difco) broth, followed by plating onto Brilliant Green Sulfa Agar (BGS) supplemented with 200 μg/ml nalidixic acid to determine the presence or absence of *Salmonella* colonies.

[#]Individual trial was analyzed by exact logistic regression via SAS LOGISTIC procedure. SAS GLIMMIX procedure was used for analysis of the two trials simultaneously (combination of the two trials) with trial as a fixed effect, except that, for groups with zero (*i.e.* the negative control), exact logistic regression was used with trial as stratum via SAS LOGISTIC procedure.NA, not applied; *P* value for trial effect = 0.09.

the regulatory region of the *ssrAB* operon, a key regulator of SPI-2 genes [4,23]. In the present study, we have examined the gene expression of *hilA, hilC,* and *hilD* in response to LAB treatment. The expression of *hilA* and *hilD* genes was significantly down-regulated by both single and mixed LAB isolates, particularly at the low dose. Translocation of the SPI-1 effectors (AvrA, SipA, SipC, SopB, SopD, SopE2, and SptP) into the host enterocytes via the type III secretion system (T3SS) is responsible, at least in part, for the intestinal invasion [24,25,26]. AvrA, a member of a family of acetyl transfereases, can dampen host inflammatory and

Table 7. Fold decrease in virulence gene expression of *Salmonella in vivo* and *in vitro*[a].

Gene	*In vivo*				*In vitro*
	Low dose LB1 (n = 3)	High dose LB1 (n = 6)	Low dose mixture (n = 6)	High dose mixture (n = 6)	LB1-ECF (n = 3)
hilA	15.99±8.95 *	8.03±2.43*	29.29±16.99*	14.54±7.16*	3.95±0.49 b[#]
hilC	7.02±2.42	1.07±0.20	24.72±7.02	4.47±1.63	3.69±0.40[#]
hilD	114.38±47.73 *	23.72±4.71*	256.61±56.91*	32.20±14.66*	1.84±0.15[#]
sopB	26.77±13.06*	13.10±2.84*	82.65±42.89*	45.60±18.21*	3.17±0.56[#]
sopD	8.20±5.01*	4.64±0.93*	18.05±6.62*	17.29±6.83*	3.29±0.65[#]
sopE2	41.19±20.26*	58.30±15.2*	186.37±61.57*	35.57±15.05*	4.13±0.40[#]
sipA	27.88±9.43*	7.48±1.32*	215.38±61.24*	28.21±8.16*	4.61±0.57[#]
sipC	27.72±9.36*	12.18±2.19*	156.46±43.54*	15.84±4.13*	**9.84±1.46**[#]
avrA	13.73±5.42*	3.80±0.87*	49.97±12.66*	6.04±1.26*	5.99±0.64[#]
sptP	20.15±6.85*	13.37±2.88*	87.08±27.48*	16.86±5.55*	1.60±0.52[#]

[a]*In vivo* gene expression: *Salmonella* cells were from the cecum of the chickens on day 3 post-infection after LAB treatments; *in vitro* gene expression: *Salmonella* cells were from the cultures that had been co-cultured for 14 h with the extracellular culture fluid (ECF) from 16 h-grown *L. zeae*LB1 cultures. Values were expressed as mean ± standard error. The fold-change of target gene was analyzed using the $2^{-\Delta\Delta Ct}$ method. The values derived from $2^{-\Delta\Delta Ct}$ represent fold changes of samples in the abundance relative to the reference groups. In the *in vivo* experiment, the reference group was the positive control chicken group (n = 5) that had been treated with *Salmonella* only. In the *in vitro* experiment, the reference samples were the *Salmonella* cultures (n = 3) that had been treated with the MRS medium instead of the ECF from *L. zeae*LB1 cultures. The reference samples in both *in vivo* and *in vitro* experiments have the $2^{-\Delta\Delta Ct}$ value of 1.

*Values in the same row indicate significant differences ($P<0.05$) compared with the positive control chicken group in the *in vivo* experiment. Values represent down-regulation (fold-decrease) of gene expression.

[#]Value for each gene represents a significant difference ($P<0.05$) between the treatment and control samples in the *in vitro* experiment. Values represent down-regulation (fold-decrease) of gene expression except for the value in bold that was up-regulated (fold-increase).

apoptotic defense [27,28]. SipA affects actin cytoskeleton, induces membrane shuffling, and promotes inflammation of the host cells. SipC is involved in actin bundling and nucleation. Through its phosphoinositide phosphatase activity, SopB participates in a broad range of events such as host membrane fission, *Salmonella*-containing vacuole maturation, and inflammation [29]. SopD is encoded outside SPI-1 and appears to be involved in membrane fission and macropinosome formation. SopE2, a guanine nucleotide exchange factor for Cdc42 of host cells, is important in membrane ruffling, bacterial entry and inflammation induction [26,30]. SptP is involved in inflammation and cytoskeleton manipulation of host cells [26]. SipA, SopB, SopD, and SopE2 have also been indicated to play roles in the late stage of *Salmonella* infection in mice [31]. Expression of avrA in *Salmonella* has been shown to increase bacterial invasion in the jejunum and colon and translocation in the spleen, liver, and gallbladder in chronically *Salmonella*-infected mice [32]. In the present study, the expression of all of these seven SPI-1 effectors was significantly down-regulated by both single and mixed LAB isolates. Compared with the corresponding high dose of LAB groups, the down-regulation was more evident at the low dose of LAB treatments except for the expression of *sopE2* by LB1 treatment only (Table 7).

Modulation of virulence gene expression in bacterial pathogens can be a mechanism underlying probiotic effects to control the infection of enteric pathogens. Previous *in vitro* studies have shown that lactobacilli and *Bifidobacterium bifidum* were able to down-regulate gene expression of *hilA* and *hilD* in *S.*Typhimurium and Enteritidis, respectively [13,14,15,16,17]. Similar *in vitro* observations have also been reported in *E. coli* O157:H7, in which *Lactobacillus acidophilus* repressed virulence gene expression and quorum sensing [33] and *Lactobacillus rhamnosus* reduced the expression of Shiga toxin genes (*stx*) [34]. The expression of eight Cag pathogenicity island genes was also down-regulated by *Lactobacillus salivarius* in a gastric epithelial cell line model [35]. *Salmonella* virulence gene expression can also be modulated by lactic acid and short-chain fatty acids (SCFAs). Lactate, propionate, and butyrate have been shown *in vitro* to down-regulate the expression of *Salmonella* virulence genes, such as *hilA, hilD, invF,* and *sipC* [36,37,38,39,40,41]. Acetate and formate were, however, reported to induce the *in vitro* expression of SPI-1 genes [36,42]. Some of our selected LAB isolates were able to produce lactic acid and SCFAs during fermentation (data not shown). It is unclear at present if the suppression of SPI-1 virulence gene expression of *Salmonella* in the chicken cecum described in the present study was caused by lactic acid and SCFAs produced by the isolates.

There is a lack of *in vivo* evidence on the reduction of *Salmonella* virulence gene expression by probiotics for control of the pathogen. The present study has generated a new piece of evidence demonstrating that the expression of intestinal infection-associated genes in *S.* Typhimurium can be down-regulated by selected LAB isolates when the pathogen was in the chicken cecum. This phenomenon coincided with an attenuation of *Salmonella* infection in the chicken spleen and liver. The evidence is further supported by our *in vitro* data, which revealed that co-culturing of ECF of *L.zeae* LB1 cultures with *Salmonella* resulted in a significant reduction in the expression of genes associated with *Salmonella* intestinal infection. These observations can thus lead to a hypothesis that metabolites from the LAB cultures are, at least in part, responsible for regulating the virulence gene expression in *Salmonella*, influencing *Salmonella* intestinal infection of chickens. Identification of the functional metabolites from LAB cultures would be the initial step to address the hypothesis, which can be facilitated by using *in vitro* assays for the virulence gene expression. Furthermore, identification of a dose response to the functional metabolites in down-regulating the virulence gene expression in *Salmonella in vivo* and in attenuating the organ infection of chickens remains critical in supporting the hypothesis.

Materials and Methods

In vitro characterization of lactic acid-producing bacterial isolates

Fourteen LAB isolates, including eight (ALB2, ALB6, CL9, L3, LB1, LB2, LB4, and S64) reported previously [18] and six used in the present study (K16, K67, S8, S33, S66, and SG2), were evaluated in triplicate *in vitro* for their tolerance to low pH and high bile salt and antibiotic resistance. The stock culture of each strain, stored at −80°C in 20% glycerol, was plated onto DeMan, Rogosa, and Sharpe (MRS) plates. Individual colonies were selected and inoculated into MRS broth, cultured at 37°C under anaerobic conditions (85% N_2, 10% CO_2, and 5% H_2) for 18 h, and the species identity of the six isolates were determined by sequencing 16S rRNA genes and comparison with the GenBank database using BLAST.

The susceptibility of the isolates to penicillin G, ciprofloxacin, tetracycline, erythromycin, ampicillin, and gentamicin was evaluated on MRS agar with MIC (Minimum Inhibition Concentration) Evaluator Strips (Oxoid, Basingstoke, UK) through gradient diffusion tests. The inhibitory zones generated by chloramphenicol and lincomycin were determined on the MRS agar using Oxoid Antimicrobial Discs (Oxoid, Basingstoke, UK). The range of antibiotics concentrations used in the test is listed in Table 3.

Tolerance to low pH was evaluated by incubating bacterial cells in simulated gastric fluid [43] with the pH values of 2.0 and 5.6, for 2 h prior to anaerobic incubation in the MRS broth at 37°C for 20 h. Tolerance to bile salt was studied by incubating the isolates in the MRS containing various concentrations (0, 0.3, 0.6, 1.5, and 1.5%) of bile salt (Catalog Number LP005, Oxoid, Nepean, ON, Canada) under anaerobic condition at 37°C for 24 h. The optical density (OD) of a sample was measured at a wavelength of 600 nm. The selected range of bile salts was based on the physiological concentration in the small intestine [44].

The effect of the ECF from a LAB culture (*L. zeae* LB1) on *in vitro* expression of *Salmonella* SPI-1 virulence genes was examined. To prepare the ECF, *L. zeae* LB1 was grown in MRS broth anaerobically at 37°C for 16 h and the ECF was recovered from the cultures (n = 3) by centrifugation (6,000 g, 10 min). After neutralized to pH 6.8–7.0 with NaOH (1 N), the ECF was sterilized through membrane filtration (0.2 μm pore size) and then mixed with the Luria–Bertani (LB) broth (1:1 ratio) that had double concentrations of each medium component. The ECF-LB mixtures were inoculated (1%) with *S.* Typhimurium P193, a nalidixic acid-resistant strain, and incubated at 37°C for 14 h prior to the treatment of *Salmonella* cells with RNAlater (Life Technologies Inc., Burlington, Canada).

Animal experiments

Newly hatched commercial female broiler chicks were obtained from Stratford Chick Hatchery (Stratford, ON, Canada). Birds were housed in floor pens containing wood shavings at the Isolation Unit of Ontario Veterinary College (University of Guelph, ON, Canada). Chickens had free access to water and a commercial starter diet without supplementation of antibiotics. The research protocol was approved by the University of Guelph Animal Care Committee and the guidelines of the Canadian Council for Animal Care were followed.

S. Typhimurium P193 was used to infect chickens according to the procedure described previously [45]. The procedure was originally introduced by Mead et al. (1989) [46] for assessment of probiotic efficacy. *Salmonella* was cultured in LB broth at 37°C for 16 h, followed by dilution with sterilized phosphate-buffered saline (PBS, pH 7.2) to a final cell count of 4×10^4 CFU per ml for chicken infection experiments. To prepare LAB inoculum cultures, each isolate was propagated twice in MRS broth and then diluted to the desired concentrations with sterilized PBS. The desired concentrations were confirmed by plating on MRS plates after a series dilution.

In Trial 1, 72 one-day-old broilers were randomly assigned to 6 treatments: 1) negative control (no LAB + no *Salmonella*), 2) positive control (no LAB + *Salmonella* 1×10^4 CFU/chick), 3) LB1 (isolate LB1 1×10^6 CFU/chick + *Salmonella* 1×10^4 CFU/chick), 4) S8 (isolate S8 1×10^6 CFU/chick + *Salmonella* 1×10^4 CFU/chick), 5) S33 (isolate S33 1×10^6 CFU/chick + *Salmonella* 1×10^4 CFU/chick), 6) S64 (isolate S64 1×10^6 CFU/chick + *Salmonella* 1×10^4 CFU/chick). Each treatment had 12 chickens in one pen. Two rooms were used, one room for the negative control birds and another room for the remaining treatments. Chickens were orally gavaged with 0.5 ml of LAB or PBS (negative control) at 1 day of age and 0.25 ml of *S.* Typhimurium P193 at 2 days of age according to the experimental design. Four days after the challenge, all birds were humanely sacrificed by carbon dioxide. Cecal digesta samples were collected aseptically for *Salmonella* counts. Livers and spleens were collected from the positive control group to examine for possible *Salmonella* infection.

To follow up our observation on *Salmonella* infection to chicken spleens and livers in Trial 1, Trials 2 and 3 were designed to investigate the effect of *Lactobacillus* isolates on protecting broilers from organ infection by *Salmonella*, including the influence of the isolates on virulence gene expression of *Salmonella* in the cecum. There were six treatments in each trial: 1) negative control (no LAB + no *Salmonella*), 2) positive control (no LAB + *Salmonella* 1×10^4 CFU/chick), 3) low dose LB1 (isolate LB1 1×10^6 CFU/chick + *Salmonella* 1×10^4 CFU/chick), 4) high dose LB1 (isolate LB1 1×10^7 CFU/chick + *Salmonella* 1×10^4 CFU/chick), 5) low dose mixed isolates (isolates LB1, S8, and S64 1×10^6 CFU/strain/chick + *Salmonella* 1×10^4 CFU/chick), and 6) high dose mixed isolates (isolates LB1, S8, and S64 1×10^7 CFU/strain/chick + *Salmonella* 1×10^4 CFU/chick). Each treatment had 14 and 28 chickens in Trials 2 and 3, respectively. The maintenance of chickens, gavage of *Lactobacillus* cultures, and challenge of *Salmonella* were similar to those in Trial 1. Cecal digesta, livers and spleens were sampled aseptically on days 3 and 4 post-infection (PI) for *Salmonella* analysis in Trials 2 and 3. In addition, cecal digesta samples were aseptically collected on days 1 and 3 PI in Trial 3 and kept immediately in RNAlater (Life Technologies Inc., Burlington, Canada) for analysis of virulence gene expression of *Salmonella*.

Detection of cecal colonization and organ infection of *Salmonella*

On the same day of sample collection, cecal digesta samples were processed by a series 1:10 dilution with sterile solution of 0.1% peptone and 0.1% Tween 80 in water and plating on Brilliant Green Sulfa Agar (BGS; BD, Sparks, MD, USA) supplemented with 200 μg/ml nalidixic acid to facilitate selection of the antibiotic-resistant challenge organism. *Salmonella* colonies are pink to red on this selective media. The plating was accomplished by an Eddy Jet Spiral Plater (Neu-tec Group, Farmingdale, NY, USA). For detecting organ infection of chickens, about 0.1 g of spleen or liver samples were homogenized with PowerLyzer (MO BIO Laboratories, Carlsbad, CA,USA) by bead beating at homogenization level 2500 for 30 sec in a tube containing 1 ml of 0.1% peptone water and 0.5 ml of beads and incubated for 16 h at 37°C in 4 ml of Selenite Brilliant Green Sulfa Enrichment (Difco) broth (Sparks, MD, USA), followed by plating onto BGS supplemented with 200 μg/ml nalidixic acid to examine the presence or absence of *Salmonella* colonies. The recovery of *Salmonella* is reported as the ratio of the number of *Salmonella* positive samples to the number of total samples tested. The sensitivity of sample preparation (including both digesta and organ samples) and plating was assessed by including a known amount of *Salmonella* cells in the samples. The detection limit of our sample preparation and plating system was determined to be 100 CFU/g sample if the enrichment procedure was not applied.

Extraction of bacterial total RNA and reverse transcription/quantitative PCR (RT-qPCR)

Bacterial total RNA was extracted using the Ambion RiboPure-Bacteria Kit (Life Technologies Corporation, Carlsbad, CA, USA) according to the manufacturer's instructions. Briefly, samples of cecal digesta or *Salmonella* pure cultures that had been treated in RNAlater were washed with 2 volumes of PBS. After centrifugation (1500 x g) at 4°C for 10 min, the pellet was transferred to a new tube containing 0.5 ml beads and 0.8 ml RNAwiz provided with the Ambion RiboPure-Bacteria Kit and subjected to bead beating with PowerLyzer (MO BIO Laboratories, Carlsbad, CA, USA) for 2 min each at homogenization level 2500, repeated once. The tubes were chilled on ice for 2 min between bead beatings. Total bacterial RNA was then extracted, washed, and eluted following the manual of the kit. The RNA quantity was measured using an ND-1000 spectrophotometer (NanoDrop Technologies, Wilmington, DE, USA).

To remove genomic DNA contamination, total bacterial RNA samples were treated with DNaseI from the Ambion TURBO DNA-free kit (Life Technologies Corporation, Carlsbad, CA, USA) according to the manufacturer's protocol. Two micrograms of total RNA was then used for synthesis of cDNA with 100 ng of random hexamers and SuperScript II reverse transcriptase from the Invitrogen SuperScript II first-strand cDNA synthesis kit (Life Technologies Corporation, Carlsbad, CA, USA) according to the manufacturer's instructions.

The qPCR assays were performed using a Stratagene MX3005 thermal cycler (Stratagene, La Jolla, CA, USA) with the following thermal cycle profile: 95°C for 3 min for initial activation of the DNA polymerase; 40 cycles of 95°C for 15 sec (denaturation), specific temperature listed in Table 8 for 30 sec (annealing) and 72°C for 30 sec (extension). A thermal melt curve was generated by heating at 95°C for 1 min, 55°C for 30 sec, and ramping back to 95°C in 0.5°C increments. The 25 μl reaction mixture contained 1.0 μl of 3-fold diluted sample cDNA, 12.5 μl of 2× iTaq SYBR Green Supermix (Bio-Rad, Hercules, CA, USA), and forward and reverse primers (Table 8). The expression levels of virulence genes were normalized using 16S rDNA as an internal housekeeping control, and fold change of target genes was calculated by the delta-delta-Ct method [47]. ΔCt represents the difference between the Ct value with the primers to a target gene and the Ct value to the housekeeping gene (16S rRNA gene). ΔΔCt represents the difference in ΔCt values between the treatment and control groups. The values derived from $2^{-\Delta\Delta Ct}$ represent fold changes of samples in abundance relative to the reference samples. The reference samples had the $2^{-\Delta\Delta Ct}$ value of 1. The samples from the positive control chicken group in the chicken trial and the samples not subjected to the ECF treatment in the *in vitro* experiment served as the reference samples, respectively.

Table 8. PCR primers.

Gene	Primers (5′-3′)	Amplicon size (bp)	Primer final concentration (nM)	Annealing temperature (°C)	Reference
16S rRNA	Forward: CAGAAGAAGCACCGGCTAACTC	87	150	60	[48]
	Reverse: GCGCTTTACGCCCAGTAATT				
hilA	Forward: CATGGCTGGTCAGTTGGAG	150	300	62	[49]
	Reverse: CGTAATTCATCGCCTAAACG				
hilC	Forward: GGACTTGTTGCCAGGGATG	241	300	62	[49]
	Reverse: TGACCATTTGCGGGTGAG				
hilD	Forward: ACTCGAGATACCGACGCAAC	129	300	62	[49]
	Reverse: CTTCTGGCAGGAAAGTCAGG				
sopB	Forward: AACCGTTCTGGGTAAACAAGAC	77	500	56	[50]
	Reverse: GGTCCGCTTTAACTTTGGCTAAC				
sopD	Forward: CTTTAAGCTTCGGTAATCATCAAAA	306	500	50	[51]
	Reverse: AAGCGTCCATCTTGATAGTAAACAG				
sopE2	Forward: GCCTGCATCAACAAACAGACA	72	500	60	[52]
	Reverse: ATACCGCCCTACCCTCAGAAG				
sipA	Forward: GGCTTGCGTGCGGAAATA	69	500	60	[53]
	Reverse: ATCGCTACATTGCGCTTTCA				
sipC	Forward: CTGTGGCTTTCAGTGGTCAG	150	500	60	[49]
	Reverse: TGCGTTGTCCGGTAGTATTTC				
avrA	Forward: GGAAACCGATCTCGAAATGA	241	500	57	[54]
	Reverse: TGCTGGTTCGAACAAAATCA				
sptP	Forward: ATGCTCGTGCCTGGTGGTGTTA	236	150	60	This study
	Reverse: ACGGTAACGGCTGGTGATCT				

Statistical analysis

Values were expressed as mean ± standard error. Tolerance to low pH and high bile salt and gene expression data were analyzed by the SAS GLM procedure and Tukey multiple comparisons. *Salmonella* counts in cecal contents were log transformed and subjected to analysis of variance and Dunnett's test for multiple comparisons. Logistic regression was used for analysis of data on *Salmonella* infection in the liver and spleen. When data from animals in Trials 2 and 3 were pooled, mixed model was employed with trial as a fixed effect.

Acknowledgments

XY and YZ were NSERC Visiting Fellows to the Canadian Federal Government Laboratories (NSERC-VF).

Author Contributions

Conceived the research: JG SS PS. Designed the experiments: XY HY JB JG SS. Performed the experiments: XY JB HY QW FY YZ. Analyzed the data: XY HY. Contributed reagents/materials/analysis tools: JG SS. Wrote the paper: XY JG.

References

1. Jackson BR, Griffin PM, Cole D, Walsh KA, Chai SJ (2013) Outbreak-associated *Salmonella enterica*serotypes and food commodities, United States, 1998-2008. Emerg Infect Dis19: 1239–1244.
2. Porwollik S, Boyd EF, Choy C, Cheng P, Florea L, et al. (2004) Characterization of *Salmonella enterica* subspecies I genovars by use of microarrays. J Bacteriol 186: 5883–5898.
3. Barrow PA, Jones MA, Thomson N (2010) *Salmonella*. In:Gyles CL, Prescott JF, Songer JG, Thoen CO, editors. Pathogenesis of bacterial infections in animals, 4th edition. Ames: Wiley-Blackwell. pp: 231–265.
4. Valdez Y, Ferreira RB, Finlay BB (2009) Molecular mechanisms of *Salmonella* virulence and host resistance. Curr Top Microbiol Immunol 337: 93–127.
5. Desin TS, Köster W, Potter AA (2013) *Salmonella* vaccines in poultry: past, present and future. Expert Rev Vaccines 12: 87–96.
6. Vandeplas S, Dubois Dauphin R, Beckers Y, Thonart P, Théwis A (2010)*Salmonella* in chicken: current and developing strategies to reduce contamination at farm level. J Food Prot 73: 774–785.
7. Chambers JR, Gong J (2011) The intestinal microbiota and its modulation for *Salmonella* control in chickens. Food Res Int 44: 3149–3159.
8. Mead GC (2000) Prospects for 'competitive exclusion' treatment to control salmonellas and other foodborne pathogens in poultry. Vet J 159: 111–123.
9. Corr SC, Hill C, Gahan CG (2009) Understanding the mechanisms by which probiotics inhibit gastrointestinal pathogens. Adv Food Nutr Res 56: 1–15.
10. Wang Y, Gu Q (2010) Effect of probiotic on growth performance and digestive enzyme activity of Arbor Acres broilers. Res Vet Sci 89: 163–167.
11. Brisbin JT, Gong J, Sharif S (2008) Interactions between commensal bacteria and the gut-associated immune system of the chicken. Anim Health Res Rev 9: 101–110.
12. Tsai YT, Cheng PC, Pan TM (2012) The immunomodulatory effects of lactic acid bacteria for improving immune functions and benefits. Appl Microbiol Biotechnol 96: 853–862.
13. Bayoumi MA, Griffiths MW (2010) Probiotics down-regulate genes in *Salmonella enterica* serovar Typhimurium pathogenicity islands 1 and 2. J Food Prot 73: 452–460.
14. Bayoumi MA, Griffiths MW (2012) *In vitro* inhibition of expression of virulence genes responsible for colonization and systemic spread of enteric pathogens using *Bifidobacterium bifidum* secreted molecules. Int J Food Microbiol 156: 255–263.
15. Das JK, Mishra D, Ray P, Tripathy P, Beuria TK, et al. (2013) *In vitro* evaluation of anti-infective activity of a *Lactobacillus plantarum* strain against *Salmonella enterica* serovar Enteritidis. Gut Pathog 5: 11. doi: 10.1186/1757-4749-5-11.
16. Nutt JD, Kubena LF, Nisbet DJ, Ricke SC (2002) Virulence response of a *Salmonella* Typhimurium *hilA*:lacZY fusion strain to spent media from pure cultures of selected bacteria and poultry cecal mixed culture. J Food Saf 22: 169–181.

17. Durant JA, Corrier DE, Stanker LH, Ricke SC (2000) *Salmonella enteritidis* hilA gene fusion response after incubation in spent media from either *S. enteritidis* or a poultry *Lactobacillus* strain. J Environ Sci Health B 35: 599–610.
18. Wang C, Wang J, Gong J, Yu H, Pacan JC, et al. (2011) Use of *Caenorhabditis elegans* for preselecting *Lactobacillus* isolates to control *Salmonella* Typhimurium. J Food Prot 74: 86–93.
19. Lewus CB, Montville TJ (1991) Detection of bacteriocins produced by lactic acid bacteria. J Microbiol Methods 13: 145–150.
20. European Food Safety Authority (EFSA) Panel on Additives and Products or Substances used in Animal Feed (FEEDAP) (2012) Guidance on the assessment of bacterial susceptibility to antimicrobials of human and veterinary importance. EFSA Journal 10: 2740.
21. European Commission (2003) Opinion of the Scientific Committee on Animal Nutrition on the criteria for assessing the safety of micro-organisms resistant to antibiotics of human clinical and veterinary importance. Available: http://ec.europa.eu/food/fs/sc/scan/out108_en.pdf. Accessed 2013 June 17.
22. Brichta-Harhay DM, Arthur TM, Bosilevac JM, Guerini MN, Kalchayanand N, et al. (2007) Enumeration of *Salmonella* and *Escherichia coli* O157:H7 in ground beef, cattle carcass, hide and faecal samples using direct plating methods. J Appl Microbiol 103: 1657–1668.
23. Bustamante VH, Martínez LC, Santana FJ, Knodler LA, Steele-Mortimer O, et al. (2008) HilD-mediated transcriptional cross-talk between SPI-1 and SPI-2. Proc Natl Acad Sci USA 105: 14591–14596.
24. Libby SJ, Halsey TA, Altier C, Potter J, Gyles CL (2004) *Salmonella*. In: Gyles CL, Prescott JF, Songer JG, Thoen CO, editors. Pathogenesis of bacterial infections in animals, 3rd edition. Ames: Blackwell Publishing. pp: 143–168.
25. Raffatellu M, Wilson RP, Chessa D, Andrews-Polymenis H, Tran QT, et al. (2005) SipA, SopA, SopB, SopD, and SopE2 contribute to *Salmonella enterica* serotype Typhimurium invasion of epithelial cells. Infect Immun 73: 146–154.
26. van der Heijden J, Finlay BB (2012) Type III effector-mediated processes in *Salmonella* infection. Future Microbiol 7: 685–703.
27. Collier-Hyams LS, Zeng H, Sun J, Tomlinson AD, Bao ZQ, et al. (2002) Cutting edge: *Salmonella* AvrA effector inhibits the key proinflammatory, anti-apoptotic *NF-kappa* B pathway. J Immunol 169: 2846–2850.
28. Wu H, Jones RM, Neish AS (2012) The *Salmonella* effector AvrA mediates bacterial intracellular survival during infection in vivo. Cell Microbiol 14: 28–39.
29. Bakowski MA, Braun V, Lam GY, Yeung T, Heo WD, et al. (2010) The phosphoinositide phosphatase SopB manipulates membrane surface charge and trafficking of the *Salmonella*-containing vacuole. Cell Host Microbe 7: 453–462.
30. Stender S, Friebel A, Linder S, Rohde M, Mirold S, et al. (2000) Identification of SopE2 from *Salmonella* Typhimurium, a conserved guanine nucleotide exchange factor for Cdc42 of the host cell. Mol Microbiol 36: 1206–1221.
31. Giacomodonato MN, Uzzau S, Bacciu D, Caccuri R, Sarnacki SH, et al. (2007) SipA, SopA, SopB, SopD and SopE2 effector proteins of *Salmonella enterica* serovar Typhimurium are synthesized at late stages of infection in mice. Microbiol 153: 1221–1228.
32. Lu R, Wu S, Liu X, Xia Y, Zhang YG, et al. (2010) Chronic effects of a *Salmonella* type III secretion effector protein AvrA *in vivo*. PLoS One 5: e10505. doi: 10.1371.
33. Medellin-Pena MJ, Wang H, Johnson R, Anand S, Griffiths MW (2007) Probiotics affect virulence-related gene expression in *Escherichia coli* O157:H7. Appl Environ Microbiol 73: 4259–4267.
34. Carey CM, Kostrzynska M, Ojha S, Thompson S (2008) The effect of probiotics and organic acids on Shiga-toxin 2 gene expression in enterohemorrhagic *Escherichia coli* O157:H7. J Microbiol Methods 73: 125–132.
35. Ryan KA, O'Hara AM, van Pijkeren JP, Douillard FP, O'Toole PW (2009) *Lactobacillus salivarius* modulates cytokine induction and virulence factor gene expression in *Helicobacter pylori*. J Med Microbiol 58: 996–1005.
36. Durant JA, Corrier DE, Ricke SC (2000) Short-chain volatile fatty acids modulate the expression of the *hilA* and *invF* genes of *Salmonella* Typhimurium. J Food Prot 63:573–578.
37. Durant JA, Corrier DE, Stanker LH, Ricke SC (2000) Expression of the hilA*Salmonella*Typhimurium gene in a poultry *Salm. enteritidis* isolate in response to lactate and nutrients.JApplMicrobiol 89:63–69.
38. Lawhon SD, Maurer R, Suyemoto M, Altier C (2002) Intestinal short-chain fatty acids alter *Salmonella* Typhimurium invasion gene expression and virulence through BarA/SirA. Mol Microbiol 46:1451–1464.
39. Gantois I, Ducatelle R, Pasmans F, Haesebrouck F, Hautefort I, et al.(2006) Butyrate specifically down-regulates *salmonella* pathogenicity island 1 gene expression. Appl Environ Microbiol72: 946–949.
40. Boyen F, Haesebrouck F, Vanparys A, Volf J, Mahu M, et al. (2008) Coated fatty acids alter virulence properties of *Salmonella* Typhimurium and decrease intestinal colonization of pigs. Vet Microbiol 132: 319–327.
41. Hung CC, Garner CD, Slauch JM, Dwyer ZW, Lawhon SD, et al. (2013) The intestinal fatty acid propionate inhibits *Salmonella* invasion through the post-translational control of HilD. Mol Microbiol 87: 1045–1060.
42. Huang Y, Suyemoto M, Garner CD, Cicconi KM, Altier C (2008) Formate acts as a diffusible signal to induce *Salmonella* invasion. J Bacteriol 190: 4233–4241.
43. Wang Q, Gong J, Huang X, Yu H, Xue F (2009) In vitro evaluation of the activity of microencapsulated carvacrol against *Escherichia coli* with K88 pili. J Appl Microbiol 107: 1781–1788.
44. Dawson PA (1998) Bile secretion and the enterohepatic circulation of bile acids. In: Feldman M, Sleisenger MH, Scharschmidt BF, editors. Sleisenger and Fordtran's gastrointestinal and liver disease: pathophysiology/diagnosis/management, 6th edition. Philadelphia: W. B. Saunders, Co. pp. 1052–1063.
45. Haghighi HR, Abdul-Careem MF, Dara RA, Chambers JR, Sharif S (2008) Cytokine gene expression in chicken cecal tonsils following treatment with probiotics and *Salmonella* infection. Vet Microbiol 126: 225–233.
46. Mead GC, Barrow PA, Hinton MH, Humbert F, Impey CS, et al. (1989) Recommended assay for treatment of chicks to prevent *Salmonella* colonization by competitive exclusion. J Food Protect 52: 500–502.
47. Livak KJ, Schmittgen TD (2001) Analysis of relative gene expression data using real-time quantitative PCR and the 2(-Delta Delta C(T)) Method. Methods 25: 402–408.
48. Botteldoorn N, Van Coillie E, Grijspeerdt K, Werbrouck H, Haesebrouck F, et al. (2006) Real-time reverse transcription PCR for the quantification of the mntH expression of *Salmonella enterica* as a function of growth phase and phagosome-like conditions. J Microbiol Methods66: 125–135.
49. Mizusaki H, Takaya A, Yamamoto T, Aizawa S (2008) Signal pathway in salt-activated expression of the *Salmonella* pathogenicity island 1 type III secretion system in *Salmonella entericas* erovar Typhimurium. J Bacteriol 190: 4624–4631.
50. Choi J, Shin D, Kim M, Park J, Lim S, et al. (2012) LsrR-mediated quorum sensing controls invasiveness of *Salmonella* Typhimurium by regulating SPI-1 and flagella genes. PLoS One 7: e37059. doi: 10.1371.
51. Lim S, Yoon H, Ryu S, Jung J, Lee M, et al. (2006) A comparative evaluation of radiation-induced DNA damage using real-time PCR: influence of base composition. Radiat Res 165: 430–437.
52. Vikram A, Jayaprakasha GK, Jesudhasan PR, Pillai SD, Patil BS (2012) Obacunone represses *Salmonella* pathogenicity islands 1 and 2 in an envZ-dependent fashion. Appl Environ Microbiol 78: 7012–7022.
53. Boyen F (2007) *Salmonella* Typhimurium infections in pigs: a closer look at the pathogenesis. Ghent: Ghent University, Belgium. PhD dissertation.
54. Wang YP, Li L, Shen JZ, Yang FJ, Wu YN (2009) Quinolone-resistance in *Salmonella* is associated with decreased mRNA expression of virulence genes *invA* and *avrA*, growth and intracellular invasion and survival. Vet Microbiol 133: 328–334.

Valuation, Categories and Attributes

Inna Galperin[1], Olav Sorenson[2]*

1 Independent scholar, Montreal, Quebec, Canada, **2** School of Management, Yale University, New Haven, Connecticut, United States of America

Abstract

Existing research on categories has only examined indirectly the value associated with being a member of a category relative to the value of the set of attributes that determine membership in that category. This study uses survey data to analyze consumers' preferences for the "organic" label versus for the attributes underlying that label. We found that consumers generally preferred products with the category label to those with the attributes required for the organic label but without the label. We also found that the value accorded to the organic label increased with the number of attributes that an individual associated with the category. Category membership nevertheless still had greater value than even that of the sum of the attributes associated with it.

Editor: Gabor Peli, Utrecht University, Netherlands

Funding: The authors thank the Michael Lee-Chin Family Institute for Corporate Citizenship at the Rotman School of Management for its generous funding. The funders had no role in study design, data collection and analysis, decision to publish, or preparation of the manuscript.

Competing Interests: The authors have declared that no competing interests exist.

* Email: olav.sorenson@yale.edu

Introduction

Socially-constructed categories – such as occupations, organizational forms and product types – play many important roles in society. They influence the ways in which people perceive and understand the world [1] and respond to social situations [2,3]. They affect the manner in which individuals and groups organize their activities and belongings. And they shape a wide variety of socio-economic outcomes, from the products that consumers buy [4,5] to the people that managers hire [6] to the activities that companies pursue [7,8].

An open question in this literature has been the relative importance of categories versus their underlying attributes in contributing to the perceived value of products, people and organizations. For example, when purchasing a computer, do consumers care about its type – perhaps a gaming machine – or do they instead mostly value a set of attributes that define that type: a fast processor, high quality video and sound processing, and a large monitor? If categories serve as cognitive shortcuts for storing and transferring information about the features (attributes) of their members [9,10], then the value of being perceived as a member would presumably equal the combined values associated with the attributes required for membership. In other words, a buyer (perhaps subconsciously) would assign values to each of the features – the CPU, graphics processors, etc. – and the value of being considered a gaming computer would simply represent the sum of these parts (because membership in the category would imply this set of components). But categories might also have value above and beyond that of the attributes associated with them [11,12]. Given two computers with identical components, consumers might then still pay more for the one labeled as a gaming machine.

Distinguishing between these two possibilities requires a research design that can assess the value of a category label separately from the values of the attributes that it has come to represent. To generate such independent assessments, we combined a conjoint survey instrument with an experimental design to assess the valuation of products assigned to the "organic" label relative to those that simply had the attributes associated with membership in this category. We found that respondents strongly preferred the organic label to its underlying attributes. In part, this valuation appeared to stem from associating the label with additional attractive features, ones not required for being classified as organic; respondents who associated the label with more features also placed a higher value on it. But in part, the organic label also appeared to have value in and of itself. We discuss the implications of our findings for the literatures relating classification to economic choices and outcomes.

The Valuation of Categories

The emerging managerial and sociological literatures on categories generally assume that groups of people with similar preferences, often referred to as audiences, construct categories to sort objects, people and organizations into sets that they find meaningful, usually in the sense that they consider the members of the set to serve as functional substitutes. Thus, for example, filmgoers might classify movies into genres – action, comedy or sci-fi – based on similarities in their appeal and themes, or consumers might classify vehicles into types – minivan, sedan or sports car – based on their shapes, engine sizes and a variety of other features. Much of the recent enthusiasm about categories, however, has not been driven by wanting to understand how people develop and represent categories cognitively but by an interest in how these categories in turn shape economic outcomes. Researchers, for example, have reported relationships between the genre classifications of movies and their box office sales [5], between the previous job titles of individuals and their odds of being hired [6], and between the industry classifications of companies and the valuation of their equities [13].

Although the idea that categories would influence economic outcomes depends on the idea that categories affect the ways in which audiences value category members relative to non-members, the nature of this relationship remains relatively unexplored. We nevertheless believe that the extensive literature on why particular objects become grouped in a category hints at some possible connections between the valuations of categories relative to their underlying attributes.

Category value = sum of attribute values

One common characterization of classification processes argues that an audience creates a category when a large proportion of the audience agrees that some set of producers or products shares a number of features that distinguishes them from other producers or products and attaches a label to the set [9,10]. Thus, as noted above, an audience might perceive certain computers with fast CPUs, high-end video processors and hi-fidelity sound, large monitors and casings with lively lights and coloring as being distinct from other computing machines and label those machines as gaming computers. The category label then essentially operates as shorthand for a set of attributes or features, and category membership depends on whether – or the extent to which – an object, individual or organization has the attributes required for membership in this set [3,10,14].

To the extent that the category label represents a set of attributes or features, one would expect the valuation accorded to membership in the category to reflect the joint value of having all of its requisite attributes [10]. In other words, the precise set of features required for membership in a category should have a single value whether enumerated or whether specified through the shortcut of the category label. Continuing on the example above, a computer considered a member of the gaming computer category would have equivalent value to one not previously encountered (and therefore not yet classified) that had all of the features expected of such a machine (fast CPU, high-end video, etc.).

Category value > sum of attribute values

Although this equivalence between the value of a category label and of its requisite attributes seems a reasonable baseline, one might expect category labels to have value above and beyond these attributes for at least three reasons:

Feature creep. In many cases, categories do not have clear mappings to a particular set of attributes. People generally do not discuss categories in terms of being defined by a set of features. Instead, they attach the category label to specific cases. If discussing universities, one might give as examples Harvard, Yale, Stanford and the University of California. Inferring what features being a university requires and being able to assess whether some newly encountered organization qualifies as one depends on identifying what these accepted members of the category have in common, such as faculty, students, classes and libraries [15–17].

This process could lead audiences to associate categories with larger sets of features than membership in those categories actually requires. Any feature that occurs more frequently among category members than it does in the population as a whole might conceivably become associated with the category, even if only a subset of those features critically distinguish category members from non-members. Seeing that all of the examples above have campuses and dormitories, some people, for example, might come to believe that being a university requires a school to have a campus and dormitories. This feature creep might in turn inflate the value attached to membership in the category. To the extent that members of the audience place positive value on these associated features, then they may come to value the category as if it implied not simply its required attributes but also all of these additional associated ones. In other words, the value that individuals would attach to being a university might include any value that they place on having a campus or on having dormitories.

When might this feature creep become most extensive and therefore contribute most to the value associated with the category label? Interestingly, exposure to a wider range of category members probably increases the number of features that an individual associates with the category. Continuing with the university example, some accepted members of the category – but not all – would have public policy schools, medical schools, African-American studies departments and so on. One effect of being exposed to all of this variety could be to conclude that only those features that all examples have are necessary to being a university. But, to the extent that audiences and individuals view items as having grades of membership (i.e. being partial members of the category) [10], another reasonable inference would be that full membership in the category requires all of these features and that the various examples – without a public policy school or without a medical school or without an African-American studies department – have high grades of membership but are nonetheless not full members of the university category. To the extent that these associated attributes in turn have positive value, one would then expect the value of the category label to increase with exposure to examples of the category.

Value creep. Categories could also come to have value above and beyond that of even their associated attributes. To the extent that audiences treat categories as a gestalt, they may form their beliefs about the value of the category in a similar manner, through association as opposed to by composition from constituent parts [16]. Rather than aggregating the values of the features that they associate with a category, audiences might value the category label through inference, perhaps averaging the values that they assign to the most salient members of the category. For example, the value that an individual assigns to being a minivan might stem not from the usefulness of three rows of seats and doors that slide open and its other features but from averaging the values associated with a Honda Odyssey, a Toyota Sienna and other examples of the vehicle type. Since each of these prototypical members probably has a number of non-requisite – in the sense of not being needed to belong to the category – but desirable features, these valuations would then implicitly incorporate not just the values of features associated with the category but also those of extraneous ones.

Consistent with this notion that audiences learn the value of category membership through association rather than through composition, producers frequently attempt to communicate the value of novel products not by enumerating all of their features but rather by relating them to established categories. Manufacturers of early computer workstations, for example, first attempted to promote their products as "smart terminals" and "mainframes on a desk" [18]. Similarly, early satellite radio providers attempted to draw analogies between their services and the established offerings of cable and satellite television services [12].

In contrast to feature creep, this value creep would probably not increase with exposure to the category. Although those with more experience with the category may have a larger number of prototypical members of the category available to them and therefore may form their beliefs about the value of the category label by averaging across a larger number of examples, this averaging would not lead to a higher or lower valuation unless limited exposure implied having an unrepresentative sample. It should, however, reduce the variance in the valuation associated with the category label (as the value converges on the population average value of the category members).

Certification. Category labels might also come to have value in excess of that accorded to their underlying attributes due to a sort of certification value. To the extent that audiences associate a category label with a set of features, they may assume that any object, individual or organization that has received the label possesses all of these features [10]. Parents, for example, might presume that a film with a PG rating has relatively little nudity or profanity. This assumption of having the requisite features could become particularly valuable in cases where membership in the category depends on a large number of features, meaning that direct examination of the features themselves would prove costly.

By contrast, audiences might discount the value of an item, even if it has all of the features required for category membership, if it has not also been assigned the category label. After all, if producers or people met the requirements for membership in a category why would they not claim membership? Imagine a movie that proclaimed itself suitable for children but that had no MPAA rating or a school that offers the same curriculum as other business schools but that does not award its graduates an MBA. Audiences may interpret information on attributes in the absence of the category label as a signal of illegitimacy, evidence that the person or producer fails to fit in the relevant category.

Empirical strategy

To gain greater insight into the relationship between categories, attributes and their valuations, we surveyed consumers to assess their preferences for hypothetical products with and without the "organic" category label.

The danger of focusing on a single category stems from distinguishing the valuation accorded to a category label from an incomplete or incorrect list of its constituent features. Even with a simple category, audiences may associate the category label with attributes not anticipated by the researcher. To address this issue, our empirical design exploited the fact that prior psychological research has found that – even within individual and within task – people shift between more automatic and more deliberative forms of information processing as a function of their psychological state.

In particular, people in positive moods tend to rely more heavily on generalized ideas, heuristics and theories, while those in negative moods more commonly focus on the specific data [19]. Speculation about the reason behind this effect stems from the notion that people interpret their mood as being informative of some aspect of their current situation [20]. Mood then points to the most useful processing style. When all is well, people feel good, the situation seems well understood and people can save time and energy by following tested scripts. A negative mood, by contrast, signals a problematic situation, which may require deviation from the routine and therefore demands attention to the details. One might therefore expect audiences to shift from treating categories as a gestalt to evaluating them more according to their constituent components when in a negative mood. By experimentally inducing such negative affect, we used this effect to understand better the relationship between the values of the category label and of its requisite features.

Setting: Organics

To test these ideas, we gathered data on the perceptions of Canadian consumers regarding the value of organic poultry and its constituent attributes. This setting has a number of advantages with respect to our research question. First and foremost, though popular understanding of the meaning of the category may diverge from its official meaning, the label organic has a clear legal definition in Canada when applied to poultry. We therefore had a basis for assessing the accuracy of audience beliefs about the category. Second, as a common category of consumption, consumers have generally had to consider these choices and therefore should have some understanding both of the category's meaning and the extent to which they personally value it and its attributes.

Background. Interest in the "organic" production of food began in the early part of the twentieth century. Around this time, a variety of factors – the invention of the Haber-Bosch process essential to producing synthetic fertilizer, the development of synthetic pesticides, and the introduction of tractors and engine-driven equipment for planting and harvesting – converged to increase the importance of economies of scale in food production. Against this backdrop, advocacy for organic farming began essentially as a social movement opposed to the increasingly industrial nature of farming and to the treatment of the production of food as more a matter of chemistry than of biology. Interestingly, early enthusiasts came primarily from the right-wing politically, conservatives hoping to preserve traditional country life and its social order [22].

Organic agriculture began to emerge from the fringes and to shift politically from the right to the left in the 1970s, when it became attached to the environmental movement. Rachel Carson's book, *Silent Spring*, published in 1962, has often been seen as helping to instigate the environmental movement. In it, she detailed many of the devastating effects of pesticides, particularly DDT, on wildlife and humans, thereby awakening concerns among the general public about the safety of the chemicals used in modern agriculture.

Demand for food made without synthetic pesticides and fertilizers has grown steadily since then. Today, worldwide sales of organic products exceeds $50 billion per year and continues to grow at a rate far above that of the food industry as a whole [23]. Organic products moreover can be found in nearly all major grocery stores in Canada and the United States. In fact, mainstream grocery stores have accounted for the majority of organic product sales in North America since 2007 [24].

Organic poultry. Although the organic designation has been attached to a plethora of products, the advantages of a clear category definition demanded that we focus on a single application. We chose to study the designation organic as applied to chicken. According to the Canadian Food Inspection Agency (CFIA), three attributes distinguish organic poultry from conventional poultry:

- Organic feed: At least 80% of the feed, mostly grain, used to feed organic poultry must come from organic sources.
- No animal byproducts: Although animal byproducts commonly serve as filler and protein sources in the feed of conventional poultry, none of the feed for organic poultry can contain animal byproducts.
- No antibiotics: Once a bird has been given antibiotics, it no longer qualifies as being organic.

Sample

To limit the potential influence of the context on our results, we gathered information from individuals engaged in a single activity: grocery shopping. This activity has the added advantage of being a context in which people must consider food categories. Three research assistants randomly intercepted individuals at five different locations – outside four grocery stores and outside one natural foods cooperative – in the greater Toronto area.

Ethics statement. Prior to participating in the survey, the interviewers explained the general purpose of the study and obtained both verbal and written consent, in the form of a signature on a consent form, from the subjects. The research assistants then only surveyed those who had provided written consent. Following completion of the survey, respondents received contact information for one of the primary investigators, so that they could follow up with questions or to request their removal from the study. The Social Sciences, Humanities and Education Research Ethics Board (REB) of the University of Toronto approved both the survey instrument and the consent protocol.

Respondents. Those who agreed to participate first had to pass several screening questions: They had to be residents of Canada, over the age of 18, who had previously purchased chicken in a grocery store. As compensation for their time, participants received five dollars in cash. A total of 576 individuals qualified on these questions and completed the survey. We excluded five surveys from the analysis—one because the respondent claimed complete indifference across all choices and four because the interviewers failed to record the responses correctly.

We conducted one-quarter of the surveys outside The Big Carrot, a local cooperative that specializes in natural and organic foods. Our intention had been to sample a set of individuals with much deeper experience with the category. Our screening questions indicated that these consumers purchased chicken roughly 15% more frequently than the grocery store shoppers ($t = 1.85$; $p \leq 0.07$). As the Big Carrot only carries organic products, these individuals also almost certainly had greater exposure to the category. Going forward, we refer to this subset of respondents as "enthusiasts" for the organic label. Table 1 provides some descriptive information about the respondents.

Each survey required roughly 15–20 minutes to complete. After reading an introductory text, respondents spent the majority of their time engaged in evaluating a set of forced comparisons in hypothetical choices, the choice task (described in detail below). Following the choice task, they answered questions relating to their beliefs about poultry and their concerns about health and food, as well as questions about their primary language, grocery shopping behavior, education and age. The research assistants also recorded the gender of each respondent.

Our approach offers something of a middle ground. Much of the psychological research on categories has been in the laboratory, evaluating either the effects of natural language categories, such as furniture, or of synthetic categories, such as patterns of dots. The sociological and managerial research on categories, meanwhile, has primarily used archival data to examine the effects of membership in categories on performance and other outcomes. Our current study has two chief advantages vis-à-vis these literatures. First, it examines a meaningful (and legitimated) category and therefore has greater external validity for the research on social categories than the extant psychological research. Second, with respect to the managerial and sociological literatures on categories, our design affords greater insight into how people actually perceive and value categories relative to attributes and therefore begins to open the black box of the socio-cognitive processes involved.

As with any research design, however, our approach also has its limitations. Given the complexity of completing the choice task, we decided that interviewers would need to guide respondents, which essentially precluded the selection of a random sample. Therefore, though the demographics of our respondents appear similar to the residents of the greater Toronto area, our results may not extrapolate to the population as a whole. Also, as discussed in the next section, the time required to complete the choice task limited the number of attributes that we could investigate.

Measures

Choice task. To understand how respondents valued the organic category relative to a subset of attributes, much of the survey asked respondents to choose between sets of paired comparisons. The forced comparison of choices has been shown to have excellent within- and out-of-sample predictive power for

Table 1. Demographics of the sample.

	All	Enthusiasts
Gender		
Male	43%	18%
Female	57%	82%
Age		
18–34	55%	27%
35–50	26%	38%
51–65	15%	27%
Over 65	4%	8%
Education		
< High school	5%	4%
High school	31%	23%
College	51%	55%
> College	13%	18%
N	571	96

actual choice [25,26]. It therefore provides an excellent method for establishing the underlying valuations that audiences place on categories and attributes.

This technique involves creating a library of potential product profiles, choosing pairs of profiles out of this library and having respondents indicate whether they prefer one or the other or feel indifferent between them. In creating these profiles, we wanted them to seem as realistic as possible, incorporating the four dimensions of information that a shopper would normally see on a package: the brand, the category label, some features and the price.

We nevertheless faced two limitations in creating our sample profiles, both a function of combinatorics. To understand the problem, imagine that one wanted to test three brands, a category label, the presence or absence of three binary attributes and four price levels. Such a combination of characteristics would produce 192 potential profiles ($=3\times2\times2\times2\times2\times4$), entailing more than 18,000 dyadic comparisons ($=192\times191/2$).

One can reduce the number of comparisons that one must sample through the use of a fractional factorial design, which selects a subset of profiles in such a way as to ensure that each dimension remains orthogonal – and therefore uncorrelated – with every other dimension. This approach has the advantage of dramatically reducing the number of choices required to estimate unbiased values but the disadvantage of precluding the estimation of at least some of the interaction effects between characteristics. However, even the most efficient fractional factorial designs would still dictate well over one thousand comparisons in the $3\times2\times2\times2\times2\times4$ example above. We therefore had to limit strictly the number of dimensions and the number of levels on each dimension.

We created our profiles by combining levels from three dimensions (Figure 1 depicts two profile cards): (1) Category/attribute, (2) Brand, and (3) Price. Beginning with category/attribute, each profile included one of four possible indications: (i) grain fed, (ii) certified organic (depicted on the left panel), (iii) no animal byproducts, and (iv) no animal byproducts or growth hormones (depicted on the right panel). We chose "grain fed" as the baseline attribute profile because it conveyed no information: all poultry have grain as the primary component of their diets. "Organic" provided one level as we wanted to compare its value to that of attributes. Of the three attributes that distinguish organic poultry from conventional poultry, we included "no animal byproducts" over the other two because including "fed organic grain" as an attribute would have limited our ability to parse the value of the label from the attribute (since this attribute carries the organic label itself) and because our discussions with the CFIA made it clear that consumers cared more about animal byproducts than about the use of antibiotics. We included the "no animal byproducts or growth hormones" dual-attribute as our final level because we had an interest in whether a placebo attribute would influence valuations and because the CFIA indicated that growth hormones represented the second-most-commonly raised public concern (despite the fact that Canada had banned them in the 1970s). Many poultry producers in Canada also include the "no growth hormones" claim on their labels despite the fact that it does not differentiate them from other producers.

For realism, each profile also included a price – \$5 or \$7 (per kilogram) – and one of two possible brand names: Maple Leaf or Rowe Farms. Both represent actual brands. Maple Leaf supplies mainstream groceries and has a positioning akin to Oscar Meyer in the United States. It did not sell organic products at the time of the survey. Rowe Farms, meanwhile, occupies an upscale niche and emphasizes its quality and connection to smaller, local farmers. However, like Maple Leaf, it also did not offer organic products.

These three dimensions produce 16 potential profiles ($2\times4\times2$). Although a complete comparison across all of these 16 profiles would have required 120 pairings, the use of a fractional factorial design allowed us to limit the choice task to 48 dyadic comparisons [27]. Even with this limited set, however, fatigue could still become a problem. To prevent this issue from influencing our results (and to eliminate other sorts of sequence effects), we rotated the order in which we presented the comparisons across the respondents. Specifically, we created a counter-balanced Latin square design, meaning that not only did the sequencing rotate but also each pairing followed every other pairing once and only once (across every group of 48 respondents).

Psychological state. We randomly assigned the negative affect condition to respondents and introduced it through the use of a prime. Before beginning the choice task, interviewers asked subjects to read and count the number of nouns in a short piece of text. Half of the respondents received the neutral prime, an account of the benefits of a heart-healthy diet (the "Mediterranean diet"). The other half of the respondents received a prime to place them in a negative mood. This text provided a factual account of the fatal, neurodegenerative disease in cattle known as bovine spongiform encephalopathy or, more colloquially, "mad-cow" disease.

For our purposes, spongiform encephalopathy has the useful property of being limited to ruminants. Poultry cannot contract it. The prime should therefore raise general concerns about health and safety but should not induce any particular preferences about poultry on the respondents. To test to see whether this manipulation worked, after the choice task, we asked respondents to indicate the degree to which they worried about (i) salmonella (a bacteria found in poultry that can cause food poisoning), (ii) their general health and (iii) the freshness of the food that they purchase (each on a four-level Likert scale). Consistent with our expectations, respondents exposed to the negative mood prime had higher levels of anxiety about their health ($t=2.1$, $p\leq.04$) and about the freshness of food ($t=2.5$, $p\leq.02$) but not about salmonella ($t=.4$, $p\leq.70$).

Estimation

The logic behind extracting valuations from the forced choices comes from considering them to be the results of linear, additive preference functions. Imagine that the utility (U) that individual, i, derives from a particular profile, j, follows equation 1:

$$U_{ij}=\alpha_i Brand_j+\beta_i Organic_j+ \gamma_{1i}Attribute_{1j}+\gamma_{2i}Attribute_{2j}-\rho_i Price_j, \quad (1)$$

where ***Brand*** takes a value of 1 for Rowe Farm (versus 0 for the Maple Leaf baseline), ***Organic*** equals 1 if the profile includes the category label, ***Price*** takes a value of 1 for the \$ 5 condition, $Attribute_1$ indicates the "no animal byproducts" attribute and $Attribute_2$ the "no animal byproducts and no hormones" dual attribute. The remaining terms – $\alpha,\beta,\gamma_1,\gamma_2$ and ρ – meanwhile capture the valuations that the individual (implicitly) assigns to these characteristics.

One can then think about the probability of preferring one profile of a pair over the other, profile j versus profile k, as being a matter of comparing the value associated with each and choosing the one that offers greater expected satisfaction:

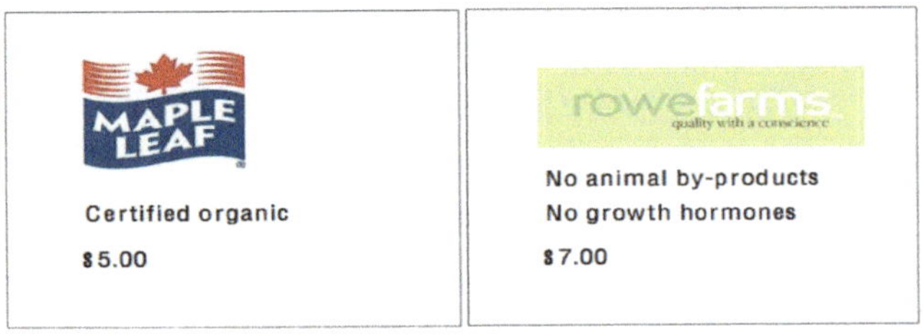

Figure 1. Two sample profile cards.

$$P(Choice = j) = f(U_j - U_k) \tag{2}$$

A number of techniques have been proposed for estimating the value coefficients, also known as partial utilities [26]. Market researchers, for example, frequently use linear optimization to derive them. Regression, however, has the benefit of allowing us to estimate standard errors.

Assuming that relative utility has a linear relationship to the probability of being chosen allowed us to estimate the coefficients with least squares regression (probit and logit regression yielded qualitatively equivalent results). In particular, we regressed a dependent variable equal to 1 if the respondent chose j, -1 if the respondent chose k and 0 if the respondent felt indifferent between the two choices, and regressed it on the difference in the characteristics vectors for profiles j and k. To accommodate potential correlations in errors within individuals across comparisons and within profiles across individuals, we report the Huber-White sandwich estimates of variance [28].

Results

Category meaning

Before turning to valuation of the category label relative to its requisite attributes, we first examined what respondents understood as the criteria for category membership. To do so, we coded the attributes mentioned in response to an open-ended question that simply asked them to describe the differences between organic and regular chicken. Table 2 reports all attributes named by at least five people (1% of the sample). The second column reports the proportion of all respondents mentioning an attribute, the third column the proportion mentioning it among enthusiasts (Big Carrot shoppers), and the final column the p-value for a t-test of the difference between the proportions for enthusiasts and non-enthusiasts.

We would begin by noting that nearly one-quarter of all respondents had no idea about the difference between organic and conventional chicken. Of those that mentioned an attribute, respondents most commonly thought that the two differed in their feed. That is correct but somewhat incomplete since these respondents did not understand the differences in the feed across the two categories. Being raised cage-free or outdoors came next in line. Interestingly, that feature does not actually differentiate organic poultry from conventional poultry in Canada. All birds are raised cage-free and none are raised outdoors (though all generally have access to the outdoors). The third-most-common belief held that organic poultry has not been fed growth hormones. As with being cage-free, while true, this characteristic also does not distinguish organic poultry from conventional poultry since Canada outlawed the use of growth hormones forty years ago. To highlight these inaccurate beliefs about the category definition, we have italicized them in the table. Note that more than half of the attributes mentioned do not distinguish organic poultry from non-organic poultry.

Much smaller proportions of the population named the actual requisite features: 11% recognized that organic poultry must receive organic feed; 6% understood that this feed could not contain animal byproducts; and 5% knew that the definition also meant that farmers could not use antibiotics in raising the animals. But not one respondent named this configuration of three distinguishing attributes as the definition, even if we generously allow the generic "difference in feed" to imply being fed organic grain.

One might nonetheless claim that this does not offer a fair test. After all, the organic category had been around for more than two decades before the Canadian government decided to codify its use as a label. Perhaps consumers had a clear understanding of the mapping of the category to attributes but the government simply did not follow it. In that case, however, even though the audience might not understand the legal definition, one would still expect a high degree of consensus in their beliefs about the attributes necessary for membership [10]. But our respondents did not even meet that lower bar. No more than one-quarter agreed on any one attribute and no more than five percent agreed on any particular combination of attributes.

Enthusiasts did not fair much better. Although only 10% of them did not mention an attribute, they actually held more inaccurate beliefs: 62% of the attributes that they mentioned – versus 51% for non-enthusiasts – do not actually distinguish organic poultry from conventional poultry ($t = 2.04$; $p \leq .04$). But they did have more consistent beliefs about these attributes: For each group – enthusiasts and non-enthusiasts – we calculated a Simpson index of attribute configurations, which essentially represents the probability that two individuals drawn at random would have the same set of beliefs [29]. It ranges from 0 to 1, with smaller values indicating greater diversity. We calculated a value of .104 for enthusiasts (more-experienced individuals) versus one of .068 for non-enthusiasts (less-experienced individuals). Individuals with greater experience with the category had more consistent beliefs about its requisite attributes ($t = 19.7$; $p < .01$). These individuals did not, however, associate the category label with a longer list of features as the feature creep conjecture would predict.

Category valuation

To assess relative valuations, we analyzed the respondents' preferences for one profile over another. Table 3 reports the results of the initial choice regressions. Model 1 estimated the utility associated with each characteristic across all respondents in the neutral treatment. The "organic" category label, the "no animal byproducts or growth hormones" attribute set, the Rowe Farms brand name and lower price all had positive utility. Because our estimation used an additive, linear model and the dependent variable ranged from -1 to $+1$ – a two-unit interval – one can directly interpret these values in terms of changes in the probability of choosing an option with a particular characteristic if one simply divides its coefficient by two. For example, the organic label increased the probability of an option being chosen by 14 percentage points ($= .280/2$) over a profile that did not contain the label. One could also scale the results by using the fact that a two-dollar change in price shifts the probability of preferring an option by 21 percentage points (dollar equivalents reported in Table 4). Hence, the average audience member attached a value of roughly \$ 1.31 (per kg) to the organic label ($= .280/.429 \times 2$).

Table 2. Beliefs about the attributes of organic poultry.

Attribute	Full sample	Enthusiasts	*p*-value
No idea	24%	10%	0.00
Difference in feed	22%	16%	0.09
Free range/cage free	*21%*	*26%*	*0.19*
No growth hormones	*21%*	*23%*	*0.65*
Fed organic grain	11%	11%	0.93
Fed grain	*10%*	*7%*	*0.31*
Not fed animal byproducts	6%	7%	0.72
No chemicals used	*6%*	*4%*	*0.38*
No antibiotics	5%	10%	0.00
Natural	*5%*	*3%*	*0.38*
Tastes better	*4%*	*4%*	*0.86*
Certification	2%	5%	0.06
Correct definition	0%	0%	1.00
N	571	96	

In this baseline condition, respondents strongly preferred the category label, organic, over the primary differentiator, no animal byproducts ($F = 328.8$, $p < .01$). They also preferred the category over the "no animal byproducts or growth hormones" attribute combination, though by a much smaller margin ($F = 3.2$, $p \leq .08$). That fact surprised us. Recall that the Canadian government bans the use of growth hormones for all poultry. The "no animal byproducts or growth hormones" condition, therefore, does not differ meaningfully from the "no animal byproducts" condition. Yet the audience clearly perceived it as different. It's worth noting, moreover, that research has found that the mere perception of even non-existent ingredients can also influence the perceived taste of foods [30]. These inequalities held even more strongly among enthusiasts: They too valued the label significantly more than either "no animal byproducts" ($F = 281.8$, $p < .01$) or "no animal byproducts or growth hormones" ($F = 37.7$, $p < .01$) but exhibited the same surprising preference for the (non-informative) "no animal byproducts or growth hormones" condition over the "no animal byproducts" condition.

Model 2 demonstrates that enthusiasts, those experienced with members of the category, valued the category more highly than those less experienced with it. The organic label increased the probability that enthusiasts would choose an option by more than twice as much as non-enthusiasts: nearly 35 percentage points (equivalent to a roughly five-dollar change in price). One might worry, however, that this difference reflects selection rather than greater exposure to category members. Maybe enthusiasts simply value the same characteristics more highly. We address this issue below.

Models 3 and 4 next shift to the issue of whether the basis for evaluation changes depending on mood. We approached the analysis conservatively, allowing the mood manipulation to influence the valuation of any characteristic—that is, we estimated fully-interacted models. Because the "main" effects essentially capture the valuations in the neutral condition, they should be (and are) identical to the first two columns. For ease of interpretation, the associated columns in Table 4 combine the main and interaction effects. The interaction effects then capture how respondents' preferences differed as a function of their mood. On average, a negative mood increased the value associated with the organic label, the "no animal byproducts" attribute, the "no animal byproducts or growth hormones" combination and the Rowe Farms brand, and decreased the attractiveness of a low price.

To the extent that the negative mood manipulation shifts participants to paying attention to the details, one would expect that the attributes would increase in valuation relative to the category label. Although in the expected direction, the evidence here appears weak: The organic designation increased less in value than the "no animal byproducts or growth hormones" condition, though the difference reached only a marginal level of significance ($F = 2.6$, $p \leq .10$). Among enthusiasts, exposure to the negative prime decreased the value of the organic label relative to that of the "no animal byproducts" condition ($F = 4.4$, $p \leq .04$) but not relative to the dual attributes ($F = 1.4$, $p \leq .24$).

However, as noted above, consumers did not appear aware of the attributes required for the organic designation. The mixed results therefore may reflect the fact that people had their own understandings of the meaning of the category label (i.e. the features that it represents). If respondents believed (even falsely) that the category encoded multiple attributes, their estimated valuations for the category may simply reflect their summed valuations of all of these attributes.

Audience-defined attributes. Although the constraints of designing a Latin square of tradeoffs did not permit an examination of the complete relationship between the category value and attributes directly, the open-ended question on the differences between organic and conventional poultry nevertheless allowed us to delve more deeply into these relationships. To address this issue, we re-estimated a series of models using respondents' reported beliefs about the distinguishing attributes (Table 2) in place of the organic label in the regression. In other words, if a respondent thought that "no growth hormones" differentiated organic from conventional fare, then we included an

Table 3. Estimated value of poultry characteristics.

	Neutral prime		Negative prime	
	All	Enthusiasts	All	Enthusiasts
	Model 1	Model 2	Model 3	Model 4
Organic	.280••	.693••	.280••	.693••
	(.017)	(.037)	(.017)	(.037)
No animal byproducts	−.027	.055	−.027	.055
	(.016)	(.036)	(.016)	(.036)
No byproducts or hormones	.250••	.471••	.250••	.471••
	(.016)	(.034)	(.016)	.034
Rowe Farms	.112••	.351••	.112••	.351••
	(.011)	(.024)	(.011)	(.024)
Price	.429••	.278••	.429••	.278••
	(.011)	(.025)	(.011)	(.025)
Negative prime			.008	.008
			(.012)	(.028)
× Organic			.042•	−.098•
			(.024)	(.053)
× No anim byprod			.041•	.014
			(.022)	(.050)
× No byproducts			.081••	−.038
or hormones			(.022)	(.048)
× Rowe Farms			.037••	.092••
			(.015)	(.033)
× Price			−.056 ••	.019
			(.016)	(.036)
Constant	−.035••	−.052••	−.035 ••	−.052••
	(.008)	(.014)	(.007)	(.020)
R^2	.12	.26	.12	.27
Observations	13,824	2,304	13,632	4,608
Individuals	288	48	571	96

Robust standard errors reported in parentheses; • $p<.10$, •• $p<.05$.

indicator variable – for beliefs about no growth hormones – to all of her product profiles that included the organic label, allowing us to estimate directly the value that respondents, on average, placed on these attributes. These models not only allow for the audience to have an understanding of the category that differs from its legal definition but also allow beliefs about these requisite attributes to vary across respondents.

In these models, the coefficient for the organic label captures the residual value attached to the label above and beyond the value of the attributes people believed that it represented. Since we could

Table 4. Valuations of characteristics (scaled in dollars).

	Neutral prime		Negative prime	
	All	Enthusiasts	All	Enthusiasts
	Model 1	Model 2	Model 3	Model 4
Organic	$1.31	$4.99	$1.73	$4.01
No animal byproducts	−$0.13	$0.40	$0.08	$0.46
No byproducts or hormones	$1.16	$3.39	$1.77	$2.92
Rowe Farms	$0.52	$2.53	$0.80	$2.98

not associate the category with attributes for those who responded that they had no idea of what differentiated organic poultry from conventional poultry ("no idea" on Table 2), we excluded them from this estimation. Dropping them allowed us to distinguish the residual effect of the category above and beyond its perceived attributes from the value of the category for those respondents who simply did not have beliefs about its attributes. Due to collinearity in the vector of belief variables, we could not estimate a coefficient for the effect of believing that organic meant not being fed animal byproducts for enthusiasts in the neutral prime. Note also that because of the small number of individuals that named it as a belief, we could not include "certification" in the vector of attributes differentiating organic and conventional poultry.

Table 5 reports the results of these regressions. We believe that a few items in this table deserve attention. First, the inclusion of these beliefs generally improved the fit of the model. People varied in their beliefs about the meaning of the category and these beliefs in turn helped to explain some of the heterogeneity across individuals in the values that they accorded to the organic label. Second, the category label had a positive and significant residual value in all four groups. Even after accounting for what people believed to be the distinguishing attributes of the category, they still valued the category label itself. Third, enthusiasts valued the category more highly, even after controlling for their potentially stronger preferences for its underlying attributes. Fourth, note that the groups valued the "no animal byproducts or hormones" dual attribute more highly than they did the category when they believed the category meant no animal byproducts or growth hormones.

These second, third and fourth findings suggest that audiences value the category label above and beyond the attributes required for membership in the category, perhaps due to feature creep, value creep or certification processes. To distinguish feature creep and certification from value creep, one can examine whether the value of the category label varied with the number of features that an individual associated with it. If the value of the category label arises from averaging the values accorded to accepted members of the category, then one would expect a relatively invariant relationship between the value of the label and its perceived attributes. But if the value of the label stems from being perceived as providing information about features not explicitly observed then its value should rise with the number of attributes the audience associates with it.

To investigate this issue, we used the responses to the open-ended question, reported in Table 2, to split individuals into three groups according to the number of features that they associated with the label: those who had no idea of the meaning (0 attributes), those who associated the category with one to three attributes, and those who associated it with four or more features. We then estimated the value of the organic label, as well as all other features, separately for each of these three groups. Although we estimated interactions between these groups and all of the attributes, Table 6 reports only the items of interest, the coefficients and standard errors for the organic label within each of these three groups. All three groups valued the category above and beyond its associated attributes, but the incremental value of the category label rose with the number of attributes that the individual associated with it, providing evidence in favor of feature creep and/or certification as central mechanisms underlying the extra value associated with category labels.

Discussion

Although the label "organic" has a clear definition for poultry in Canada, Canadian consumers exhibited little understanding of the distinguishing characteristics necessary to qualify for the label. In fact, many of the attributes they believed to be conditions for qualification are common to both organic and conventional poultry. Not only did the audiences not understand the "organic" definition, but they did not even display any substantial degree of consensus over its meaning. Enthusiasts – those with greater experience with the category – fared little better.

Despite their limited understanding of the meaning of the category, consumers nevertheless always preferred products with the "organic" label to those meeting its legal definition (but without the label), as well as to those with the attributes that they believed organics to have (but without the label). Those with more experience with the category and who associated more attributes with the category valued it even more highly.

These findings seem difficult to reconcile with the idea that categories serve as an efficient cognitive shorthand for sets of attributes [9,31]. If categories simply mapped onto attribute sets, then one would expect audiences to understand their definitions and to value the label equivalently to the set of attributes that it represented. The findings do, however, fit with the expectations that one would have if categories represented an alternate means of organizing the world [32].

These results also seem surprising in light of recent evidence suggesting that audiences prefer crisp categories – those with clear boundaries – over more lenient ones – those with more ambiguous definitions [17,33]. We would note, however, that these ideas about the advantage of crispness have been in terms of competition among categories. The organic label does not have any real competitors at the moment and therefore neither consumers nor producers can opt for a label with greater precision.

More broadly, category-level competition may have some interesting and somewhat counter-intuitive effects on the value of category labels. By selecting more lenient labels out of the system, competition may produce categories with more homogenous members, thereby producing categories less prone to feature creep, to value creep and to the need for certification. By doing so, category-level competition may interestingly limit the value of the label to being little more than the sum of the values associated with its underlying features.

Although our results provide evidence that the organic label has acquired value above and beyond that of its associated attributes, this finding represents but a single category. In thinking about how the premium accorded to the label might vary from one category to the next, we have two immediate expectations. First, we would expect a positive association between the value of the label and the complexity of the category. To the extent that audiences cannot enumerate the relevant attributes and would probably not even have the ability to examine them if they could, one would expect an even greater reliance on the category label in judgments of valuation.

Second, we would expect a positive association between the premium associated with a category label and its legitimacy for two reasons. On the one hand, the fact that a category label has been generally accepted may limit the perceived need for examining the meaning of and for understanding the label [34]. Audiences therefore might have a high degree of consensus on membership in the category while simultaneously not agreeing on the rules for membership. On the other hand, to the extent that audiences infer the value of the label from its associations, one might expect these associations to expand as audiences become more experienced with the category and consequently develop deeper associations between it and various attributes—ironically, from a dispersion of understandings about the category meaning rather than a sharpening of them.

To the extent that category labels do acquire a value of their own that potentially increases with legitimacy, it raises interesting issues for industry dynamics. Entrants – particularly those with novel products or organizational forms – face liabilities of newness due to the difficulty of developing reliable and accountable internal processes [35,36]. If the category label has value above and beyond the attributes of the organizations, products and services being classified, it places entrants between a rock and a hard place. Failure to conform to the operations and offerings of incumbents – not just having all of the features of the incumbents but also, just as crucially, not having additional ones – may lead to entrants being perceived as less than full members of the category and therefore being viewed by consumers as offering less valuable goods and services. But entering with products identical to those already available dooms them to competing on price and quality against established players with greater scale and experience.

Table 5. Estimated value based on self-reported category meaning.

	Neutral prime		Negative prime	
	Non-enthusiasts	Enthusiasts	Non-enthusiasts	Enthusiasts
	Model 5	Model 6	Model 7	Model 8
Organic	.222••	.641••	.431••	.586••
	(.046)	(.092)	(.042)	(.088)
Meaning of organic				
Difference in feed	.005	−.365••	−.175••	.148
	(.048)	(.102)	(.044)	(.103)
Free range/cage free	.003	.262••	−.126••	−.098
	(.042)	(.097)	(.043)	(.096)
No growth hormones	.053	.110	.009	−.064
	(.044)	(.119)	(.042)	(.109)
Fed organic grain	−.070	.279••	−.267••	.271••
	(.054)	(.125)	(.055)	(.095)
Fed grain	−.148••	−.313•	.008	−.079
	(.051)	(.176)	(.053)	(.112)
Not fed animal byproducts	.050		.010	.018
	(.075)		(.058)	(.087)
No chemicals used	.107	−.028	−.010	−1.30••
	(.074)	(.150)	(.058)	(.137)
No antibiotics	.114	.169	.158•	.489••
	(.080)	(.113)	(.083)	(.115)
Natural	.054	.029	.066	−.242
	(.088)	(.196)	(.063)	(.291)
Tastes better	−.046	.591••	−.033	.257•
	(.102)	(.134)	(.080)	(.134)
No animal byproducts	−.022	.068•	−.006	.090
	(.020)	(.037)	(.020)	(.036)
No byproducts or hormones	.275••	.504••	.332••	.455••
	(.020)	(.034)	(.020)	.035
Rowe Farms	.112••	.409••	.137••	.446••
	(.014)	(.024)	(.014)	(.024)
Price	.460••	.284••	.371••	.248••
	(.014)	(.026)	(.014)	(.026)
Constant	−.039••	−.055••	−.024••	−.046••
	(.011)	(.020)	(.011)	(.020)
R^2	.14	.33	.12	.30
Observations	8,208	2,016	8,304	2,112
Individuals	171	42	173	44

Robust standard errors reported in parentheses; • $p < .10$, •• $p < .05$.

Table 6. Estimated value of category based on extensiveness of category beliefs.

	Organic	
	β	SE
No idea (0 attributes)	.139	.034
1–3 attributes	.321	.019
4+ attributes	.522	.132

Given this bind, it's perhaps not surprising that entrepreneurial entry in many industries coincides with attempts to establish novel categories. When evaluated as a minicomputer, the machines that eventually become known as computer workstations could not compete on price or performance [18]. Software companies constantly struggle to define spaces that allow them to highlight their novel features without violating the expectations associated with a class of program [33]. When successful, these attempts, perhaps depending on the functional substitutability of the product being introduced, may either lead to the emergence of a new industry or the partitioning of an existing one [11].

Acknowledgments

We thank Mark Bielby of the Canadian Food Inspection Agency for his time and patience, Natasza Ararile, Melanie Gogol and Rachel Stewart for their able research assistance, and Daniel Armanios, Anne Bowers, Greta Hsu, Balázs Kovács, George Newman, Gábor Péli, Peter Roberts, two anonymous reviewers, and seminar participants at Tilburg University and the University of Toronto for their feedback on earlier versions of this paper.

Author Contributions

Conceived and designed the experiments: IG. Performed the experiments: IG. Analyzed the data: OS. Wrote the paper: IG OS.

References

1. Whorf BL (1956) Language, Thought and Reality: Selected Writings of Benjamin Lee Whorf. Oxford: Technology Press of MIT.
2. Durkheim E (1984) The Division of Labor in Society. New York: Free Press.
3. Zerubavel E (1991) The Fine Line: Making Distinctions in Everyday Life. New York: Free Press.
4. Loken B, Ward J (1990) Alternative approaches to understanding the determinants of typicality. Journal of Consumer Research 17: 111–126.
5. Hsu G, Hannan MT, Koçak O (2009) Multiple category memberships in markets: An integrative theory and two empirical tests. American Sociological Review 74: 150–169.
6. Leung MD (2014) Dilettante or Renaissance Man? How the order of job experiences affects hiring in an external labor market. American Sociological Review 79: 136–158.
7. White HC (1981) Where do markets come from? American Journal of Sociology 87: 517–547.
8. Zuckerman EW (2000) Focusing the corporate product: Securities analysts and de-diversification. Administrative Science Quarterly 45: 591–619.
9. Tversky A (1977) Features of similarity. Psychological Review 84: 327–352.
10. Hannan MT, Polos L, Carroll GR (2007) Logics of Organization Theory: Audiences, Codes, and Ecologies. Princeton University Press.
11. Carroll GR, Swaminathan A (2000) Why the microbrewery movement? Organizational dynamics of resource partitioning in the U.S. brewing industry. American Journal of Sociology 106: 715–762.
12. Navis C, Glynn MA (2010) How new market categories emerge: Legitimacy, identity, and en-trepreneurship in satellite radio, 1990–2005. Administrative Science Quarterly 55: 439–471.
13. Zuckerman EW (1999) The categorial imperative: Securities analysts and the illegitimacy discount. American Journal of Sociology 104: 1398–1438.
14. Rosch E, Mervis CB, Gray WD, Johnson DM, Boyes-Braem P (1976) Basic objects in natural categories. Cognitive Psychology 8: 382–439.
15. Murphy G, Medin DL (1985) The role of theories in conceptual coherence. Psychological Review 92: 289–316.
16. Medin DL (1989) Concepts and conceptual structure. American Psychologist 44: 1469–1481.
17. Pontikes E, Hannan MT (2014) An ecology of social categories. Sociological Science 1: in press.
18. Sorenson O (1997) The complexity catastrophe in the computer industry: Interdependence and adaptability in organizational evolution. Unpublished dissertation, Stanford University.
19. Bless H (2000) Feeling and Thinking: The Role of Affect in Social Cognition, New York: Cambridge University Press, chapter The interplay of affect and cognition: The mediating role of general knowledge structures. pp. 201–222.
20. Schwarz N (1990) Feelings as information: Informational and motivational functions of affective states. In: Sorrentino RM, Higgins ET, editors, Handbook of Motivation and Cognition: Foundations of Social Behavior, New York: Guilford, volume 2. pp. 527–561.
21. Heckman J (2006) A history of organic farming: Transitions from Sir Albert Howard's *War in the Soil* to USDA National Organic Program. Renewable Agriculture and Food Systems 21: 143–150.
22. Conford P (2001) The Origins of the Organic Movement. Glasgow: Floris Books.
23. Willer H, Kilcher L, editors (2011) The World of Organic Agriculture – Statistics and Emergining Trends 2011. Bonn: IFOAM.
24. Willer H, Kilcher L, editors (2008) The World of Organic Agriculture – Statistics and Emergining Trends 2011. Bonn: IFOAM.
25. Green PE, Srinivasan V (1978) Conjoint analysis in consumer research: Issues and outlook. Journal of Consumer Research 5: 103–123.
26. Green PE, Srinivasan V (1990) Conjoint analysis in marketing: New developments with implications for research and practice. Journal of Marketing 54: 3–19.
27. Green PE (1974) On the design of choice experiments involving multifactor alternatives. Journal of Consumer Research 1: 61–68.
28. White H (1980) A heteroskedasticity-consistent covariance matrix estimator and a direct test for heteroskedasticity. Econometrica 48: 817–838.
29. Simpson E (1949) Measurement of diversity. Nature 163: 688.
30. Wansink B, Park SB (2002) Sensory suggestiveness and labeling: Do soy labels bias taste? Journal of Sensory Studies 17: 483–491.
31. Fiske ST, Pavelchak MA (1986) The Handbook of Motivation and Cognition: Foundations of Social Behavior, Guilford Press, chapter Category-based versus piecemeal-based affective responses: Developments in schema-triggered affect.
32. Medin DL, Schaffer MM (1978) Context theory of classification learning. Psychological Review 85: 207–238.
33. Pontikes E (2012) Fitting in or starting new? invention, leniency, and category emergence in the software industry, 1990–2002. Working paper, University of Chicago.
34. Hsu G, Hannan MT (2005) Identities, genres, and organizational forms. Organization Science 16: 474–490.
35. Stinchcombe AL (1965) Handbook of Organizations, Rand McNally, chapter Social structure and organizations. pp. 142–193.
36. Hannan MT, Freeman J (1984) Structural inertia and organizational change. American Sociological Review 49: 149–164.

PERMISSIONS

All chapters in this book were first published in PLOS ONE, by The Public Library of Science; hereby published with permission under the Creative Commons Attribution License or equivalent. Every chapter published in this book has been scrutinized by our experts. Their significance has been extensively debated. The topics covered herein carry significant findings which will fuel the growth of the discipline. They may even be implemented as practical applications or may be referred to as a beginning point for another development.

The contributors of this book come from diverse backgrounds, making this book a truly international effort. This book will bring forth new frontiers with its revolutionizing research information and detailed analysis of the nascent developments around the world.

We would like to thank all the contributing authors for lending their expertise to make the book truly unique. They have played a crucial role in the development of this book. Without their invaluable contributions this book wouldn't have been possible. They have made vital efforts to compile up to date information on the varied aspects of this subject to make this book a valuable addition to the collection of many professionals and students.

This book was conceptualized with the vision of imparting up-to-date information and advanced data in this field. To ensure the same, a matchless editorial board was set up. Every individual on the board went through rigorous rounds of assessment to prove their worth. After which they invested a large part of their time researching and compiling the most relevant data for our readers.

The editorial board has been involved in producing this book since its inception. They have spent rigorous hours researching and exploring the diverse topics which have resulted in the successful publishing of this book. They have passed on their knowledge of decades through this book. To expedite this challenging task, the publisher supported the team at every step. A small team of assistant editors was also appointed to further simplify the editing procedure and attain best results for the readers.

Apart from the editorial board, the designing team has also invested a significant amount of their time in understanding the subject and creating the most relevant covers. They scrutinized every image to scout for the most suitable representation of the subject and create an appropriate cover for the book.

The publishing team has been an ardent support to the editorial, designing and production team. Their endless efforts to recruit the best for this project, has resulted in the accomplishment of this book. They are a veteran in the field of academics and their pool of knowledge is as vast as their experience in printing. Their expertise and guidance has proved useful at every step. Their uncompromising quality standards have made this book an exceptional effort. Their encouragement from time to time has been an inspiration for everyone.

The publisher and the editorial board hope that this book will prove to be a valuable piece of knowledge for researchers, students, practitioners and scholars across the globe.

LIST OF CONTRIBUTORS

Timothy P. Robinson
Livestock Systems and Environment Research Theme (LSE), International Livestock Research Institute (ILRI), Nairobi, Kenya
Animal Production and Health Division (AGA), Food and Agriculture Organization of the United Nations (FAO), Rome, Italy

Giulia Conchedda, Valentina Ercoli, Elisa Palamara, Giuseppina Cinardi and Laura D'Aietti
Animal Production and Health Division (AGA), Food and Agriculture Organization of the United Nations (FAO), Rome, Italy

G. R. William Wint
Environmental Research Group Oxford (ERGO) - Department of Zoology, University of Oxford, Oxford, United Kingdom

Marius Gilbert
Biological Control and Spatial Ecology, Université Libre de Bruxelles, Brussels, Belgium
Fonds National de la Recherche Scientifique, Brussels, Belgium

Simon I. Hay
Spatial Ecology and Epidemiology Group - Department of Zoology, University of Oxford, Oxford, United Kingdom
Fogarty International Center, National Institutes of Health, Bethesda, Maryland, United States of America

Thomas P. Van Boeckel
Biological Control and Spatial Ecology, Université Libre de Bruxelles, Brussels, Belgium
Fonds National de la Recherche Scientifique, Brussels, Belgium
Department of Ecology and Evolutionary - Biology Department, Princeton University Princeton, New Jersey, United States of America
Princeton Environmental Institute, Princeton, New Jersey, United States of America

Anandan Paldurai, Sa Xiao, Shin-Hee Kim, Sachin Kumar, Baibaswata Nayak, Sweety Samal and Siba K. Samal
Virginia-Maryland Regional College of Veterinary Medicine, University of Maryland, College Park, Maryland, United States of America

Peter L. Collins
Laboratory of Infectious Diseases, National Institute of Allergy and Infectious Diseases, Bethesda, Maryland, United States of America

Karen Staines, Lawrence G. Hunt, John R. Young and Colin Butter
The Pirbright Institute, Compton, United Kingdom

Stephanie Smith, Jennifer Fox, Yongjun Choi and Kyungjae Myung
Genome Instability Section, Genetics and Molecular Biology Branch, National Human Genome Research Institute, National Institutes of Health, Bethesda, Maryland, United States of America

Marco Mejia, Wanvipa Ruangpradit and Mark Muller
Department of Molecular Biology and Microbiology, College of Medicine, University of Central Florida, Orlando, Florida, United States of America

Alihossein Saberi and Shunichi Takeda
Department of Radiation Genetics Kyoto University, Medical School, Kyoto, 606-8501 Japan

Kyungho Choi
Department of Environmental Health School of Public Hearth, Seoul National University, Seoul, Korea

Lei Li
Department of Experimental Radiation Oncology, The University of Texas MD Anderson Cancer Center, Houston, Texas, United States of America
Department of Genetics, The University of Texas MD Anderson Cancer Center, Houston, Texas, United States of America

Yucai Wang
Department of Experimental Radiation Oncology, The University of Texas MD Anderson Cancer Center, Houston, Texas, United States of America
The University of Texas Graduate School of Biomedical Sciences at Houston, Houston Texas, United States of America

Eric A. Hendrickson and Sehyun Oh
Department of Biochemistry, Molecular Biology and Biophysics, University of Minnesota Medical School, Minneapolis, Minnesota, United States of America

Sunmi Kim
Genome Instability Section, Genetics and Molecular Biology Branch, National Human Genome Research Institute, National Institutes of Health, Bethesda, Maryland, United States of America
Department of Radiation Genetics Kyoto University, Medical School, Kyoto, 606-8501 Japan
Department of Environmental Health School of Public Hearth, Seoul National University, Seoul, Korea

Martin J. Sergeant, Chrystala Constantinidou and Mark J. Pallen
Division of Microbiology and Infection, Warwick Medical School, University of Warwick, Coventry, United Kingdom

Tristan A. Cogan
School of Clinical Veterinary Science, Bristol, United Kingdom

Michael R. Bedford
AB Vista Feed Ingredients, Marlborough, United Kingdom

Charles W. Penn
Institute of Microbiology and Infection, University of Birmingham, Birmingham, United Kingdom

Sangsu Shin, Young Min Choi and Kichoon Lee
Department of Animal Sciences, The Ohio State University, Columbus, Ohio, United States of America

Jae Yong Han
World Class University Biomodulation Major, Department of Agricultural Biotechnology, Research Institute for Agriculture and Life Sciences, College of Agriculture and Life Sciences, Seoul National University, Seoul, Korea

Dragana Stanley
Central Queensland University, School of Medical and Applied Sciences, Rockhampton, Queensland, Australia
Australian Animal Health Laboratory, CSIRO Biosecurity Flagship, Geelong, Victoria, Australia
Poultry Cooperative Research Centre, University of New England, Armidale, New South Wales, Australia

Robert J. Moore
Australian Animal Health Laboratory, CSIRO Biosecurity Flagship, Geelong, Victoria, Australia
Poultry Cooperative Research Centre, University of New England, Armidale, New South Wales, Australia

Shu-Biao Wu, Nicholas Rodgers and Robert A. Swick
Poultry Cooperative Research Centre, University of New England, Armidale, New South Wales, Australia
School of Environmental and Rural Science, University of New England, Armidale, New South Wales, Australia

Fatemeh Ameri Sefideh, Mi Jin Moon, Seongsik Yun, Jong-Ik Hwang and Jae Young Seong
Graduate School of Medicine, Korea University, Seoul, Republic of Korea

Sung In Hong
Department of East-West Integrated Medicine, College of Oriental Medicine, Gachon University, Incheon, Republic of Korea

Frank R. Morrissey-Wettey, Helen Craig and Antony P. Jackson
Department of Biochemistry, Hopkins Building, University of Cambridge, Cambridge, United Kingdom

Alison Downing and Richard Talbot
Roslin Institute, Roslin, Midlothian, Scotland, United Kingdom

Alena Pance
The Wellcome Trust Sanger Institute, Hinxton, Cambridge, United Kingdom

Stefanie Kaufmann
Department of Genome Oriented Bioinformatics, Technische Universität München, Freising, Bavaria, Germany

Dmitrj Frishman
Department of Genome Oriented Bioinformatics, Technische Universität München, Freising, Bavaria, Germany
Institute of Bioinformatics and Systems Biology, German Research Center for Environmental Health, Neuherberg, Bavaria, Germany
Department of Bioinformatics, St Petersburg State Polytechnical University, St Petersburg, Russia

Olivier Leymarie, Christophe Chevalier, Luc Jouneau, Ronan Le Goffic and Bruno Da Costa
Unité de Virologie et Immunologie Moléculaires, Unitéde Recherche UR892, Institut National de la Recherche Agronomique, Jouy-en-Josas, France

Carissa Embury-Hyatt and Yohannes Berhane
National Centre for Foreign Animal Disease, Canadian Food Inspection Agency, Winnipeg, Manitoba, Canada

Marco Moroldo
Centre de Ressources Biologiques pour la Génomique des Animaux Domestiques et d'Intérêt Economique, Institut National de la Recherche Agronomique, Jouy-en-Josas, France

Bernard Delmas and Hana M. Weingartl
National Centre for Foreign Animal Disease, Canadian Food Inspection Agency, Winnipeg, Manitoba, Canada
Department of Medical Microbiology, University of Manitoba, Winnipeg, Manitoba, Canada

Kyle E. Godden, Jeremy P. Landry, Natalya Slepneva, Paola V. Migues and Maria Pompeiano
Department of Psychology, McGill University, Montreal, Quebec, Canada

Lawrence K. Silbart
Department of Animal Science, The University of Connecticut, Storrs, Connecticut, United States of America
Department of Pathobiology and Veterinary Sciences, The University of Connecticut, Storrs, Connecticut, United States of America
Center of Excellence for Vaccine Research, The University of Connecticut, Storrs, Connecticut, United States of America
Department of Allied Health Sciences, The University of Connecticut, Storrs, Connecticut, United States of America

Frank Zappulla
Department of Pathobiology and Veterinary Sciences, The University of Connecticut, Storrs, Connecticut, United States of America

Sanjukta Majumder
Department of Animal Science, The University of Connecticut, Storrs, Connecticut, United States of America Center of Excellence for Vaccine Research, The University of Connecticut, Storrs, Connecticut, United States of America

Keiji Kinoshita, Makoto Mizutani and Takao Namikawa
Avian Bioscience Research Center, Graduate School of Bioagricultural Sciences, Nagoya University, Nagoya, Japan

Yoichi Matsuda
Avian Bioscience Research Center, Graduate School of Bioagricultural Sciences, Nagoya University, Nagoya, Japan
Laboratory of Animal Genetics, Department of Applied Molecular Biosciences, Graduate School of Bioagricultural Sciences, Nagoya University, Nagoya, Japan

Toyoko Akiyama and Ai Shinomiya
Department of Biology, Keio University, Yokohama, Japan

Akira Ishikawa
Laboratory of Animal Genetics, Department of Applied Molecular Biosciences, Graduate School of Bioagricultural Sciences, Nagoya University, Nagoya, Japan

Hassan Hassan Younis
Laboratory of Animal Genetics, Department of Applied Molecular Biosciences, Graduate School of Bioagricultural Sciences, Nagoya University, Nagoya, Japan
Department of Poultry Production, Faculty of Agriculture, Kafr El-Sheikh University, Kafr El-Sheikh, Egypt

Masaoki Tsudzuki
Laboratory of Animal Breeding and Genetics, Graduate School of Biosphere Science, Hiroshima University, Higashi-Hiroshima, Japan
Japanese Avian Bioresource Project Research Center, Hiroshima University, Higashi-Hiroshima, Japan

Beatrix Agnvall and Per Jensen
IFM Biology, AVIAN Behaviour and Genomics group, Linköping University, Linköping, Sweden

Daniel Nätt
IFM Biology, AVIAN Behaviour and Genomics group, Linköping University, Linköping, Sweden
Department of Clinical and Experimental Medicine, Laboratory of Integrative and Behavioral Neuroscience, Linköping University, Linköping, Sweden

Juliana L. Bernardoni, Leijiane F. Sousa and Ana M. Moura-da-Silva
Laboratório de Imunopatologia, Instituto Butantan, São Paulo, SP, Brazil

Russolina B. Zingali
Laboratório de Hemostasia e Venenos, Instituto de Bioquímica Médica, Universidade Federal do Rio de Janeiro, Rio do Janeiro, RJ, Brazil

Luciana S. Wermelinger
Laboratório de Hemostasia e Venenos, Instituto de Bioquímica Médica, Universidade Federal do Rio de Janeiro, Rio do Janeiro, RJ, Brazil
Laboratório de Fisiopatologia da Trombose, Faculdade de Farmácia, Universidade Federal do Rio de Janeiro, Rio do Janeiro, RJ, Brazil

Aline S. Lopes and Solange M. T. Serrano
Laboratório Especial de Toxinologia Aplicada, Instituto Butantan, São Paulo, SP, Brazil
Center of Toxins, Immune-Response and Cell Signaling (CeTICS), FAPESP, São Paulo, SP, Brazil

Benedito C. Prezoto
Laboratório de Farmacologia, Instituto Butantan, São Paulo, SP, Brazil

Xiaojian Yang, Hai Yu, Qi Wang, Fugui Yin, Yonggang Zhang, Parviz Sabour and Joshua Gong
Guelph Food Research Centre, Agriculture and Agri-Food Canada, Guelph, Ontario, Canada

Jennifer Brisbin and Shayan Sharif
Department of Pathobiology, University of Guelph, Guelph, Ontario, Canada

Inna Galperin
Independent scholar, Montreal, Quebec, Canada

Olav Sorenson
School of Management, Yale University, New Haven, Connecticut, United States of America

Index